Clinical Asthma: Theory and Practice

Clinical Asthma: Theory and Practice

Editor: Jordan Long

AMERICAN
MEDICAL PUBLISHERS
www.americanmedicalpublishers.com

AMERICAN
MEDICAL PUBLISHERS
www.americanmedicalpublishers.com

Cataloging-in-Publication Data

Clinical asthma : theory and practice / edited by Jordan Long.
p. cm.
Includes bibliographical references and index.
ISBN 979-8-88740-587-2
1. Asthma. 2. Asthma--Treatment. 3. Bronchi—Diseases. 4. Lungs—Diseases, 5. Respiratory allergy. I. Long, Jordan.
RC591.C55 2023
616.238--dc23

American Medical Publishers,
41 Flatbush Avenue,
1st Floor, New York,
NY 11217, USA

ISBN 979-8-88740-587-2 (Hardback)

Contents

Preface

This book has been an outcome of determined endeavour from a group of educationists in the field. The primary objective was to involve a broad spectrum of professionals from diverse cultural background involved in the field for developing new researches. The book not only targets students but also scholars pursuing higher research for further enhancement of the theoretical and practical applications of the subject.

Asthma refers to a type of long-term inflammatory disease which affects the airways of the lungs. It occurs due to extra mucus blocking the airways causing them to swell and narrow down. It is identified by easily activated bronchospasms, recurrent and variable symptoms, as well as reversible airflow obstruction. This disease can affect both children and adults in various ways and with varied levels of severity. There are various signs and symptoms of asthma, including chest tightness, episodes of wheezing, shortness of breath and coughing. It can be caused by a variety of factors such as respiratory infections, allergies, and genetic and environmental factors like exposure to allergens and air pollution. Breathing tests, health history inquiries and physical examinations are used to diagnose it. There is no treatment for asthma, but it can be managed by biologic treatments, anti-inflammatory drugs, and bronchodilators. This book explores all the important clinical aspects of asthma in the present day scenario. It is appropriate for students as well as for experts seeking detailed information about this medical condition.

It was an honour to edit such a profound book and also a challenging task to compile and examine all the relevant data for accuracy and originality. I wish to acknowledge the efforts of the contributors for submitting such brilliant and diverse chapters in the field and for endlessly working for the completion of the book. Last, but not the least; I thank my family for being a constant source of support in all my research endeavours.

Editor

1

Difficult vs. Severe Asthma: Definition and Limits of Asthma Control in the Pediatric Population

*Amelia Licari, Ilaria Brambilla, Alessia Marseglia, Maria De Filippo, Valeria Paganelli and Gian L. Marseglia**

Department of Pediatric, Fondazione IRCCS Policlinico San Matteo, University of Pavia, Pavia, Italy

Correspondence:
Gian L. Marseglia
gl.marseglia@smatteo.pv.it

Evaluating the degree of disease control is pivotal when assessing a patient with asthma. Asthma control is defined as the degree to which manifestations of the disease are reduced or removed by therapy. Two domains of asthma control are identified in the guidelines: symptom control and future risk of poor asthma outcomes, including asthma attacks, accelerated decline in lung function, or treatment-related side effects. Over the past decade, the definition and the tools of asthma control have been substantially implemented so that the majority of children with asthma have their disease well controlled with standard therapies. However, a small subset of asthmatic children still requires maximal therapy to achieve or maintain symptom control and experience considerable morbidity. Childhood uncontrolled asthma is a heterogeneous group and represents a clinical and therapeutic challenge requiring a multidisciplinary systematic assessment. The identification of the factors that may contribute to the gain or loss of control in asthma is essential in differentiating children with difficult-to-treat asthma from those with severe asthma that is resistant to traditional therapies. The aim of this review is to focus on current concept of asthma control, describing monitoring tools currently used to assess asthma control in clinical practice and research, and evaluating comorbidities and modifiable and non-modifiable factors associated with uncontrolled asthma in children, with particular reference to severe asthma.

Keywords: asthma control and severity, severe asthma, difficult to treat asthma, asthma, treatment adherence, severe asthma risk factors

INTRODUCTION

Asthma is one of the most common chronic diseases affecting all age groups, with up to 20% of children aged 6–7 years experiencing severe wheezing episodes within a year (1). Childhood asthma is currently defined as a clinical umbrella syndrome encompassing symptoms such as wheezing, shortness of breath, chest tightness, and cough, ranging in severity from mild symptoms to life-threatening attacks (2). In this context, several pathophysiologic components (traits) have been identified in children such as airflow limitation, eosinophilic airway inflammation, airway infection and impaired airway defenses, some of which being treatable (2). The primary goal of asthma management and treatment is to achieve the control of symptoms and underlying airway inflammation, aiming at minimizing the risk of future asthma attacks and medication-related side effects, and preventing the progression of obstructive lung damage during growth and then later in life (3).

International guidelines emphasize the importance of evaluating asthma control, rather than asthma severity, in order to guide asthma management decisions (3–5). Asthma control is defined as the degree to which manifestations of the disease are reduced or removed by therapy (6, 7). Two components of asthma control are identified in the guidelines: symptom control and risk. Symptom control domain refers to daytime symptoms and nighttime symptoms (i.e., cough, wheeze, exercise limitation), reliever use (short-acting β2 agonists, SABA) for the treatment of symptoms, and deviation from normal levels of activity (i.e., playing, sleeping, attending work or school), preserving normal or near-normal lung function, and meeting patient and parent expectations. Future risk of poor asthma outcomes domain includes preventing severe asthma attacks (requiring systemic corticosteroids, emergency medical treatment or hospitalization), loss of lung function or impairment of normal lung growth in childhood, and adverse effects caused by medication use (3–7). Asthma severity reflects the intrinsic "activity" of the disease and should be typically assessed both prior to beginning treatment with controller medications, and then at regular intervals to determine degree of responsiveness to treatment. Thus, asthma severity is usually defined from the level of treatment needed to achieve and maintain adequate control (7).

Over the past decade, the definition and the tools of asthma control have been substantially implemented so that the majority of children with asthma have their disease well controlled with standard therapies. However, a small subset of asthmatic children (<5% of all pediatric asthma) still requires maximal therapy to achieve or maintain symptom control and experience considerable morbidity (8–11). The identification of the factors that may contribute to the gain or loss of control in asthma is essential in differentiating children with difficult-to-treat asthma from those with severe asthma that is resistant to traditional therapies. The aim of this review is to focus on current concept of asthma control, describing monitoring tools currently used to assess asthma control in clinical practice and research, and evaluating comorbidities and modifiable and non modifiable factors associated with uncontrolled asthma in children, with particular reference to severe asthma.

ASSESSMENT OF ASTHMA CONTROL

Evaluating asthma control starts with taking a detailed history of frequency of asthma symptoms, sleep disturbances, limitation of activity, and frequency of reliever use in the past 4 weeks. Treatment issues (adherence to therapy and inhaler technique) as well as comorbidities (i.e., nasal disease, eczema, food allergy, obesity, etc.) and factors that may complicate care should be also periodically reviewed (3).

Asthma attacks are characterized by an acute worsening of asthma symptoms in response to a trigger such as allergen exposure, viral infection, environmental irritants (including pollution and cigarette smoke) or a combination of these. Given that asthma attacks can occur also on the background of seemingly good control and normal lung function (12), the concepts of acute asthma attacks and asthma baseline control, although overlapping, are not the same.

Symptom Control

Common tools for monitoring asthma available in a clinical practice setting can be distinguished in subjective measures, such as asthma diaries and questionnaires-based composites asthma scores, and objective measures, including spirometry, bronchial hyperreactivity tests and biomarkers of airways inflammation (7).

Subjective Measures

Subjective measures of asthma control include asthma diaries and asthma symptom questionnaires; moreover, visual analog scale (VAS) may be introduced in assessing patient's airways obstruction perception. These tools were initially introduced in clinical research; nevertheless, they are spreading also in clinical practice, since they enable the physicians to strictly monitor their patients' symptoms trends. Each of these tools presents pros and cons, that are briefly reported also in **Table 1**.

Asthma diaries are created to obtain data regarding asthma-related events on a daily basis. So far asthma diaries validated for clinical practice or for clinical trials are the Pediatric Asthma Diary (PAD) (13), the Pediatric Asthma Caregiver Diary (PACD) (14), the daytime and nocturnal asthma symptom diary scales (15) and the Asthma Control Diary (ACD) (16). Asthma diaries collect data day-to-day, so that they do not depend on patient recall. This feature enables the physician to monitor asthma-related events in real time and to promptly adjust therapy. The main concern regarding paper diaries is represented by the risk of missing large amounts of data, since this kind of diaries can be retrospectively filled-in by the patient, either with invented data or with false data. In order to solve this problem, the diaries should be administered day-by-day through telematics-primed device, for instance telephone-administered diaries or online diaries (17–19). This solution has been already adopted in allergic rhinitis (20): as a matter of fact, the MASK-rhinitis study collected symptoms referred by patients, by means of a user-friendly smartphone application; so similar "apps" might be developed in order to be administered to asthmatic patients. Each asthma diary collects a large amount of data for each patient, so another concern about this tool regards the way to evaluate and analyse data derived from asthma diaries in clinical trials. Mixed model analyses should be adopted in order to report the large amount of longitudinal data collected by asthma diaries (21). Furthermore, there is not a standardized method to account for outcome data from asthma diaries: some studies used either "symptom-free days" (22) or "symptom days" (23) so as to obtain information about cost-benefit analysis. Other studies reported the proportion of patients with at least one event or the rate of annual events (24). Both these methods reveal the efficacy of medication in the population level, although a small number of patients may be responsible for a large number of events. Another method to report diaries-derived data is "time to first event" (25), which can estimate the impact of treatment on disease progression.

Asthma symptom questionnaires are intended to monitor asthma-related events over a period between 1 and 4 weeks.

TABLE 1 | Subjective measures of asthma control.

	Pros	Cons
Asthma Diaries	Do not depend on patient recall Monitor asthma-related events in real time	They can be retrospectively filled in Each diary collects large amount of data Lack of a standardized method to account for outcome data
Asthma Symptom Questionnaires		
ACQ, ACT, cACT, TRACK	Changes in composites asthma scores correlate to clinical deterioration and to the need of step-up therapy Provide data easy to analyze	Depend on patient recall Focus on a small-time window
CASI	Identify differences between patients who could seem similar only on the basis of their clinical symptoms Useful in clinical research to test impact of additional treatment in the context of standard care	Need for additional studies to validate the application of this tool Its role in clinical practice is unclear It does not include some relevant aspects of disease control
APGAR	Provides a wider spectrum of information than other questionnaires, about features that can be crucial in therapeutic planning It is linked to a care algorithm, which can help the physician to undertake a therapy	Need for additional studies to validate the application of this tool in clinical practice or in clinical research
VAS	Quick and feasible tool for "real-life" monitoring VAS <6 is a reliable marker of uncontrolled asthma Provides information about symptom perception	Need for additional studies to validate the application of this tool in clinical practice or in clinical research

ACQ, Asthma Control Questionnaire; ACT, Asthma Control Test; APGAR, Activities, Persistent, triGGers, Asthma medications, Response to therapy; cACT, Childhood Asthma Control Test; CASI, Composite Asthma Severity Index; TRACK, Test for Respiratory and Asthma Control in Kids; VAS, Visual Analog Scale.

They can be administered only to patients (i.e. Asthma Control Questionnaire–ACQ; Asthma Control Test–ACT), or both to patients and their caregivers (i.e., Childhood Asthma Control Test–ACT), or only to caregivers (i.e., Asthma Therapy Assessment Questionnaire–ATAQ; Test for Respiratory and Asthma Control in Kids–TRACK). Their items usually include the frequency and impact of daytime symptoms, nocturnal symptoms, limitation of normal activities; some questionnaires include also questions about exercise induced-dyspnea (cACT and TRACK) and just one questionnaire evaluate also a measure of lung function (ACQ) (7). From all these data, each questionnaire elaborates a composite score, which express the level of asthma control. Four questionnaires (ACQ, ACT, cACT, TRACK) provide a cut-off value that enables the physician to distinguish between uncontrolled vs. controlled asthma, while ACT and ATAQ have a cut-off value to identify poorly controlled asthma (7). In clinical practice it may be useful to monitor for each patient how the answer to a specific question changes, so as to understand whether the disease is under control or not. Some changes in composites asthma scores correlate to clinical deterioration in asthma control and, consequently, to the need of a step-up of therapy (26). In clinical trials asthma questionnaires are more useful than asthma diaries because their provided data are more easily analyzable than those derived from asthma diaries. As a matter of fact, they have been used to assess the efficacy of different treatments (27, 28).

The answers given to asthma questionnaires depend on patient recall. Moreover, the questionnaires focus on a small-time window, which can not entirely reflect the level of disease control, because patients could improve their adherence to therapy just before clinical visit, recent events or recent period of bad control may bias reporting of the whole recall period and the trend of disease attacks can be inconstant through different seasons. In c-ACT, that is administered both to patients and to their caregivers, usually children give lower scores to asthma control than those given by their parents; in addition to that, some studies demonstrated that the correlation between c-ACT score and forced expiratory volume in the first second (FEV_1) and forced vital capacity (FVC) is stronger in newly diagnosed asthma, while it becomes weaker in patients who undergo treatment for asthma (29).

VAS is a measurement instrument designed as 10 cm–long ruler, on which the patient is asked to put a mark corresponding to his symptom perception, considering that "0" represents "severe airflow obstruction perception," while "10" represents "no respiratory symptoms." VAS has been already introduced in some allergic conditions (such as rhinitis) as a quick, achievable instrument to monitor in "real-life" setting whether the disease is under control or not (30). Recently VAS has been suggested as a useful tool also for evaluating asthma symptoms perception: there are some evidence that a VAS <6 is a reliable marker of uncontrolled asthma in adults (31) and that, in children with bronchial obstruction, poor VAS scores well correlate with respiratory function decrease; moreover, after bronchodilation test, children with initial bronchial obstruction usually report a significant improvement in VAS scores (32). However, the perception of dyspnea has been little studied in severe pediatric asthma (33) and additional studies are needed to validate the application of this tool in clinical research and then in clinical practice.

Composite Asthma Severity Index (CASI) is a subjective measure based on multiple aspects of asthma severity, such as impairment, risk and treatment. It accounts for five domains of disease, which include symptoms (day symptoms and night symptoms), controller medication use, lung function tests and asthma attacks. The final score can go from 0 to 20: the higher it is, the more severe the disease is quantified (34). CASI estimates asthma severity by means of the level of medication needed to obtain the present clinical situation, in addition to impairment features and future risk measures. This peculiarity enables the examiner to identify differences between patients who, otherwise, could seem similar only on the basis of their clinical symptoms. Therefore, it is useful for clinical research, since it is sensitive in discriminating among treatment groups even in a well-controlled population, and it can detect the effect of a specific intervention in addition to guidelines-based treatment (35). However, this score needs to be validated on a larger population and its feasibility in clinical practice is unclear. Finally, it does not include some relevant aspects of disease control (i.e. quality of life and economic costs of asthma) (35).

The Asthma APGAR is a newly introduced tool for primary assessment of asthma. The acronym "APGAR" stands for "Activities, Persistent, triGGers, Asthma medications, Response to therapy," it consists in a sequence of questions regarding not only the number of asthma attacks, the presence of diurnal or nocturnal symptoms or the limitation of normal activities due to asthma symptoms, but also the triggers of attacks, the way and the frequency with which the patients take their medicine and whether they think their medicines work or not. Its main distinctive feature is that it gathers a wider spectrum of information than other questionnaires: it mainly focuses on some peculiar aspects of the disease, which are not investigated by means of other questionnaires, but which can be pivotal for tailoring therapy (36). APGAR's questionnaire is also linked to a care algorithm, which is thought to help the physician to undertake a therapy, while all of the other questionnaires so far adopted only give the physician a simple score. Further evidences are needed to validate this tool as a reliable instrument in clinical research and/or in clinical practice.

Beyond electro-monitoring devices, mobile phone-based apps, gadgets and wearable devices, another tool assessing the degree of asthma disease control may be represented by Telemedicine. According to the American Telemedicine Association definition, it consists in "the remote delivery of health care services and clinical information using telecommunications technology" (37). It makes use of internet monitoring, text messages, email reminders. Its efficacy in controlling asthma is still unclear, and it may be cost-effective in rural communities or in underserved areas.

Objective Measures

No objective gold-standard measure is currently available to diagnose asthma. Among objective measures commonly used to diagnose and monitor asthma, we can identify lung function tests, airway hyperresponsiveness (AHR) tests (**Table 2**) and biomarkers of airways inflammation.

Lung function tests, particularly spirometry, are objective, noninvasive, and extremely helpful in the diagnosis and follow-up of patients with asthma. Examination of the FVC, FEV_1, and forced expiratory flow rate over 25%−75% of the FVC (FEF_{25-75}) is a reliable way to detect baseline airway obstruction. An obstructive airflow pattern is defined by a reduced FEV_1 (<0.80), a reduced FEV_1/FVC ratio (normally >0.75 to 0.80, and usually >0.90 in children) and a concavity of the expiratory flow volume loop during a spirometry test (38). FEV_1/FVC ratio is the most sensitive tool to assess the airflow obstruction and it is related to asthma severity; as a matter of fact, it can predict asthma-related morbidity and mortality even when FEV_1 is still normal (39). However, younger children may have briefer exhalation times and/or lower lung volumes than adults, so that their FEV_1 may be comparable to their FVC and, consequently, their FEV_1/FVC ratio may result normal even in case of airways obstruction (40). FEF_{25-75} has been proposed as a sensitive indicator of small airway obstruction and a better indicator of a response to bronchodilators and AHR than either FEV_1 or FVC; it can be considered normal when it is ≥70% of predicted FEF_{25-75} (41). Unfortunately, its great variability makes it unreliable as exclusive tool to assess airflow obstruction. In patients affected by asthma, it decreases earlier than other spirometry parameters and is able to predict long-term asthma persistence (42).

TABLE 2 | Obejctive measures of lung function.

	Pros	Cons
Spirometry	Objective, noninvasive, helpful for diagnosis and follow-up FEV_1/FVC ratio can predict asthma-related morbidity and mortality even when FEV_1 is still normal FEF_{25-75} is a sensitive indicator of small airway obstruction and a better indicator of a response to bronchodilators	It relies on patients' ability to carry out the test (unlikely applicable in children younger than 6 years old) Children may have briefer exhalation times and/or lower lung volumes than adults, consequently, their FEV_1/FVC ratio may result normal even in case of airways obstruction Its great variability makes it unreliable as exclusive tool to assess airflow obstruction
PEF	Useful information about obstruction in the large central airways	The test is extremely effort-dependent
AHR	Objective, replicable, useful for diagnosis Exercise-induced bronchoconstriction is more specific than other provocation tests in detecting asthma among pediatric population	Unlikely applicable in young children It relies on patients' ability to carry out the test

AHR, airway hyperresponsiveness; FEF_{25-75}, forced expiratory flow rate over 25–75% of the FVC; FEV_1, forced expiratory volume in the first second; FVC, forced vital capacity; PEF, peak of expiratory flow.

Documentation of reversibility of air flow obstruction following inhalation of a bronchodilator is central to the definition of asthma. After bronchodilation, an improvement of at least 12% and 200 mL in the FEV_1 is considered a positive response and is indicative of reversible air flow obstruction; however, in children, an improvement of 10% may be adequate to indicate significant improvement. It has been proved that the persistence of a significant degree of bronchodilator responsiveness despite regular treatment according to guidelines may represent a marker of worse asthma control (43, 44). Higher bronchodilator reversibility has been added as an additional independent risk factor for asthma attacks in both adults and children in 2018 update of the Global Strategy for Asthma Management and Prevention (3). Besides, reversible or partially reversible airflow obstruction seems to be a distinctive spirometry feature of pediatric severe asthma clinical phenotypes, as demonstrated by the results from severe asthma cohort studies (45, 46).

Although spirometry is still considered the gold standard for use in diagnosing and monitoring change in airway function in patients with asthma, other modalities may have particular application in both younger and older children. The Forced Oscillation Technique (FOT) is a lung function modality based on the application of an external oscillatory signal in order to determine the mechanical response of the respiratory system. The method is noninvasive and requires minimal patient cooperation, which makes it suitable for use in young pediatric patients. In the context of asthma, FOT may be more sensitive than spirometry in identifying disturbances of peripheral airways and assessing the level of asthma control or the effectiveness of therapy at the long term (47). Further research is required to determine the exact role of FOT as an objective monitoring tool in pediatric asthma.

Measuring peak of expiratory flow (PEF) may provide some useful information about obstruction in the large central airways. An exaggerated variability in PEF (morning-to-evening more than 20%) can confirm the diagnosis of asthma; however, the test is extremely effort-dependent and should not be used alone to diagnose asthma. Variability in PEF was suggested as an indicator of poor asthma control (48); however, studies evaluating the efficacy of PEF monitoring for improving various outcome measures in childhood asthma have yielded conflicting results (49–51).

AHR can be demonstrated either by direct inhaled agents (i.e., methacholine) or by indirect stimulants (i.e., exercise). Provocation tests with direct inhaled agents result positive if they cause a 20% fall in baseline FEV_1, but they are not routinely used in pediatric population (52). Exercise challenge testing consists in assessing the FEV_1 variations after 6–8 min of treadmill exercise; a decrease in FEV_1 of more than 10% is diagnostic of exercise induced bronchoconstriction (53). There is some evidence that exercise-induced bronchoconstriction is more specific than other provocation tests in detecting asthma among pediatric population (54).

Airway inflammation is the hallmark of disease pathophysiology in asthma. Currently bronchoscopy, bronchial biopsy, and bronchoalveolar lavage (BAL) are considered the gold standard to assess airway inflammation and remodeling in asthma; however, the invasiveness of these diagnostic methods limits their use in pediatric age in daily clinical practice. Over the last 10 years, there has been an explosion of interest in the research of non-invasive biomarkers to assess of airway inflammation. Biomarkers for asthma have potential utility for distinguishing the inflammatory and/or molecular pattern or "endotype," predict and monitor responsiveness to specific treatments, and assess of the risk of disease progression (55). Thus, the identification of non-invasive methods to study and monitor disease inflammation represents a relevant challenging field of research in childhood asthma. Most of the current established biomarkers available in clinical practice are related to allergic eosinophilic (Th2-high) inflammation. These include blood or sputum eosinophils, serum IgE, and fractional exhaled nitric oxide (FeNO) (55). Single and combination biomarkers are now being recommended for use in the assessment of children with asthma, in particular with severe asthma, and have been extensively reviewed elsewhere (55). Among these, fractional exhaled NO (FeNO) monitoring has a validated role in current clinical practice as a biomarker useful in asthma diagnosis, monitoring control, and predicting asthma attacks (56, 57). Its measurement is simple, safe, and well tolerated, and it has been standardized in school-aged children (58, 59). In pediatric asthma, FeNO is now recognized as a surrogate marker of eosinophilic airway inflammation and it is used to identify children with allergic asthma that are likely to respond to ICS treatment (60). Multiple studies have demonstrated that an increased FeNO value at baseline or increasing FeNO values during ICS reduction accurately predict an asthma attack (60). According to the cut-off values published in the American Thoracic Society (ATS) guidelines, a FeNO of > 35 ppb suggests a likely response to ICS, while a FeNO of <20 ppb in children indicates a less likely responsiveness to ICS treatment (61). Although FeNO-guided treatment has been associated with significantly fewer asthma attacks and lower attack rate than treatment based on current guidelines in childhood asthma, it not routinely recommended for the general asthma population at present (62). Identifying the populations most likely to benefit from FeNO-guided treatment, as well as establishing the optimal frequency of monitoring FeNO, still require further studies.

Risk Factors for Poor Asthma Outcomes

The evaluation of symptom control should be always combined with the assessment of risk factors of adverse outcome in children with asthma, both at diagnosis and periodically thereafter.

First of all, having uncontrolled asthma symptoms, experiencing more than 1 episode of asthma attack in last year and/or admission to intensive care unit for asthma are the main independent risk factors for future attacks (63–67); other risk factors that are potentially modified have been recently updated and include: (i) high SABA use (more than 3 canisters/year) (68) and inadequate inhaled corticosteroids (ICS) therapy (not prescribed, poor adherence, incorrect inhaler technique) (69, 70); (ii) low FEV_1 (even if normal spirometry does not exclude severe asthma in children) (71, 72) and higher bronchodilator reversibility (44); (iii) viral infections (rhinovirus and other respiratory viruses), allergen exposure in atopic children, tobacco smoke exposure and outdoor air pollution

(65). Eosinophilic airway inflammation has been associated with risk of attacks that can be prevented with corticosteroid treatment (2). Blood eosinophils and FeNO have been identified as indirect measures of eosinophilic airway inflammation both in adults and children. These reliable biomarkers may provide a better perspective on risk of attacks and the likely response to treatment with corticosteroids than traditional physiological measures as lung function and asthma symptoms (2). However, blood eosinophilia and elevated FeNO have been recognized as risk factors for acute attacks mainly in adults with allergic asthma taking ICS (3). Overall, it has also been recently established that the presence of any of these mentioned conditions increases the risk of asthma attacks, even if the patient has few asthma symptoms (3).

The severity of asthma attack is a risk marker of both subsequent attacks and mortality from asthma (73). A recent revision of risk factors for severe asthma attacks identified nonwhite race, psycho-social stress and obesity as additional clinical predictors in children (67). Furthermore, cadherin-related family member 3 (CDHR3) has been identified as a novel susceptibility gene for recurrent severe asthma attacks in children ages 2–6 years: in particular, variants of CDH3 seem to alter the integrity of airway epithelium and subsequently promote entry and replication of respiratory viruses (74). However, with the exception of history of one recent severe attack, no current clinical or biological markers has been shown to be highly predictive of severe asthma attacks in children (67). Finally, the recent UK National Review of Asthma Deaths (NRAD) identified the conditions at high risk for death from asthma: (i) a single severe attack; (ii) recent discharge from hospital after an acute asthma attack; (iii) use of hospital urgent care facilities in the previous year; (iv) utilization of more than 6 canisters of SABA/year; and (v) failure to attend follow-up appointments[1]. Thus, an asthma attack (even one) should be carefully considered a significant immediate red flag signaling a high risk of future attacks and asthma deaths, in particular in primary care. Moreover, considering that NRAD reported that around 60% of those who died from asthma were classified as "mild to moderate," the definition of severity by level of treatment should need to be questioned. All these mentioned factors should be added to the conventional definitions of risk as "high risk factors" with the aim to improve care and hopefully reduce the number of deaths.

Early growth characteristics such as pre-term birth, low birth weight and greater infant weight gain have been recently added to the list of risk factors of poor asthma outcomes, all being determinants of airflow limitation and associated with increased risk of childhood asthma (3, 75).

Children with uncontrolled asthma, in particular if treated with high-dose ICS and oral corticosteroids (OCS), may experience medication side-effects (i.e. local and systemic side-effects) (76, 77). The risk factors for medication side-effects include frequent use of oral steroids, long-term, high-dose and/or potent ICS use, or concomitant use of P450 inhibitors (such as ritonavir, ketoconazole, itraconazole) that can markedly increase both bioavailability and decrease clearance of most of the ICS (3). Ongoing monitoring of medication side-effects should be an essential component of a comprehensive childhood asthma management program.

[1] Data from National Review of Asthma Deaths' (2014) Available online at: https://www.rcplondon.ac.uk/projects/outputs/why-asthma-still-kills.

UNCONTROLLED ASTHMA: DIFFICULT VS. SEVERE ASTHMA IN CHILDREN

The actual asthma management is control-based, including evaluation of symptom control and risk domains; therapeutic strategies are based on a stepwise approach and adjusted in a continuous cycle involving assessment, treatment and review (3). Asthma severity should be determined before the patient is treated, while the assessment of asthma control should be performed after treatment has been instituted; then, both of them should be re-determined at every visit. Step up and step down of treatment should be adapted to every patient in order to maintain asthma control with the minimum dose of medication. The frequency of the assessment of asthma control is variable and depends on disease activity but typically is every 1–6 months. Patients with asthma may be classified into three broad categories as well controlled, partly controlled, or uncontrolled, according to established criteria (**Table 3**) (3).

Identifying children and adolescents with uncontrolled severe asthma is important because they potentially need close monitoring and additional treatment with advanced biological therapies (78–82). Although accounting for <5% of all pediatric asthma (83), uncontrolled severe asthma carries the majority of morbidity and accounts for nearly 50% of all asthma healthcare costs, and even mortality (8). Children with persistent uncontrolled asthma, despite maximal therapy, are defined as having problematic severe asthma, an umbrella term comprising asthma-mimicking conditions, asthma that is difficult-to-treat because of comorbidities, improper inhaler technique or poor therapeutic adherence, and other environmental factors, and true severe therapy-resistant asthma, as defined by the latest European Respiratory Society/American Thoracic Society (ERS/ATS) definition (8, 84, 85): after confirming a diagnosis of asthma

TABLE 3 | Levels of asthma symptom control (to assess retrospectively in the past 4 weeks). adapted from Global Initiative for Asthma (3).

	Well-controlled	Partly controlled	Uncontrolled
Daytime asthma symptoms more than twice a week	None of these	1 or 2 of these	3 or 4 of these
Night waking due to asthma			
Need for reliever* for symptoms more than twice a week			
Limitation of activity due to asthma			

**Excluding before exercise.*

and addressing comorbidities, true severe therapy-resistant asthma is that which requires treatment with high dose inhaled glucocorticoids plus a second controller and/or systemic glucocorticoids to prevent asthma from becoming 'uncontrolled' or which remains 'uncontrolled' despite this therapy (8). The identification of the factors that may contribute to the gain or loss of control in asthma is essential in differentiating children with difficult-to-treat asthma from those with severe asthma that is resistant to traditional therapies.

Monitoring and Managing Comorbidities

Once alternative diagnoses have been excluded and the diagnosis of asthma confirmed, the contribution of comorbid conditions to disease severity should be evaluated. Childhood asthma is associated with several comorbidities (**Table 4**), variably presenting and depending on the age of the subject (86–89). Observations from severe asthma international registries and cohort studies highlighted a distinct picture for pediatric age. In the National Heart, Lung and Blood Institute's Severe Asthma Research Program (SARP) the highest prevalence of comorbid conditions, namely sinus disease, gastroesophageal reflux and obesity, has been found in only 20% of children studied (clustered as "Group 3") (90). In the Unbiased Biomarkers for the Prediction of Respiratory Disease Outcomes (U-BIOPRED), around 65% of school-aged children with severe asthma had a diagnosis of concomitant allergic rhinitis, while 40% of children reported food allergy (91). Unlike upper airway pathology, the relationship between gastroesophageal reflux and asthma is still a matter of debate and there is not enough evidence to support causality; besides, it has been demonstrated that treating reflux does not actually improve asthma outcomes (92). Likewise, the relationship between food allergy and respiratory symptoms is still unclear.

Dysfunctional breathing has been reported as common in some asthma cohort; however, the available data suggest that 5.3% or more of children with asthma have dysfunctional breathing and that, unlike in adults, it is associated with poorer asthma control (93). Besides, the results of an observational cohort study conducted on 71 children with problematic asthma reported that 15% of them has dysfunctional breathing, including hyperventilation and vocal cord dysfunction (94). Although it is not possible to draw conclusive estimates on the prevalence of comorbidities in childhood severe asthma, it is well established that the presence of one and/or more comorbid conditions contributes to the loss of asthma control and may complicate the assessment of asthma and potentially impact on its management, outcome and healthcare expenditure (8, 86, 88). Thus, addressing comorbidities is an essential step in the approach to the child with uncontrolled asthma.

Adherence to Treatment

Determining if the child is receiving the prescribed controller medication with the adequate inhaler technique is another essential cornerstone of the management of childhood asthma. Poor adherence to treatment is common in asthmatic children, as well as in adults, with reported rates varying from 30 to 70% (85, 94, 95) and it should be considered in all children with uncontrolled asthma. Medication issues do not only concern about therapeutic adherence, but also affect management of prescriptions, parental supervision, and use of inhaler devices (70, 94, 96). These are all potentially modifiable factors that have been associated with loss of asthma control (97). Interventions to improve patient adherence have been tested in several clinical trials and demonstrated a variable efficacy (94). Identifying non-adherent patients and establishing an educational intervention can be complex and time-consuming and require an integrated strategy in everyday clinical practice including regular follow-up assessment at the doctor office, effective patient-centered behavioral interventions, improvement of doctor-patient communication, and new instruments of control such as electronic monitoring (85).

Review of Environmental Factors

Ongoing exposure to environmental factors is an important cause of poor asthma control in some patients (98). For patients with severe asthma who have an allergic component to their disease, allergen control measures will have an important effect. Potential triggers should be identified during evaluation and need renewed strategies for control. Common inhalant allergens that can contribute to poor asthma control and cause attacks include animal allergens (both pets and pests: cats, dogs, rodents), house dust mites, cockroaches, indoor and outdoor fungi and outdoor plant allergens (tree, grass, ragweed pollen) (99–101). In particular, home and school exposures to pets, house dust mites, mold are associated with severe asthma attacks in children, supporting the importance of atopy in this population (98).

Fungal exposure and sensitization have been recently associated with a sub-phenotype of childhood asthma characterized by increased disease severity, AHR, airway eosinophilic inflammation, more exacerbations and relative

TABLE 4 | Asthma comorbidities in childhood.

Comorbid Conditions	Potential mechanism contributing to worsen asthma
Obesity	Mechanical effects on lung functions; pro-inflammatory state contributing to airway inflammation; corticosteroid resistance
Gastroesophageal reflux	Direct contamination of the lower airway; esophago-bronchial reflex; reduced efficiency of the lower esophageal sphincter due to altered configuration of the diaphragm during respiratory disease
Food allergy	Unclear (consider anaphylaxis at rest and on exercise in the differential diagnosis)
Rhinosinusitis	Shared complex inflammatory mechanisms between upper and lower airways, according to the "United Airways Disease" concept
Upper Airway Obstruction/Sleep Disordered Breathing	Obesity-associated (common); increased neutrophilic inflammation of the airways
Dysfunctional Breathing	Unclear (also consider vocal cord dysfunction and other hyperventilation syndromes in the differential diagnosis)

steroid resistance (102). Severe asthma with fungal sensitization (SAFS) is a recognized subphenotype of severe asthma in both children and adults. SAFS is defined as severe, therapy-resistant asthma with fungal sensitization demonstrated by a positive skin prick test response or specific IgE to at least one of 7 fungi (i.e., Aspergillus fumigatus, Alternaria alternata, Cladosporium herbarum, Penicillium chrysogenum, Candida albicans, Trichophyton mentagrophytes, or Botrytis cinerea), with IgE <1,000 and with negative IgG Aspergillus serology (102). Little is known about the mechanisms mediating this subphenotype. Recent evidence suggests a role for innate epithelial cytokine IL-33 in the pathogenesis of SAFS, as higher levels of IL-33 have been found on BAL and airway samples from children with SAFS compared to children without SAFS (102). Till date there are no guidelines for the diagnosis and treatment of SAFS in pediatric population: reduction of environmental fungal exposure in the home and antifungal therapy have been anecdotally successful in some children.

There are also non-allergic factors that potentially contribute to asthma such as exposure to tobacco smoke (including active and passive smoking, as well as vaping), environmental pollution and other irritants (i.e., incense, joss sticks, air fresheners and other aerosol sprays) (103). Tobacco smoke exposure is common in children with asthma and it has been reported in 25% of cases in a cohort of children having problematic severe asthma (94); it is also associated with loss of asthma control, higher incidence of respiratory infections, increased likehood of asthma attack-related hospitalizations (104–107); furthermore, it was found that parental (passive) smoking impairs histone deacetylase-2 function, which could contribute to increased corticosteroid-resistant inflammation in children with severe asthma (108). In addition, exposure to tobacco smoke exacerbates inflammatory airway responses to allergens (109). Exposures at home, daycare, school and/or work should be reviewed.

Evaluation of Psychosocial Factors

Asthma attacks may be triggered by both acute and chronic stress, through a supposed effect of enhancement of allergic eosinophilic airway inflammatory response (110). Among psychosocial issues, anxiety and depression have been more frequently reported in children with persistent and severe asthma rather than mild or intermittent asthma, and in their families (94, 111, 112). Given the complexity of relationship between these two entities, it is yet to be determined whether anxiety and depression are the cause or result of severe asthma; however, both should be treated on their individual merits.

CONCLUSIONS

Over the past 10 years, there has been an increasing interest on the concept of asthma control, with development and validation of new and promising "asthma control tools."

Uncontrolled persistent asthma in children represents a clinical challenge and requires a multidisciplinary systematic assessment, including the assessment of comorbid conditions, treatment- related issues, environmental exposures and psychosocial factors. The presence or absence of these factors may contribute to the gain or loss of control and differentiate children with difficult-to-treat asthma from those with true severe therapy-resistant asthma. Finally, the early identification of modifiable factors contributing to childhood uncontrolled asthma is essential to avoid a further and useless escalation of treatment; likewise, addressing a correct diagnosis of true severe therapy-resistant asthma avoids deferring of invasive testing and advanced biological therapies.

AUTHOR CONTRIBUTIONS

All authors made substantial contribution to the conception of the work, reviewed the literature on the subject, and drafted the final version of the manuscript; AL, VP, and GM revised it critically for important intellectual content. All authors finally approved the version to be published and agreed to be accountable for all aspects of the work in ensuring that questions related to the accuracy or integrity of any part of the work are appropriately investigated and resolved.

REFERENCES

1. Lai CK, Beasley R, Crane J, Foliaki S, Shah J, Weiland S, et al. Global variation in the prevalence and severity of asthma symptoms: phase three of the International Study of Asthma and Allergies in Childhood (ISAAC). *Thorax* (2009) 64:476–83. doi: 10.1136/thx.2008.106609
2. Pavord ID, Beasley R, Agusti A, Anderson GP, Bel E, Brusselle G, et al. After asthma: redefining airways diseases. *Lancet* (2018) 391:350–400. doi: 10.1016/S0140-6736(17)30879-6
3. Global Initiative for Asthma. *GINA Guidelines 2018. Global Strategy for Asthma Management and Prevention*. (2018) Available online at: http://www.ginasthma.org/
4. National Asthma Education and Prevention Program. Expert Panel Report 3 (EPR-3). Guidelines for the diagnosis and management of asthma—summary report 2007. *J Allergy Clin Immunol.* (2007) 120:S94–S138. doi: 10.1016/j.jaci.2007.09.043
5. British Thoracic Society. *Scottish Intercollegiate Guidelines Network. British Guideline on the Management of Asthma*. (2016) Available from https://www.brit-thoracic.org.uk/standards-of-care/guidelines/btssign-british-guideline-on-the-management-of-asthma/
6. Taylor DR, Bateman ED, Boulet LP, Boushey HA, Busse WW, Casale TB, et al. A new perspective on concepts of asthma severity and control. *Eur Respir J* (2008) 32:545–54. doi: 10.1183/09031936.00155307
7. Dinakar C, Chipps BE. Clinical tools to assess asthma control in children. *Pediatrics* (2017) 139:e20163438. doi: 10.1542/peds.2016-3438
8. Chung KF, Wenzel SE, Brozek JL, Bush A, Castro M, Sterk PJ, et al. International ERS/ATS guidelines on definition, evaluation and treatment of severe asthma. *Eur Respir J.* (2014) 43:343–73. doi: 10.1183/09031936.00202013
9. Licari A, Marseglia GL. Current and future challenges in pediatric severe asthma. *Curr Med Res Opin* (2018) 34:943–44. doi: 10.1080/03007995.2018.1439463
10. Montella S, Baraldi E, Cazzato S, Aralla R, Berardi M, Brunetti LM, et al. Severe asthma features in children: a case-control online survey. *Ital J Pediatr.* (2016) 42:9. doi: 10.1186/s13052-016-0217-z

11. Licari A, Castagnoli R, Denicolò C, Rossini L, Seminara M, Sacchi L, et al. Omalizumab in children with severe allergic asthma: the italian real-life experience. *Curr Respir Med Rev.* (2017) 13:36–42. doi: 10.2174/1573398X13666170426094536
12. Reddel HK, Busse WW, Pedersen S, Tan WC, Chen YZ, Jorup C, et al. Should recommendations about starting inhaled corticosteroid treatment for mild asthma be based on symptom frequency: a post-hoc efficacy analysis of the START study. *Lancet* (2017) 389:157–166. doi: 10.1016/S0140-6736(16)31399-X
13. Santanello NC, Davies G, Galant SP, Pedinoff A, Sveum R, Seltzer J, et al. Validation of an asthma symptom diary for interventional studies. *Arch Dis Child* (1999) 80:414–20.
14. Santanello NC, Demuro-Mercon C, Davies G, Ostrom N, Noonan M, Rooklin A, et al. Validation of a pediatric asthma caregiver diary. *J Allergy Clin Immunol.* (2000) 106:861–6.
15. Santanello NC, Barber BL, Reiss TF, Friedman BS, Juniper EF, Zhang J. Measurement characteristics of two asthma symptom diary scales for use in clinical trials. *Eur Respir J.* (1997) 10:646–51.
16. Juniper EF, O'Byrne PM, Ferrie PJ, King DR, Roberts JN. Measuring asthma control. Clinic questionnaire or daily diary? *Am J Respir Crit Care Med.* (2000) 162:1330–4.
17. Reddel HK, Ware SI, Salome CM, Jenkins CR, Woolcock AJ. Pitfalls in processing home electronic spirometric data in asthma. *Eur Respir J.* (1998) 12:853–8.
18. Reddel HK, Toelle BG, Marks GB, Ware SI, Jenkins CR, Woolcock AJ. Analysis of adherence to peak flow monitoring when recording of data is electronic. *BMJ* (2002) 324:146–7. doi: 10.1136/bmj.324.7330.146
19. Koop A, Mösges R. The use of handheld computers in clinical trials. *Control Clin Trials* (2002) 23:469–80. doi: 10.1016/S0197-2456(02)00224-6
20. Bousquet J, Schunemann HJ, Fonseca J, Samolinski B, Bachert C, Canonica GW, et al. MACVIA-ARIA Sentinel NetworK for allergic rhinitis (MASK-rhinitis): the new generation guideline implementation. *Allergy* (2015) 70:1372–92. doi: 10.1111/all.12686
21. Lambert PC, Burton PR, Abrams KR, Brooke AM. The analysis of peak expiratory flow data using a three-level hierarchical model. *Stat Med.* (2004) 23:3821–39. doi: 10.1002/sim.1951
22. Tasche MJ, van der Wouden JC, Uijen JH, Ponsioen BP, Bernsen RM, van Suijlekom-Smit LW, et al. Randomised placebo- controlled trial of inhaled sodium cromoglycate in 1-4-year-old children with moderate asthma. *Lancet* (1997) 350:1060–4.
23. O'Byrne PM, Barnes PJ, Rodriguez-Roisin R, Runnerstrom E, Sandstrom T, Svensson K, et al. Low dose inhaled budesonide and formoterol in mild persistent asthma: the OPTIMA randomized trial. *Am J Respir Crit Care Med.* (2001) 164:1392–7. doi: 10.1164/ajrccm.164.8.2104102
24. American Lung Association Asthma Clinical Research Centers, Mastronarde JG, Anthonisen NR, Castro M, Holbrook JT, Leone FT, et al. Efficacy of esomeprazole for treatment of poorly controlled asthma. *N Engl J Med.* (2009) 360:1487–99. doi: 10.1056/NEJMoa0806290
25. Szefler SJ, Baker JW, Uryniak T, Goldman M, Silkoff PE. Comparative study of budesonide inhalation suspension and montelukast in young children with mild persistent asthma. *J Allergy Clin Immunol.* (2007) 120:1043–50. doi: 10.1016/j.jaci.2007.08.063
26. Chipps BE, Zeiger RS, Dorenbaum A, Borish L, Wenzel SE, Miller DP, et al. Assessment of asthma control and asthma exacerbations in the epidemiology and natural history of asthma: outcomes and treatment regimens (TENOR) observational cohort. *Curr Respir Care Rep* (2012) 1:259–69. doi: 10.1007/s13665-012-0025-x
27. Arets HG, Kamps AW, Brackel HJ, Mulder PG, Vermue NA, van der Ent CK. Children with mild asthma: do they benefit from inhaled corticosteroids? *Eur Respir J* (2002) 20:1470–5. doi: 10.1183/09031936.02.00292702
28. Bateman ED, Boushey HA, Bousquet J, Busse WW, Clark TJ, Pauwels RA, et al. Can guideline-defined asthma control be achieved? The gaining optimal asthma control study. *Am J Respir Crit Care Med.* (2004) 170:836–44. doi: 10.1164/rccm.200401-033OC
29. Piacentini GL, Peroni DG, Bodini A, Bonafiglia E, Rigotti E, Baraldi E, et al. Childhood Asthma Control Test and airway inflammation evaluation in asthmatic children. *Allergy* (2009) 64:1753–7. doi: 10.1111/j.1398-9995.2009.02068.x
30. Gani F, Lombardi C, Barrocu L, Landi M, Ridolo E, Bugiani M, et al. The control of allergic rhinitis in real life: a multicenter cross-sectional Italian study. *Clin Mol Allergy* (2018) 16:4. doi: 10.1186/s12948-018-0082-y
31. Ciprandi G, Schiavetti I, Ricciardolo FL. Symptom perception and asthma control. *Postgrad Med.* (2015) 127:738–43. doi: 10.1080/00325481.2015.1074033
32. Tosca MA, Silvestri M, Rossi GA, Ciprandi G. Perception of bronchodilation assessed by Visual Analogue Scale in children with asthma. *Allergol Immunopathol (Madr)* (2013) 41:359–63. doi: 10.1016/j.aller.2012.06.002
33. Schweitzer C, Marchal F. Dyspnoea in children. Does development alter the perception of breathlessness? *Respir Physiol Neurobiol.* (2009) 167:144–53. doi: 10.1016/j.resp.2008.12.001
34. Krouse RZ, Sorkness CA, Wildfire JJ, Calatroni A, Gruchalla R, Hershey GKK, et al. Minimally important differences and risk levels for the Composite Asthma Severity Index. *J Allergy Clin Immunol.* (2017) 139:1052–55. doi: 10.1016/j.jaci.2016.08.041
35. Wildfire JJ, Gergen PJ, Sorkness CA, Mitchell HE, Calatroni A, Kattan M, et al. Development and validation of the Composite Asthma Severity Index–an outcome measure for use in children and adolescents. *J Allergy Clin Immunol.* (2012) 129:694–701. doi: 10.1016/j.jaci.2011.12.962
36. Yawn BP, Wollan PC, Rank MA, Bertram SL, Juhn Y, Pace W. Use of asthma APGAR tools in primary care practices: a cluster-randomized controlled trial. *Ann Fam Med.* (2018) 16:100–110. doi: 10.1370/afm.2179
37. Data from FAQs. *ATA Main [Internet].* (2018) Available online at: https://www.americantelemed.org/about/telehealth-faqs-
38. Pellegrino R, Viegi G, Brusasco V, Crapo RO, Burgos F, Casaburi R, et al. Interpretative strategies for lung function tests. *Eur Respir J.* (2005) 26:948–68. doi: 10.1183/09031936.05.00035205
39. Mannino DM, Buist AS, Petty TL, Enright PL, Redd SC. Lung function and mortality in the United States: data from the First National Health and Nutrition Examination Survey follow up study. *Thorax* (2003) 58:388–93. doi: 10.1136/thorax.58.5.388
40. Raywood E, Lum S, Aurora P, Pike K. The bronchodilator response in preschool children: a systematic review. *Pediatr Pulmonol.* (2016) 51:1242–50. doi: 10.1002/ppul.23459
41. Marseglia GL, Cirillo I, Vizzaccaro A, Klersy C, Tosca MA, La Rosa M, et al. Role of forced expiratory flow at 25-75% as an early marker of small airways impairment in subjects with allergic rhinitis. *Allergy Asthma Proc.* (2007) 28:74–8.
42. Siroux V, Boudier A, Dolgopoloff M, Chanoine S, Bousquet J, Gormand F, et al. Forced midexpiratory flow between 25% and 75% of forced vital capacity is associated with long-term persistence of asthma and poor asthma outcomes. *J Allergy Clin Immunol.* (2016) 137:1709–16.e6. doi: 10.1016/j.jaci.2015.10.029
43. Galant SP, Morphew T, Newcomb RL, Hioe K, Guijon O, Liao O. The relationship of the bronchodilator response phenotype to poor asthma control in children with normal spirometry. *J Pediatr.* (2011) 158:953–9.e1. doi: 10.1016/j.jpeds.2010.11.029
44. Pongracic JA, Krouse RZ, Babineau DC, Zoratti EM, Cohen RT, Wood RA, et al. Distinguishing characteristics of difficult-to-control asthma in inner-city children and adolescents. *J Allergy Clin Immunol.* (2016) 138:1030–41. doi: 10.1016/j.jaci.2016.06.059
45. Sorkness RL, Teague WG, Penugonda M, Fitzpatrick AM, National Institutes of Health, National Heart, Lung, and Blood Institute's Severe Asthma Research Program. Sex dependence of airflow limitation and air trapping in children with severe asthma. *J Allergy Clin Immunol.* (2011) 127:1073–4. doi: 10.1016/j.jaci.2010.12.1079
46. Fitzpatrick AM, Moore WC. Severe asthma phenotypes-how should they guide evaluation and treatment? *J Allergy Clin Immunol Pract.* (2017) 5:901–8. doi: 10.1016/j.jaip.2017.05.015
47. Skylogianni E, Douros K, Anthracopoulos MB, Fouzas S. The forced oscillation technique in paediatric respiratory practice. *Paediatr Respir Rev.* (2016) 18:46–51. doi: 10.1016/j.prrv.2015.11.001
48. Kaminsky DA, Wang LL, Bates JH, Thamrin C, Shade DM, Dixon AE, et al. Fluctuation analysis of peak expiratory flow and its association with treatment failure in asthma. *Am J Respir Crit Care Med.* (2017) 195:993–9. doi: 10.1164/rccm.201601-0076OC

49. Goldberg S, Springer C, Avital A, Godfrey S, Bar-Yishay E. Can peak expiratory flow measurements estimate small airway function in asthmatic children? *Chest* (2001) 120:482–8. doi: 10.1378/chest.120.2.482
50. Yoos HL, Kitzman H, McMullen A, Henderson C, Sidora K. Symptom monitoring in childhood asthma: a randomized clinical trial comparing peak expiratory flow rate with symptom monitoring. *Ann Allergy Asthma Immunol.* (2002) 88:283–91. doi: 10.1016/S1081-1206(10)62010-8
51. Wensley D, Silverman M. Peak flow monitoring for guided self-management in childhood asthma: a randomized controlled trial. *Am J Respir Crit Care Med.* (2004) 170:606–12. doi: 10.1164/rccm.200307-1025OC
52. Park GM, Han HW, Kim JY, Lee E, Cho HJ, Yoon J, et al. Association of symptom control with changes in lung function, bronchial hyperresponsiveness, and exhaled nitric oxide after inhaled corticosteroid treatment in children with asthma. *Allergol Int* (2016) 65:439–443. doi: 10.1016/j.alit.2016.03.011
53. Crapo RO, Casaburi R, Coates AL, Enright PL, Hankinson JL, Irvin CG, et al. Guidelines for methacholine and exercise challenge testing-1999. This official statement of the American Thoracic Society was adopted by the ATS Board of Directors, July 1999. *Am J Respir Crit Care Med.* (2000) 161:309–29. doi: 10.1164/ajrccm.161.1.ats11-99
54. Carlsen KH, Engh G, Mørk M, Schrøder E. Cold air inhalation and exercise-induced bronchoconstriction in relationship to metacholine bronchial responsiveness: different patterns in asthmatic children and children with other chronic lung diseases. *Respir Med.* (1998) 92:308–15.
55. Licari A, Castagnoli R, Brambilla I, Marseglia A, Tosca MA, Marseglia GL, et al. Asthma endotyping and biomarkers in childhood asthma. *Pediatr Allergy Immunol Pulmonol.* (2018) 31:1–12. doi: 10.1089/ped.2018.0886
56. Pijnenburg MW, De Jongste JC. Exhaled nitric oxide in childhood asthma: a review. *Clin Exp Allergy* (2008) 38:246–59. doi: 10.1111/j.1365-2222.2007.02897.x
57. Gomersal T, Harnan S, Essat M, Tappenden P, Wong R, Lawson R, et al. A systematic review of fractional exhaled nitric oxide in the routine management of childhood asthma. *Pediatr Pulmonol* (2016) 51:316–28. doi: 10.1002/ppul.23371
58. Baraldi E, de Jongste JC, European Respiratory Society/American Thoracic Society (ERS/ATS) Task Force. Measurement of exhaled nitric oxide in children, 2001. *Eur Respir J.* (2002) 20:223-237. doi: 10.1183/09031936.02.00293102
59. Horváth I, Barnes PJ, Loukides S, Sterk PJ, Högman M, Olin AC, et al. A European Respiratory Society technical standard: exhaled biomarkers in lung disease. *Eur Respir J* (2017) 49:1600965. doi: 10.1183/13993003.009 65-2016
60. Spahn JD, Malka J, Szefler SJ. Current application of exhaled nitric oxide in clinical practice. *J Allergy Clin Immunol.* (2016) 138:1296–8. doi: 10.1016/j.jaci.2016.09.002
61. Dweik RA, Boggs PB, Erzurum SC, Irvin CG, Leigh MW, Lundberg JO, et al. An official ATS clinical practice guideline: interpretation of exhaled nitric oxide levels (FENO) for clinical applications. *Am J Respir Crit Care Med.* (2011) 184:602–15. doi: 10.1164/rccm.9120-11ST
62. Petsky HL, Kew KM, Chang AB. Exhaled nitric oxide levels to guide treatment for children with asthma. *Cochrane Database Syst Rev.* (2016) 11:CD011439. doi: 10.1002/14651858.CD011439.pub2
63. Turner MO, Noertjojo K, Vedal S, Bai T, Crump S, Fitzgerald JM. Risk factors for near-fatal asthma. A case-control study in hospitalized patients with asthma. *Am J Respir Crit Care Med.* (1998) 157:1804–9. doi: 10.1164/ajrccm.157.6.9708092
64. Haselkorn T, Fish JE, Zeiger RS, Szefler SJ, Miller DP, Chipps BE, et al. Consistently very poorly controlled asthma, as defined by the impairment domain of the Expert Panel Report 3 guidelines, increases risk for future severe asthma exacerbations in The Epidemiology and Natural History of Asthma: outcomes and Treatment Regimens (TENOR) study. *J Allergy Clin Immunol.* (2009) 124:895–902.e1-4. doi: 10.1016/j.jaci.2009. 07.035
65. Forno E, Celedón JC. Predicting asthma exacerbations in children. *Curr Opin Pulm Med.* (2012) 18:63–9. doi: 10.1097/MCP.0b013e32834db288
66. Carroll CL, Uygungil B, Zucker AR, Schramm CM. Identifying an at-risk population of children with recurrent near-fatal asthma exacerbations. *J Asthma* (2010) 47:460–4. doi: 10.3109/02770903.2010.481344
67. Puranik S, Forno E, Bush A, Celedón JC. Predicting severe asthma exacerbations in children. *Am J Respir Crit Care Med.* (2017) 195:854–9. doi: 10.1164/rccm.201606-1213PP
68. Patel M, Pilcher J, Reddel HK, Pritchard A, Corin A, Helm C, et al. Metrics of salbutamol use as predictors of future adverse outcomes in asthma. *Clin Exp Allergy* (2013) 43:1144–51. doi: 10.1111/cea.12166
69. Ernst P, Spitzer WO, Suissa S, Cockcroft D, Habbick B, Horwitz RI, et al. Risk of fatal and near-fatal asthma in relation to inhaled corticosteroid use. *JAMA* (1992) 268:3462–4.
70. Melani AS, Bonavia M, Cilenti V, Cinti C, Lodi M, Martucci P, et al. Inhaler mishandling remains common in real life and is associated with reduced disease control. *Respir Med* (2011) 105:930–8. doi: 10.1016/j.rmed.2011.01.005
71. Fuhlbrigge AL, Kitch BT, Paltiel AD, Kuntz KM, Neumann PJ, Dockery DW, et al. FEV1 is associated with risk of asthma attacks in a pediatric population. *J Allergy Clin Immunol.* (2001) 107:61–7. doi: 10.1067/mai.2001.111590
72. Bossley CJ, Fleming L, Ullmann N, Gupta A, Adams A, Nagakumar P, et al. Assessment of corticosteroid response in pediatric patients with severe asthma by using a multidomain approach. *J Allergy Clin Immunol.* (2016) 138:413–420.e6. doi: 10.1016/j.jaci.2015.12.1347
73. Levy ML, Winter R. Asthma deaths: what now? *Thorax* (2015) 70:209–210. doi: 10.1136/thoraxjnl-2015-206800
74. Bønnelykke K, Sleiman P, Nielsen K, Kreiner-Møller E, Mercader JM, Belgrave D, et al. A genome-wide association study identifies CDHR3 as a susceptibility locus for early childhood asthma with severe exacerbations. *Nat Genet* (2014) 46:51–5. doi: 10.1038/ng.2830
75. den Dekker HT, Sonnenschein-van der Voort AMM, de Jongste JC, Anessi-Maesano I, Arshad SH, Barros H, et al. Early growth characteristics and the risk of reduced lung function and asthma: a meta-analysis of 25,000 children. *J Allergy Clin Immunol.* (2016) 137:1026–35. doi: 10.1016/j.jaci.2015. 08.050
76. Kaur S, Singh V. Asthma and medicines-long-term side-effects, monitoring and dose titration. *Indian J Pediatr.* (2018). doi: 10.1007/s12098-017-2553-4. [Epub ahead of print].
77. Raissy HH, Kelly HW. Benefits and risks of long-term asthma management in children: where are we heading? *Drug Saf.* (2017) 40:201–10. doi: 10.1007/s40264-016-0483-0
78. Licari A, Marseglia A, Caimmi S, Castagnoli R, Foiadelli T, Barberi S, et al. Omalizumab in children. *Paediatr Drugs* (2014) 16:491–502. doi: 10.1007/s40272-014-0107-z
79. Licari A, Marseglia G, Castagnoli R, Marseglia A, Ciprandi G. The discovery and development of omalizumab for the treatment of asthma. *Expert Opin Drug Discov.* (2015) 10:1033–42. doi: 10.1517/17460441.2015.1048220
80. Ciprandi G, Marseglia GL, Castagnoli R, Valsecchi C, Tagliacarne C, Caimmi S, et al. From IgE to clinical trials of allergic rhinitis. *Expert Rev Clin Immunol.* (2015) 11:1321–33. doi: 10.1586/1744666X.2015.10 86645
81. Licari A, Castagnoli R, Panfili E, Marseglia A, Brambilla I, Marseglia GL. An update on anti-ige therapy in pediatric respiratory diseases. *Curr Respir Med Rev.* (2017) 13:22–9. doi: 10.2174/1573398X13666170616110738
82. Licari A, Castagnoli R, Brambilla I, Marseglia A, Tosca MA, Marseglia GL, et al. New approaches for identifying and testing potential new anti-asthma agents. *Expert Opin Drug Discov.* (2018) 13:51–63. doi: 10.1080/17460441.2018.1396315
83. Lang A, Carlsen KH, Haaland G, Devulapalli CS, Munthe-Kaas M, Mowinckel P, et al. Severe asthma in childhood: assessed in 10 year olds in a birth cohort study. *Allergy* (2008) 63:1054–60. doi: 10.1111/j.1398-9995.2008.01672.x
84. Bush A, Fleming L, Saglani S. Severe asthma in children. *Respirology* (2017) 22:886–97. doi: 10.1111/resp.13085
85. Ramratnam SK, Bacharier LB, Guilbert TW. Severe asthma in children. *J Allergy Clin Immunol Pract.* (2017) 5:889–98. doi: 10.1016/j.jaip.2017.04.031
86. de Groot EP, Duiverman EJ, Brand PL. Comorbidities of asthma during childhood: possibly important, yet poorly studied. *Eur Respir J.* (2010) 36:671–8. doi: 10.1183/09031936.00185709
87. Licari A, Castagnoli R, Denicolò CF, Rossini L, Marseglia A, Marseglia GL. The nose and the lung: united airway disease? *Front Pediatr.* (2017) 5:44. doi: 10.3389/fped.2017.00044

88. Licari A, Brambilla I, De Filippo M, Poddighe D, Castagnoli R, Marseglia GL. The role of upper airway pathology as a co-morbidity in severe asthma. *Expert Rev Respir Med.* (2017) 11:855–65. doi: 10.1080/17476348.2017.1381564
89. Peters U, Dixon AE, Forno E. Obesity and asthma. *J Allergy Clin Immunol.* (2018) 141:1169–79. doi: 10.1016/j.jaci.2018.02.004
90. Fitzpatrick AM, Teague WG, Meyers DA, Peters SP, Li X, Li H, et al. Heterogeneity of severe asthma in childhood: confirmation by cluster analysis of children in the National Institutes of Health/National Heart, Lung, and Blood Institute Severe Asthma Research Program. *J Allergy Clin Immunol.* (2011) 127:382–389.e1-13. doi: 10.1016/j.jaci.2010.11.015
91. Fleming L, Murray C, Bansal AT, Hashimoto S, Bisgaard H, Bush A, et al. The burden of severe asthma in childhood and adolescence: results from the paediatric U-BIOPRED cohorts. *Eur Respir J.* (2015) 46:1322–33. doi: 10.1183/13993003.00780-2015
92. Writing Committee for the American Lung Association Asthma Clinical Research Centers, Holbrook JT, Wise RA, Gold BD, Blake K, Brown ED, et al. Lansoprazole for children with poorly controlled asthma: a randomized controlled trial. *JAMA* (2012) 307:373–81. doi: 10.1001/jama.2011.2035
93. Barker NJ, Jones M, O'Connell NE, Everard ML. Breathing exercises for dysfunctional breathing/hyperventilation syndrome in children. *Cochrane Database Syst Rev.* (2013) 12:CD010376. doi: 10.1002/14651858.CD010376.pub2
94. Bracken M, Fleming L, Hall P, Van Stiphout N, Bossley C, Biggart E, et al. The importance of nurse-led home visits in the assessment of children with problematic asthma. *Arch Dis Child* (2009) 94:780–4. doi: 10.1136/adc.2008.152140
95. Chan AHY, Stewart AW, Foster JM, Mitchell EA, Camargo CA Jr, Harrison J. Factors associated with medication adherence in school-aged children with asthma. *ERJ Open Res.* (2016) 2:00087-2015. doi: 10.1183/23120541.00087-2015
96. Levy ML, Hardwell A, McKnight E, Holmes J. Asthma patients' inability to use a pressurised metered-dose inhaler (pMDI) correctly correlates with poor asthma control as defined by the Global Initiative for Asthma (GINA) strategy: a retrospective analysis. *Prim Care Respir J.* (2013) 22: 406–11. doi: 10.4104/pcrj.2013.00084
97. Klok T, Kaptein AA, Duiverman EJ, Brand PL. Long-term adherence to inhaled corticosteroids in children with asthma: observational study. *Respir Med.* (2015) 109:1114–9. doi: 10.1016/j.rmed.2015.07.016
98. Sala KA, Carroll CL, Tang YS, Aglio T, Dressler AM, Schramm CM. Factors associated with the development of severe asthma exacerbations in children. *J Asthma* (2011) 48:558–64. doi: 10.3109/02770903.2011.585411
99. Platts-Mills TA, Carter MC. Asthma and indoor exposure to allergens. N Engl J Med (1997) 336:1382. doi: 10.1056/NEJM199705083361909
100. Pongracic JA, O'Connor GT, Muilenberg ML, Vaughn B, Gold DR, Kattan M, et al. Differential effects of outdoor versus indoor fungal spores on asthma morbidity in inner-city children. *J Allergy Clin Immunol* (2010) 125:593. doi: 10.1016/j.jaci.2009.10.036
101. Darrow LA, Hess J, Rogers CA, Tolbert PE, Klein M, Sarnat SE. Ambient pollen concentrations and emergency department visits for asthma and wheeze. *J Allergy Clin Immunol.* (2012) 130:630–38.e4. doi: 10.1016/j.jaci.2012.06.020
102. Castanhinha S, Sherburn R, Walker S, Gupta A, Bossley CJ, Buckley J, et al. Pediatric severe asthma with fungal sensitization is mediated by steroid-resistant IL-33. *J Allergy Clin Immunol.* (2015) 136:312–22.e7. doi: 10.1016/j.jaci.2015.01.016
103. Rottier BL, Eber E, Hedlin G, Turner S, Wooler E, Mantzourani E, et al. Monitoring asthma in childhood: management-related issues. *Eur Respir Rev.* (2015) 24:194–203. doi: 10.1183/16000617.00003814
104. Kit BK, Simon AE, Brody DJ, Akinbami LJ. US prevalence and trends in tobacco smoke exposure among children and adolescents with asthma. *Pediatrics* (2013) 131:407–14. doi: 10.1542/peds.2012-2328
105. Akinbami LJ, Kit BK, Simon AE. Impact of environmental tobacco smoke on children with asthma, United States, 2003-2010. *Acad Pediatr.* (2013) 13:508–16. doi: 10.1016/j.acap.2013.07.003
106. Howrylak JA, Spanier AJ, Huang B, Peake RW, Kellogg MD, Sauers H, et al. Cotinine in children admitted for asthma and readmission. *Pediatrics* (2014) 133:e355-62. doi: 10.1542/peds.2013-2422
107. Lang JE, Dozor AJ, Holbrook JT, Mougey E, Krishnan S, Sweeten S, et al. Biologic mechanisms of environmental tobacco smoke in children with poorly controlled asthma: results from a multicenter clinical trial. *J Allergy Clin Immunol Pract.* (2013) 1:172–80. doi: 10.1016/j.jaip.2012.11.006
108. Kobayashi Y, Bossley C, Gupta A, Akashi K, Tsartsali L, Mercado N, et al. Passive smoking impairs histone deacetylase-2 in children with severe asthma. *Chest* (2014) 145:305–12. doi: 10.1378/chest.13-0835
109. Diaz-Sanchez D, Rumold R, Gong H Jr. Challenge with environmental tobacco smoke exacerbates allergic airway disease in human beings. *J Allergy Clin Immunol.* (2006) 118:441–6. doi: 10.1016/j.jaci.2006.04.047.
110. Liu LY, Coe CL, Swenson CA, Kelly EA, Kita H, Busse WW. School examinations enhance airway inflammation to antigen challenge. *Am J Respir Crit Care Med.* (2002) 165:1062–7. doi: 10.1164/ajrccm.165.8.2109065
111. Kohlboeck G, Koletzko S, Bauer C-P, von Berg A, Berdel D, Krämer U, et al. Association of atopic and non-atopic asthma with emotional symptoms in school children. *Pediatr Allergy Immunol.* (2013) 24:230–6. doi: 10.1111/pai.12056
112. Goodwin RD, Fergusson DM, Horwood LJ. Asthma and depressive and anxiety disorders among young persons in the community. *Psychol Med.* (2004) 34:1465–74.

2

Severe Asthma—Perspectives from Adult and Pediatric Pulmonology

Louise Fleming [1] and Liam Heaney [2]*

[1] National Heart and Lung Institute, Imperial College, London and Royal Brompton Hospital, London, United Kingdom,
[2] Centre for Experimental Medicine, School of Medicine, Dentistry and Biomedical Sciences, Institute for Health Sciences, Queens University Belfast, Belfast, United Kingdom

***Correspondence:**
Louise Fleming
l.fleming@rbht.nhs.uk

Both adults and children with severe asthma represent a small proportion of the asthma population; however, they consume disproportionate resources. For both groups it is important to confirm the diagnosis of severe asthma and ensure that modifiable factors such as adherence have, as far as possible, been addressed. Most children can be controlled on inhaled corticosteroids and long term oral corticosteroid use is rare, in contrast to adults where steroid related morbidity accounts for a large proportion of the costs of severe asthma. Atopic sensitization is very common in children with severe asthma as are other atopic conditions such as allergic rhinitis and hay fever which can impact on asthma control. In adults, the role of allergic driven disease, even in those with co-existent evidence of sensitization, is unclear. There is currently an exciting pipeline of novel biologicals, particularly directed at Type 2 inflammation, which afford the possibility of improved asthma control and reduced treatment side effects for people with asthma. However, not all drugs will work for all patients and accurate phenotyping is essential. In adults the terms T2 high and T2 low asthma have been coined to describe groups of patients based on the presence/absence of eosinophilic inflammation and T-helper 2 (TH_2) cytokines. Bronchoscopic studies in children with severe asthma have demonstrated that these children are predominantly eosinophilic but the cytokine patterns do not fit the T2 high paradigm suggesting other steroid resistant pathways are driving the eosinophilic inflammation. It remains to be seen whether treatments developed for adult severe asthma will be effective in children and which biomarkers will predict response.

Keywords: asthma, children, adults, adherance, type 2 inflammation, biological therapies

INTRODUCTION

Most children and adults diagnosed with asthma can achieve good symptom control on a low dose of correctly administered inhaled steroids with or without additional controller medication. However, there remains a small but significant proportion with ongoing symptoms and/or frequent attacks despite high intensity treatment. This group consume a high proportion of healthcare resources in terms of treatment costs and hospital admissions, as well as the wider societal costs of time of work and school. Direct healthcare costs are mostly due to prescribed medication for asthma and corticosteroid induced morbidity, particularly in adults (1, 2). In both adults and children, it is essential to firstly confirm the diagnosis of severe asthma in order to implement appropriate management. This article will outline the definition of severe asthma, before exploring the similarities and differences between adults and children in terms of demographics, pathophysiology and management.

DEFINITION OF SEVERE ASTHMA

Many terms, including difficult; problematic; therapy resistant and refractory asthma have been used interchangeably with severe asthma. Over the past 20 years national and international organizations have sought to clarify these differences and refine the definitions and nomenclature. The European Respiratory Society (ERS)/American Thoracic Society (ATS) guidelines 2016 (3) set out a framework for the diagnosis of severe asthma in adults and children and more recently the Global Initiative for Asthma (GINA) has produced a useful guide for the diagnosis and management of "Difficult-to-treat" and Severe Asthma in adolescents and adults (4). Only those with a confirmed diagnosis of asthma, prescribed high dose treatment, who have ongoing poor control (or who require a high level of treatment to maintain control) once modifiable factors have been addressed are classified as severe asthma. The diagnosis of asthma is covered elsewhere in this supplement and will not be dealt with further here but identification and addressing poor medication adherence, comorbidities and psychosocial issues is a critical aspect of determining if severe asthma is present and will be discussed below. High intensity standard treatment is generally defined for both adults and children as high dose inhaled corticosteroids (ICS) plus at least one additional controller medication (long acting beta agonist (LABA), theophylline or leukotriene receptor antagonist (LRTA) (5, 6). The definition of high dose ICS is usually stratified by age: children under 5 (or 6) years; between 5 (or 6) to 12 years; and over 12 years. Children and young people (CYP) over 12 years are often included in the adult classification. The rationale for such an approach is likely based on drug licensing studies. Most Phase 3/4 adult studies include adolescent patients but these data are rarely reported separately (or indeed include sufficient adolescents for meaningful subgroup analysis). The definition of "high dose" varies between guidelines. The ERS/ATS and British Thoracic Society (BTS)/Scottish Intercollegiate Guidelines Network (SIGN) guidelines use cut offs of $\geq$1,000 mcg/day fluticasone propionate (FP) or equivalent for adults and $\geq$500 mcg/day FP equivalent for children whereas GINA uses lower cut points of >500 mcg FP/day for 12 years and older and >400 mcg for children aged 6–11 years (3, 5, 6). Given the flat dose response curve of ICS, there is little additional benefit from stepping up to very high doses in most patients (7) and therefore the GINA thresholds are probably more appropriate. Furthermore, adolescence is an important time of growth and development and most pediatricians are judicious in their use of very high (i.e., adult) doses of ICS in teenagers, preferring to stick with the pediatric thresholds.

PREVALENCE OF SEVERE ASTHMA

Estimates of the prevalence of severe asthma vary depending on the definition used. It is widely quoted that 5–10% of the asthmatic population have severe asthma, but this will include a significant number of patients with ongoing poor adherence, untreated co-morbidities or mis-diagnosis. In a Dutch study, 17.4% of the adult asthma population had "difficult to control" asthma (poor asthma control despite prescription of high intensity treatment) but after excluding non-adherence and poor inhaler technique, only 3.6% had severe refractory asthma (8). In adults referred with severe asthma, when evaluated systematically with a multi-disciplinary team, high rates of mis-diagnosis and comorbid disease are identified (9, 10). In children the numbers are likely even lower. A study which defined severity on the basis on symptoms, exacerbation frequency and spirometry found that 13% of children with asthma were classified as "severe persistent asthma" (11). However, "difficult to control asthma" would have been a more appropriate label for this group. Of children with difficult to control asthma referred to a specialist severe asthma clinic less than half were assessed as having severe asthma (12). Improvements in assessment of those children, particularly adherence monitoring has seen that figure fall to around 20% (13), suggesting that <2.5% of children with asthma have severe refractory asthma. Severity in pre-school children is even harder to estimate, particularly given the challenges of asthma diagnosis. In the Manchester Asthma and Allergy birth cohort approximately 6% of children with a history of wheeze were classified as severe (14).

DIFFERENTIATING SEVERE REFRACTORY ASTHMA FROM MILDER ASTHMA

The umbrella term problematic severe asthma or difficult to treat asthma covers all those with ongoing poor control despite high intensity treatment (5, 15, 16). A significant proportion of this group will have improved control once modifiable factors such as adherence, allergen exposure and psychosocial issues are addressed, and co-morbidities identified and managed appropriately (9, 12, 17). Those with ongoing poor control despite attention to these basics of asthma management are considered to have severe asthma, although it is accepted there is overlap between these groups (18).

POOR ADHERENCE TO MEDICATION

Poor adherence to ICS, for both adults and children is the most common reason for treatment failure and poor asthma control (19, 20). In adults, 65% of patients with "difficult to control" asthma and prone to exacerbation and referred for specialist assessment in the UK, collected <80% of their inhaled preventive medication (21, 22). Medication issues including poor adherence (from prescription records), poor technique and inappropriate device were assessed as contributing to poor asthma control in half of children with seemingly severe asthma referred to a tertiary center (12). Identification of poor adherence to inhaled treatment as the primary clinical problem can be difficult. Physician assessment and patient self-report overestimate adherence when compared with objective or surrogate measures such as prescription records (21, 23). Whilst prescription or dispensing records are helpful, these still overestimate adherence as patients may pick up their inhalers and not use them or use them incorrectly. In children, there is a reliance on parents to request and collect prescriptions; and the child must actually take the medication. A US study which sought to determine if azithromycin or montelukast was an inhaled steroid sparing treatment (MARS trial), was abandoned as most of the children were adequately controlled when adherence was addressed under close medical supervision (24). Objective measures for monitoring inhaled medication are available but have been slow to be implemented in routine clinical care. In both adults and children monitoring adherence to inhaled corticosteroids, aligned with biological response—including suppression of fractional exhaled nitric oxide (FeNO) with monitored treatment—can be used to identify patients with poor prior adherence to inhaled corticosteroids who are likely to achieve substantial benefit from optimized inhaled treatment (13, 23, 25, 26). In addition, this approach can identify those subjects who are unlikely to suppress markers of type-2 biology (FeNO and blood eosinophils) with optimized inhaled treatment alone, and would potentially be candidates for biologic (27, 28). Collectively, these studies have shown that at least 50% of adult and 80% of pediatric patients who would qualify for novel biologic therapies based on their exacerbation history and inflammatory biomarkers are simply not taking regular inhaled anti-inflammatory treatment.

However, having identified that adherence is the primary problem, we still need to define the best intervention to change non-adherent behavior in the medium to long-term and there is unlikely to be a "one size fits all" solution. In adults and children there are a number of factors that can influence adherence, both intentional and unintentional (29): The device must be age appropriate and use demonstrated by an appropriately trained team member (30). Unfortunately, even among healthcare professionals, inhaler technique skills are poor (31). A metered dose inhaler (MDI) should always be used with a spacer in children, and all but the youngest children should be able to use a spacer with mouth piece. In children, an additional complexity is the need to engage parents and caregivers in their child's asthma management. The use of remote directly observed therapy using a Smartphone and associated App has demonstrated that children's inhaler technique is generally inadequate, even when use has recently been demonstrated by a specialist children's asthma nurse (32). Ongoing and continued education is needed, particularly as parents often over estimate their child's technique (33). Furthermore, supervision by parents is often poor; 20% of children aged 7 years are not supervised and by 11 years this figure rises to over 50% (34). Interestingly rates of adherence are equally poor among preschool children; younger school aged children and adolescents (13, 35).

Mobile text messaging in chronic disease management improves adherence rates and simple reminder systems have also been shown to improve inhaled maintenance treatment in asthma, suggesting the gains are potentially large in this population (36–38).

Multiple pharmaceutical companies are now involved with digital technologies and "smart inhalers." Monitoring of inhaled treatment may potentially become available across a number of inhaler platforms for asthma patients.

CO-MORBIDITIES

In both adults and children, co-morbidities and psychosocial factors, such as atopy, obesity, gastroesophageal reflux (GER), rhinitis, anxiety disorders, depression, and dysfunctional breathing can negatively impact on asthma control, medication adherence, mimic the symptoms of asthma and contribute to the complexity of asthma management in those with both severe and difficult to treat asthma (10, 18, 39). These should be regarded as "treatable traits" which can be identified and targeted as part of a comprehensive disease management approach (40–44). **Table 1** [adapted from Porsbjerg and Menzies-Gow (39)] summarizes these extrapulmonary traits and potential management strategies. The prevalence and importance of many of these comorbidities is much better described in adults than children with asthma (39, 53). Identifying and addressing these multiple factors is critically important because factors such as psychological dysfunction can be a major driver of recurrent exacerbation in this population (60).

The majority of children (>80%) with asthma are sensitized to at least one aeroallergen, and those with severe asthma are likely to have multiple sensitisations (46, 61). In adults, atopy defined by positivity to skin prick testing or specific IgE measurement in severe asthma cohorts is between 60 and 80% (45, 57, 62), with higher prevalence noted in research cohorts. However, atopy with sensitization to aeroallergens is common in non-asthmatic subjects and in many adults with severe asthma, the role of allergic driven disease even in those with co-existent evidence of sensitization, is unclear. Other atopic conditions such as allergic rhinitis and hay fever are common in children (46) and have been shown to impact on asthma control (63). Chronic rhinosinusitis and nasal polyposis is common in adults, although not children and indeed the presence of nasal polyps in children should be a red flag for an alternative diagnosis such as cystic fibrosis or primary ciliary dyskinesia (9, 45).

Gastro-esophageal reflux (GER) and asthma frequently co-exist in children and adults with asthma (64); however, there is inconsistent evidence of a "cause and effect" relationship between the two GER is associated with asthma symptoms and poor control (65) however, a study of lansoprazole in children with proven GER showed no impact on asthma control (66). A Cochrane review concluded that treatment of GER did not result in an improvement in asthma symptoms in adults or children (67). However, it is possible that non-acid reflux may be important and explain the relationship between symptoms and lack of treatment effect (68).

TABLE 1 | Comorbidities in children and adults with severe asthma.

Clinical Trait	Adults	Children	Management
Obesity	Patients with severe asthma have a higher BMI than healthy controls and up to 40% are obese (45)	Children with severe asthma have a higher BMI although few children with severe asthma are clinically obese (46)	Weight loss programme; bariatric surgery
Depression and anxiety	Anxiety and depression found up to 27% of patients with difficult asthma (9, 47)	High levels of anxiety in both children with severe asthma and their caregivers	Psychological support
Breathing pattern disorder (BPD); including vocal cord dysfunction (VCD)	BPD common in difficult asthma, 19–52% (39, 48); VCD reported in up to 50% (49, 50)	One study in children found only 6% of children with severe asthma had BPD; this is likely an underestimate (51), prevalence of VCD unknown	Physiotherapy for BPD and EILO; speech and language therapy for VCD; surgery for supraglottic EILO in selected cases
Chronic rhinosinusitis and nasal polyps	Approximately 50% of severe asthma patients have chronic rhinosinusitis; and over 30% nasal polyps (45, 52)	Rare in children; nasal polyps suggest an alternative diagnosis such as cystic fibrosis or primary ciliary dyskinesia	Sinus rinses, nasal steroids, surgery
Allergic rhinitis	Allergic sensitization common in severe asthma (approximately 70–80%; and up to 60% report symptoms of allergic rhinitis (although this is similar in milder asthma) Ref Shaw UBIO	Allergic sensitization and allergic rhinitis common in children (up to 80%) (53)	Anti-histamines, nasal steroids
Obstructive sleep apnoea (OSA)	Common in severe asthma, up to 92% in one cohort (54), 31% in SARP (55)	Reported prevalence of 63% in poorly controlled asthma secondary to adeno-tonsillar hypertrophy (56)	CPAP, weight loss, adenotonsillectomy (children)
Gastro-esophageal reflux	Common in severe asthma, 17–74% (45, 57, 58)	Diagnosed in 20% of children with severe asthma, although unrelated to any measures of asthma severity (46, 59)	Proton pump inhibitors; little evidence to suggest an impact on asthma symptoms

Obesity is a growing global health problem and can impact on asthma diagnosis, control and exacerbation severity in both adults and children (69, 70). In children the strength of this relationship appears less strong than in adults, although this may in part be because it has been less well-studied (71). There are a number of plausible mechanisms for this relationship: deconditioning leading to breathlessness may mimic asthma symptoms leading to an erroneous asthma diagnosis or assessment of control; lung mechanics are altered in obesity with pulmonary restriction and lower functional residual capacity and ventilatory reserve which can have secondary effects on airway smooth muscle shortening during bronchoconstriction; dysynaptic lung growth (increased in lung volume and airway length but not caliber has been shown to be more common on obese children and associated with worse disease severity and poor response to steroids (72–74). Obesity is also associated with systemic inflammation and IL-6 may be a potential mediator of T2 low asthma (and hence steroid resistance) in some obese patients (75). Furthermore, an adult-onset obese female phenotype has been identified with a link to non-eosinophilic airway inflammation (76). Data from small randomized controlled trials show that weight loss improves asthma control, quality of life and lung function but the overall level of evidence of benefit is low (77, 78) and bariatric surgery has been shown to have a positive effect on asthma outcomes (79–81). The relationship between asthma severity and obesity is further confounded by the fact that steroids lead to weight gain. Thus, it can be difficult to untangle whether obesity is driving asthma symptoms (via the mechanisms described above) or whether persistent symptoms and attacks lead to increased steroid use, causing obesity. Furthermore, weight loss is hindered by steroid use.

Anxiety and depression are both associated with increased exacerbation frequency, poorer asthma control and quality of life (60, 82, 83). A negative life event can increase the risk of an asthma attack within a short time of that event and the effect is magnified if there is a background of chronic stress (84, 85). The precise mechanisms underlying the relationship between stress and severity are not known, however an increased T-helper 2 (TH_2) cytokine response has been associated with higher chronic stress and perceived threat in children (86). It may also be that psychological factors such as anxiety and depression along with other mental health conditions may affect a patient's ability to self-manage their asthma and impact on other behaviors such as smoking and poor adherence.

Dysfunctional breathing (DB) is common in adult patients with severe asthma with a reported prevalence of 19–52% (39, 48). There is good evidence that breathing retraining can improve asthma control and quality of life (87, 88). Much less is known about DB in children. A single study assessing dysfunctional breathing in a pediatric severe asthma clinic found that only 5.4% were found to have a breathing pattern disorder (51). It is likely that DB in under-recognized in children and in the broader population of children with difficult to treat to asthma the prevalence is likely much higher. A more comprehensive review of this topic can be found elsewhere in this supplement.

SMOKING

Although active cigarette smoking does not appear to be related to the development of adult onset asthma, it is associated with asthma severity, frequent exacerbations and lung function decline (89, 90). Active smoking has been shown to reduce expression of histone deacetylase (HDAC2) via phosoinositide-3-kinase activation, leading to reduced glucocorticoid sensitivity (91). The same has also been found in children with severe asthma exposed to second hand smoke (92).

THE PATHOBIOLOGY OF SEVERE ASTHMA AND ASTHMA PHENOTYPES

Both pediatric and adult severe asthma are characterized by heterogeneity in clinical expression and underlying pathobiological features (**Table 2**).

In contrast to adults, where a female preponderance is very consistently seen, there is a male preponderance in childhood (47, 97). The increasing proportion of women with severe asthma through the life course is particularly seen in adolescence and around the time of the menopause suggesting a link with female sex hormones (98).

T2 HIGH AND T2 LOW ASTHMA

In 1958, Dr. Harry Morrow Brown published a seminal paper in the Lancet, which demonstrated that the clinical response to corticosteroids in adults with chronic persistent asthma was associated with the presence of eosinophils in sputum (99). This study was performed after the United Kingdom Medical Research Council subcommittee on clinical trials in asthma reported no advantage of cortisone acetate in the treatment of chronic asthma, which was a result which many, including Dr. Morrow Brown, found surprising (99). This outcome may have been due in part to the study design and reported outcomes but also in part to the inclusion of a heterogeneous patient population with a clinical diagnosis of asthma. Many years later, a study in adults using sputum samples induced with hypertonic saline also demonstrated that patients with asthma and a sputum eosinophil count $\geq$3% had a greater response to inhaled corticosteroids (ICS) compared to those with an eosinophil count <3% (100). Woodruff et al. (101) subsequently demonstrated that an IL-13 derived epithelial gene signature (periostin, serpin B2, and CCLA1) was associated with airway eosinophilia and upregulation of T-helper 2 (TH_2) cytokines IL-5 and IL-13 but importantly this was only seen in 50% of asthmatics who had withdrawn ICS. Further, reintroduction of ICS was again associated with an improvement in lung function in subjects with evidence of eosinophilia and upregulation of type-2 cytokines, but which importantly was not seen in those subjects without evidence of airway type-2 inflammation/eosinophilia. The authors coined the terms TH_2-high and TH_2–low asthma and reinvigorated the debate about non-eosinophilic asthma and importantly asthma, which is not responsive to ICS. The classical paradigm was that this process was predominantly driven by TH_2 cells however it is now recognized that there are other cellular sources of these cytokines and innate lymphoid cells and mast cells are potential sources of these pro-inflammatory cytokines (102, 103).

Asthma in children is predominantly an atopic disorder. Children with severe asthma are characterized by multiple aeroallergen sensitization, food allergy, high exhaled nitric oxide and progressive loss of lung function throughout childhood (47, 97, 104). Childhood severe asthma is predominantly eosinophilic with increased luminal (bronchoalveolar lavage) and tissue eosinophils (105). However, inflammatory phenotypes based on sputum are not stable in children (106). Furthermore, bronchoscopic studies have demonstrated an absence of TH_2 cytokines (105, 107) suggesting that airway eosinoplhia in children is mediated by relatively steroid resistance pathways. IL-33 remains elevated despite maximal steroid therapy (108, 109) and increased levels of innate lymphoid cells (ILCs) in children with severe asthma suggests a possible therapeutic target (110). Few studies in children have targeted eosinophils. The only study in children that based management on sputum eosinophils did not show a significant reduction in exacerbations (111), in contrast to benefit demonstrated in adult studies as described above (112).

Bronchoscopic studies in adults have provided rich evidence for underlying pathobiology of adult severe asthma and potential endotypes. Mechanistic studies in children are hampered by ethical constraints: samples from healthy controls have to be opportunistically collected from those having bronchoscopy for upper airway problems or a general anesthetic for an unrelated procedure and it is not possible to repeat bronchoscopies to assess the airway response to an intervention or challenge.

Recent data suggests that steroid resistant type-2 biology in adults is associated with older patients. There is likely to be a degree of overlap but our understanding of inhaled steroid resistant disease has been hampered by our prior failure to measure effective drug delivery in mechanistic studies (25, 113).

NON-T2 MECHANISMS IN SEVERE ASTHMA

A study using data form the National Asthma Research Programme in the United States demonstrated that subjects with mild to moderate asthma and no evidence of sputum eosinophilia (defined as sputum eosinophil count <2%) had no improvement in lung function with ICS but showed evidence of a bronchodilator response consistent with asthma (114). This study also identified that in ICS naive subjects 47% have no evidence of sputum eosinophilia in serial samples taken at various points over a 1-year period but this proportion increased to 72% in subjects currently taking ICS treatment. Taken together, these data suggests that substantial groups of patients with mild and moderate asthma have little evidence of type-2 cytokine driven airway eosinophilia (T2-low asthma) and by extension are likely to have little response to either initiation or escalation ICS treatment. Unfortunately, many patients who are unresponsive to inhaled steroids have their doses relentlessly increased, with no clinical benefit but substantial risk of harm.

McGrath et al. (114) also reported that the patients with non-eosinophilic mild asthma had less bronchial hyperresponsiveness than those with airways eosinophilia and Arron et al. (115) also

TABLE 2 | Comparison of phenotypes in adults and children with severe asthma.

Phenotype	Description	Adults	Pediatrics	Therapy
T2 high	High levels TH_2 cytokines (IL4, IL5, and IL13); biomarkers include airway and blood eosinophils, FENO, and periostin	More severe disease with higher risk of asthma attacks	Children with severe asthma are predominantly eosinophilic, although TH_2 cytokines may not be elevated	Steroid sensitive, anti IgE or anti IL4, IL5, or IL13
T2 low	Low levels of eosinophils, often associated with airway neutrophilia	Patients tend to be older; associated with low FEV_1 and air trapping, poor steroid response	Little evidence for T_2 low asthma in children; airway neutrophils may be protective; airway neutrophilia associated with infection	Macrolide antibiotics may have some benefit
Persistent airflow limitation	Low FEV_1 or FEV_1/FVC post bronchodilator, post steroid trial	40–60% with severe asthma, older age, longer asthma duration, smoking (93)	25% of children with severe asthma have PAL; associated with increase in airway smooth muscle (94–96)	Optimize long acting bronchodilators, down titrate steroids to lowest dose to control symptoms
Atopic	Sensitisation to aeroallergens and elevated IgE	Associated with early onset asthma persisting into adulthood	Most children are atopic and have co-morbid atopic diseases	Steroid responsive; T_2 targeted therapies as above

demonstrated an inverse relationship between an IL13-high gene signature (T2-high asthma) and bronchial hyperresponsiveness suggesting that T2-low/non-eosinophilic disease is associated with less physiological abnormalities. This is supported by data which suggest that non-eosinophilic asthma is associated with lower risk of asthma exacerbation and there is strong evidence that surrogate biomarkers of type-2 airways inflammation (blood eosinophil count, FeNO, serum ECP, and serum periostin) are all prognostic biomarkers for exacerbation (116–118). In addition, elevated blood eosinophil count and FeNO have consistently been associated with a higher exacerbation rate in the placebo arms of clinical trials in patients with severe asthma unselected on the basis of a pre-stipulated biomarker threshold (119–121) This would suggest that within severe asthma populations, defined using usual diagnostic and treatment criteria, there are subjects with little evidence of active T2-driven disease (type-2 biomarker low), who are persistently symptomatic and defined as uncontrolled asthma, but who have a comparatively low exacerbation risk. However, it is important to comment that severe asthma exacerbations still occur in these symptom high type-2 biomarker low patients albeit at a much lower rate.

It is recognized that ICS will down-regulate type-2 inflammation and related biomarkers (122, 123) and is thus an important confounder in subjects with more severe asthma on ICS treatment raising two important issues—firstly, whether true T2-low asthma exists in more severe asthma, when corticosteroids are down titrated and secondly, what is the mechanism of persistent symptoms in subjects with asthma when type-2 corticosteroid responsive asthma is not present. As discussed above, "true" T2-low asthma appears to be relatively common in mild asthmatic subjects but is generally associated with mild symptoms, less bronchial hyperresponsiveness and a lower risk of asthma exacerbation compared to subjects with T2-high disease. Intuitively, it seems improbable that this group of patients would be progressed to high dose ICS treatment, however if symptoms are persistent and not ICS responsive as appears to be the case, it is possible that some of these patients may be escalated to high intensity treatment to try and improve their symptoms. The issue of whether true T2-low asthma exists in severe asthma is currently being explored in the RASP-UK programme, where patients are having corticosteroids "down titrated" if their biomarkers of T2-driven disease are low (124).

The neutrophilic phenotype is not seen consistently in children (106) and there is evidence to suggest that airway neutrophils may be protective (125) and very little is known about T2 low asthma in children (if it exists at all).

Non-atopic clinical phenotypes described in adults including those associated with sensitivity to non-steroidal anti-inflammatories and nasal polyposis are rare in childhood.

AIRWAY REMODELING

Airway remodeling starts early in childhood asthma. Although no differences in reticular basement membrane (RBM) thickness were seen in infants with respiratory symptoms with or without evidence of reversible airflow obstruction at a median 1 year of age (126) by a median of 3 years there were significant differences between those with troublesome wheeze and healthy controls (127) and by school age the changes were consistent with those seen in adult severe asthma (128). Interestingly, only increased airway smooth muscle in pre-schoolers predicted the persistence of asthma at school age (129). Almost a quarter of children with severe asthma have persistent airflow limitation (PAL), defined as post systemic post-bronchodilator z score ≤ -1.96 for FEV_1 (94, 97). In adults this rises to almost 50% and is associated with older age, longer duration of asthma symptoms and airway eosinophilia (93). In children there appears to be no association between PAL and eosinophilic inflammation although there is evidence of an increase in airway smooth muscle surface area and mass in those with PAL (95, 96).

MANAGEMENT

As previously discussed, the first stage of management is the confirmation of the diagnosis of severe asthma and the comprehensive assessment and modification of co-morbidities and factors driving persistent symptoms and asthma attacks. For who remain poorly controlled following this assessment and remain on high intensity conventional treatment (high dose ICS as defined above, plus additional add on treatments including LABA, LRTA or theophylline or maintenance OCS) there is an exciting pipeline of targeted treatments which predominantly target the type-2 cytokine axis including IL-4, IL-5, and IL-13 causing IgE production and eosinophilic inflammation (130, 131).

Omalizumab, the monoclonal antibody to IgE, was the first biologic licensed in the United Sates (US) in 2003 in adults and children (>12 years) and by 2009 it was approved in the US and Europe for all patients with asthma from the age of 6 years. The last 3 years have seen an acceleration in the number of Phase 2 and 3 studies and the licensing of new drugs. The choice of biologic depends on the patient's age, weight, IgE evaluation (both total and specific), degree of eosinophilia and route of administration. The Global initiative for Asthma (GINA) has recently produced a pocket guide to aid the physician in determining the most appropriate treatment for the individual (4).

OMALIZUMAB

Omalizumab is a recombinant antibody to IgE that diminishes free IgE levels and prevents IgE binding to mast cells and basophils, thus inhibiting degranulation and release of proinflammatory mediators. Studies in adults and children have demonstrated benefit, particularly in terms of reduction in exacerbations (132). The dose is based on IgE level and weight. Approximately 25% of children have an IgE level outside the licensed range and for those at the upper end of the range it may entail 2 weekly injections (97) and additionally adults may not qualify without sensitization to an aeroallergen. The frequency of these scheduled visits must be balanced against a reduction in attacks and hence unscheduled time off school and work. In children omalizumab has also been used seasonally to attenuate the September peak in asthma attacks (133) and this approach showed greatest utility in children on the higher treatment steps. In a randomized withdrawal study, after long-term treatment with omalizumab, patients on omalizumab did better than those randomized to placebo suggesting continuation of omalizumab results in continued benefit and does not support a disease modifying effect of this treatment (134).

DRUGS TARGETING IL-5—MEPOLIZUMAB, RESLIZUMAB, AND BENRALIZUMAB

Mepolizumab is a humanized monoclonal antibody to IL-5 that inhibits eosinophilic maturation and activation. The DREAM and MENSA studies recruited patients with recurrent asthma exacerbations and evidence of eosinophilic inflammation despite high doses of inhaled glucocorticoids and demonstrated a reduction in asthma attacks in those randomized to mepolizumab (135, 136). In subjects with increased blood eosinophil levels, greater efficacy was seen with additional improvements in lung function and symptoms. Although adolescents were recruited for the licensing studies the data were not reported separately and there are no specific pediatric randomized controlled trials. The results of an open label pharmacokinetics and pharmacodynamics study in children aged 6–12 years are awaited (137). Despite this, mepolizumab has recently been licensed by the European Medicines Agency (EMA) for use in patients with severe asthma from 6 years of age. Two further drugs targeting the IL-5 axis have recently been licensed by the EMA for adults: reslizumab and benralizumab. Reslizumab has a similar mode of action to mepolizumab. It binds to IL-5 thus reducing IL-5 mediated maturation and trafficking of eosinophils from the bone marrow as well as inhibiting mediator release and eosinophil apoptosis. It is given by 4 weekly intravenous infusion and demonstrated a significant reduction in exacerbations in the reslizumab arm compared to placebo (138). It is licensed by the Food and Drug Administration (FDA) and EMA for use in adults only and notably studies using a fixed sub-cutaneous dose of 110 mg were negative (139, 140). Benralizumab binds to the IL-5 receptor and in addition to inhibiting growth and activation of eosinophils benralizumab also binds to the Fc receptor on natural killer cells and induces antibody dependent cell mediated cytotoxicity leading to apoptosis of eosinophils. In clinical trials benralizumab led to decreased exacerbations, improved lung function and enhanced quality of life (141, 142). It is theoretically more effective than other IL-5 blockers which allow IL-5 independent migration of eosinophils into the tissue, although superior efficacy was not evident in clinical trials to date and the results of targeting the IL-5 axis seem broadly consistent with reduced exacerbation rates (rescue OCS $\geq$ 3 days) by approximately 50% and more modest improvements in symptoms and asthma-related quality of life measured and lung function (143). Benralizumab and mepolizumab have also been shown to reduce oral corticosteroid dose compared to placebo with a parallel reduction in exacerbation rate in adult subjects with severe asthma on maintenance oral corticosteroids (144, 145). It also has the advantage of being given every 8 weeks after the initial three, four weekly injections. The FDA have licensed benralizumab for use as an add on treatment for patients with eosinophilic asthma aged 12 years and above. In Europe it has been licensed by the EMA for use in adults only.

DUPILUMAB

Dupilumab binds to the IL-4 receptor-α blocking signaling of IL-4 and IL-13, thus reducing IgE production and eosinophil recruitment. Phase 3 studies have demonstrated a significant reduction in severe exacerbations (47.7% reduction for 200 mg dupilumab compared to placebo, $p < 0.001$) and additionally demonstrated lung function improvement which was evident early after treatment initiation (at week 12, FEV_1 increased 0.14 liters compared to placebo, $p < 0.001$) (120). Dupilumab treatment also resulted in a significant reduction in OCS in adult subjects with severe asthma on maintenance OCS treatment (70.1% with dupilumab vs. 41.9% in the placebo group ($p < 0.001$) with a 59% lower exacerbation rate than placebo and mean increase in FEV1 of mean 0.22 liters more than placebo (146). It was licensed in October 2018 by the FDA and in May 2019 by the EMA for use in patients with severe eosinophilic asthma from 12 years of age. It also has a license for treatment of severe atopic eczema and will clearly be a useful treatment in patients with both conditions.

It is disappointing that no data from pediatric specific randomized controlled trials have been presented for mepolizumab, reslizumab, benralizumab or dupilumab and there has been no separate analysis of the adolescents recruited for these studies (likely because of insufficient numbers for meaningful subgroup analysis). Given the challenges recruiting to the MARS trial as discussed above (24), and the inference that there are relatively small number of children who have uncontrolled asthma when adherent with standard of care inhaled treatment, it is acknowledged that the feasibility of any such study is challenging and the need for international collaboration essential (147, 148). None-the-less the majority of these drugs have been licensed by the FDA and EMA for 12 years and older and in the case of mepolizumab by the EMA for use from the age of 6 years. In view of the limited add on choices for children with severe asthma, the addition of an increasing number of biologics is to be welcomed. It will be important to use "real-world" outcome data to identify if similar efficacy is seen in pediatric cohorts and to identify markers of response (149). In addition, it has become clear that there is substantial overlap in the populations for these new biologic therapies and randomized pragmatic head to head comparisons between the various biologics will potentially identify which patients should be treated with each drug (149, 150).

SUMMARY

There is heterogeneity both within and between pediatric and adult severe asthma. Although there is overlap between the two there are a number of differences in clinical expression and disease mechanisms in children and adults. The impact of the growing lung and developing immune system is likely to account for some of the observable differences however, much remains poorly understood, including the natural history of asthma; adult onset vs. childhood onset disease; and the impact of early life influences (including in utero). Studies such as the Unbiased Biomarkers for the PREDiction of respiratory outcomes (U-BIOPRED) marks a step change in asthma research. Cohorts of preschool, school aged and adults with severe asthma (45, 46) were recruited to this multi-omics study which aims to define phenotypes and endotypes of severe adult and pediatric asthma and preschool wheeze and compare these groups across the life course. In the meantime, there remain a number of unmet needs in the management of severe asthma. Expensive biologics are available to only the minority of patients with severe asthma globally; there is an ongoing disease burden both in terms of asthma related morbidity and mortality and corticosteroids, the mainstay of treatment for many, have an unacceptable side effect profile. Finally, there is the absence to date of any disease modifying treatments. The window of opportunity for such an intervention is likely to lie in very early childhood and therefore to improve the care of all patients with severe disease, there needs to be investment and a focus on research in young children.

AUTHOR CONTRIBUTIONS

All authors listed have made a substantial, direct and intellectual contribution to the work, and approved it for publication.

REFERENCES

1. Barry LE, Sweeney J, O'Neill C, Price D, Heaney LG. The cost of systemic corticosteroid-induced morbidity in severe asthma: a health economic analysis. *Respir Res.* (2017) 18:129. doi: 10.1186/s12931-017-0614-x
2. O'Neill S, Sweeney J, Patterson CC, Menzies-Gow A, Niven R, Mansur AH, et al. The cost of treating severe refractory asthma in the UK: an economic analysis from the British Thoracic Society Difficult Asthma Registry. *Thorax.* (2015) 70:376–8. doi: 10.1136/thoraxjnl-2013-204114
3. Chung KF, Wenzel SE, Brozek JL, Bush A, Castro M, Sterk PJ, et al. International ERS/ATS guidelines on definition, evaluation and treatment of severe asthma. *Eur Respir J.* (2014) 43:343–73. doi: 10.1183/09031936.00202013
4. Difficult-to-treat and Severe Asthma in Adolescent and Adult Patients. *Diagnosis and Management. A GINA Pocket Guide for Health Professionals.* (2018). Available online at: https://ginasthma.org/wp-content/uploads/2018/11/GINA-SA-FINAL-wms.pdf
5. Global Initiative for Asthma. *Global Strategy for Asthma Management and Prevention.* (2018). Available online at: www.ginasthma.org (accessed December 15, 2018).
6. Asthma. *British Guideline on the Management of Asthma.* (2016).
7. Kankaanranta H, Lahdensuo A, Moilanen E, Barnes PJ. Add-on therapy options in asthma not adequately controlled by inhaled corticosteroids: a comprehensive review. *Respir Res.* (2004) 5:17. doi: 10.1186/1465-9921-5-17
8. Hekking PP, Wener RR, Amelink M, Zwinderman AH, Bouvy ML, Bel EH. The prevalence of severe refractory asthma. *J Allergy Clin Immunol.* (2015) 135:896–902. doi: 10.1016/j.jaci.2014.08.042
9. Heaney LG, Conway E, Kelly C, Johnston BT, English C, Stevenson M, et al. Predictors of therapy resistant asthma: outcome of a systematic evaluation protocol. *Thorax.* (2003) 58:561–6. doi: 10.1136/thorax.58.7.561
10. Robinson DS, Campbell DA, Durham SR, Pfeffer J, Barnes PJ, Chung KF, et al. Systematic assessment of difficult-to-treat asthma. *Eur Respir J.* (2003) 22:478–83. doi: 10.1183/09031936.03.00017003

11. Carroll WD, Lenney W, Child F, Strange RC, Jones PW, Whyte MK, et al. Asthma severity and atopy: how clear is the relationship? *Arch Dis Child.* (2006) 91:405–9. doi: 10.1136/adc.2005.088278
12. Bracken M, Fleming L, Hall P, Van SN, Bossley C, Biggart E, et al. The importance of nurse-led home visits in the assessment of children with problematic asthma. *Arch Dis Child.* (2009) 94:780–4. doi: 10.1136/adc.2008.152140
13. Jochmann A, Artusio L, Jamalzadeh A, Nagakumar P, Delgado-Eckert E, Saglani S, et al. Electronic monitoring of adherence to inhaled corticosteroids: an essential tool in identifying severe asthma in children. *Eur Respir J.* (2017) 50:1700910. doi: 10.1183/13993003.00910-2017
14. Belgrave DCM, Simpson A, Semic-Jusufagic A, Murray CS, Buchan I, Pickles A, et al. Joint modeling of parentally reported and physician-confirmed wheeze identifies children with persistent troublesome wheezing. *J Allergy Clin Immunol.* (2013) 132:575–83.e12. doi: 10.1016/j.jaci.2013.05.041
15. Currie GP, Douglas JG, Heaney LG. Difficult to treat asthma in adults. *BMJ.* (2009) 338:b494. doi: 10.1136/bmj.b494
16. Lodrup Carlsen KC, Hedlin G, Bush A, Wennergren G, de Benedictis FM, De Jongste JC, et al. Assessment of problematic severe asthma in children. *Eur Respir J.* (2011) 37:432–40. doi: 10.1183/09031936.00091410
17. Bush A, Saglani S. Management of severe asthma in children. *Lancet.* (2010) 376:814–25. doi: 10.1016/S0140-6736(10)61054-9
18. Bush A, Fleming L, Saglani S. Severe asthma in children. *Respirology.* (2017) 22:886–97. doi: 10.1111/resp.13085
19. Bender B, Milgrom H, Apter A. Adherence intervention research: what have we learned and what do we do next? *J Allergy Clin Immunol.* (2003) 112:489–94. doi: 10.1016/S0091-6749(03)00006-X
20. Heaney LG, Horne R. Non-adherence in difficult asthma: time to take it seriously. *Thorax.* (2012) 67:268–70. doi: 10.1136/thoraxjnl-2011-200257
21. Gamble J, Stevenson M, McClean E, Heaney LG. The prevalence of non-adherence in difficult asthma. *Am J Respir Crit Care Med.* (2009) 180:817–22. doi: 10.1164/rccm.200902-0166OC
22. Murphy AC, Proeschal A, Brightling CE, Wardlaw AJ, Pavord I, Bradding P, et al. The relationship between clinical outcomes and medication adherence in difficult-to-control asthma. *Thorax.* (2012) 67:751–3. doi: 10.1136/thoraxjnl-2011-201096
23. Lee J, Tay TR, Radhakrishna N, Hore-Lacy F, Mackay A, Hoy R, et al. Nonadherence in the era of severe asthma biologics and thermoplasty. *Eur Respir J.* (2018) 51:1701836. doi: 10.1183/13993003.01836-2017
24. Strunk RC, Bacharier LB, Phillips BR, Szefler SJ, Zeiger RS, Chinchilli VM, et al. Azithromycin or montelukast as inhaled corticosteroid-sparing agents in moderate-to-severe childhood asthma study. *J Allergy Clin Immunol.* (2008) 122:1138–44. doi: 10.1016/j.jaci.2008.09.028
25. Heaney LG, Busby J, Bradding P, Chaudhuri R, Mansur AH, Niven R, et al. Remotely monitored therapy and nitric oxide suppression identifies nonadherence in severe asthma. *Am J Respir Crit Care Med.* (2019) 199:454–64. doi: 10.1164/rccm.201806-1182OC
26. McNicholl DM, Stevenson M, McGarvey LP, Heaney LG. The utility of fractional exhaled nitric oxide suppression in the identification of nonadherence in difficult asthma. *Am J Respir Crit Care Med.* (2012) 186:1102–8. doi: 10.1164/rccm.201204-0587OC
27. Bender BG. Sorting out nonadherence and airway inflammation in treatment escalation for severe asthma. *Am J Respir Crit Care Med.* (2019) 199:400–2. doi: 10.1164/rccm.201811-2144ED
28. Fleming L, Koo M, Bossley CJ, Nagakumar P, Bush A, Saglani S. The utility of a multidomain assessment of steroid response for predicting clinical response to omalizumab. *J Allergy Clin Immunol.* (2016) 138:292–4. doi: 10.1016/j.jaci.2015.12.1317
29. Horne R, Weinman J, Barber N, Elliott RA, Morgan M. Compliance, adherence and concordance. In: KTG Harding, editor. *Pharmacy Practice.* London: Taylor & Francis (2001). p. 47–67.
30. Szefler SJ, Chmiel JF, Fitzpatrick AM, Giacoia G, Green TP, Jackson DJ, et al. Asthma across the ages: knowledge gaps in childhood asthma. *J Allergy Clin Immunol.* (2014) 133:3–13; quiz 4. doi: 10.1016/j.jaci.2013.10.018
31. Plaza V, Giner J, Rodrigo GJ, Dolovich MB, Sanchis J. Errors in the use of inhalers by health care professionals: a systematic review. *J Allergy Clin Immunol Pract.* (2018) 6:987–95. doi: 10.1016/j.jaip.2017.12.032
32. Shields MD, F AL, Rivey MP, McElnay JC. Mobile direct observation of therapy (MDOT) - A rapid systematic review and pilot study in children with asthma. *PLoS ONE.* (2018) 13:e0190031. doi: 10.1371/journal.pone.0190031
33. Winkelstein ML, Huss K, Butz A, Eggleston P, Vargas P, Rand C. Factors associated with medication self-administration in children with asthma. *Clin Pediatr.* (2000) 39:337–45. doi: 10.1177/000992280003900603
34. Orrell-Valente JK, Jarlsberg LG, Hill LG, Cabana MD. At what age do children start taking daily asthma medicines on their own? *Pediatrics.* (2008) 122:e1186–92. doi: 10.1542/peds.2008-0292
35. Klok T, Kaptein AA, Duiverman EJ, Brand PL. It's the adherence, stupid (that determines asthma control in preschool children)! *Eur Respir J.* (2014) 43:783–91. doi: 10.1183/09031936.00054613
36. Morton RW, Elphick HE, Rigby AS, Daw WJ, King DA, Smith LJ, et al. STAAR: a randomised controlled trial of electronic adherence monitoring with reminder alarms and feedback to improve clinical outcomes for children with asthma. *Thorax.* (2016) 72:347–54. doi: 10.1136/thoraxjnl-2015-208171
37. Thakkar J, Kurup R, Laba TL, Santo K, Thiagalingam A, Rodgers A, et al. Mobile telephone text messaging for medication adherence in chronic disease: a meta-analysis. *JAMA Intern Med.* (2016) 176:340–9. doi: 10.1001/jamainternmed.2015.7667
38. Tran N, Coffman JM, Sumino K, Cabana MD. Patient reminder systems and asthma medication adherence: a systematic review. *J Asthma.* (2014) 51:536–43. doi: 10.3109/02770903.2014.888572
39. Porsbjerg C, Menzies-Gow A. Co-morbidities in severe asthma: clinical impact and management. *Respirology.* (2017) 22:651–61. doi: 10.1111/resp.13026
40. Agusti A, Bel E, Thomas M, Vogelmeier C, Brusselle G, Holgate S, et al. Treatable traits: toward precision medicine of chronic airway diseases. *Eur Respir J.* (2016) 47:410–9. doi: 10.1183/13993003.01359-2015
41. Fingleton J, Hardy J, Beasley R. Treatable traits of chronic airways disease. *Curr Opin Pulm Med.* (2018) 24:24–31. doi: 10.1097/MCP.0000000000000445
42. McDonald VM, Fingleton J, Agusti A, Hiles SA, Clark VL, Holland AE, et al. Treatable Traits: a new paradigm for 21(st) century management of chronic airway diseases. *Eur Respir J.* (2019) 53:1802058. doi: 10.1183/13993003.02058-2018
43. Tay TR, Hew M. Comorbid "treatable traits" in difficult asthma: current evidence and clinical evaluation. *Allergy.* (2018) 73:1369–82. doi: 10.1111/all.13370
44. McDonald VM, Hiles SA, Godbout K, Harvey ES, Marks GB, Hew M, et al. Treatable traits can be identified in a severe asthma registry and predict future exacerbations. *Respirology.* (2019) 24:37–47. doi: 10.1111/resp.13389
45. Shaw DE, Sousa AR, Fowler SJ, Fleming LJ, Roberts G, Corfield J, et al. Clinical and inflammatory characteristics of the European U-BIOPRED adult severe asthma cohort. *Eur Respir J.* (2015) 46:1308–21. doi: 10.1183/13993003.00779-2015
46. Fleming L, Murray C, Bansal AT, Hashimoto S, Bisgaard H, Bush A, et al. The burden of severe asthma in childhood and adolescence: results from the paediatric U-BIOPRED cohorts. *Eur Respir J.* (2015) 46:1322–33. doi: 10.1183/13993003.00780-2015
47. Chipps BE, Szefler SJ, Simons FE, Haselkorn T, Mink DR, Deniz Y, et al. Demographic and clinical characteristics of children and adolescents with severe or difficult-to-treat asthma. *J Allergy Clin Immunol.* (2007) 119:1156–63. doi: 10.1016/j.jaci.2006.12.668
48. Heaney LG, Robinson DS. Severe asthma treatment: need for characterising patients. *Lancet.* (2005) 365:974–6. doi: 10.1016/S0140-6736(05)71087-4
49. Low K, Lau KK, Holmes P, Crossett M, Vallance N, Phyland D, et al. Abnormal vocal cord function in difficult-to-treat asthma. *Am J Respir Crit Care Med.* (2011) 184:50–6. doi: 10.1164/rccm.201010-1604OC
50. Tay TR, Radhakrishna N, Hore-Lacy F, Smith C, Hoy R, Dabscheck E, et al. Comorbidities in difficult asthma are independent risk factors for frequent exacerbations, poor control and diminished quality of life. *Respirology.* (2016) 21:1384–90. doi: 10.1111/resp.12838
51. Barker NJ, Jones M, O'Connell NE, Everard ML. Breathing exercises for dysfunctional breathing/hyperventilation syndrome in children. *Cochrane Database Syst Rev.* (2013) 2013:CD010376. doi: 10.1002/14651858.CD010376.pub2

52. ten Brinke A, Grootendorst DC, Schmidt JT, De Bruine FT, van Buchem MA, Sterk PJ, et al. Chronic sinusitis in severe asthma is related to sputum eosinophilia. *J Allergy Clin Immunol.* (2002) 109:621–6. doi: 10.1067/mai.2002.122458
53. de Groot EP, Duiverman EJ, Brand PL. Comorbidities of asthma during childhood: possibly important, yet poorly studied. *Eur Respir J.* (2010) 36:671–8. doi: 10.1183/09031936.00185709
54. Julien JY, Martin JG, Ernst P, Olivenstein R, Hamid Q, Lemiere C, et al. Prevalence of obstructive sleep apnea-hypopnea in severe versus moderate asthma. *J Allergy Clin Immunol.* (2009) 124:371–6. doi: 10.1016/j.jaci.2009.05.016
55. Teodorescu M, Broytman O, Curran-Everett D, Sorkness RL, Crisafi G, Bleecker ER, et al. Obstructive sleep apnea risk, asthma burden, and lower airway inflammation in adults in the severe asthma research program (SARP) II. *J Allergy Clin Immunol Pract.* (2015) 3:566–75.e1. doi: 10.1016/j.jaip.2015.04.002
56. Kheirandish-Gozal L, Dayyat EA, Eid NS, Morton RL, Gozal D. Obstructive sleep apnea in poorly controlled asthmatic children: effect of adenotonsillectomy. *Pediatr Pulmonol.* (2011) 46:913–8. doi: 10.1002/ppul.21451
57. Heaney LG, Brightling CE, Menzies-Gow A, Stevenson M, Niven RM, et al. Refractory asthma in the UK: cross-sectional findings from a UK multicentre registry. *Thorax.* (2010) 65:787–94. doi: 10.1136/thx.2010.137414
58. Moore WC, Meyers DA, Wenzel SE, Teague WG, Li H, Li X, et al. Identification of asthma phenotypes using cluster analysis in the severe asthma research program. *Am J Respir Crit Care Med.* (2009) 181:315–23. doi: 10.1164/ajrccm-conference.2009.179.1_MeetingAbstracts.A2522
59. Tanner N FL, Li A, Bush A. Airway inflammation in severe asthmatics with gastro-oesophageal reflux. *Eur Respir Soc.* (2017) 50:4504. doi: 10.1183/1393003.congress-2017.PA4504
60. ten Brinke A, Sterk PJ, Masclee AA, Spinhoven P, Schmidt JT, Zwinderman AH, et al. Risk factors of frequent exacerbations in difficult-to-treat asthma. *Eur Respir J.* (2005) 26:812–8. doi: 10.1183/09031936.05.000 37905
61. Frith J, Fleming L, Bossley C, Ullmann N, Bush A. The complexities of defining atopy in severe childhood asthma. *Clin Exp Allergy.* (2011) 41:948–53. doi: 10.1111/j.1365-2222.2011.03729.x
62. Teague WG, Phillips BR, Fahy JV, Wenzel SE, Fitzpatrick AM, Moore WC, et al. Baseline features of the severe asthma research program (SARP III) cohort: differences with age. *J Allergy Clin Immunol Pract.* (2018) 6:545–54.e4. doi: 10.1016/j.jaip.2017.05.032
63. de Groot EP, Nijkamp A, Duiverman EJ, Brand PL. Allergic rhinitis is associated with poor asthma control in children with asthma. *Thorax.* (2012) 67:582–7. doi: 10.1136/thoraxjnl 2011-201168
64. Leggett JJ, Johnston BT, Mills M, Gamble J, Heaney LG. Prevalence of gastroesophageal reflux in difficult asthma: relationship to asthma outcome. *Chest.* (2005) 127:1227–31. doi: 10.1016/S0012-3692(15)34471-8
65. Thakkar K, Boatright RO, Gilger MA, El-Serag HB. Gastroesophageal reflux and asthma in children: a systematic review. *Pediatrics.* (2010) 125:e925–30. doi: 10.1542/peds.2009-2382
66. Writing Committee for the American Lung Association Asthma Clinical Research C, Holbrook JT, Wise RA, Gold BD, Blake K, Brown ED, et al. Lansoprazole for children with poorly controlled asthma: a randomized controlled trial. *JAMA.* (2012) 307:373–81. doi: 10.1001/jama.2011.2035
67. Gibson PG, Henry RL, Coughlan JL. Gastro-oesophageal reflux treatment for asthma in adults and children. *Cochrane Database Syst Rev.* (2003) 2003:CD001496. doi: 10.1002/14651858.CD001496
68. Pacheco-Galvan A, Hart SP, Morice AH. Relationship between gastro-oesophageal reflux and airway diseases: the airway reflux paradigm. *Arch Bronconeumol.* (2011) 47:195–203. doi: 10.1016/S1579-2129(11)70046-5
69. Pradeepan S, Garrison G, Dixon AE. Obesity in asthma: approaches to treatment. *Curr Allergy Asthma Rep.* (2013) 13:434–42. doi: 10.1007/s11882-013-0354-z
70. Akerman MJ, Calacanis CM, Madsen MK. Relationship between asthma severity and obesity. *J Asthma.* (2004) 41:521–6. doi: 10.1081/JAS-120037651
71. Ahmadizar F, Vijverberg SJ, Arets HG, de Boer A, Lang JE, Kattan M, et al. Childhood obesity in relation to poor asthma control and exacerbation: a meta-analysis. *Eur Respir J.* (2016) 48:1063–73. doi: 10.1183/13993003.00766-2016
72. Ali Z, Ulrik CS. Obesity and asthma: a coincidence or a causal relationship? A systematic review. *Respir Med.* (2013) 107:1287–300. doi: 10.1016/j.rmed.2013.03.019
73. Shore SA, Fredberg JJ. Obesity, smooth muscle, and airway hyperresponsiveness. *J Allergy Clin Immunol.* (2005) 115:925–7. doi: 10.1016/j.jaci.2005.01.064
74. Forno E, Weiner DJ, Mullen J, Sawicki G, Kurland G, Han YY, et al. Obesity and airway dysanapsis in children with and without asthma. *Am J Respir Crit Care Med.* (2017) 195:314–23. doi: 10.1164/rccm.201605-1039OC
75. Peters MC, McGrath KW, Hawkins GA, Hastie AT, Levy BD, Israel E, et al. Plasma interleukin-6 concentrations, metabolic dysfunction, and asthma severity: a cross-sectional analysis of two cohorts. *Lancet Respir Med.* (2016) 4:574–84. doi: 10.1016/S2213-2600(16)30048-0
76. Amelink M, de Nijs SB, de Groot JC, van Tilburg PM, van Spiegel PI, Krouwels FH, et al. Three phenotypes of adult-onset asthma. *Allergy.* (2013) 68:674–80. doi: 10.1111/all.12136
77. Adeniyi FB, Young T. Weight loss interventions for chronic asthma. *Cochrane Database Syst Rev.* (2012) 2012:CD009339. doi: 10.1002/14651858.CD009339.pub2
78. Freitas PD, Ferreira PG, Silva AG, Stelmach R, Carvalho-Pinto RM, Fernandes FL, et al. The role of exercise in a weight-loss program on clinical control in obese adults with asthma. a randomized controlled trial. *Am J Respir Crit Care Med.* (2017) 195:32–42. doi: 10.1164/rccm.201603-0446OC
79. Boulet LP, Turcotte H, Martin J, Poirier P. Effect of bariatric surgery on airway response and lung function in obese subjects with asthma. *Respir Med.* (2012) 106:651–60. doi: 10.1016/j.rmed.2011.12.012
80. Moreira A, Bonini M, Garcia-Larsen V, Bonini S, Del Giacco SR, Agache I, et al. Weight loss interventions in asthma: EAACI evidence-based clinical practice guideline (part I). *Allergy.* (2013) 68:425–39. doi: 10.1111/all.12106
81. Heaney LG, Conway E, Kelly C, Gamble J. Prevalence of psychiatric morbidity in a difficult asthma population: relationship to asthma outcome. *Respir Med.* (2005) 99:1152–9. doi: 10.1016/j.rmed.2005.02.013
82. Eisner MD, Katz PP, Lactao G, Iribarren C. Impact of depressive symptoms on adult asthma outcomes. *Ann Allergy Asthma Immunol.* (2005) 94:566–74. doi: 10.1016/S1081-1206(10)61135-0
83. Mancuso CA, Wenderoth S, Westermann H, Choi TN, Briggs WM, Charlson ME. Patient-reported and physician-reported depressive conditions in relation to asthma severity and control. *Chest.* (2008) 133:1142–8. doi: 10.1378/chest.07-2243
84. Sandberg S, Jarvenpaa S, Penttinen A, Paton JY, McCann DC. Asthma exacerbations in children immediately following stressful life events: a Cox's hierarchical regression. *Thorax* (2004) 59:1046–51. doi: 10.1136/thx.2004.024604
85. Sandberg S, Paton JY, Ahola S, McCann DC, McGuinness D, Hillary CR, et al. The role of acute and chronic stress in asthma attacks in children. *Lancet.* (2000) 356:982–7. doi: 10.1016/S0140-6736(00)02715-X
86. Chen E, Hanson MD, Paterson LQ, Griffin MJ, Walker HA, Miller GE. Socioeconomic status and inflammatory processes in childhood asthma: the role of psychological stress. *J Allergy Clin Immunol.* (2006) 117:1014–20. doi: 10.1016/j.jaci.2006.01.036
87. Bruton A, Lee A, Yardley L, Raftery J, Arden-Close E, Kirby S, et al. Physiotherapy breathing retraining for asthma: a randomised controlled trial. *Lancet Respir Med.* (2018) 6:19–28. doi: 10.1016/S2213-2600(17)30474-5
88. Thomas M, Bruton A, Little P, Holgate S, Lee A, Yardley L, et al. A randomised controlled study of the effectiveness of breathing retraining exercises taught by a physiotherapist either by instructional DVD or in face-to-face sessions in the management of asthma in adults. *Health Technol Assess.* (2017) 21:1–162. doi: 10.3310/hta21530
89. Silverman RA, Boudreaux ED, Woodruff PG, Clark S, Camargo CA, Jr. Cigarette smoking among asthmatic adults presenting to 64 emergency departments. *Chest.* (2003) 123:1472–9. doi: 10.1378/chest.123.5.1472
90. Siroux V, Pin I, Oryszczyn MP, Le Moual N, Kauffmann F. Relationships of active smoking to asthma and asthma severity in the EGEA study.

Epidemiological study on the Genetics and Environment of Asthma. *Eur Respir J.* (2000) 15:470–7. doi: 10.1034/j.1399-3003.2000.15.08.x

91. Ito K, Lim S, Caramori G, Chung KF, Barnes PJ, Adcock IM. Cigarette smoking reduces histone deacetylase 2 expression, enhances cytokine expression, and inhibits glucocorticoid actions in alveolar macrophages. *FASEB J.* (2001) 15:1110–2. doi: 10.1096/fj.00-0432fje
92. Kobayashi Y, Bossley C, Gupta A, Akashi K, Tsartsali L, Mercado N, et al. Passive smoking impairs histone deacetylase-2 in children with severe asthma. *Chest.* (2014) 145:305–12. doi: 10.1378/chest.13-0835
93. ten Brinke A, Zwinderman AH, Sterk PJ, Rabe KF, Bel EH. Factors associated with persistent airflow limitation in severe asthma. *Am J Respir Crit Care Med.* (2001) 164:744–8. doi: 10.1164/ajrccm.164.5.2011026
94. A Nayeem SS, A Bush, LP Silveira, C Bossley, L Fleming. Clinical and pathogical characteristics of severely asthmatic children with persistent airflow limitation. *Thorax.* (2017) 72:A45–6. doi: 10.1136/thoraxjnl-2017-210983.78
95. Regamey N, Ochs M, Hilliard TN, Muhlfeld C, Cornish N, Fleming L, et al. Increased airway smooth muscle mass in children with asthma, cystic fibrosis, and non-cystic fibrosis bronchiectasis. *Am J Respir Crit Care Med.* (2008) 177:837–43. doi: 10.1164/rccm.200707-977OC
96. Tillie-Leblond I, de Blic J, Jaubert F, Wallaert B, Scheinmann P, Gosset P. Airway remodeling is correlated with obstruction in children with severe asthma. *Allergy.* (2008) 63:533–41. doi: 10.1111/j.1398-9995.2008.01656.x
97. Bossley CJ, Saglani S, Kavanagh C, Payne DN, Wilson N, Tsartsali L, et al. Corticosteroid responsiveness and clinical characteristics in childhood difficult asthma. *Eur Respir J.* (2009) 34:1052–9. doi: 10.1183/09031936.00186508
98. McCleary N, Nwaru BI, Nurmatov UB, Critchley H, Sheikh A. Endogenous and exogenous sex steroid hormones in asthma and allergy in females: a systematic review and meta-analysis. *J Allergy Clin Immunol.* (2018) 141:1510–3.e8. doi: 10.1016/j.jaci.2017.11.034
99. Morrow Brown H. Treatment of chronic asthma with prednisolone significance of eosinophils in the sputum. *Lancet.* (1958) 272:1245–7. doi: 10.1016/S0140-6736(58)91385-0
100. Green RH, Brightling CE, McKenna S, Hargadon B, Parker D, Bradding P, et al. Asthma exacerbations and sputum eosinophil counts: a randomised controlled trial. *Lancet.* (2002) 360:1715–21. doi: 10.1016/S0140-6736(02)11679-5
101. Woodruff PG, Modrek B, Choy DF, Jia G, Abbas AR, Ellwanger A, et al. T-helper type 2-driven inflammation defines major subphenotypes of asthma. *Am J Respir Crit Care Med.* (2009) 180:388–95. doi: 10.1164/rccm.200903-0392OC
102. Ray A, Raundhal M, Oriss TB, Ray P, Wenzel SE. Current concepts of severe asthma. *J Clin Invest.* (2016) 126:2394–403. doi: 10.1172/JCI84144
103. Saglani S. Innate helper cells: a novel cell type essential in the initiation of asthma? Thorax. (2011) 66:834–5. doi: 10.1136/thoraxjnl-2011-200510
104. Fitzpatrick AM, Gaston BM, Erzurum SC, Teague WG. Features of severe asthma in school-age children: atopy and increased exhaled nitric oxide. *J Allergy Clin Immunol.* (2006) 118:1218–25. doi: 10.1016/j.jaci.2006.08.019
105. Bossley CJ, Fleming L, Gupta A, Regamey N, Frith J, Oates T, et al. Pediatric severe asthma is characterized by eosinophilia and remodeling without T(H)2 cytokines. *J Allergy Clin Immunol.* (2012) 129:974–82. doi: 10.1016/j.jaci.2012.01.059
106. Fleming L, Tsartsali L, Wilson N, Regamey N, Bush A. Sputum inflammatory phenotypes are not stable in children with asthma. *Thorax.* (2012) 67:675–81. doi: 10.1136/thoraxjnl-2011-201064
107. Fitzpatrick AM, Teague WG, Meyers DA, Peters SP, Li X, Li H, et al. Heterogeneity of severe asthma in childhood: confirmation by cluster analysis of children in the National Institutes of Health/National Heart, Lung, and Blood Institute Severe Asthma Research Program. *J Allergy Clin Immunol.* (2011) 127:382–9 e1–13. doi: 10.1016/j.jaci.2010.11.015
108. Castanhinha S, Sherburn R, Walker S, Gupta A, Bossley CJ, Buckley J, et al. Pediatric severe asthma with fungal sensitization is mediated by steroid-resistant IL-33. *J Allergy Clin Immunol.* (2015) 136:312–22.e7. doi: 10.1016/j.jaci.2015.01.016
109. Saglani S, Lui S, Ullmann N, Campbell GA, Sherburn RT, Mathie SA, et al. IL-33 promotes airway remodeling in pediatric patients with severe steroid-resistant asthma. *J Allergy Clin Immunol.* (2013) 132:676–85.e13. doi: 10.1016/j.jaci.2013.04.012
110. Nagakumar P, Denney L, Fleming L, Bush A, Lloyd CM, Saglani S. Type 2 innate lymphoid cells in induced sputum from children with severe asthma. *J Allergy Clin Immunol.* (2016) 137:624–6.e6. doi: 10.1016/j.jaci.2015.06.038
111. Fleming L, Wilson N, Regamey N, Bush A. The use of non-invasive markers of inflammation to guide management in children with severe asthma. *Am J Respir Crit Care Med.* (2009) 179:A1305. doi: 10.1164/ajrccm-conference.2009.179.1_MeetingAbstracts.A1305
112. Petsky HL, Cates CJ, Kew KM, Chang AB. Tailoring asthma treatment on eosinophilic markers (exhaled nitric oxide or sputum eosinophils): a systematic review and meta-analysis. *Thorax.* (2018) 73:1110–9. doi: 10.1136/thoraxjnl-2018-211540
113. Peters MC, Kerr S, Dunican EM, Woodruff PG, Fajt ML, Levy BD, et al. Refractory airway type 2 inflammation in a large subgroup of asthmatic patients treated with inhaled corticosteroids. *J Allergy Clin Immunol.* (2019) 143:104–13.e14. doi: 10.1016/j.jaci.2017.12.1009
114. McGrath KW, Icitovic N, Boushey HA, Lazarus SC, Sutherland ER, Chinchilli VM, et al. A large subgroup of mild-to-moderate asthma is persistently noneosinophilic. *Am J Respir Crit Care Med.* (2012) 185:612–9. doi: 10.1164/rccm.201109-1640OC
115. Arron JR, Scheerens H, Matthews JG. Redefining approaches to asthma: developing targeted biologic therapies. *Adv Pharmacol.* (2013) 66:1–49. doi: 10.1016/B978-0-12-404717-4.00001-9
116. Heaney LG, Djukanovic R, Woodcock A, Walker S, Matthews JG, Pavord ID, et al. Research in progress: Medical Research Council United Kingdom Refractory Asthma Stratification Programme (RASP-UK). *Thorax.* (2016) 71:187–9. doi: 10.1136/thoraxjnl-2015-207326
117. Malinovschi A, Fonseca JA, Jacinto T, Alving K, Janson C. Exhaled nitric oxide levels and blood eosinophil counts independently associate with wheeze and asthma events in National Health and Nutrition Examination Survey subjects. *J Allergy Clin Immunol.* (2013) 132:821–7 e1–5. doi: 10.1016/j.jaci.2013.06.007
118. Mogensen I, Alving K, Bjerg A, Borres MP, Hedlin G, Sommar J, et al. Simultaneously elevated exhaled nitric oxide and serum-eosinophil cationic protein relate to recent asthma events in asthmatics in a cross-sectional population-based study. *Clin Exp Allergy.* (2016) 46:1540–8. doi: 10.1111/cea.12792
119. Wenzel S, Castro M, Corren J, Maspero J, Wang L, Zhang B, et al. Dupilumab efficacy and safety in adults with uncontrolled persistent asthma despite use of medium-to-high-dose inhaled corticosteroids plus a long-acting beta2 agonist: a randomised double-blind placebo-controlled pivotal phase 2b dose-ranging trial. *Lancet.* (2016) 388:31–44. doi: 10.1016/S0140-6736(16)30307-5
120. Castro M, Corren J, Pavord ID, Maspero J, Wenzel S, Rabe KF, et al. Dupilumab efficacy and safety in moderate-to-severe uncontrolled asthma. *N Engl J Med.* (2018) 378:2486–96. doi: 10.1056/NEJMoa1804092
121. Corren J, Parnes JR, Wang L, Mo M, Roseti SL, Griffiths JM, et al. Tezepelumab in adults with uncontrolled asthma. *N Engl J Med.* (2017) 377:936–46. doi: 10.1056/NEJMoa1704064
122. Evans PM, O'Connor BJ, Fuller RW, Barnes PJ, Chung KF. Effect of inhaled corticosteroids on peripheral blood eosinophil counts and density profiles in asthma. *J Allergy Clin Immunol.* (1993) 91:643–50. doi: 10.1016/0091-6749(93)90270-P
123. Smith AD, Cowan JO, Brassett KP, Filsell S, McLachlan C, Monti-Sheehan G, et al. Exhaled nitric oxide: a predictor of steroid response. *Am J Respir Crit Care Med.* (2005) 172:453–9. doi: 10.1164/rccm.200411-1498OC
124. Hanratty CE, Matthews JG, Arron JR, Choy DF, Pavord ID, Bradding P, et al. A randomised pragmatic trial of corticosteroid optimization in severe asthma using a composite biomarker algorithm to adjust corticosteroid dose versus standard care: study protocol for a randomised trial. *Trials.* (2018) 19:5. doi: 10.1186/s13063-017-2384-7
125. Andersson CK, Adams A, Nagakumar P, Bossley C, Gupta A, De Vries D, et al. Intraepithelial neutrophils in pediatric severe asthma are associated with better lung function. *J Allergy Clin Immunol.* (2017) 139:1819–29.e11. doi: 10.1016/j.jaci.2016.09.022

126. Saglani S, Malmstrom K, Pelkonen AS, Malmberg LP, Lindahl H, Kajosaari M, et al. Airway remodeling and inflammation in symptomatic infants with reversible airflow obstruction. *Am J Respir Crit Care Med.* (2005) 171:722–7. doi: 10.1164/rccm.200410-1404OC
127. Saglani S, Payne DN, Zhu J, Wang Z, Nicholson AG, Bush A, et al. Early detection of airway wall remodeling and eosinophilic inflammation in preschool wheezers. *Am J Respir Crit Care Med.* (2007) 176:858–64. doi: 10.1164/rccm.200702-212OC
128. Payne DN, Rogers AV, Adelroth E, Bandi V, Guntupalli KK, Bush A, et al. Early thickening of the reticular basement membrane in children with difficult asthma. *Am J Respir Crit Care Med.* (2003) 167:78–82. doi: 10.1164/rccm.200205-414OC
129. O'Reilly R, Ullmann N, Irving S, Bossley CJ, Sonnappa S, Zhu J, et al. Increased airway smooth muscle in preschool wheezers who have asthma at school age. *J Allergy Clin Immunol.* 2012. doi: 10.1016/j.jaci.2012.08.044
130. Pepper AN, Renz H, Casale TB, Garn H. Biologic Therapy and Novel Molecular Targets of Severe Asthma. *J Allergy Clin Immunol Pract.* (2017) 5:909–16. doi: 10.1016/j.jaip.2017.04.038
131. Fajt ML, Wenzel SE. Biologic therapy in asthma: entering the new age of personalized medicine. *J Asthma.* (2014) 51:669–76. doi: 10.3109/02770903.2014.910221
132. Normansell R, Walker S, Milan SJ, Walters EH, Nair P. Omalizumab for asthma in adults and children. *Cochrane Database Syst Rev.* (2014) 1:CD003559. doi: 10.1002/14651858.CD003559.pub4
133. Teach SJ, Gill MA, Togias A, Sorkness CA, Arbes SJ, Jr., Calatroni A, et al. Preseasonal treatment with either omalizumab or an inhaled corticosteroid boost to prevent fall asthma exacerbations. *J Allergy Clin Immunol.* (2015) 136:1476–85. doi: 10.1016/j.jaci.2015.09.008
134. Ledford D, Busse W, Trzaskoma B, Omachi TA, Rosen K, Chipps BE, et al. A randomized multicenter study evaluating Xolair persistence of response after long-term therapy. *J Allergy Clin Immunol.* (2017) 140:162–9 e2. doi: 10.1016/j.jaci.2016.08.054
135. Pavord ID, Korn S, Howarth P, Bleecker ER, Buhl R, Keene ON, et al. Mepolizumab for severe eosinophilic asthma (DREAM): a multicentre, double-blind, placebo-controlled trial. *Lancet.* (2012) 380:651–9. doi: 10.1016/S0140-6736(12)60988-X
136. Ortega HG, Liu MC, Pavord ID, Brusselle GG, FitzGerald JM, Chetta A, et al. Mepolizumab treatment in patients with severe eosinophilic asthma. *N Engl J Med.* (2014) 371:1198–207. doi: 10.1056/NEJMoa1403290
137. Asthma. *Pharmacokinetics and Pharmacodynamics of Mepolizumab Administered Subcutaneously in Children.* (2018). Available online at: https://clinicaltrials.gov/ct2/show/NCT02377427 (accessed March 15, 2019).
138. Castro M, Zangrilli J, Wechsler ME, Bateman ED, Brusselle GG, Bardin P, et al. Reslizumab for inadequately controlled asthma with elevated blood eosinophil counts: results from two multicentre, parallel, double-blind, randomised, placebo-controlled, phase 3 trials. *Lancet Respir Med.* (2015) 3:355–66. doi: 10.1016/S2213-2600(15)00042-9
139. Asthma. An *Efficacy and Safety Study of Reslizumab Subcutaneous in Patients With Oral Corticosteroid Dependent Asthma and Elevated Blood Eosinophils*. (2018). Available online at: https://clinicaltrials.gov/ct2/results?cond=&term=NCT02501629+&cntry=&state=&city=&dist= (accessed March 15, 2019).
140. Asthma. *Study of Reslizumab in Participants With Uncontrolled Asthma and Elevated Blood Eosinophils.* (2018). Available online at: https://clinicaltrials.gov/ct2/results?cond=&term=NCT02452190&cntry=&state=&city=&dist= (accessed March 15, 2019).
141. Bleecker ER, FitzGerald JM, Chanez P, Papi A, Weinstein SF, Barker P, et al. Efficacy and safety of benralizumab for patients with severe asthma uncontrolled with high-dosage inhaled corticosteroids and long-acting beta2-agonists (SIROCCO): a randomised, multicentre, placebo-controlled phase 3 trial. *Lancet.* (2016) 388:2115–27. doi: 10.1016/S0140-6736(16)31324-1
142. FitzGerald JM, Bleecker ER, Nair P, Korn S, Ohta K, Lommatzsch M, et al. Benralizumab, an anti-interleukin-5 receptor alpha monoclonal antibody, as add-on treatment for patients with severe, uncontrolled, eosinophilic asthma (CALIMA): a randomised, double-blind, placebo-controlled phase 3 trial. *Lancet.* (2016) 388:2128–41. doi: 10.1016/S0140-6736(16)31322-8
143. Farne HA, Wilson A, Powell C, Bax L, Milan SJ. Anti-IL5 therapies for asthma. *Cochrane Database Syst Rev.* (2017) 9:CD010834. doi: 10.1002/14651858.CD010834.pub3
144. Bel EH, Wenzel SE, Thompson PJ, Prazma CM, Keene ON, Yancey SW, et al. Oral glucocorticoid-sparing effect of mepolizumab in eosinophilic asthma. *N Engl J Med.* (2014) 371:1189–97. doi: 10.1056/NEJMoa1403291
145. Nair P, Wenzel S, Rabe KF, Bourdin A, Lugogo NL, Kuna P, et al. Oral glucocorticoid-sparing effect of benralizumab in severe asthma. *N Engl J Med.* (2017) 376:2448–58. doi: 10.1056/NEJMoa1703501
146. Rabe KF, Nair P, Brusselle G, Maspero JF, Castro M, Sher L, et al. Efficacy and Safety of Dupilumab in Glucocorticoid-Dependent Severe Asthma. *N Engl J Med.* (2018) 378:2475–85. doi: 10.1056/NEJMoa1804093
147. Liu NM, van Aalderen W, Carlsen KCL, Coleman C, Chalmers JD, Cunningham S, et al. Severe Paediatric Asthma Collaborative in Europe (SPACE): protocol for a European registry. *Breathe.* (2018) 14:93–8. doi: 10.1183/20734735.002018
148. Rusconi F, Fernandes RM, Pijnenburg MWH, Grigg J, Collaboration SCR, European Lung Foundation severe asthma patient advisory g. The Severe Paediatric Asthma Collaborative in Europe (SPACE) ERS Clinical Research Collaboration: enhancing participation of children with asthma in therapeutic trials of new biologics and receptor blockers. *Eur Respir J.* (2018) 52:1801665. doi: 10.1183/13993003.01665-2018
149. Saglani S, Bush A, Carroll W, Cunningham S, Fleming L, Gaillard E, et al. Biologics for paediatric severe asthma: trick or TREAT? *Lancet Respir Med.* (2019) 7:294–6. doi: 10.1016/S2213-2600(19)30045-1
150. Pilette C, Brightling C, Lacombe D, Brusselle G. Urgent need for pragmatic trial platforms in severe asthma. *Lancet Respir Med.* (2018) 6:581–3. doi: 10.1016/S2213-2600(18)30291-1

3

Severe Asthma and Allergy: A Pediatric Perspective

Stefania Arasi [1], Federica Porcaro [2], Renato Cutrera [2] and Alessandro G. Fiocchi [1]*

[1] Pediatric Allergology Unit, Bambino Gesù Hospital (IRCCS), Rome, Italy, [2] Pediatric Pulmonology & Respiratory Intermediate Care Unit, Sleep and Long-Term Ventilation Unit, Department of Pediatrics, Bambino Gesù Children's Hospital, Rome, Italy

***Correspondence:**
Stefania Arasi
stefania.arasi@opbg.net

Severe asthma in children is associated with significant morbidity and lung function decline. It represents a highly heterogeneous disorder with multiple clinical phenotypes. As its management is demanding, the social and economic burden are impressive. Several co-morbidities may contribute to worsen asthma control and complicate diagnostic and therapeutic management of severe asthmatic patients. Allergen sensitization and/or allergy symptoms may predict asthma onset and severity. A better framing of "allergen sensitization" and understanding of mechanisms underlying progression of atopic march could improve the management and the long-term outcomes of pediatric severe asthma. This review focuses on the current knowledge about interactions between severe asthma and allergies.

Keywords: allergy, allergic rhinitis, atopic dermatitis, children, difficult-to-treat asthma, food allergy, severe asthma

INTRODUCTION

Atopic sensitization is a well-established, but not exclusive, risk factor for severe asthma both in children (1, 2) and adults (3), all over the world (1–4). Although its role in determining asthma severity has been considered limited in the past years, some reports confirm that allergy may play a significant role especially in childhood, when early atopic sensitization is crucial to determine the severity of disease.

Though most asthmatic children achieve symptoms' control through occasional bronchodilator (BD) use or low to medium dose of inhaled corticosteroids (ICSs), a small but significant subset of patients remains with uncontrolled asthma despite treatment with high-dose inhaled glucocorticoids (**Table 1**) or requiring such a treatment to remain well-controlled (5). This group of children with chronic symptoms and episodic exacerbation requiring short-acting beta$_2$ agonists (SABA) is defined as affected by "difficult-to-treat asthma." This definition includes poorly-controlled asthma due to at least one of the following: an incorrect diagnosis; comorbidities; poor adherence to therapy because of adverse psychological or environmental factors (6). "Severe asthma" is considered a specific subset of "difficult-to-treat asthma." It is characterized by the need of higher intensity therapy in order to maintain symptom control or uncontrolled symptoms despite such therapy (6), proper diagnosis (7), and management of comorbidities and correction of unsuitable behavior for control disease.

In 2014, a task force of the European Respiratory Society (ERS) and the American Thoracic Society (ATS) updated the definition of severe asthma in pediatric patients. According to the latter, children affected by severe asthma require treatment with high-dose ICSs and either a long-acting beta-agonist (LABA) or a leukotriene antagonist for the previous year or systemic corticosteroids for at least 50% of the previous year to prevent uncontrolled asthma or asthma that remains uncontrolled despite this therapy (5).

TABLE 1 | High-dose ICD dosages for children (mcg/d) according to Global Initiative for Asthma (GINA) guidelines.

Drug name	GINA (6–11 y)	GINA (>12 y)
Beclomethasone dipropionate (HFA)	>200	>400
Budesonide (DPI)	>400	>800
Budesonide (nebules)	>1,000	
Ciclesonide (HFA)	>160	>320
Fluticasone propionate (DPI)	>400	>500
Fluticasone propionate (HFA)	>500	>500
Mometasone furoate (DPI)	>440	>440

DPI, dry powder inhalers; HFA, hydrofluoroalkane.

TABLE 2 | Characteristics of severe bronchial asthma in children and adults.

Characteristics	Pediatric asthma	Adult-onset asthma
IgE-sensitization	+++	+
Poly-sensitization	+++	+
High specific IgE levels	+++	+
Clinical heterogeneity (i.e., multiple phenotypes)	+++	+++
Severe non-allergic obese female prevalent phenotype	–	+++
Severe non-allergic eosinophilic phenotype (nasal polyposis, sputum eosinophilia, and aspirin sensitivity)	–	+++

In a birth cohort study, the prevalence of severe asthma has been estimated about 0.5 and 4.5% in all 10-year-olds and current asthmatic children when assessed in 10 year olds, respectively (8). Notwithstanding, it is associated with a significant economic burden related to more and severe symptoms needing of adjunctive medical resource use and higher health costs (9). Furthermore, the increased number of parent's working days lost during child asthma exacerbations is accompanied by less global economic productivity (10).

Since only a small percentage of asthmatic patients is affected by severe asthma, this clinical entity is still poorly known even if associated with notable morbidity. Both in children and adults, severe asthma is a heterogeneous disorder with multiple clinical phenotypes (11). However, elegant cluster analyses have shown that the role of atopic sensitization might be more important in the pathogenesis of severe asthma specifically in childhood onset asthma: more than 85% of children with severe asthma are severely atopic (12). In contrast, severe adult-onset asthma is a distinct phenotype that is usually not characterized by atopic sensitization, but often associated with nasal polyposis and sputum eosinophilia (13, 14). A brief overview of characteristics and differences between pediatric and adult-onset severe asthma is provided in **Table 2**.

Though it is well-recognized that atopic sensitization is an important risk factor mainly for pediatric asthma, the role of allergy in children affected by severe asthma is still under debate. This review aims to focus the role of allergy in pediatric severe asthma.

THE ATOPIC MARCH

Though atopic manifestations may persist for several years and then resolve over time (15), in atopic children, adolescents, and adults allergy manifestations may evolve according to a predetermined sequence, characterized by the progression from atopic dermatitis (AD) to allergic rhinitis (AR) and asthma (16–18).

Therefore, it seems that atopic predisposition represents a major risk factor for developing all atopic diseases in patients for which the progression from AD to asthma defines the well-known "atopic march" (19). However, the temporal presentation of allergic diseases may differ from the usual progression of the atopic march due to genetic influences and environmental factors (20).

Foremost, allergens may penetrate easier a defective skin barrier, therefore leading to transcutaneous sensitization and subsequentially initiating the atopic march (21). Indeed, IgE sensitization to food or airborne allergens is a significant cofactor to induce the progression of the atopic march in patients with AD (22–24). Moreover, it is widely described that the risk of developing asthma in patients with AD is strictly related to both the clinical expression of IgE sensitization and the severity of eczema (25–27).

It seems that transcutaneous IgE-sensitization may precede airway sensitization (28) and that IgE-associated AD might represent the first step of the atopic march and, therefore, it may predict the upcoming development of allergic diseases, including food allergy, AR, and asthma (please see **Figure 1**) (28). Since AR is a further major risk factor for bronchial hyper-reactivity and asthma, it can precede asthma onset in the natural history of the atopic march (29–31).

ALLERGIC COMORBIDITIES

Several factors and co-morbidities may contribute to worsen asthma control and complicate diagnostic and therapeutic management of severe asthmatic patients (**Figure 2**) (32).

Atopic Dermatitis

Several studies reported that family history of atopy, early onset AD, higher initial severity of atopic eczema, hens' egg sensitization and male sex are associated with an increased risk of asthma in childhood (33). Furthermore, the percentage of patients with severe asthma and concomitant eczema is greater than expected and close relationship between asthma and atopic dermatitis severity has been reported (34).

Abbreviations: ABPA, allergic bronchopulmonary aspergillosis; AERD, aspirin exacerbated respiratory disease; AD, atopic dermatitis; AIT, allergen specific immunotherapy; AR, allergic rhinitis; ATS, American Thoracic Society; BD, bronchodilator; ERS, European Respiratory Society; FA, food allergy; HDM, house dust mites; ICS, inhaled corticosteroid; IgE, immunoglobulin E; LABA, long-acting beta2-agonist; MAAS, Manchester Asthma and Allergy Study; MAS, Multicentre Allergy Study; NSAIDs, non-steroidal anti-inflammatory drugs; SABA, short-acting beta2-agonist; SAFS, Severe asthma with fungal sensitization.

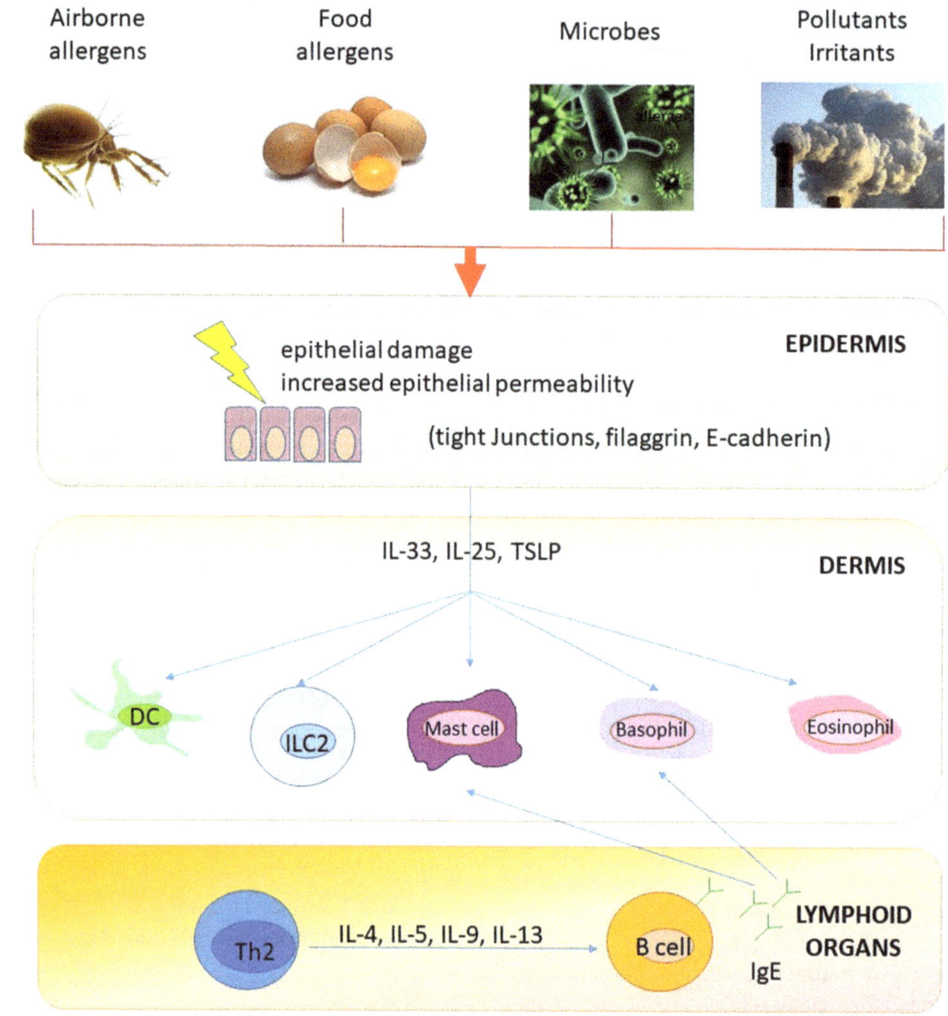

FIGURE 1 | A model of epithelial barrier damage and skin IgE-sensitization. Impaired skin barrier (e.g., eczema) promotes foreign antigen (e.g., airborne and food allergens) penetration and activation of innate and specific immune responses. Epithelial cell-derived cytokines (such as TSLP, IL-33, and IL-25) license antigen presenting cells (i.e., dendritic cells) to drive type 2 immune responses and stimulate several cell types (including basophils, eosinophils, mast cells, and ILCs) to start and maintain allergic inflammation also in regional draining lymph nodes (e.g., B-cell IgE skewing). Furthermore, T cells circulate back to infiltrate the skin or are distributed peripherally to other end organs to initiate diverse atopic disorders. DC, dendritic cells; Ig, Immunoglobulin; IL, interleukin; ILC, Innate Lymphoid cells; Th, T helper cells; TSLP, thymic stromal lymphopoietin.

Therefore, as AD and the subsequent atopic march mostly present in early infancy, primary, and secondary prevention should be attempted as early as possible to prevent asthma symptoms onset (35).

Allergic Rhinitis

Allergic rhinitis is almost ubiquitous in children with asthma living in urban areas. The presence of allergic sensitization to inhalant allergens and rhinitis symptoms is typically associated with early onset of severe asthma (36). Patients with AR report poorer asthma control, more exacerbations and emergency visits (37) and have more difficulty in achieving symptom control (38).

Perennial allergic rhinitis with seasonal exacerbations is considered the most severe phenotype and most likely to be associated with difficult-to-control asthma (39).

This means that treating coexisting allergic rhinitis could improve asthma control and reduce healthcare resource utilization (40).

Food Allergy

Respiratory symptoms as clinical manifestation of IgE-mediated food allergy (FA), usually, occur immediately after exposure to the offensive food and are accompanied by skin and/or gastrointestinal manifestations. Food allergen exposure occurs usually by ingestion, but the inhalation of food proteins (through dust or aerosolized particles) may also trigger respiratory symptoms (41).

Among patients with FA, asthmatic symptoms are more frequent in children, and especially in those with concomitant atopic dermatitis. In addition to respiratory symptoms occurring

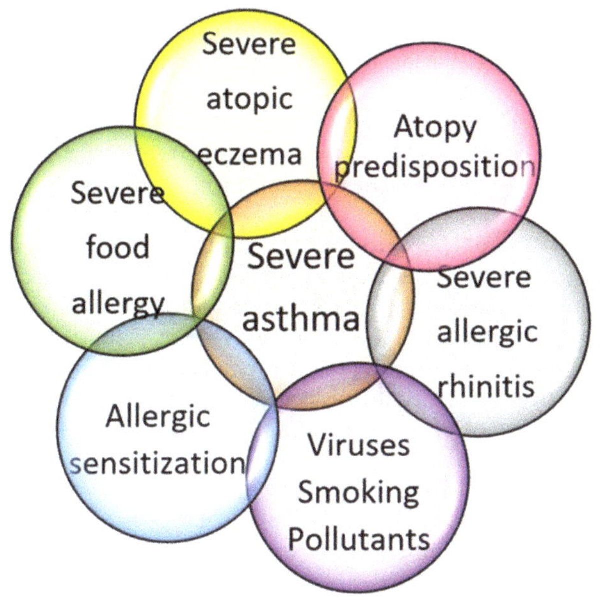

FIGURE 2 | Factors contributing to severe asthma development in childhood.

as a presentation of FA, patients with FA are at increased risk for developing asthma and often severe asthma as expression of progression of the atopic march. Symptomatic FA and food allergen sensitization are associated with asthma development both in younger and older children: it was reported that this association is stronger among children with multiple or severe FAs (42–44). Moreover, children with FA develop asthma earlier and at a higher prevalence than children without FA. The opposite is also true, as asthma is a risk factor for the persistence of food allergy (45–47).

Food allergy and food sensitization can be also considered as important markers to predict asthma severity. Indeed, it is reported that children with FA and sensitization to at least one food (e.g., egg, milk, soy, peanut, wheat, and fish) had worse lung function (48), higher rates of hospitalization, emergency department visits, use of systemic glucocorticoids (49), or need of mechanical ventilation for severe asthma exacerbation (50, 51).

Aspirin Sensitization

Aspirin-exacerbated respiratory disease (AERD) is a chronic medical condition, usually in adults and adolescents, consisting of three clinical features: sinus disease with recurrent nasal polyps, asthma, and sensitivity to aspirin and other non-steroidal anti-inflammatory drugs (NSAIDs). Even though asthma is not always present in AERD, asthma symptoms develop 1–3 years after the development of rhinitis or later. When present, asthma is severe and difficult to treat and often characterized by increased residual volume and diminished diffusing capacity due to increased airway remodeling (52).

ROLE OF ATOPIC SENSITIZATION IN SEVERE ASTHMA

Previous studies showed that atopic sensitization is a major risk factor for severe asthma in children (53–55). Overall, the expression "atopic sensitization" refers to the positivity either of serum allergen-specific IgE (sIgE) or a positive skin prick test (SPT) to allergen extracts. Arbitrary cut-off points have been set: levels of sIgE >0.35 KU/l (56) and a mean wheal diameter ≥3 mm (SPT) (57). Though these tests are highly sensitive, their mere positivity do not mean itself clinical disease. Quantification of atopic sensitization increases the specificity in relation to childhood asthma presence and severity (4), and asthma persistence in adulthood (58–60). The severity of asthma correlates with both sIgE levels and the number of sensitizations, also on the molecular level. The number of component-specific sensitizations correlate with disease severity in **grass** allergic children (61) as well as in **house dust mites** allergic (HDM) pediatric patients. In the Multicentre Allergy Study (MAS) cohort, a birth cohort started in 1990 in Germany, the number of HDM-component specific sensitizations increased with disease severity and with age. Sensitization to Der p 1 and Der p 23 before the age of 5 years was predictive of asthma at school age (62). Similarly, in the Manchester Asthma and Allergy Study (MAAS) birth cohort, asthmatic children were characterized by more complex molecular patterns of IgE sensitization to grass and mite molecules (Der p 1 and Der p 2) (63). In a French study, atopic sensitization to Der p 2 and Der f 2 was more common in severe asthma. In a cohort of 300 asthmatic children (age range, 4–12 years), higher levels of Der p 1 and pet allergen [cat (Fel d 1), dog (Can f 1)] were found to be associated with greater asthma severity (64). Similarly, in **latex** allergy sensitization to 3 (5, 6.01/6.02) of the 12 recombinant natural rubber antigens so far known was strongly linked with asthma (65).

Fungal Allergy

Fungal allergy drives asthma severity, too (66). Sensitization to molds has been estimated: 7–20% in the general asthma population; 35–75% in severe asthma patients; 54–91% in life-threatening asthma population (67–69). The severity of exacerbation relates to the different fungi species: in particular, Aspergillus or Alternaria or *Cladosporium* spp. sensitization has been linked to severe asthma (70, 71).

Long-term or uncontrolled fungal infections are associated with a poor controlled asthma, bronchiectasis, and chronic allergic bronchopulmonary aspergillosis (ABPA) (71). The term "Severe asthma with fungal sensitization" (SAFS), introduced by Denning et al. (71), describes a specific phenotype in patients with persistent severe asthma (despite standard treatment) and evidence of fungal sensitization, and do not meet the criteria for ABPA. An EAACI Task Force sets the total IgE cut-off at <1,000 IU/ml for SAFS and >1,000 IU/ml for ABPA, a specific endotypes of asthma, with a genetic predisposition.

ROLE OF VIRUSES, SMOKING, AND POLLUTANTS

In poli-sensitized asthmatics, daily exposure to allergens combined with other enhancing factors, such as viral infections, smoking (even tertiary one), and/or environmental pollution, influences the asthma course and severity (**Figure 2**). There is robust evidence concerning the synergistic effect of **viral**

lower respiratory tract infections (LRTI) and IgE sensitization on asthma development, particularly in children predisposed to atopy (72) and asthma exacerbation (73). Increased risks of asthma inception in atopic predisposed children include: the type of virus (more than 10-fold increased risk for asthma development with rhinovirus compared to 5-fold with respiratory syncytial virus); the severity of viral LRTI; and the age during viral LRTI (74). The risk of hospital admission due to asthma exacerbation is increased by the interaction among respiratory viral infections in combination with atopic sensitization and exposure to allergens (75).

Cigarette Smoking

Cigarette smoking itself may influence asthma severity, through different patho-mechanisms (76). There is evidence that smoking increases itself serum IgE levels, especially in male adults (77), and rises the risk of IgE sensitization, mainly to occupational allergens (78). Nevertheless, in severe asthmatic patients, the complex association between cigarette smoking and allergy remains currently controversial.

Data reports that children exposed to **air pollution** are at major to develop IgE sensitization to inhalant allergens (79, 80). However, the immunological mechanisms underlying this link remain to be better clarified. Notwithstanding, some data suggest that ultrafine carbon black particles may induce maturation of dendritic cells *in vitro* (81), which might then facilitate sensitization to airborne allergens. On the other side, airborne pollutants may modulate the inflammatory cellular response in the lungs, thereby lowering the threshold for sensitization.

PREVENTION STRATEGIES

As widely described above and resumed in **Table 2**, children with early onset atopy, high specific IgE-sensitization and multiple IgE-sensitizations are at increased risk for developing severe asthma in childhood. In addition, it is well-established that severe allergic diseases more frequently coexist (**Figure 2**).

Based on these premises, it is reasonable that prevention strategies and proper treatments of atopic diseases could prevent occurrence of severe asthma and viceversa. However, asthma development depends on complex and still not fully known interception of genes and environment. Therefore, effective primary prevention strategies for asthma, and especially for severe asthma in children, -though highly desirable- might be difficult to be identified both at population and individual level.

Primary Prevention

Some studies have suggested that maternal consumption of allergenic food (such us cow's milk, peanut, or fish) and vitamin D and E intake during pregnancy could be associated to decreased risk of allergy and wheezing in their offspring, respectively (82–84).

Conflicting results have been reported about the beneficial effect of maternal breastfeeding on pediatric asthma development (85). The role of prebiotics, probiotics, and synbiotic interventions (86) and other dietary supplements (such as nucleosides and nucleotides) (87) is under investigation. Overall, the level of evidence remains currently low or even very low because of the risk of bias, heterogeneity among studies, imprecision, and inconsistency of results, as well as indirectness of available research.

Instead, there is stronger evidence concerning maternal smoking and tobacco post-natal exposition. They are both associated to increased risk of asthma in offspring (88).

Atopic Dermatitis

Since the epithelium plays an important role in protecting against the development of allergic diseases and the occurrence of transcutaneous IgE-sensitization may precede airway sensitization (**Figure 1**), proactive emollient therapy able to make stronger the epithelial barrier may prevent or delay the development of IgE-sensitization in children affected by AD (89).

Allergic Rhinitis

It is well-known that AR and asthma often coexist. As they share genetic background, chronic airway inflammation pathway and similar triggers (allergen exposure, viral infections, cold air, and air pollution) (90), treatment of rhinitis can be beneficial for preventing severe asthma exacerbations.

The role of exposure to airborne allergens on AR and asthma is well-established and strict avoidance of the culprit allergen(s) is desirable though it is often hard or even impossible. Symptomatic drugs for AR, such as H1-antihistamines and intranasal corticosteroids are not recommended for asthma management (40). However, data suggest that the use of H1-antihistamines in AR children is associated with delayed asthma development (91) and improvement of asthma outcomes (92). Similarly, a significant reduction of asthma symptom scores and rescue medication use has been reported for patients with AR and coexisting asthma by using intranasal corticosteroid therapy (93). Moreover, anti-leukotrienes target both upper and lower airways and could be beneficial in patients with asthma and concomitant AR (94).

Biological drugs—such as anti-IgE therapy (i.e., omalizumab) and antibody against the α-subunit of receptor for IL-4 and IL-13 (i.e., dupilumab)- have been approved for a few specific phenotypes of severe asthmatic patients at different ages (**Table 3**). They could be beneficial on both diseases: severe asthma and severe AR (95, 96). Notwithstanding, allergen immunotherapy (AIT) is considered the only etiological treatment able to prevent asthma development (97), to improve asthma symptoms in AR affected children (98), and to prevent new sensitizations in already sensitized patients (99). Furthermore, since adverse events are more common during the escalation or build-up phases of AIT, omalizumab has been suggested as "add-on therapy" to AIT (100). Nevertheless, larger studies are needed to identify patients who would benefit the addition of omalizumab to AIT, as well as optimal dosing strategies and duration treatment (101).

Food Allergy

Strict avoidance of the culprit food(s) represents currently the standard therapeutic option for FA (102). However, accidental exposure is possible and related to severe adverse events. Allergen

TABLE 3 | Main biological targeted treatments for severe asthma in children.

Drug (trade name), dosage	Mechanism of action	Suggested population	Adverse effects
APPROVED			
Omalizumab (Xolair), s.c. injections every 2–4 wks, depending on body weight and IgE levels	Anti- IgE; binds Fc receptor of free circulating IgE and downloads IgE production	Age >6 yrs; 30 UI < IgE < 700 UI* ; positive skin test or elevated specific IgE level toward a perennial	Anaphylaxis (~0.2% pts); monitor for helmintic infection
Mepolizumab (Nucala), 100 mg in pts aged 12 yrs or older (40 mg in pts aged 6–11 yrs) by s.c. injections every 4 wks	Anti- IL-5; binds circulating IL-5	Age >12 yrs; eosinophlic asthma	Zoster (rare); avoid if active helminithic infection
UNDER INVESTIGATION			
Reslizumab (Cinqair), approved for adults (3 mg/kg by i.v. injections every 4 wks)	Anti- IL-5; binds circulating IL-5	Eosinophilic asthma	Anaphylaxis (rare); avoid if active helmintic infection
Dupilumab (Dupixent), approved for adults with atopic dermatitis	Anti- IL-4 and anti-IL-13; binds common α-subunit of receptor for IL-4 and IL-13	Eosinophlic asthma	Eosinophilia (rare); avoid live vaccines; avoid if active helmintic infection

*IL, interleukin; i.v., intravenous; pt, patient; s.c., subcutaneous; wk, week; yr, year. *Upper limit varies according to body weight and regulatory authorities.*

specific immunotherapy (AIT) alone or combined with adjuvants (including probiotics and anti-IgE monoclonal antibodies) is nowadays the only active treatment for FA (103). Nevertheless, it is highly demanding, especially in patients with a severe phenotype, who usually have allergies to multiple foods and concomitant severe asthma. For these severe patients, biologicals might be a better potential therapy alone or in combination with AIT (104, 105). However, more data are needed.

AERD

Careful avoidance of aspirin and other NSAIDs is mandatory in patients affected by AERD in order to prevent asthmatic exacerbations. The use of acetaminophen or selective COX-2 inhibitors should be encouraged as alternative drugs. Furthermore, the addition of a leukotriene receptor antagonist (e.g., montelukast) and 5-lipoxygenase inhibitors (e.g., zileuton) to standard asthma treatment have been shown to be effective in improving asthma outcomes (106). Aspirin desensitization is currently the only causative treatment in AERD affected patients improving both upper and lower airway symptoms; however, only a very small percentage of patients benefit from this therapeutic option (107). Biologic therapies (such as anti-IgE, anti-IL-5 monoclonal antibodies, IL-4α receptor antagonist, and anti-thymic stromal lymphopoietin) could be promising therapeutic options for AERD patients given their effectiveness in nasal polyposis and asthma (108).

Unfortunately, there is currently lack of data about any specific role of the treatment of allergic comorbidities in preventing the development of severe asthma in atopic children.

OPTIMIZING TREATMENT OF SEVERE ASTHMA

The current guideline-based drug therapy of pediatric severe asthma is based primarily on data extrapolated from adult studies. High dose of inhalant **corticosteroids** (or oral corticosteroids) combined with a second controller (such as a LABA or leukotriene modifier/theophylline) are the mainstay of treatment (5).

However, the current challenge facing physicians and researchers is to provide a "**personalized medicine**," which is tailored to the diverse patho-mechanisms underlying clinical presentations (109).

Allergen Specific Immunotherapy

AIT has been demonstrated to have beneficial effects in the management of childhood allergic asthma, including effects on symptom control, medication use, and airway hyperresponsiveness (110). However, trials involve children with mild-moderate allergic asthma, and studies specifically examining the efficacy of AIT in children with severe asthma are missing. Notwithstanding, the majority of studies involved monosensitized patients, whereas most children with severe asthma are polysensitized, mainly in Southern Europe. In addition, allergen immunotherapy should be commenced in patients with well-controlled asthma, a situation which is less common among children with severe asthma. Since 2003, several **targeted therapies** have been approved for severe asthma and others are still under investigation (**Table 3**). Furthermore, they could be beneficial in other allergic comorbidities. However, their cost is often expensive. Therefore, a precise identification and selection of good responders is pivotal.

A **regular longitudinal assessment** of outcomes of children with severe asthma is pivotal. Follow-up appointments should be devoted not only to reduce maintenance therapy to the minimal amount required to achieve control of asthma symptoms, but also to assess the atopic status of the patient and any concomitant atopic co-morbidities and, therefore, address any modifiable factors (including allergen exposure, basics of inhaler technique, and adherence).

CONCLUSIONS

Asthma is a common disease in childhood with a minority of affected children having severe asthma. Several data suggest that allergies may play a key role in children with severe asthma. Many children with severe asthma have coexisting allergic disease(s). Allergies to foods, molds, pollens, and pets have been associated with both asthma inception and severe asthma exacerbations. A better understanding of interactions between asthma and allergy and mechanistic implications of cofactors, such as virus infections, pollution, and smoking will allow the development of novel therapeutic targets and, therefore, additional strategies for improving disease control.

AUTHOR CONTRIBUTIONS

SA and FP wrote the first draft of the manuscript. AF and RC critically reviewed the manuscript. All authors read and approved the final manuscript.

REFERENCES

1. Addo-Yobo EO, Custovic A, Taggart SC, Craven M, Bonnie B, Woodcock A. Risk factors for asthma in urban Ghana. *J Allergy Clin Immunol.* (2001)108:363–8. doi: 10.1067/mai.2001.117464
2. Al-Mousawi MS, Lovel H, Behbehani N, Arifhodzic N, Woodcock A, Custovic A. Asthma and sensitization in a community with low indoor allergen levels and low petkeeping frequency. *J Allergy Clin Immunol.* (2004) 114:1389–94. doi: 10.1016/j.jaci.2004.09.005
3. Caminati M, Pham DL, Bagnasco D, Canonica GW. Type 2 immunity in asthma. *World Allergy Organ J.* (2018) 11:13. doi: 10.1186/s40413-018-0192-5
4. Stevens W, Addo-Yobo E, Roper J, Woodcock A, James H, Platts-Mills T, et al. Differences in both prevalence and titre of specific immunoglobulin E among children with asthma in affluent and poor communities within a large town in Ghana. *Clin Exp Allergy* (2011) 41:1587–94. doi: 10.1111/j.1365-2222.2011.03832.x
5. Chung KF, Wenzel SE, Brozek JL, Bush A, Castro M, Sterk PJ, et al. International ERS/ATS guidelines on definition, evaluation and treatment of severe asthma. *Eur Respir J.* (2014) 43:343–73. doi: 10.1183/09031936.00202013
6. Guilbert TW, Bacharier LB, Fitzpatrick AM. Severe asthma in children. *J Allergy Clin Immunol Pract.* (2014) 2:489–500. doi: 10.1016/j.jaip.2014.06.022
7. Gherasim A, Dao A, Bernstein JA. Confounders of severe asthma: diagnoses to consider when asthma symptoms persist despite optimal therapy. *World Allergy Organ J.* (2018) 11:29. doi: 10.1186/s40413-018-0207-2
8. Lang A, Carlsen KH, Haaland G, Devulapalli CS, Munthe-Kaas M, Mowinckel P, et al. Severe asthma in childhood: assessed in 10-year olds in a birth cohort study. *Allergy* (2008) 63:1054–60. doi: 10.1111/j.1398-9995.2008.01672.x
9. Flórez-Tanus Á, Parra D, Zakzuk J, Caraballo L, Alvis-Guzmán N. Health care costs and resource utilization for different asthma severity stages in Colombia: a claims data analysis. *World Allergy Organ J.* (2018) 11:26. doi: 10.1186/s40413-018-0205-4
10. Sullivan SD, Rasouliyan L, Russo PA, Kamath T, Chipps BE; TENOR Study Group. Extent, patterns, and burden of uncontrolled disease in severe or difficult-to-treat asthma. *Allergy* (2007) 62:126–33. doi: 10.1111/j.1398-9995.2006.01254.x
11. Schatz M, Hsu JW, Zeiger RS, Chen W, Dorenbaum A, Chipps BE, et al. Phenotypes determined by cluster analysis in severe or difficult-to-treat asthma. *J Allergy Clin Immunol.* (2014) 133:1549–56. doi: 10.1016/j.jaci.2013.10.006
12. Bossley CJ, Fleming L, Gupta A, Regamey N, Frith J, Oates T, et al. Pediatric severe asthma is characterized by eosinophilia and remodeling without T(H)2 cytokines. *J Allergy Clin Immunol.* (2012) 129:974–82. doi: 10.1016/j.jaci.2012.01.059
13. Amelink M, de Groot JC, de Nijs SB, Lutter R, Zwinderman AH, Sterk PJ, et al. Severe adult-onset asthma: a distinct phenotype. *J Allergy Clin Immunol.* (2013) 132:336–41. doi: 10.1016/j.jaci.2013.04.052
14. Hekking PP, Loza MJ, Pavlidis S, de Meulder B, Lefaudeux D, Baribaud F, et al. U-BIOPRED Study Group. Pathway discovery using transcriptomic profiles in adult-onset severe asthma. *J Allergy Clin Immunol.* (2018) 141:1280–90. doi: 10.1016/j.jaci.2017.06.037
15. Spergel JM. Epidemiology of atopic dermatitis and atopic march in children. *Immunol Allergy Clin N Am.* (2010) 30:269–80. doi: 10.1016/j.iac.2010.06.003
16. Bergmann, RL, Bergmann KE, Lau-Schadensdorf S, Luck W, Dannemann A, Bauer CP, et al. Atopic diseases in infancy: the German Multicenter Atopy Study (MAS-90). *Pediatr Allergy Immunol.* (1994) 5:19–25. doi: 10.1111/j.1399-3038.1994.tb00343.x
17. Wahn, U. What drives the allergic march? *Allergy* (2000) 55:591–99. doi: 10.1034/j.1398-9995.2000.00111.x
18. Høst, A. Frequency of cow's milk allergy in childhood. *Ann Allergy Asthma Immunol.* (2002) 89:33–7. doi: 10.1016/S1081-1206(10)62120-5
19. Spergel JM, Paller AS. Atopic dermatitis and the atopic march. *J Allergy Clin Immunol.* (2003) 112:S118–27. doi: 10.1016/j.jaci.2003.09.033
20. Ricci G, Patrizi A, Baldi E, Menna G, Tabanelli M, Masi M. Long-term follow-up of atopic dermatitis: retrospective analysis of related risk factors and association with concomitant allergic diseases. *J Am Acad Dermatol.* (2006) 55:765–71. doi: 10.1016/j.jaad.2006.04.064
21. Hogan MB, Peele K, Wilson NW. Skin barrier function and its importance at the start of the atopic march. *J Allergy (Cairo)* (2012) 2012:901940. doi: 10.1155/2012/901940
22. Warner JO. A double-blinded, randomized, placebo-controlled trial of cetirizine in preventing the onset of asthma in children with atopic dermatitis: 18 months' treatment and 18 months' post-treatment follow-up. *J Allergy Clin Immunol.* (2001) 108:929–37. doi: 10.1067/mai.2001.120015
23. Novembre E, Cianferoni A, Lombardi E, Bernardini R, Pucci N, Vierucci A. Natural history of "intrinsic" atopic dermatitis. *Allergy* (2001) 56:452–3. doi: 10.1034/j.1398-9995.2001.056005452.x
24. Wuthrich B, Schmid-Grendelmeier P. Natural course of AEDS. *Allergy* (2002) 57:267–8. doi: 10.1034/j.1398-9995.2002.1n3572.x
25. Filipiak-Pittroff B, Schnopp C, Berdel D, Naumann A, Sedlmeier S, Onken A, et al. Predictive value of food sensitization and filaggrin mutations in children with eczema. *J Allergy Clin Immunol.* (2011) 128:1235–41. doi: 10.1016/j.jaci.2011.09.014
26. Marenholz I, Kerscher T, Bauerfeind A, Esparza-Gordillo J, Nickel R, Keil T, et al. An interaction between filaggrin mutations and early food sensitization improves the prediction of childhood asthma. *J Allergy Clin Immunol.* (2009) 123:911–6. doi: 10.1016/j.jaci.2009.01.051
27. Gustafsson D, Sjöberg O, Foucard T. Development of allergies and asthma in infants and young children with atopic dermatitis - a prospective follow-up to 7 years of age. *Allergy* (2000) 55:240–5. doi: 10.1034/j.1398-9995.2000.00391.x
28. Dohi M, Okudaira H, Sugiyama H, Tsurumachi K, Suko M, Nakagawa T. Bronchial responsiveness to mite allergen in atopic dermatitis without asthma. *Int Arch Allergy Immunol.* (1990) 92: 138–42. doi: 10.1159/000235204
29. Leynaert B, Neukirch C, Kony S, Guénégou A, Bousquet J, Aubier M, et al. Association between asthma and rhinitis according to atopic sensitization in a population-based study. *J Allergy Clin Immunol.* (2004) 113:86–93. doi: 10.1016/j.jaci.2003.10.010
30. Ciprandi G, Cirillo I, Vizzaccaro A, Milanese M, Tosca MA. Airway function and nasal inflammation in seasonal allergic rhinitis and asthma. *Clin Exp Allergy* (2004) 34:891–6. doi: 10.1111/j.1365-2222.2004.01970.x
31. Spergel JM. Atopic march: link to upper airways. *Curr Opin Allergy Clin Immunol.* (2005) 5:17–21. doi: 10.1097/00130832-200502000-00005

32. Bonner K, Roberts G. Does allergy explain why some children have severe asthma? *Clin Exp Allergy* (2018) 48:1594–605. doi: 10.1111/cea.13234
33. Amat F, Soria A, Tallon P, Bourgoin-Heck M, Lambert N, Deschildre A, et al. New insights into the phenotypes of atopic dermatitis linked with allergies and asthma in children: an overview. *Clin Exp Allergy* (2018) 48:919–34. doi: 10.1111/cea.13156
34. Lee JK, Han D. Atopic dermatitis is an important comorbidity in severe asthma. *Ann Allergy Asthma Immunol.* (2018) 120:661–71. doi: 10.1016/j.anai.2018.02.026
35. Czarnowicki T, Krueger JG, Guttman-Yassky E. Novel concepts of prevention and treatment of atopic dermatitis through barrier and immune manipulations with implications for the atopic march. *J Allergy Clin Immunol.* (2017) 139:1723–34. doi: 10.1016/j.jaci.2017.04.004
36. Moore WC, Meyers DA, Wenzel SE, Teague WG, Li H, Li X, et al. Identification of asthma phenotypes using cluster analysis in the Severe Asthma Research Program. *Am J Respir Crit Care Med.* (2010) 181:315–23. doi: 10.1164/rccm.200906-0896OC
37. Bousquet J, Gaugris S, Kocevar VS, Zhang Q, Yin DD, Polos PG, et al. Increased risk of asthma attacks and emergency visits among asthma patients with allergic rhinitis: a subgroup analysis of the improving asthma control trial. *Clin Exp Allergy* (2005) 35:723–7. doi: 10.1111/j.1365-2222.2005.02251.x
38. Valovirta E, Pawankar R. Survey on the impact of comorbid allergic rhinitis in patients with asthma. *BMC Pulm Med.* (2006) 6:S3. doi: 10.1186/1471-2466-6-S1-S3
39. Togias A, Gergen PJ, Hu JW, Babineau DC, Wood RA, Cohen RT, et al. Rhinitis in children and adolescents with asthma: ubiquitous, difficult to control, and associated with asthma outcomes. *J Allergy Clin Immunol.* (2018) doi: 10.1016/j.jaci.2018.07.041. [Epub ahead of print].
40. Bousquet J, Khaltaev N, Cruz AA, Denburg J, Fokkens WJ, Togias A, et al. Allergic Rhinitis and its Impact on Asthma (ARIA) 2008. *Allergy* (2008) 63:8–160. doi: 10.1111/j.1398-9995.2007.01620.x
41. Sampson HA, Aceves S, Bock SA, James J, Jones S, Lang D, et al. Food allergy: a practice parameter update-2014. *J Allergy Clin Immunol.* (2014) 134:1016–25. doi: 10.1016/j.jaci.2014.05.013
42. Rhodes HL, Sporik R, Thomas P, Holgate ST, Cogswell JJ. Early life risk factors for adult asthma: a birth cohort study of subjects at risk. *J Allergy Clin Immunol.* (2001) 108:720–5. doi: 10.1067/mai.2001.119151
43. Pham MN, Wang J. Management of food allergies and asthma in schools. *Ann Allergy Asthma Immunol.* (2018) 121:391–9. doi: 10.1016/j.anai.2018.07.028
44. Sherenian MG, Singh AM, Arguelles L, Balmert L, Caruso D, Wang X, et al. Association of food allergy and decreased lung function in children and young adults with asthma. *Ann Allergy Asthma Immunol.* (2018) 121:588–93. doi: 10.1016/j.anai.2018.07.037
45. Fiocchi A. Incremental prognostic factors associated with cow's milk allergy outcomes in infant and child referrals: the Milan Cow's Milk Allergy Cohort study. *Ann Allergy Asthma Immunol.* (2008) 101:166–73. doi: 10.1016/S1081-1206(10)60205-0
46. Wood RA, Sicherer SH, Vickery BP, Jones SM, Liu AH, Fleischer DM, et al. The natural history of milk allergy in an observational cohort. *J Allergy Clin Immunol.* (2013) 131:805–12. doi: 10.1016/j.jaci.2012.10.060
47. Sicherer SH, Wood RA, Vickery BP, Jones SM, Liu AH, Fleischer DM, et al. The natural history of egg allergy in an observational cohort. *J Allergy Clin Immunol.* (2014) 133:492–9. doi: 10.1016/j.jaci.2013.12.1041
48. Friedlander JL, Sheehan WJ, Baxi SN, Kopel LS, Gaffin JM, Ozonoff A, et al. Food allergy and increased asthma morbidity in a School-based Inner-City Asthma Study. *J Allergy Clin Immunol Pract.* (2013) 1:479–84. doi: 10.1016/j.jaip.2013.06.007
49. Wang J, Visness CM, Sampson HA. Food allergen sensitization in inner-city children with asthma. *J Allergy Clin Immunol.* (2005) 115:1076–80. doi: 10.1016/j.jaci.2005.02.014
50. Roberts G, Patel N, Levi-Schaffer F,Habibi P, Lack G. Food allergy as a risk factor for life-threatening asthma in childhood: a case-controlled study. *J Allergy Clin Immunol.* (2003) 112:168–74. doi: 10.1067/mai.2003.1569
51. Berns SH, Halm EA, Sampson HA, Sicherer SH, Busse PJ, Wisnivesky JP. Food allergy as a risk factor for asthma morbidity in adults. *J Asthma* (2007) 44:377–81. doi: 10.1080/02770900701364031
52. Kennedy JL, Stoner AN, Borish L. Aspirin-exacerbated respiratory disease: prevalence, diagnosis, treatment, and considerations for the future. *Am J Rhinol Allergy* (2016) 30:407–13. doi: 10.2500/ajra.2016.30.4370
53. Fitzpatrick AM, Teague WG, Meyers DA, Peters SP, Li X, Li H, et al. Heterogeneity of severe asthma in childhood: confirmation by cluster analysis of children in the National Institutes of Health/National Heart, Lung, and Blood Institute Severe Asthma Research Program. *J Allergy Clin Immunol.* (2011) 127:382–9. doi: 10.1016/j.jaci.2010.11.015
54. Lee E, Kim YH, Cho HJ, Yoon J, Jung S, Yang SI, et al. Clinical phenotypes of bronchial hyperresponsiveness in school-aged children. *Ann Allergy Asthma Immunol.* (2018) 121:434–43. doi: 10.1016/j.anai.2018.05.033
55. Lu KD, Phipatanakul W, Perzanowski MS, Balcer-Whaley S, Matsui EC. Atopy, but not obesity is associated with asthma severity among children with persistent asthma. *J Asthma* (2016) 53:1033–44. doi: 10.3109/02770903.2016.1174259
56. Heinzerling LM, Burbach GJ, Edenharter G, Bachert C, Bindslev-Jensen C, Bonini S, et al. GA(2)LEN skin test study I: GA(2) LEN harmonization of skin prick testing: novel sensitization patterns for inhalant allergens in Europe. *Allergy* (2009) 64:1498–506. doi: 10.1111/j.1398-9995.2009.02093.x
57. Johansson SG, Hourihane JO, Bousquet J, Bruijnzeel-Koomen C, Dreborg S, Haahtela T, et al. A revised nomenclature for allergy. An EAACI position statement from the EAACI nomenclature task force. *Allergy* (2001) 56:813–24. doi: 10.1034/j.1398-9995.2001.t01-1-00001.x
58. Lodrup Carlsen KC, Soderstrom L, Mowinckel P, Haland G, Pettersen M, Munthe Kaas MC, et al. Asthma prediction in school children; the value of combined IgE antibodies and obstructive airways disease severity score. *Allergy* (2010) 65:1134–40. doi: 10.1111/j.1398-9995.2010.02344.x
59. Sly PD, Boner AL, Bjorksten B, Bush A, Custovic A, Eigenmann PA, et al. Early identification of atopy in the prediction of persistent asthma in children. *Lancet* (2008) 372:1100–110. doi: 10.1016/S0140-6736(08)61451-8
60. Soto-Quiros M, Avila L, Platts-Mills TA, Hunt JF, Erdman DD, Carper H, et al. High titers of IgE antibody to dust mite allergen and risk for wheezing among asthmatic children infected. *J Allergy Clin Immunol.* (2012) 129:1499–505. doi: 10.1016/j.jaci.2012.03.040
61. Hatzler L, Panetta V, Lau S, Wagner P, Bergmann RL, Illi S, et al. Molecular spreading and predictive value of preclinical IgE response to Phleum pratense in children with hay fever. *J Allergy Clin Immunol.* (2012) 130:894–901. doi: 10.1016/j.jaci.2012.05.053
62. Posa D, Perna S, Resch Y, Lupinek C, Panetta V, Hofmaier S, et al. Evolution and predictive value of IgE responses toward a comprehensive panel of house dust mite allergens during the first 2 decades of life. *J Allergy Clin Immunol.* (2017) 139:541–9. doi: 10.1016/j.jaci.2016.08.014
63. Custovic A, Sonntag HJ, Buchan IE, Belgrave D, Simpson A, Prosperi MCF. Evolution pathways of IgE responses to grass and mite allergens throughout childhood. *J Allergy Clin Immunol.* (2015) 136:1645–52. doi: 10.1016/j.jaci.2015.03.041
64. Gent JF, Belanger K, Triche EW, Bracken MB, Beckett WS, Leaderer BP. Association of pediatric asthma severity with exposure to common household dust allergens. *Environ Res.* (2009) 109:768–74. doi: 10.1016/j.envres.2009.04.010
65. Vandenplas O, Froidure A, Meurer U, Rihs HP, Rifflart C, Soetaert S, et al. The role of allergen components for the diagnosis of latex-induced occupational asthma. *Allergy* (2016) 71:840–9. doi: 10.1111/all.12872
66. Masaki K, Fukunaga K, Matsusaka M, Kabata H, Tanosaki T, Mochimaru T, et al. Characteristics of severe asthma with fungal sensitization. *Ann Allergy Asthma Immunol.* (2017) 119:253–7. doi: 10.1016/j.anai.2017.07.008
67. Larenas-Linnemann D, Baxi S, Phipatanakul W, Environmental Allergens Workgroup. Clinical evaluation and management of patients with suspected fungus sensitivity. *J Allergy Clin Immunol Pract.* (2016) 4:405–14. doi: 10.1016/j.jaip.2015.10.015
68. Black PN, Udy AA, Brodie SM. Sensitivity to fungal allergens is a risk factor for life-threatening asthma. *Allergy* (2000) 55:501–4. doi: 10.1034/j.1398-9995.2000.00293.x

69. Vicencio AG, Santiago MT, Tsirilakis K, Stone A, Worgall S, Foley EA, et al. Fungal sensitization in childhood persistent asthma is associated with disease severity. *Pediatr Pulmonol.* (2014) 49:8–14. doi: 10.1002/ppul.22779
70. Tham R, Dharmage SC, Taylor PE, Katelaris CH, Vicendese D, Abramson MJ, et al. Outdoor fungi and child asthma health service attendances. *Pediatr Allergy Immunol.* (2014) 25:439–49. doi: 10.1111/pai.12257
71. Denning DW, Pashley C, Hartl D, Wardlaw A, Godet C, Del Giacco S, et al. Fungal allergy in asthma-state of the art and research needs. *Clin Transl Allergy* (2014) 4:14. doi: 10.1186/2045-7022-4-14
72. Jackson DJ, Gangnon RE, Evans MD, Roberg KA, Anderson EL, Pappas TE, et al. Wheezing rhinovirus illnesses in early life predict asthma development in high-risk children. *Am J Respir Crit Care Med.* (2008) 178:667–72. doi: 10.1164/rccm.200802-309OC
73. Kusel MM, de Klerk NH, Kebadze T, Vohma V, Holt PG, Johnston SL, et al. Early-life respiratory viral infections, atopic sensitization, and risk of subsequent development of persistent asthma. *J Allergy Clin Immunol.* (2007) 119:1105–10. doi: 10.1016/j.jaci.2006.12.669
74. Martorano LM, Grayson MH. Respiratory viral infections and atopic development: from possible mechanisms to advances in treatment. *Eur J Immunol.* (2018) 48:407–14. doi: 10.1002/eji.201747052
75. Kim CK, Callaway Z, Gern JE. Viral infections and associated factors that promote acute exacerbations of asthma. *Allergy Asthma Immunol Res.* (2018) 10:12–17. doi: 10.4168/aair.2018.10.1.12
76. Polosa R, Thomson NC. Smoking and asthma: dangerous liaisons. *Eur Respir J.* (2013) 41:716–26. doi: 10.1183/09031936.00073312
77. Oryszczyn MP, Annesi-Maesano I, Charpin D, Paty E, Maccario J, Kauffmann F. Relationships of active and passive smoking to total IgE in adults of the Epidemiological Study of the Genetics and Environment of Asthma, Bronchial Hyperresponsiveness, and Atopy (EGEA). *Am J Respir Crit Care Med.* (2000) 161:1241–6. doi: 10.1164/ajrccm.161.4.9905027
78. Cockcroft DW. Environmental causes of asthma. *Semin Respir Crit Care Med.* (2018) 39:12–18. doi: 10.1055/s-0037-1606219
79. Bowatte G, Lodge CJ, Knibbs LD, Lowe AJ, Erbas B, Dennekamp M, et al. Traffic-related air pollution exposure is associated with allergic sensitization, asthma, and poor lung function in middle age. *J Allergy Clin Immunol.* (2017) 139:122–9. doi: 10.1016/j.jaci.2016.05.008
80. Bowatte G, Lodge C, Lowe AJ, Erbas B, Perret J, Abramson MJ, et al. The influence of childhood traffic-related air pollution exposure on asthma, allergy and sensitization: a systematic review and a meta-analysis of birth cohort studies. *Allergy* (2015) 70:245–56. doi: 10.1111/all.12561
81. Brandt EB, Biagini Myers JM, Acciani TH, Ryan PH, Sivaprasad U, Ruff B, et al. Exposure to allergen and diesel exhaustparticles potentiates secondary allergen-specific memory responses, promoting asthma susceptibility. *J Allergy Clin Immunol.* (2015) 136:295–303. doi: 10.1016/j.jaci.2014.11.043
82. Bunyavanich S, Rifas-Shiman SL, Platts-Mills TA, Workman L, Sordillo JE, Camargo CA Jr, et al. Peanut, milk, and wheat intake during pregnancy is associated with reduced allergy and asthma in children. *J Allergy Clin Immunol.* (2014) 133:1373–82. doi: 10.1016/j.jaci.2013.11.040
83. Best KP, Gold M, Kennedy D, Martin J, Makrides M. Omega-3 long-chain PUFA intake during pregnancy and allergic disease outcomes in the offspring: a systematic review and meta-analysis of observational studies and randomized controlled trials. *Am J Clin Nutr.* (2016) 103:128–43. doi: 10.3945/ajcn.115.111104
84. Chawes BL, Bonnelykke K, Stokholm J, Vissing NH, Bjarnadóttir E, Schoos AM, et al. Effect of vitamin D3 supplementation during pregnancy on risk of persistent wheeze in the offspring: a randomized clinical trial. *JAMA* (2016) 315:353–61. doi: 10.1001/jama.2015.18318
85. Chan-Yeung M, Becker A. Primary prevention of childhood asthma and allergic disorders. *Curr Opin Allergy Clin Immunol.* (2006) 6:146–51. doi: 10.1097/01.all.0000225150.91661.34
86. Forsberg A, West CE, Prescott SL, Jenmalm MC. Pre- and probiotics for allergy prevention: time to revisit recommendations? *Clin Exp Allergy* (2016) 46:1506–21. doi: 10.1111/cea.12838
87. Hawkes JS, Gibson RA, Roberton D, Makrides M. Effect of dietary nucleotide supplementation on growth and immune function in term infants: a randomized controlled trial. *Eur J Clin Nutr.* (2006) 60:254–64. doi: 10.1038/sj.ejcn.1602310
88. Burke H, Leonardi-Bee J, Hashim A, Pine-Abata H, Chen Y, Cook DG, et al. Prenatal and passive smoke exposure and incidence of asthma and wheeze: systematic review and meta-analysis. *Pediatrics* (2012) 129:735–44. doi: 10.1542/peds.2011-2196
89. Shaker M, Murray RGP, Mann JA. The ins and outs of an 'outside-in' view of allergies: atopic dermatitis and allergy prevention. *Curr Opin Pediatr.* (2018) 30:576–81. doi: 10.1097/MOP.0000000000000646
90. Bousquet J, Van Cauwenberge P, Khaltaev N, Aria Workshop Group, World Health Organization. Allergic rhinitis and its impact on asthma. *J Allergy Clin Immunol.* (2001) 108(Suppl. 5):S147–334. doi: 10.1067/mai.2001.118891
91. Bustos GJ, Bustos D, Bustos GJ, Romero O. Prevention of asthma with ketotifen in preasthmatic children: a three-year follow-up study. *Clin Exp Allergy* (1995) 25:568–73. doi: 10.1111/j.1365-2222.1995.tb01096.x
92. Crystal-Peters J, Neslusan C, Crown WH, Torres A. Treating allergic rhinitis in patients with comorbid asthma: the risk of asthma-related hospitalizations and emergency department visits. *J Allergy Clin Immunol.* (2002) 109:57–62. doi: 10.1067/mai.2002.120554
93. Lohia S, Schlosser RJ, Soler ZM. Impact of intranasal corticosteroids on asthma outcomes in allergic rhinitis: a meta-analysis. *Allergy* (2013) 68:569–79. doi: 10.1111/all.12124
94. Price DB, Swern A, Tozzi CA, Philip G, Polos P. Effect of montelukast on lung function in asthma patients with allergic rhinitis: analysis from the COMPACT trial. *Allergy* (2006) 61:737–42. doi: 10.1111/j.1398-9995.2006.01007.x
95. Humbert M, Boulet LP, Niven RM, Panahloo Z, Blogg M, Ayre G. Omalizumab therapy: patients who achieve greatest benefit for their asthma experience greatest benefit for rhinitis. *Allergy* (2009) 64:81–4. doi: 10.1111/j.1398-9995.2008.01846.x
96. GINA 217. Available online at: https://ginasthma.org/wp-content/uploads/2018/04/wms-GINA-2018-report-V1.3-002.pdf
97. Halken S, Larenas-Linnemann D, Roberts G, Calderón M, Angier E, Pfaar O, et al. EAACI Guidelines on Allergen Immunotherapy: Prevention of allergy. *Pediatr Allergy Immunol.* (2017) 28:728–45. doi: 10.1111/pai.12807
98. Kristiansen M, Dhami S, Netuveli G, Halken S, Muraro A, Roberts G, et al. Allergen immunotherapy for the prevention of allergy: a systematic review and meta-analysis. *Pediatr Allergy Immunol.* (2017) 28:18–29. doi: 10.1111/pai.12661
99. Nolte H, Hébert J, Berman G, Gawchik S, White M, Kaur A, et al. Randomized controlled trial of ragweed allergy immunotherapy tablet efficacy and safety in North American adults. *Ann Allergy Asthma Immunol.* (2013) 110:450–6. doi: 10.1016/j.anai.2013.03.013
100. Lombardi C, Canonica GW, Passalacqua G. Allergen immunotherapy as add-on to biologic agents. *Curr Opin Allergy Clin Immunol.* (2018) 18:502–8. doi: 10.1097/ACI.0000000000000479
101. Dantzer JA, Wood RA. The use of omalizumab in allergen immunotherapy. *Clin Exp Allergy* (2018) 48:232–40. doi: 10.1111/cea.13084
102. Emons JAM, Gerth van Wijk R. Food allergy and asthma: is there a link? *Curr Treat Options Allergy* (2018) 5:436–44. doi: 10.1007/s40521-018-0185-1
103. Nurmatov U, Dhami S, Arasi S, Pajno GB, Fernandez-Rivas M, Muraro A, et al. Allergen immunotherapy for IgE-mediated food allergy: a systematic review and meta-analysis. *Allergy* (2017) 72:1133–47. doi: 10.1111/all.13124
104. Arasi S, Mennini M, Valluzzi R, Riccardi C, Fiocchi A. Precision medicine in food allergy. *Curr Opin Allergy Clin Immunol.* (2018) 18:438–43. doi: 10.1097/ACI.0000000000000465
105. Wood RA, Kim JS, Lindblad R, Nadeau K, Henning AK, Dawson P, et al. A randomized, double-blind, placebo-controlled study of omalizumab combined with oral immunotherapy for the treatment of cow's milk allergy. *J Allergy Clin Immunol.* (2016) 137:1103–10. doi: 10.1016/j.jaci.2015.10.005
106. Lee RU, Stevenson DD. Aspirin-exacerbated respiratory disease: evaluation and management. *Allergy Asthma Immunol Res.* (2011) 3:3–10. doi: 10.4168/aair.2011.3.1.3
107. Cho K-S, Soudry E, Psaltis AJ, Nadeau KC, McGhee SA, Nayak JV, et al. Long-term sinonasal outcomes of aspirin desensitization in aspirin exacerbated

respiratory disease. *Otolaryngol Head Neck Surg.* (2014) 151:575–81. doi: 10.1177/0194599814545750
108. Tsetsos N, Goudakos JK, Daskalakis D, Konstantinidis I, Markou K. Monoclonal antibodies for the treatment of chronic rhinosinusitis with nasal polyposis: a systematic review. *Rhinology* (2018) 56:11–21. doi: 10.4193/Rhin17.156
109. Arasi S, Corsello G, Villani A, Pajno GB. The future outlook on allergen immunotherapy in children: 2018 and beyond. *Ital J Ped.* (2018) 44:80. doi: 10.1186/s13052-018-0519-4
110. Dhami S, Kakourou A, Asamoah F, Agache I, Lau S, Jutel M, et al. Allergen immunotherapy for allergic asthma: a systematic review and meta-analysis. *Allergy* (2017) 72:1825–48. doi: 10.1111/all.13208

4

Transition for Adolescents and Young Adults with Asthma

Adelaide LIndsay Withers [1*†] *and Ruth Green* [2†]

[1] *Department of Respiratory Medicine, Perth Children's Hospital, Perth, WA, Australia,* [2] *Glenfield Hospital, Leicester, United Kingdom*

Correspondence:
Adelaide LIndsay Withers
adelaide.withers@health.wa.gov.au

† *These authors have contributed equally to this work*

Asthma is a complex, heterogenous medical condition which is very common in children and adults. The transition process from pediatric to adult health care services can be a challenge for young people with chronic medical conditions. The significant changes in physical and mental health during this time, as well as the many unique developmental and psychosocial challenges that occur during adolescence can complicate and impede transition if not adequately addressed and managed. The transition period can also be a challenging time for health professionals to assess readiness for transition and manage some of the complications which are particularly common during this time, including poor adherence to therapy, smoking, drug use, and emerging mental health conditions. The natural history, presentation, symptoms, and management of asthma is often significantly different when comparing pediatric and adult practice. In addition, management in infants, toddlers, school aged children, and adolescents differs significantly, offering an additional challenge to pediatric physicians managing asthmatic children and young people. Despite these challenges, if the transition process for young people with asthma is planned and performed in a formalized manner, many of these issues can be addressed, allowing the transition to occur smoothly despite changes that may occur in medical and psychosocial domains.

Keywords: asthma, transition, transition process, asthma phenotype, asthma management, adolescent, young adult

INTRODUCTION

Transition is "the purposeful, planned movement of adolescents and young adults with chronic physical and medical conditions from child-centered care to adult-oriented health care systems" (1). In 1993 the Society for Adolescent Medicine published standards of care for transition, the goals being to provide a transition process that was coordinated, uninterrupted, psychosocially sound, developmentally appropriate, and comprehensive (1). In 2011 the American Academy of Pediatrics (AAP) with endorsement of the American Academy of Family Physicians (AAFP) and American College of Physician (ACP) published a clinical report that described preparation for transition, the process of transition and tracking of transition as well as appropriate follow up post transition (2). This document was updated in 2018 (3, 4). The purpose of these documents was to highlight the importance of planning for transition and to provide a framework or model for transitioning adolescent and young adult patients from pediatric to adult care in a standardized and effective manner.

Asthma is the most common chronic medical condition in children, affecting over 7 billion children in the United States of America (5) and about 300 million people worldwide (6). Although the underlying pathology (reversible obstruction of the small airways) is similar in asthma at any age, there can be marked differences in presentation, triggers, phenotype and treatment when considering asthma in children, adolescents and adults. The changes that occur in an individual during adolescence include physical, emotional, and psycho-social. The influence these changes exert upon pathophysiology, presentation, prognosis, and treatment of asthma must be carefully considered during the transition from pediatric to adult health care. For example, poor adherence to treatment is very common during adolescence as there is increasing independence and individuation, as a consequence more frequent asthma exacerbations may occur. Therefore, transitioning patients with asthma must be a carefully planned process, with consideration of the significant changes in all domains of a young person's life and the effects these changes exert upon their asthma.

NATURAL HISTORY OF ASTHMA

Patterns of wheezing are often quite variable in childhood in contrast to adults where there tends to be more stability in type, frequency and triggers of exacerbations. Viral induced wheeze is extremely common in the first year of life due to small airway caliber and the presence of multiple episodes of viral induced wheeze is not necessarily an indicator of future asthma (6). It is known that wheezing in the first year of life, even if episodes are severe, does not always predict persistence of wheezing at 10 years of age (7). Toddlers and pre-schoolers who wheeze tend to either have episodic viral induced wheeze or multiple trigger wheeze (commonly associated with personal and/or family history of atopy) (8). Viral induced wheeze (and asthma) tend to improve with age and increase in size of airway caliber, however young children who wheeze with atopy and/or a family history of asthma are at risk of persistent wheeze later in childhood (6, 9–11). The Tucson Children's Respiratory Study demonstrated that persistent wheezing in childhood is likely to persist at least to early adulthood (12). Despite asthma in children being strongly linked to atopy, the association between atopy and asthma extends beyond childhood, as atopic individuals without wheeze and/or airway hyperresponsiveness at 12 years of age can still develop asthma as adults (13).

Adolescence is a time where asthma may change significantly. Studies that have followed adolescents in a longitudinal fashion until adulthood have focused on asthma remission, persistence, relapse and new onset adult asthma (6). Although cross sectional studies have demonstrated that significant changes occur in the asthmatic population in adolescents, individual factors that influence prognosis have not been identified (14). Longitudinal studies of adolescents and young adults have demonstrated that bronchial hyperreactivity as a child is a strong predictor of persistence of asthma in adult life (15–18), however these studies have not allowed description of an accurate asthma "phenotype" in adolescents and young adults (14). Interestingly, the higher incidence of asthma in boys compared to girls tends to reverse after adolescence with asthma becoming more common in women than men (11, 14, 19, 20). This may be related to male sex being a risk factor for late onset atopy and female sex a risk factor for later onset bronchial hyperreactivity (14). However, as Xuan et al. (13) point out, this observation could be also caused by a higher rate of onset of asthma in puberty in females or a lower remission rate of asthma in females after puberty. It may also reflect better response to treatment in childhood in males with increased likelihood of resolution (6).

Remission of asthma can occur during adolescence (14, 21–23), with some reporting that "most" children have remission in adolescence and early adulthood (6, 24, 25). To the contrary, Xuan et al. (13) demonstrated in their longitudinal cohort of young adults recruited at ages 8–10 that onset of wheeze during follow up was more common than remission (12.4 vs. 5.6%) and the prevalence of wheeze increased by 6% in a 10 year follow-up period. Importantly, even if asthma truly remits, it is not known if remission of symptoms is the same as resolution of underlying airway pathology (6). The observations of a longitudinal Dutch cohort suggest that underlying airway pathology does not resolve despite remission of symptoms, as asymptomatic patients still had abnormal lung function and/or persisting airway hyperresponsiveness (26).

Between 3–5% of people who wheeze in childhood continue to wheeze as adults (6, 24). As demonstrated by the Tucson Children's Respiratory Study, persistent wheezing in childhood is likely to persist into early adulthood, with airway hyperresponsiveness at 6 years of age predicting the presence of asthma at 22 years (11). Other groups have demonstrated that persistent asthma in adulthood was associated with lower lung function in childhood, persistence of airway hyperresponsiveness, atopy by the age of 13 and early smoking as a young adult (27–29). In severe asthmatic adults, 69% reported asthma symptoms were present before the age of 20 years (8).

Asthma which has resolved in childhood may relapse later in life, even if asymptomatic as adolescents or young adults (6, 24, 27, 30). Relapse of symptoms in adulthood was associated with smoking (particularly in those who were not atopic), asymptomatic airway hyperresponsiveness at 13 years of age and atopy (24, 27).

Knowledge regarding asthma with the onset in adolescence or young adulthood is limited (13). Although new onset bronchial hyperresponsiveness is unusual in adolescence, the appearance of asthma in previous well adolescents and young adults is described (13). Adult onset asthma generally has a poorer prognosis and poorer response to treatment when compared to childhood onset asthma. In a longitudinal cohort study of young adults with asthma, of those who wheezed at any time, 7.8% had developed airway hyperresponsiveness after the age of 8–12 years (13). Atopy at ages 8–12 and parental history of asthma were also predictors of late onset wheeze and female sex a predictor of late onset airway hyperresponsiveness (13). However, it has been postulated that recall of childhood symptoms as an adult may be poor, and that adult onset asthma may actually represent a relapse rather than true adult onset of asthma (6). This is supported by the findings of the Tucson Children's Respiratory Study, where 63% of participants reporting "new" symptoms as adults had already reported symptoms as children (11). The effect of cigarette smoking must also be taken into account for adults with the onset of asthma (6). In addition, new onset adult asthma may be a different phenotype as individuals are more likely to be female, obese, non-atopic and smokers (31–33).

PEDIATRIC, ADOLESCENT, AND ADULT ASTHMA—DIFFERENCES AND SIMILARITIES

Marked differences exist when comparing asthma in children, adolescents and adults. Even when considering children with asthma as a group, significant heterogeneity exists when comparing toddlers, school aged children and teenagers. To further complicate matters, asthma during the adolescent and young adult period has unique features and from an epidemiological perspective, the transition period from childhood asthma to young adult asthma is poorly understood (14). For these reasons, asthma is best thought of as a heterogenous, complex syndrome rather than a single disease (6, 34).

Phenotyping is not commonly applied to pediatric asthma as it does not tend to be particularly useful, in contrast to adult asthma (8, 35). Phenotypes can be defined in various ways, such as disease severity, presence of atopy or inflammation, temporal patterns of symptoms, response to treatments or triggers (6). When phenotypes are applied to children with wheeze and/or asthma, children frequent move between groups when they are young (34), making phenotypes less useful for prognostication. This is not surprising given the variability in the natural history, persistence and remission/relapse of asthma during childhood and adolescence. In addition, phenotyping in adults often relies on biomaterials sampled from the lower airways, which is often not available in children (6). Phenotyping by atopic status is not useful in preschool children as presence of atopy is often unclear, there is poor correlation between atopy and wheeze in this age group and atopy does not predict response to inhaled steroids (8). When considering severe asthma, older children with severe asthma tend to be male, highly atopic and are usually not completely steroid responsive which is in contrast to severe adult asthmatics who tend to be females, atopy is less common and neutrophilic inflammation is common (8).

It is known that asthma in early life is a risk factor for asthma and COPD in later life (27, 36–38). Although children who wheeze in early infancy often don't go on to develop asthma in childhood, they too have been shown to be at risk of developing COPD in adult life (6).

Therefore, it is difficult to say how similar pediatric and adult asthma are overall, given the complexities of early wheeze phenotypes, but the demonstration that many children with severe asthma continue to have severe asthma as adults (8, 11, 39) suggests that *severe asthma* may be similar in these different age groups. Prevalence of severe asthma in childhood ranges widely depending on location from 2.1% (40) of children in Sweden with asthma to 5% (41) in the U.S.A, 8.8% in Spain (42) and 36% in Canada (43). Therefore, given the heterogeneity in early viral induced wheeze and preschool wheeze, the authors estimate that approximately 10% of cases with adult asthma and childhood asthma have the same condition.

GENERAL CONSIDERATIONS FOR ADOLESCENT AND YOUNG ADULT HEALTH CARE

Some general considerations when seeing adolescent and young adult patients with medical conditions include seeing adolescents without their parents, increasing autonomy, confidentiality, consent, puberty/contraception/sexual health, poor adherence to medical treatment, mental health concerns, substance use and screening for risk taking behaviors (44). It is important to note that the following considerations not only apply in the pediatric health care system, but after transition to adult services. In addition, addressing these issues may prove very useful for adult physicians to help in building rapport, particularly during the first few appointments with a new patient who has just transitioned to adult services. Following the same principles of age and developmentally appropriate adolescent and young adult health care in adult services ensures continuity of care standards and demonstrates the commitment of the adult health professionals to providing individualized care that is tailored to age and maturity of the young adult.

As a pediatric patient enters adolescence, ideally at least some of the consultation should occur with the patient on their own (44). As adult patients will often be seen on their own, it is good to prepare young people to be able to provide relevant history and information for their appointment. This can be particularly challenging for pediatric physicians when they have known the patient since infancy, and are used to taking the majority of history from the parents (44). This concept can also prove very challenging to parents. Parents may worry their concerns won't be voiced by their child, that "secrets" may be withheld from them or that their child is unable to take responsibility for their own health care. Parents should be reassured that this is a normal, routine part of health care for all young people, and an excellent way to start preparing for future transition. Young people with cystic fibrosis have indicated that they wish to be seen at least partly on their own between the ages of 13–16 as they have private issues they wish to discuss with their doctor (45). Of concern, some young people indicated they were never offered the opportunity to be seen on their own (45). Gently introducing the idea of being seen alone for part of the consultation around the age of 12–13 is useful, with the parent present initially to provide any additional information about the medical concerns (while encouraging the adolescent to answer the questions), then some time with the adolescent alone to build rapport (44). After a rapport is built and confidentiality is discussed, screening for adolescent issues can occur at subsequent appointments. Explaining to the young person that seeing them alone is important as there may be health concerns they may not want to discuss with their parents present, and normalizing the process as part of becoming independent and assuming responsibility for their own health care (44). Discussing confidentiality is imperative so that parents and patients are aware of this concept and exceptions to confidentiality (discussed below).

Confidentiality is of the utmost importance when seeing an adolescent or young adult patient alone, and it must be clear that they understand the exceptions to confidentiality (if someone is hurting them, they are in danger of hurting themselves or hurting someone else) (44). It is also helpful to explain that sometimes health information will need to be shared with other members of the medical team, but that this would only happen with permission from the adolescent. It is particularly important to discuss confidentiality prior to undertaking an adolescent health screen, as information may be disclosed which would require a breach of confidentiality (for example, disclosure of sexual abuse or suicidal ideation). The need to disclose this information and break confidentiality can be extremely damaging to the therapeutic relationship if the young person feels they have been betrayed or punished for disclosing this information. Clear discussion of the limits of confidentiality is therefore essential in maintaining the therapeutic relationship.

Providing consent for medical procedures will vary based on local laws. Under common law in Australia and the UK, adolescents under the age of 16 can provide informed consent without parental knowledge if they are deemed by the treating doctor to have sufficient understanding of the proposed treatment, consequences of accepting or rejecting treatment and alternative options (44). The gravity of the situation must be considered; as clearly there is a significant difference between a 14-year-old providing consent for antibiotics for a skin infection vs. providing consent for a chemotherapy. If there is any doubt seeking legal advice and advice from an ethics committee is advisable, particularly when there may be child protection concerns, questions about capacity of an adolescent to provide valid consent in the context of intellectual disability, mental health concerns, suicidal ideation or disagreement between the adolescent and their parents/legal guardian. In addition, clear documentation of conversations and decisions about providing consent, the adolescent's understanding of risks and benefits of treatment etc. must be recorded in the medical notes.

Adolescent health screening is not only an important part of providing age appropriate medical care but can assist in establishing a rapport with a young person. This is particularly important when an adult physician is meeting an adolescent patient for the first time, as it helps to establish who the young person is, their interests, their family and living situation and any health risk factors that may be present. Given the very personal nature of some of the questions, it is best to start with topics such as whom they live with before moving to topics such as drug use and sexuality. This may need to occur over a number of visits, particularly when meeting a young person for the first time. This process is often straightforward for pediatric physicians as they will usually know the adolescent quite well, but paradoxically it can complicate health screening as young people may be more reluctant to disclose risk taking behaviors to a doctor they know well for fear of disappointing their doctor or fear of their parents being informed. Often honest responses are obtained by normalizing the process ("we ask everyone your age these questions") and normalizing their situation ("lots of people your age drink alcohol, do your friends drink? What about you?"). A useful acronym to perform an adolescent health screen is HEARDDSS (home environment, education, activities they participate in, relationships with friends, family and opposite/same sex, drug use including smoking, alcohol and illicit drugs, depression, sexuality and suicide risk/risk taking behaviors) (44).

Generally by the time transition is occurring, adolescents will have completed growth and puberty but this is not always the case in chronic medical conditions. It is important to be sensitive as pubertal delay and short stature can be extremely distressing to young people, particularly if they look noticeably different and younger than their peers. Regular assessment of height and weight at each visit is essential and monitoring pubertal status with Tanner staging on a growth chart is most easily done by getting the adolescent to self-identify the picture that looks most like them. If significant pubertal delay and/or short stature are evident, assessment of bone age should be performed as well as screening for other medical causes of pubertal delay/short stature such as coeliac disease and thyroid dysfunction. Referral to an endocrinologist should be considered, particularly for those on high dose inhaled or oral steroids or complex medical conditions, as augmentation of puberty and/or Growth Hormone may be considered.

Following on from this, contraceptive needs should always be addressed, particularly when pregnancy may have an adverse effect on the underlying medical condition (for example cystic fibrosis and Type 1 Diabetes). Discussion about planning for future pregnancies, impact of pregnancy on the medical condition and potential side effects/contraindications of various methods of contraception should be discussed from early puberty. Consideration should be given to offering genetic counseling in inherited diseases when adolescents are in established puberty, and "safer sex" should always be encouraged to minimize risk of unwanted pregnancy and sexually transmitted diseases.

Adolescence is naturally a time of testing limits and boundaries, and often risk taking behavior such as experimentation with smoking and drug/alcohol use occurs (44). There is conflicting evidence regarding whether young people with chronic medical conditions are more or less likely than their peers to smoke or use drugs/alcohol (46, 47). Smoking can be particularly difficult to address, as adolescents will often want to experiment with their peers to fit in and minimize differences between themselves and their "well" peers. As adolescents often do not have the cognitive capacity to understand future consequences as a result of their current actions, explaining how smoking reduces lung function in the long term is unlikely to be successful in dissuading them not to smoke. Immediate consequences, particularly when related to appearance (such as yellow nails and teeth from smoking or missing out on a party as they require admission) may act as a deterrent to smoking (44).

Depression and anxiety can emerge or worsen in adolescence, particularly when there is a chronic medical condition. Mental health problems can have a negative effect on health outcomes, health related quality of life and adherence to treatment (44).

Depression is common in adolescents, with the incidence of major depression estimated between 3 and 5% (48, 49), unsurprisingly with a higher incidence (up to three times) in adolescents with a chronic medical condition (48–51). Chronic medical conditions are also known to increase the risk of suicide attempts, particularly in females (52, 53). It is important to screen for and refer on to appropriate services if there are concerns about emerging depression, anxiety or suicidal ideation, and recognize how these conditions can affect medical outcomes and adherence to treatment.

Adherence to medical treatment can be particularly challenging in the adolescent period for a number of reasons. Mean adherence rates for long term treatments in adolescents with a chronic medical condition are reported between 33 and 94% (44). Adherence is known to decrease in adolescence in those with chronic medical conditions (54, 55). Adolescents naturally test limits and boundaries and wish to become independent. Often part of developing autonomy includes adolescents not wishing to be "told" what to do, and this includes taking medications, doing airway clearance, physiotherapy and attending appointments. Barriers to adherence include a wish to rebel, lack of time, school commitments, not wanting to seem different to peers, forgetting, disagreement with the physician and feeling that treatments don't work. Non-adherence to treatment can impede transition, and occasionally a young person will purposefully stop taking their treatment to delay transition (unfortunately this may have the opposite effect and the pediatric team may transition out of sheer frustration) (44, 56). Pediatric physicians may also wish to delay transition as they do not feel confident the young person is adherent enough to manage their medical condition in the adult system. Non-adherence is best addressed with patience and over time, exploring in a sensitive and non-judgemental manner the barriers to adherence. Again, it can be helpful to normalize that non-adherence is common, trying to solve the problem together by offering choices, acknowledging the treatment burden and minimizing unnecessary or duplications of treatments. Focusing on the "most important" treatment can be helpful, as well as setting review dates for treatment and setting realistic goals. In some situations, the only way forward is to continue to reassure the young person that you will continue to see them and stick with them throughout the process regardless of whether they are adherent or not. Outlining issues with adherence with the adult team is crucial so that continuity of care after transition can be assured and that patients do not "fall through the gaps" if they fail to attend future appointments with adult services. This can become a particular problem as the pediatric health care system is often more accommodating when it comes to poor attendance, whereas adult services simply may not have the capacity to repeatedly book non-attenders.

MODELS OF TRANSITION

Although many different models for transition have been proposed, the Society for Adolescent Medicine position statement highlights the lack of published research comparing the different models of transition, in particular whether certain models performed better for specific medical conditions/illness severity or even if a formalized transition program actually improved health care outcomes (1). A review by Wright et al. (57) as well as the AAP report also highlighted the paucity of randomized control trials comparing different models of transition, as the majority of transition related research comprises interventional studies. Despite the existence of numerous models for transition, many share the core components of being well-prepared, starting transition early, familiarization with the adult health care system prior to transition and use of joint pediatric/adult clinics. Models draw on frameworks, concepts, and core components such as the AAP transition theory framework core principles of (3);

1. Importance of transition being youth focused
2. Emphasis on self-determination, self-management and family/caregiver engagement
3. Acknowledging individual difficulties and complexities
4. Recognizing vulnerabilities and the need for a population health approach
5. Importance of shared accountability and care co-ordination between pediatric and adult centers
6. Recognition of the influence of cultural beliefs, attitudes and socio-economic status
7. Emphasis on achieving health equality, eliminating disparities
8. Parents/caregivers to support young people to develop health knowledge and skills.

The Six Core Elements of Transition 2.0 are elements of a transition that must be present for it to be considered successful (4, 57, 58). These core elements are establishing a transition policy, tracking the transition process, administering transition readiness tools/checklists, planning for, transfer to and integration into adult care (58).

Combinations of these components appear in various forms in the majority of the proposed models for transition. Published models exist for transition in primary care/general pediatric care (for example the Medicaid Managed Care Plan and Health Practice Transformation Model) and for mental health care (European Union-Funded Transition Project) (57). Other models have been published for specific medical conditions, such as sickle cell anemia, renal transplant recipients and type 1 diabetes (57). Again, although the models are different, they all incorporate various aspects of the Six Core Elements of Transition 2.0 and include clinic based transition models, multi-disciplinary team models, transition co-ordinator models, patient developed transition curriculum and web based/mobile health interventions (57). Readers are directed to the excellent and comprehensive review by Wright et al. (57) for discussion and critical evaluation of the various models.

In 2016 a Cochrane review of intervention studies for transition models only included 4 small studies ($n = 261$ patients) and was unable to make conclusions regarding the effectiveness of various models in managing the chronic medical conditions during the transition process, healthcare outcomes or healthcare utilization (59). However, the review by Wright et al. (57) highlights the importance of a nominated individual to act as the "transition co-ordinator" and facilitate the process as a common component of the models that were felt to be the most effective in their review. Although lack of provision of extra staffing and financial incentives for providing transition services has been identified as a barrier to implementing and sustaining transition programs, many of these effective models were able to perform effectively without extra staff or financial incentives (57).

In addition, the needs of a health care service (specifically education and resources) to provide an effective transition program need to be considered prior to choosing and implementing a transition model, based on the suitability of that particular model within the constraints of the health care system.

There are many considerations when choosing a model to use when implementing a transition program, and this highlights the importance of critical evaluation of transition models when determining effectiveness. The lack of published evidence comparing different models, particularly interventional studies, is a barrier to successful implementation of transition models and highlights the need for more research in this area.

GENERAL CONSIDERATIONS FOR TRANSITION

Table 1 for a summary of issues to be considered during transition. The general focus of pediatric health care can be very different to adult health care. Whereas, pediatric health care tends to be developmentally focused and family centered, development, growth, and family concerns are not commonly primary concerns for adult physicians (56). However, adult health care places an emphasis on autonomy, employment and reproductive health, which are often ignored in pediatric medicine, particularly as pediatricians may struggle with their patient's increased independence, autonomy and "adult" behaviors (56). This struggle of balancing the adolescent's need for increasing autonomy and individuation with the need for adherence to treatment is a struggle not only for pediatricians but parents. Transition can be complicated by a chronic illness as it can be difficult for parents to "let go" and allow the young person to assume primary responsibility for their medical treatment and develop their independence but at the same time ensure adherence to treatment remains optimal and medical management is continued. This struggle is often unconsciously reinforced by the pediatric health care system, which encourages family centered care and is at risk of "infantilising" the young adult (44). This can impede the transition process, particularly as it has been demonstrated that pediatric physicians are often reluctant to "let go" of their patients, and may consciously or unconsciously reinforce the idea that the adult health care system is a frightening environment (44). On the contrary, adult physicians may find it difficult to act in a manner they deem paternalistic when a young adult has not gained the necessary independence to demonstrate autonomy with their medical care, or feel frustrated with receiving patients whom they feel were "mollycoddled" or "treated as babies" by the pediatric system.

Barriers within the healthcare system to implementing a sustainable transition process include lack of infrastructure for co-ordination (particularly at adult healthcare sites), lack of financial reward with increased workload to implement programs and lack of electronic or shareable medical records (58). The difficult with multiple interfaces for entering and storing healthcare information can present a particular challenge, as it can significantly impede communication between pediatric and adult sites. It is useful to have a standard format for transition documents to be prepared by the pediatric service. If regular transitions are occurring to the same adult service, involving the adult physicians in designing a template for exactly which information they need and which formats will be compatible with their record system will reduce the risk of poor handover or loss of medical records.

Engagement of adult physicians in the transition process is essential to ensuring a successful transition, but can present a significant barrier (3). Adult physicians may require a significant amount of education regarding medical conditions that were traditionally considered "pediatric" diseases, with children not surviving to adolescence or adulthood, such as metabolic disorders, cystic fibrosis and congenital heart disease. Adult physicians may understandably feel overwhelmed at providing care to these very complex patients when they may not be familiar with their underlying medical condition, let alone the numerous challenges individuals with these conditions may face in young adulthood. Similarly, a unique challenge exists when there are no equivalent adult services for specific pediatric conditions, particularly those with inborn errors of metabolism, complex neuro-behavioral disorders, cerebral palsy and developmental disorders.

Although some adolescents wish to transition early as they find attending a pediatric center embarrassing, many find transition to be a distressing time due to loss of familiarity, particularly those who have been seen at the same center by the same team for many years. Preparation for transition to adult services should start early and young people and their families should be well-informed of the proposed timeline for the process. The age of transition varies between centers and should be individualized to the young person, however, generally will take place between the ages of 16–18, or when completing secondary education. This is a time of great change in all domains of a young person's life (44). Therefore, a transition checklist is very useful, ensuring all aspects of the transition have been covered (which may include a physical visit to the new site, ensuring the process for obtaining prescriptions is known, how to get to the new appointment and how to seek medical review or emergency review). Particularly for complex patients who require tertiary level care or a dedicated team, having prior appointments with the adult team or even joint appointments prior to transition can be extremely useful to familiarize the young person and their family with the new team and facilities. Young people have reported a tour of the adult facility, joint sessions and a familiar face from the pediatric team joining the first adult appointment are very reassuring (60).

Guidelines and standards for the transition process have been published for a wide range of medical conditions, including diabetes (61), congenital heart disease (62), and cystic fibrosis (63). The transition from being a dependent child to an

TABLE 1 | Considerations for transition.

Considerations for transition	Pediatric perspective	Adult perspective	Organizational perspective
Preparation for transition (young person and their family)	Start transition process early Normalize the transition process Joint clinics Regular assessment of readiness for transition See the young person on their own Encourage their independence and assuming responsibility for healthcare	Meet the young person prior to formal transition Normalize the transition process Joint clinics Adolescent health screen to build rapport Organize tour of adult site	Encourage joint clinics Consider formalized transition pathway/process Appoint a specific transition co-ordinator Facilitate visit to adult site
Poor adherence to treatment	Open and honest discussion about barriers to poor adherence Problem solving with the young adult Focus on immediate consequences, personal appearance Screening for depression	Open and honest discussion about barriers to poor adherence Problem solving with the young adult Focus on immediate consequences, personal appearance Screening for depression	Consider formalized transition pathway/process Appoint a specific transition co-ordinator
Avoiding being lost to follow-up	Ensure formal transition to adult team with letters and good communication Consider booking a final appointment/phone consult after seeing adult team to ensure everything is in place	Ensure clear communication with pediatric team as to when adult team will be taking over Ensure adult team knows contact details for young person and correct address to send appointment to Consider a written handout about arranging appointments or urgent review	Establish a "safety net"—transition co-ordinator or respiratory nurse to ensure follow-up has occurred
Clinical deterioration during transition process	Ensure follow-up with adult team occurs Address poor adherence as much as possible Delay transition if a major change in clinical status occurs Flag young people with complex issues to inform adult team May require several joint appointments Ensure verbal and written handover for all medical and allied health services Assess medical knowledge and understanding for the young person prior to transition	Close liaison with pediatric team to cover all outstanding issues Be prepared to attend more than one joint appointment	Have a "Transition Checklist" to ensure nothing is missed

independent adult is not always smooth, and becomes more complex when there is a chronic medical condition (44). The transition process must be well-planned and must not be rushed, and careful consideration of adolescent issues as well as medical issues must be addressed prior to handing over medical care to an adult physician (56, 64, 65). As well as managing general adolescent issues, transitioning a young person with asthma (particularly severe or poorly controlled asthma) offers some unique challenges. Specific considerations for transitioning the asthmatic patient with to adult heath care services is discussed in more detail below.

SPECIFIC CONSIDERATIONS FOR TRANSITIONING PATIENTS WITH ASTHMA

There is very little published literature specifically examining the transition process in adolescents and young adults with asthma (66). This is surprising given asthma is the most common chronic medical condition in children (5), and highlights the need for further research to determine optimal care for adolescents transition with asthma. For the majority of young people and adolescents with well-controlled asthma, transitioning to adult services is unlikely to be a difficult process. Indeed those already being managed very well in general practice/primary practice do not require transition at all as they can remain with their primary care provider, ensuring excellent continuity. If there is any concern about deterioration of asthma control in young adulthood, an opinion from an adult respiratory specialist could be sought, while the general practitioner maintains primary management with specialist reviews as required.

Those well-managed by general pediatricians are likely to be able to transition to ongoing care in general practice, and liaison with a suitable general practitioner should be encouraged early on to ensure they are comfortable with the transition plan. A study of the transition process for adolescents with asthma at a children's hospital asthma/allergy clinic found that young people with mild/moderate asthma were managed equally effectively regardless of whether they transitioned to primary or specialist care (66). All patients in this study with severe asthma were transitioned to specialist adult asthma services (66). It is important that adolescents with asthma do have ongoing follow-up, even if their asthma is mild, as childhood asthma is a risk factor for developing chronic obstructive pulmonary disease

(COPD) in later life (27, 36, 37). In addition, asthma can recur in adult life despite remission as a teenager (30).

Adolescents who require tertiary level care are more likely to have difficult to control or severe asthma and may have other considerations which complicate the transition process (particularly poor adherence to treatment, exposure to cigarette smoke, mental health concerns or additional medical conditions). These complicating factors are common in asthmatic adolescents. For example, in a study of adolescents with asthma, 25% were reported to be poorly adherent to treatment (66). Of particular concern is adolescents with asthma who smoke or are exposed to passive smoke from peers. A study of Swedish adolescents with asthma found that 8% reported being smokers and 28% were exposed to passive smoke at home or by their peers (66). The incidence of depression in individuals with asthma is higher than the general population and depression in asthmatics may be more common than in other chronic medical conditions (67). In addition, depression may increase morbidity and mortality associated with asthma (67). These concerns that may complicate transition should be identified and managed if possible prior to transition and handed over to the adult team for ongoing management.

The vast majority of adolescents requiring tertiary level care for their asthma would be expected to require tertiary level respiratory care as an adult, especially those requiring frequent hospital and/or intensive care admissions. This is reinforced in the study above, where all adolescents with severe asthma required transition to specialist adult respiratory services (66). If a tertiary adult respiratory service is not available, an adult respiratory physician with an interest in asthma could be considered to take over ongoing care. In more remote locations visiting respiratory services may be available, with a local doctor taking primary responsibility for ongoing care. Young people who are likely to require ongoing hospital admissions for exacerbations of asthma should be referred to a service that is able to manage emergency presentations, admissions and provide frequent review. In these cases, a suitable service with experience in managing difficult asthma should be identified early on and liaison should occur prior to transition, particularly if there is the possibility of a joint appointment or meeting the adult team prior to transition. Development of a specific center-based transition pathway for adolescents with difficult or severe asthma is encouraged to formalize the process and ensure nothing is missed.

Adolescent and young adult patients with frequent asthma exacerbations requiring presentation and management in emergency departments present additional challenges during the transition period. A review of care transition within the emergency department back to primary care identified that those who presented to ED often received improper management of exacerbations at home, and families required education and support to transition safely back to primary care (5). Although these findings are presented in the context of the emergency department, they highlight the need for excellent communication, care coordination and patient education to ensure a successful transition, regardless of the health care providers involved. It also highlights the need to specifically consider the high care needs of asthmatic patients who are frequent presenters at emergency services, and the value of involving the emergency department in planning for transition and ensuring access to adult emergency services as part of preparing for the transition process.

A common concern in chronic medical conditions is deterioration of stability during the transition process and loss to follow-up by adult services (44). This may delay the transition process, particularly if the pediatric service is not confident the young adult has acquired the skills to manage their medical condition or seek help appropriately if unwell. Bergstrom et al. (66) studied 150 adolescents with asthma during the transition process to identify risk factors for deterioration of asthma control during and after transition. They found that it was rare for pulmonary function to deteriorate during and up to 5 years post transition (66). In addition, the majority of those with reduced FEV1 at the time of transition had improved pulmonary function at follow-up (66) which is encouraging. Poor adherence to medical treatment and female gender predicted persisting bronchial hyper responsiveness and chronic symptoms (66), therefore this groups of patients may require more frequent monitoring during and post transition.

Untreated or poorly controlled asthma can be associated with pubertal delay (68–71), and the associated emotional distress secondary to pubertal delay can contribute to poorer asthma control and poor adherence to treatment (68). This is particularly the case as there is some evidence inhaled corticosteroids may contribute to pubertal delay (69) hence adolescent patients may be reluctant to use them. However, untreated or poorly treated asthma delays puberty on average by 1.3 years (71) and discussing this information may encourage adherence to treatment. Many young people with asthma are concerned about short stature and may attribute this to chronic use of inhaled corticosteroids, however in severe or poorly controlled asthma pubertal delay itself is more likely to explain the apparent growth failure rather than suppression from corticosteroids (71). Reassurance that treating asthma and better adherence to treatment may improve the pubertal delay and short stature may assist in encouraging adherence to treatment. Pubertal status and stature should be monitored closely in all adolescent patients with asthma, particularly those on high dose inhaled corticosteroids or oral steroids.

Prior to transition, contraception and sexual history should always be discussed. Although the majority of detailed discussion will be with female patients, sexual history should also be discussed with males and an open discussion about which form of contraception they use is encouraged. When choosing contraception to avoid unwanted pregnancy in asthmatic adolescents, a number of considerations are necessary. Firstly, barrier contraception is the only method offering any protection against sexually transmitted diseases, and barrier contraceptives should be used in combination with a more effective form of contraception for avoiding pregnancy. Second, if adherence to treatment is a challenge, a reliable form of contraception that doesn't rely on remembering to take medication should be chosen, such as a hormonal implant or intra-uterine device. In particular the Progesterone Only Pill should be avoided as efficacy is dependent upon taking it regularly and at the same time each day. Thirdly, contraception should be encouraged, particularly in severe asthmatics, as asthma exacerbations during pregnancy have been shown to be associated with low birthweight babies (72) and oral contraception use in pregnancy has been shown to reduce the risk of asthma exacerbations (73). Although preconception and obstetric care of the asthmatic women is beyond the scope of this article, readers are directed to resources such as the Australian Asthma Handbook section on pregnancy and preconception considerations (74) (available from http://www.asthmahandbook.org.au). Although there appears to be a significant association between maternal ingestion of Paracetamol during pregnancy and subsequent risk of asthma in offspring (75), non-causal explanations have not been able to be excluded (76), and a significant number of confounders exist, particularly family history of asthma and atopy. The large Norwegian Mother and Child Cohort Study found that prenatal exposure to Paracetamol was associated with a small increase (13%) in the risk of developing asthma when accounting for confounders (77). Given infants of asthmatic mothers will already be at a higher risk of developing asthma given family history of asthma and/or atopy, it may be prudent to advise adolescent and young adult women of childbearing age to avoid Paracetamol while pregnant or planning a pregnancy.

Financial concerns after transition are more likely to be a concern for young adults, as adolescents will often live in the family home. Scal et al. (78) found that adolescents with asthma were more likely to have a usual care provider and private health insurance than young adults with asthma, with young adults facing increased financial barriers to accessing health care after transition. Of concern, these young adults reported more unmet health care needs and delays in receiving health care due to financial constraints (78). Other barriers to accessing appropriate health care for asthma in both adolescents undergoing transition and young adults post transition were difficulties with transportation, frustration at long wait times at physician offices, difficulties arranging appointments (especially by telephone) and inconvenient physician office hours (78). Addressing these concerns may require social work involvement and provision of financial assistance to ensure continued access to health care post transition.

Gibson-Scipio et al. (79) highlighted the additional challenges for young adults with asthma who are transitioning and are not Caucasian. For example, it is known that asthma morbidity and mortality rates are higher in those individuals who are not Caucasian (80). In addition, African American youth are less likely to discuss transition or engage in the transition process than Caucasian youth (81). In their study, Gibson-Scipio et al. (79) found that African American youth with asthma often did not use preventer medications and lacked understanding of the inflammatory nature of asthma that required preventer medication even when symptoms were well-controlled. Nearly half expressed that they didn't want to inform their peers of their medical condition as it was a sign of "weakness" and most felt routine visits for asthma were unnecessary (79). Although these concerns are unlikely to be limited to adolescents who are not Caucasian, it raises the importance of ensuring transition is well-planned and there is a good understanding of the medical condition, particularly in those groups with a higher risk of morbidity and poor ongoing engagement.

The importance of health education and assessing understanding of the underlying medical condition cannot be overstated, particularly when preparing for transition. Although this is important for all patients with asthma, it is particularly important in non-Caucasian adolescents who are at higher risk of poorer health outcomes and poor understanding of the their asthma and treatments (79, 82). Holley et al. (83) demonstrated that understanding of the medical condition and treatments was essential for allowing adolescents to develop self-management skills and improve adherence to treatment. Lack of knowledge about asthma was identified by adolescents as a significant barrier to adherence to treatment (83). Particularly important focuses for education were triggers, how to recognize symptoms indicating an exacerbation and the seriousness of asthma (83). Other groups describe the importance of educating about treatments, how they work and why to use them as key to encouraging self-management of asthma by adolescent patients (83–85). Correct inhaler technique is essential, particularly as few children use their inhalers in the correct way (86). Volerman et al. (86) highlight the need for careful assessment and direct observation of inhaler technique, given parents and children will over-estimate their skills in delivering inhaled medications effectively. If poor inhaler technique can be corrected prior to transition, it may contribute to better inhaler technique in adult patients, as up to 90% of adults with asthma and COPD do not use their inhalers correctly (87, 88). It is essential that people with asthma carry their inhalers at all times, and for young people there can be barriers to carrying their inhalers and using them at school (89), such poor knowledge of how to assemble the inhaler in an emergency (90). These results emphasize the importance of practical asthma education including careful assessment of inhaler technique, assembly of devices and discussing practical strategies for carrying devices at school to ensure rescue medications are used effectively. Other strategies for education written action plans for daily management (very common in pediatrics), formal asthma education with an asthma nurse and partnering with schools and housing authorities (82). Transition presents an opportunity for assessment of asthma knowledge, particularly treatments and identifying exacerbations, and encouraging the adolescent to be able to self-manage in preparation for transition. Importantly, it has been demonstrated that health education regarding asthma treatment can improve remove health literacy barriers, improving asthma self-management and treatment adherence (91). Therefore, the importance of regular asthma education with a focus on practical assessment prior to and after transition (and on an ongoing basis in adult health care) cannot be overstated.

A SUGGESTED APPROACH FOLLOWING TRANSITION TO ADULT SERVICES

For those young adults who do require transition to specialist adult asthma services, the transfer of their care provides an opportunity for a detailed review of their asthma, starting with a careful reassessment of the diagnosis. For most patients a review of the pediatric case notes will identify objective evidence supporting the diagnosis, for example presence of variable airflow obstruction and/or airway hyper responsiveness, often along with markers of airway inflammation such as elevated FeNO, blood or airway eosinophilia. In the absence of this evidence, or where the pattern of symptoms or exacerbations has changed, it may be helpful to organize further investigations such as methacholine or histamine challenge testing, induced sputum, FeNO, and in selected cases to consider CT imaging or bronchoscopy. These investigations will not only help to confirm that asthma is still the primary condition driving their morbidity, but also help to characterize the underlying asthma phenotype and to determine which are the active treatable traits that require attention (11, 42, 43). Identification of an eosinophilic inflammation predominant phenotype, for example, may direct the clinician to consider targeted anti-eosinophil therapies such as anti-IL5 treatment (44, 45). As adolescent patients transfer to adult services and start to take more individual responsibility for their own healthcare, non-adherence to treatment is a particularly important issue (46). Transfer to adult services should prompt a full medication review including an assessment of the patients' beliefs and understanding of the rationale for treatment, their current and anticipated adherence pattern, use of rescue medication including any inappropriate reliance on short acting B2 agonists, inhaler technique and presence and understanding of a personalized asthma action plan for exacerbations. A review of inhaler device and treatment doses will often also be appropriate. Similarly it is important to remember that patients are often undergoing significant changes in their psychosocial circumstances such moving away to university or starting full time employment and it will be important to consider the impact that these lifestyle changes will have on the patient's asthma. With appropriate initial support from the multidisciplinary asthma team most patients can accept increasing responsibility for managing their own asthma following transition. For some young adults, particularly those with the most severe asthma who have had a history of frequent hospital admissions, more time will be needed to lessen the need for the input of parents and other carers, but wherever possible the goal should be independent asthma self-management with support from the specialist asthma team.

AUTHOR CONTRIBUTIONS

All authors listed have made a substantial, direct and intellectual contribution to the work, and approved it for publication.

REFERENCES

1. Blum RW, Garell D, Hodgman CH, Jorissen TW, Okinow NA, Orr DP, et al. Transition from child-centred care to adult health-care systems for adolescents with chronic conditions. A position paper of the Society for Adolescent Medicine. *J Adolesc Health.* (1993) 14:570–6. doi: 10.1016/1054-139X(93)90143-D
2. White PH, Cooley WC. Supporting the health care transition from adolescence to adulthood in the medical home. *Pediatrics.* (2011) 128:182–200. doi: 10.1542/peds.2011-0969
3. White PH, Cooley WC. Supporting the health care transition from adolescence to adulthood in the medical home. *Pediatrics.* (2018) 142:e20182587. doi: 10.1542/peds.2018-2587
4. White PH, Cooley WC. Supporting the health care transition from adolescence to adulthood in the medical home. *Pediatrics.* (2018) 142:e20182587. *Pediatrics.* (2019) 143:e20183610. doi: 10.1542/peds.2018-3610
5. Martin MA, Press VG, Nyenhuis SM, Krishnan JA, Erwin K, Mosnaim G, et al. Care transition interventions for children with asthma in the emergency department. *J Allergy Clin Immunol.* (2016) 138:1518–25. doi: 10.1016/j.jaci.2016.10.012
6. Fuchs O, Bahmer T, Rabe KF, von Mutius E. Asthma transition from childhood into adulthood. *Lancet Respir Med.* (2017) 5:224–34. doi: 10.1016/S2213-2600(16)30187-4
7. Devulapalli CS, Carlsen KC, Haland G, Munthe-Kaas MC, Pettersen M, Mowinckel P, et al. Severity of obstructive airways disease by age 2 years predicts asthma at 10 years of age. *Thorax.* (2008) 63:8–13. doi: 10.1136/thx.2006.060616
8. Bush A, Menzies-Gow A. Phenotypic differences between pediatric and adult asthma. *Proc Am Thorac Soc.* (2009) 6:712–9. doi: 10.1513/pats.200906-046DP
9. Depner M, Fuchs O, Genuneit J, Karvonen AM, Hyvarinen A, Kaulek V, et al. Clinical and epidemiologic phenotypes of childhood asthma. *Am J Respir Crit Care Med.* (2014) 189:129–38. doi: 10.1164/rccm.201307-1198OC
10. Henderson J, Granell R, Heron J, Sherriff A, Simpson A, Woodcock A, et al. Associations of wheezing phenotypes in the first 6 years of life with atopy, lung function and airway responsiveness in mid-childhood. *Thorax.* (2008) 63:974–80. doi: 10.1136/thx.2007.093187
11. Stern DA, Morgan WJ, Halonen M, Wright AL. Wheezing and bronchial hyper-responsiveness in early childhood as predictors of newly diagnosed asthma in early adulthood: a longitudinal birth-cohort study. *Lancet.* (2008) 372:1058–64. doi: 10.1016/S0140-6736(08)61447-6
12. Albuali WH, Singh RN, Fraser DD, Seabrook JA, Kavanagh BP, Parshuram CS, et al. Have changes in ventilation practice improved outcome in children with acute lung injury? *Pediatr Crit Care Med.* (2007) 8:324–30. doi: 10.1097/01.PCC.0000269390.48450.AF
13. Xuan W, Marks GB, Toelle BG, Belousova E, Peat JK, Berry G, et al. Risk factors for onset and remission of atopy, wheeze, and airway hyperresponsiveness. *Thorax.* (2002) 57:104–9. doi: 10.1136/thorax.57.2.104
14. Russell G. Asthma in the transition from childhood to adulthood. *Thorax.* (2002) 57:96–7. doi: 10.1136/thorax.57.2.96
15. Kelly WJ, Hudson I, Phelan PD. Childhood asthma in adult life: a further study at 28 years of age. *BMJ.* (1987) 294:1059–62. doi: 10.1136/bmj.294.6579.1059
16. Phelan PD. Hyperresponsiveness as a determinant of the outcome in childhood asthma. *Am Rev Respir Dis.* (1991):1463–6; discussion 6–7. doi: 10.1164/ajrccm/143.6.1463
17. Roorda RJ, Gerritsen J, Van Aalderen WM, Schouten JP, Veltman JC, Weiss ST, et al. Risk factors for the persistence of respiratory symptoms in childhood asthma. *Am Rev Respir Dis.* (1993) 148 (6 Pt 1):1490–5. doi: 10.1164/ajrccm/148.6_Pt_1.1490
18. Ulrik CS, Backer V, Hesse B, Dirksen A. Risk factors for development of asthma in children and adolescents: findings from a longitudinal population study. *Respir Med.* (1996) 90:623–30. doi: 10.1016/S0954-6111(96)90021-9
19. Fagan JK, Scheff PA, Hryhorczuk D, Ramakrishnan V, Ross M, Persky V. Prevalence of asthma and other allergic diseases in an adolescent population: association with gender and race. *Ann Allergy Asthma Immunol.* (2001) 86:177–84. doi: 10.1016/S1081-1206(10)62688-9
20. de Marco R, Locatelli F, Sunyer J, Burney P. Differences in incidence of reported asthma related to age in men and women. A retrospective analysis of the data of the European Respiratory Health Survey. *Am J Respir Crit Care Med.* (2000) 162:68–74. doi: 10.1164/ajrccm.162.1.9907008

21. Martin AJ, Landau LI, Phelan PD. Natural history of allergy in asthmatic children followed to adult life. *Med J Aust.* (1981) 2:470–4.
22. Blair H. Natural history of childhood asthma. 20-year follow-up. *Arch Dis Child.* (1977) 52:613–9. doi: 10.1136/adc.52.8.613
23. Cserhati E, Mezei G, Kelemen J. Late prognosis of bronchial asthma in children. *Respiration.* (1984) 46:160–5. doi: 10.1159/000194685
24. Strachan DP, Butland BK, Anderson HR. Incidence and prognosis of asthma and wheezing illness from early childhood to age 33 in a national British cohort. *BMJ.* (1996) 312:1195–9. doi: 10.1136/bmj.312.7040.1195
25. Jenkins MA, Hopper JL, Bowes G, Carlin JB, Flander LB, Giles GG. Factors in childhood as predictors of asthma in adult life. *BMJ.* (1994) 309:90–3. doi: 10.1136/bmj.309.6947.90
26. Vonk JM, Postma DS, Boezen HM, Grol MH, Schouten JP, Koeter GH, et al. Childhood factors associated with asthma remission after 30 year follow up. *Thorax.* (2004) 59:925–9. doi: 10.1136/thx.2003.016246
27. Sears MR, Greene JM, Willan AR, Wiecek EM, Taylor DR, Flannery EM, et al. A longitudinal, population-based, cohort study of childhood asthma followed to adulthood. *N Engl J Med.* (2003) 349:1414–22. doi: 10.1056/NEJMoa022363
28. Tai A, Tran H, Roberts M, Clarke N, Gibson AM, Vidmar S, et al. Outcomes of childhood asthma to the age of 50 years. *J Allergy Clin Immunol.* (2014) 133:1572–8 e3. doi: 10.1016/j.jaci.2013.12.1033
29. Andersson M, Hedman L, Bjerg A, Forsberg B, Lundback B, Ronmark E. Remission and persistence of asthma followed from 7 to 19 years of age. *Pediatrics.* (2013) 132:e435–42. doi: 10.1542/peds.2013-0741
30. Taylor DR, Cowan JO, Greene JM, Willan AR, Sears MR. Asthma in remission: can relapse in early adulthood be predicted at 18 years of age? *Chest.* (2005) 127:845–50. doi: 10.1378/chest.127.3.845
31. Sood A, Qualls C, Schuyler M, Arynchyn A, Alvarado JH, Smith LJ, et al. Adult-onset asthma becomes the dominant phenotype among women by age 40 years. The longitudinal CARDIA study. *Ann Am Thorac Soc.* (2013) 10:188–97. doi: 10.1513/AnnalsATS.201212-115OC
32. Burgess JA, Walters EH, Byrnes GB, Giles GG, Jenkins MA, Abramson MJ, et al. Childhood adiposity predicts adult-onset current asthma in females: a 25-yr prospective study. *Eur Respir J.* (2007) 29:668–75. doi: 10.1183/09031936.00080906
33. Castro-Rodriguez JA, Holberg CJ, Morgan WJ, Wright AL, Martinez FD. Increased incidence of asthmalike symptoms in girls who become overweight or obese during the school years. *Am J Respir Crit Care Med.* (2001) 163:1344–9. doi: 10.1164/ajrccm.163.6.2006140
34. Spycher BD, Kuehni CE. Asthma phenotypes in childhood: conceptual thoughts on stability and transition. *Eur Respir J.* (2016) 47:362–5. doi: 10.1183/13993003.02011-2015
35. Hirose M, Horiguchi T. Asthma phenotypes. *J Gen Fam Med.* (2017) 18:189–94. doi: 10.1002/jgf2.7
36. Vonk JM, Jongepier H, Panhuysen CI, Schouten JP, Bleecker ER, Postma DS. Risk factors associated with the presence of irreversible airflow limitation and reduced transfer coefficient in patients with asthma after 26 years of follow up. *Thorax.* (2003) 58:322–7. doi: 10.1136/thorax.58.4.322
37. de Marco R, Marcon A, Jarvis D, Accordini S, Almar E, Bugiani M, et al. Prognostic factors of asthma severity: a 9-year international prospective cohort study. *J Allergy Clin Immunol.* (2006) 117:1249–56. doi: 10.1016/j.jaci.2006.03.019
38. McGeachie MJ, Yates KP, Zhou X, Guo F, Sternberg AL, Van Natta ML, et al. Patterns of growth and decline in lung function in persistent childhood asthma. *N Engl J Med.* (2016) 374:1842–52. doi: 10.1056/NEJMoa1513737
39. Gupta A, Bazari F, Holloway E, Bossley C, Payne D, Wilson N, et al. Progression of paediatric difficult asthma five years after initial assessment. *Am J Respir Crit Care Med.* (2009) 179:a4840. doi: 10.1164/ajrccm-conference.2009.179.1_MeetingAbstracts.A4840
40. Nordlund B, Melen E, Schultz ES, Gronlund H, Hedlin G, Kull I. Prevalence of severe childhood asthma according to the WHO. *Respir Med.* (2014) 108:1234–7. doi: 10.1016/j.rmed.2014.05.015
41. Guilbert TW, Bacharier LB, Fitzpatrick AM. Severe asthma in children. *J Allergy Clin Immunol Pract.* (2014) 2:489–500. doi: 10.1016/j.jaip.2014.06.022
42. Plaza-Martin AM, Vennera MC, Galera J, Herraez L, Group PS. Prevalence and clinical profile of difficult-to-control severe asthma in children: results from pneumology and allergy hospital units in Spain. *Allergol Immunopathol.* (2014) 42:510–7. doi: 10.1016/j.aller.2014.02.003
43. Garner R, Kohen D. Changes in the prevalence of asthma among Canadian children. *Health Rep.* (2008) 19:45–50.
44. Withers AL. Management issues for adolescents with cystic fibrosis. *Pulm Med.* (2012) 2012:134132. doi: 10.1155/2012/134132
45. Zack J, Jacobs CP, Keenan PM, Harney K, Woods ER, Colin AA, et al. Perspectives of patients with cystic fibrosis on preventive counseling and transition to adult care. *Pediatr Pulmonol.* (2003) 36:376–83. doi: 10.1002/ppul.10342
46. Segal TY. Adolescence: what the cystic fibrosis team needs to know. *J R Soc Med.* (2008) 101 (Suppl. 1):S15–27. doi: 10.1258/jrsm.2008.s18005
47. Suris JC, Parera N. Sex, drugs and chronic illness: health behaviours among chronically ill youth. *Eur J Public Health.* (2005) 15:484–8. doi: 10.1093/eurpub/cki001
48. Quittner AL, Barker DH, Snell C, Grimley ME, Marciel K, Cruz I. Prevalence and impact of depression in cystic fibrosis. *Curr Opin Pulm Med.* (2008) 14:582–8. doi: 10.1097/MCP.0b013e3283121cf1
49. Bhatia SK, Bhatia SC. Childhood and adolescent depression. *Am Fam Physician.* (2007) 75:73–80.
50. Evans DL, Charney DS, Lewis L, Golden RN, Gorman JM, Krishnan KR, et al. Mood disorders in the medically ill: scientific review and recommendations. *Biol Psychiatry.* (2005) 58:175–89. doi: 10.1016/j.biopsych.2005.05.001
51. Cadman D, Boyle M, Szatmari P, Offord DR. Chronic illness, disability, and mental and social well-being: findings of the Ontario Child Health Study. *Pediatrics.* (1987) 79:805–13.
52. Greydanus D, Patel D, Pratt H. Suicide risk in adolescents with chronic illness: implications for primary care and specialty pediatric practice: a review. *Dev Med Child Neurol.* (2010) 52:1083–7. doi: 10.1111/j.1469-8749.2010.03771.x
53. Suris JC, Parera N, Puig C. Chronic illness and emotional distress in adolescence. *J Adolesc Health.* (1996) 19:153–6. doi: 10.1016/1054-139X(95)00231-G
54. Fiese BH, Everhart RS. Medical adherence and childhood chronic illness: family daily management skills and emotional climate as emerging contributors. *Curr Opin Pediatr.* (2006) 18:551–7. doi: 10.1097/01.mop.0000245357.68207.9b
55. Helgeson VS, Novak SA. Illness centrality and well-being among male and female early adolescents with diabetes. *J Pediatr Psychol.* (2007) 32:260–72. doi: 10.1093/jpepsy/jsl018
56. Viner R. Transition from paediatric to adult care. Bridging the gaps or passing the buck? *Arch Dis Child.* (1999) 81:271–5. doi: 10.1136/adc.81.3.271
57. Wright C, Steinway C, Jan S. The genesis of systems of care for transition to adulthood services: emerging models in primary and subspecialty care. *Curr Opin Pediatr.* (2018) 30:303–10. doi: 10.1097/MOP.0000000000000608
58. McManus M, White P, Pirtle R, Hancock C, Ablan M, Corona-Parra R. Incorporating the six core elements of health care transition into a medicaid managed care plan: lessons learned from a pilot project. *J Pediatr Nurs.* (2015) 30:700–13. doi: 10.1016/j.pedn.2015.05.029
59. Campbell F, Biggs K, Aldiss SK, O'Neill PM, Clowes M, McDonagh J, et al. Transition of care for adolescents from paediatric services to adult health services. *Cochrane Database Syst Rev.* (2016) 4:CD009794. doi: 10.1002/14651858.CD009794.pub2
60. Brumfield K, Lansbury G. Experiences of adolescents wtih cystic fibrosis durings teir transition from paediatric to adult health care: a qualitative study of young Australian adults. *Disabil Rehab.* (2004) 26:223–34. doi: 10.1080/09638280310001644924
61. Nakhla M, Bell LE, Wafa S, Dasgupta K. Improving the transition from pediatric to adult diabetes care: the pediatric care provider's perspective in Quebec, Canada. *BMJ Open Diabetes Res Care.* (2017) 5:e000390. doi: 10.1136/bmjdrc-2017-000390
62. Sable C, Foster E, Uzark K, Bjornsen K, Canobbio MM, Connolly HM, et al. Best practices in managing transition to adulthood for adolescents with congenital heart disease: the transition process and medical and psychosocial issues: a scientific statement from the American Heart Association. *Circulation.* (2011) 123:1454–85. doi: 10.1161/CIR.0b013e3182107c56
63. Al-Yateem N. Guidelines for the transition from child to adult cystic fibrosis care. *Nurs Child Young People.* (2013) 25:29–34. doi: 10.7748/ncyp2013.06.25.5.29.e175
64. Couriel J. Asthma in adolescence. *Paediatr Respir Rev.* (2003) 4:47–54. doi: 10.1016/S1526-0542(02)00309-3

65. American Academy of Pediatrics, American Academy of Family Physicians, American College of Physicians-American Society of Internal Medicine. A consensus statement on health care transitions for young adults with special health care needs. *Pediatrics.* (2002) 110 (6 Pt 2):1304–6.
66. Bergstrom SE, Sundell K, Hedlin G. Adolescents with asthma: consequences of transition from paediatric to adult healthcare. *Respir Med.* (2010) 104:180–7. doi: 10.1016/j.rmed.2009.09.021
67. Zielinski TA, Brown ES, Nejtek VA, Khan DA, Moore JJ, Rush AJ. Depression in asthma: prevalence and clinical implications. *Prim Care Companion J Clin Psychiatry.* (2000) 2:153–8. doi: 10.4088/PCC.v02n0501
68. Balfour-Lynn L. Effect of asthma on growth and puberty. *Pediatrician.* (1987) 14:237–41.
69. Dakhel AKA, Alqeaid FAR, Alkhuzayyim FMA. Association between bronchial asthma and pubertal delay in pediatric patients. *Egypt J Hospital Med.* (2018) 70:245–50. doi: 10.12816/0043084
70. Wolthers OD. Growth problems in children with asthma. *Horm Res.* (2002) 57 (Suppl. 2):83–7. doi: 10.1159/000058107
71. Doull IJ. The effect of asthma and its treatment on growth. *Arch Dis Child.* (2004) 89:60–3. doi: 10.1136/adc.2003.014365
72. Murphy VE, Clifton VL, Gibson PG. Asthma exacerbations during pregnancy: incidence and association with adverse pregnancy outcomes. *Thorax.* (2006) 61:169–76. doi: 10.1136/thx.2005.049718
73. Nwaru BI, Sheikh A. Hormonal contraceptives and asthma in women of reproductive age: analysis of data from serial national Scottish Health Surveys. *J R Soc Med.* (2015) 108:358–71. doi: 10.1177/01410768155 88320
74. NAC. *Australian Asthma Handbook, Version 2.0.* Melbourne, VIC: NAC (2019).
75. Fan G, Wang B, Liu C, Li D. Prenatal paracetamol use and asthma in childhood: a systematic review and meta-analysis. *Allergol Immunopathol.* (2017) 45:528–33. doi: 10.1016/j.aller.2016.10.014
76. Andersen AB, Farkas DK, Mehnert F, Ehrenstein V, Erichsen R. Use of prescription paracetamol during pregnancy and risk of asthma in children: a population-based Danish cohort study. *Clin Epidemiol.* (2012) 4:33–40. doi: 10.2147/CLEP.S28312
77. Magnus MC, Karlstad O, Haberg SE, Nafstad P, Davey Smith G, Nystad W. Prenatal and infant paracetamol exposure and development of asthma: the Norwegian Mother and Child Cohort Study. *Int J Epidemiol.* (2016) 45:512–22. doi: 10.1093/ije/dyv366
78. Scal P, Davern M, Ireland M, Park K. Transition to adulthood: delays and unmet needs among adolescents and young adults with asthma. *J Pediatr.* (2008) 152:471–75.e1. doi: 10.1016/j.jpeds.2007.10.004
79. Gibson-Scipio W, Gourdin D, Krouse HJ. Asthma self-management goals, beliefs and behaviors of Urban African American adolescents prior to transitioning to adult health care. *J Pediatr Nurs.* (2015) 30:e53–61. doi: 10.1016/j.pedn.2015.06.012
80. Lara M, Akinbami L, Flores G, Morgenstern H. Heterogeneity of childhood asthma among Hispanic children: Puerto Rican children bear a disproportionate burden. *Pediatrics.* (2006) 117:43–53. doi: 10.1542/peds.2004-1714
81. Lotstein DS, Kuo AA, Strickland B, Tait F. The transition to adult health care for youth with special health care needs: do racial and ethnic disparities exist? *Pediatrics.* (2010) 126 (Suppl. 3):S129–36. doi: 10.1542/peds.2010-1466F
82. Volerman A, Chin MH, Press VG. Solutions for asthma disparities. *Pediatrics.* (2017) 139:e20162546. doi: 10.1542/peds.2016-2546
83. Holley S, Walker D, Knibb R, Latter S, Liossi C, Mitchell F, et al. Barriers and facilitators to self-management of asthma in adolescents: an interview study to inform development of a novel intervention. *Clin Exp Allergy.* (2018) 48:944–56. doi: 10.1111/cea.13141
84. Rhee H, Belyea MJ, Ciurzynski S, Brasch J. Barriers to asthma self-management in adolescents: relationships to psychosocial factors. *Pediatr Pulmonol.* (2009) 44:183–91. doi: 10.1002/ppul.20972
85. Buston KM, Wood SF. Non-compliance amongst adolescents with asthma: listening to what they tell us about self-management. *Fam Pract.* (2000) 17:134–8. doi: 10.1093/fampra/17.2.134
86. Volerman A, Toups MM, Hull A, Press VG. Does inhaler technique align with confidence among African-American children and their parents? *Ann Allergy Asthma Immunol.* (2019) 123:100–1. doi: 10.1016/j.anai.2019.04.012
87. Cochrane MG, Bala MV, Downs KE, Mauskopf J, Ben-Joseph RH. Inhaled corticosteroids for asthma therapy: patient compliance, devices, and inhalation technique. *Chest.* (2000) 117:542–50. doi: 10.1378/chest.117.2.542
88. Lavorini F, Magnan A, Dubus JC, Voshaar T, Corbetta L, Broeders M, et al. Effect of incorrect use of dry powder inhalers on management of patients with asthma and COPD. *Respir Med.* (2008) 102:593–604. doi: 10.1016/j.rmed.2007.11.003
89. Toups MM, Press VG, Volerman A. National analysis of state health policies on students' right to self-carry and self-administer asthma inhalers at school. *J Sch Health.* (2018) 88:776–84. doi: 10.1111/josh.12681
90. Sridharan G, Spalding A, Press VG, Volerman A. Barriers and facilitators to self-carry of inhalers in school: a qualitative study of children with asthma. Conference Abstract 195 A:3327. *Am J Respir Crit Care Med.* (2017) 195.
91. Paasche-Orlow MK, Riekert KA, Bilderback A, Chanmugam A, Hill P, Rand CS, et al. Tailored education may reduce health literacy disparities in asthma self-management. *Am J Respir Crit Care Med.* (2005) 172:980–6. doi: 10.1164/rccm.200409-1291OC

5

The Burden of Pediatric Asthma

Giuliana Ferrante[1] *and Stefania La Grutta*[1,2]*

[1] *Department of Science for Health Promotion and Mother and Child Care, University of Palermo, Palermo, Italy,* [2] *National Research Council of Italy, Institute of Biomedicine and Molecular Immunology, Palermo, Italy*

Correspondence:
Stefania La Grutta
stefania.lagrutta@ibim.cnr.it

Asthma is the most common chronic disease in children, imposing a consistent burden on health system. In recent years, prevalence of asthma symptoms became globally increased in children and adolescents, particularly in Low-Middle Income Countries (LMICs). Host (genetics, atopy) and environmental factors (microbial exposure, exposure to passive smoking and air pollution), seemed to contribute to this trend. The increased prevalence observed in metropolitan areas with respect to rural ones and, overall, in industrialized countries, highlighted the role of air pollution in asthma inception. Asthma accounts for 1.1% of the overall global estimate of "Disability-adjusted life years" (DALYs)/100,000 for all causes. Mortality in children is low and it decreased across Europe over recent years. Children from LMICs particularly suffer a disproportionately higher burden in terms of morbidity and mortality. Global asthma-related costs are high and are usually are classified into direct, indirect and intangible costs. Direct costs account for 50–80% of the total costs. Asthma is one of the main causes of hospitalization which are particularly common in children aged < 5 years with a prevalence that has been increased during the last two decades, mostly in LMICs. Indirect costs are usually higher than in older patients, including both school and work-related losses. Intangible costs are unquantifiable, since they are related to impairment of quality of life, limitation of physical activities and study performance. The implementation of strategies aimed at early detect asthma thus providing access to the proper treatment has been shown to effectively reduce the burden of the disease.

Keywords: asthma, burden, children, cost, epidemiology, prevalence, morbidity, mortality

INTRODUCTION

Asthma is the most prevalent chronic respiratory disease worldwide, affecting more than 300 million people of all ethnic groups throughout all ages (1). It is the most common chronic disease in children, imposing an increasingly consistent burden on health system (2). Despite the various asthma phenotypes described in children, this condition is overall recognized as a chronic inflammatory disease of the airways characterized by variable symptoms of wheeze, breathlessness, chest tightness and/or cough associated with expiratory airflow limitation that may resolve spontaneously or in response to medication (3).

The understanding of the global burden of pediatric asthma has increased over the last two decades thanks to national and international studies on general populations. In defining asthma prevalence, epidemiological surveys have focused on self-reported (or parent-reported) symptoms by using standardized questionnaires, rather than on doctor diagnosis.

In particular, wheezing has been considered the most important symptom in the identification of asthma (4). The International Study of Asthma and Allergies in Childhood (ISAAC) consisted of 3 phases. Phase I was conducted during the period 1991–1995 in children and adolescents aged 6–7 and 13–14 years, respectively, in 56 countries throughout the world (5); Phase III, including 237 centers in 98 countries, was performed 5 years later, in order to examine changes in prevalence of symptoms after Phase I (6). Data on respiratory health in the younger age group were obtained from questionnaires fulfilled by parents, whereas the older age group was able to self-complete the questionnaires, which were constructed in order to be accessible to people from different countries and income levels. This accurate methodology explains the high response rate with 721.601 children involved in Phase One and 1.187.496 in Phase Three. The Italian part of ISAAC, the SIDRIA (Italian acronym for Studi Italiani sui Disturbi Respiratori nell'Infanzia e l'Ambiente) Study, was performed in two different phases between 1994 and 2002 and provided information on the epidemiology of childhood asthma in Italy, basing on questionnaires including the ISAAC core module (7, 8). Data collected from these surveys contributed to improve knowledge in the epidemiology of childhood asthma through a standardized approach. A survey to examine variations in prevalence rates of childhood asthma, wheeze and wheeze with asthma in Europe has been recently carried out (9), but further studies are needed for a more comprehensive and ongoing assessment of disease prevalence, morbidity and hospitalization all over the world (10).

GLOBAL AND TIME TRENDS OF ASTHMA IN CHILDREN

Overall, "asthma ever" was more common in High-Income Countries (HICs), even though the highest prevalence of severe symptoms among children with current (past 12 months) wheeze were found in Low- and Middle-Income Countries (LMICs) (**Figure 1**) (11). Conspicuous variations in the lifetime prevalence of asthma have been reported between countries all over the world (6). Between ISAAC Phase One and Phase Three prevalence of asthma symptoms became globally increased in children and adolescents ranging from 11.1 to 11.6% and from 13.2 to 13.7%, respectively (12). Generally, prevalence of "asthma ever" significantly increased in children and adolescents, probably due to a greater awareness of this condition and changes in diagnostic practice. However also host (genetics, atopy) and environmental factors (microbial exposure, exposure to passive smoking, and air pollution), seemed to contribute to the observed increasing trends. In particular, lifetime prevalence of asthma remained the same or even decreased in HICs, whereas it increased in many LMICs, especially in Eastern European as well as in Latin American and Northern African countries (6, 13). In Europe, increased prevalence has been reported in children (12).

Between SIDRIA Phase One and Phase Two, prevalence of "asthma ever" tended toward a stabilization in children, ranging from 9.1 to 9.5%, whereas in adolescents it increased from 9.1 to 10.4%. Prevalence of "current wheeze" resulted to be little increased in children, ranging from 7.8 to 8.6%, whereas it slightly decreased in adolescents, ranging from 10.5 to 9.7%. Noteworthy, asthma prevalence in adolescents increased only in those living in large metropolitan areas, with a percent prevalence change of 3.3% (14). Prevalence of asthma symptoms in migrant children was found to increase with the number of years of living in Italy, with risk of lifetime asthma and current wheeze very similar to Italian children (15). This finding adds further evidence to the critical role that environmental exposures may play in the development of asthma in childhood. Lastly, prevalence of asthma was found to be higher in males as in children as in adolescents, whereas asthma was more common in girls after puberty. These gender differences might be attributed to a narrower airways caliber in males than females in early life due to the effects of different hormonal factors (7).

RISK FACTORS FOR ASTHMA IN CHILDHOOD

Genetics and Epigenetics

Differences in asthma prevalence observed in vary ethnic groups all over the world may be explained by differences in the genetic susceptibility. Although the specific contribution of genetics to asthma has not thoroughly clarified, a large number of genetic markers reliably associated with asthma and airway inflammation have been identified to date. Particularly, different polymorphisms in the 17q21 locus have been found to be associated with asthma. This is considered one of the strongest loci for asthma, even though its function is still not known. Risk alleles of some single nucleotide polymorphisms (SNPs) in this locus were associated with an increased number of CD4+ cells as well as with the number of eosinophils in the airway wall biopsies of asthmatics, suggesting the involvement of these genes in the Th2 pathway in asthma (16). A new locus associated with time to asthma onset was identified at position 16q12 (17). A recent study found novel genetic factors to potentially explain sex-specific asthma effects during childhood (18). Moreover, a SNP on chromosome 8 was associated with early lung function decline (19). No specific models of genetic transmission have been identified so far.

A multi-factorial model characterized by complex relationships between genes and environment has been instead proposed. In this context, greater and greater interest on epigenetics has been focused in recent years, finding that environmental exposures are able to modulate genes expression in a complex interaction that may be even transferred from mother to child (20). More recently, traffic related air pollution's influence on asthma was showed to be associated with DNA demethylation of a CpG site in the promoter region of the Ten-eleven translocation 1 gene, a possible biomarker for childhood asthma (21).

Atopy

Data from epidemiological studies showed the strong link between asthma and atopy. Indeed, the family history of atopy is considered one of the most relevant risk factors for developing asthma. The relationship between allergic sensitization and

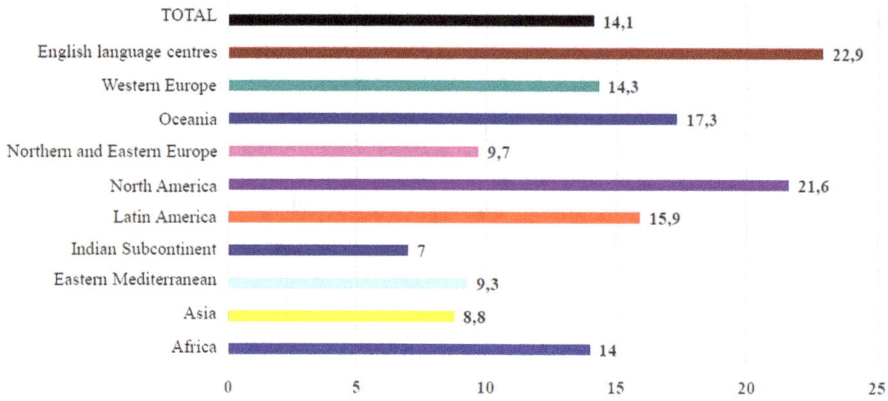

FIGURE 1 | Prevalence of current wheezing in adolescents 13–14 years: data from ISAAC Phase III.

asthma onset has been well-documented (22, 23). However, the causal relationship between individual allergen exposure and the development of symptoms has been not clearly delineated, probably due to the complexity of interactions between timing and dose of exposure and genetic predisposition. Almost 60% of schoolchildren with asthma are allergic, mainly to perennial allergens such as house dust mites, animal dander and molds. These indoor allergens play an important role in eliciting asthma exacerbations, by increasing airway inflammation and bronchial hyper-responsiveness (24). Lastly, it was recently showed that aeroallergen sensitization before the age of 5 years significantly increased the risk of asthma with persistence into adolescence (25).

Microbial Exposure

A reduced microbial exposure since early life through improved sanitation and increased rates of immunization have been linked to the increased prevalence of asthma observed in childhood. Changes in environment and/or lifestyle have been suggested to alter the development of the immune system increasing the risk of asthma in genetically susceptible subjects, basing on the so called "hygiene hypothesis." Accordingly, children raised in modern environment with a scanty natural microbial burden may be prone to develop allergic diseases in view of an under-stimulation of the immune system. Indeed, recent evidences showed that exposure to some microbes can protect from atopy, whereas others seem to promote allergic diseases. The timing of exposure to as well as the properties of the infectious agent, in addition to the genetic susceptibility of the host, may influence the future development of asthma (26). There is evidence for a critical role of respiratory virus infections in early life for asthma development. In particular, Respiratory Syncytial Virus (RSV) and Human Rhinovirus (HRV) are most frequently associated with wheezing episodes in preschool children and with asthma development in the next years. Approximately 50% of the infants with lower respiratory tract infections caused by RSV during the first 12 months of life developed persistent asthma at school age (27). In children at high risk for development of asthma, HRV-induced wheezing in infancy resulted to be the strongest predictor of doctor diagnosed asthma at age 6 years (28, 29). In addition to viral causes, some studies suggested that infections by atypical bacterial, such as *Mycoplasma pneumoniae* and *Chlamydia pneumonia*, may play a role in inducing and exacerbating asthma (30, 31).

Environmental Exposure

The increased asthma prevalence in metropolitan areas with respect to rural ones and, overall, in industrialized countries, highlighted the role of air pollution in asthma inception (14). Exposure to both outdoor and indoor pollutants has been associated with increased asthma exacerbations, rates of hospitalization and reduced lung function (32–34). Even though a cross-sectional study on 5 European birth cohorts recently showed no associations between air pollutants exposure and asthma prevalence (35), a European population-based birth cohort study on more than 14,000 children found that increasing exposure to nitric dioxide (NO_2) and particulate matter with a diameter of less than 2.5 μm ($PM_{2.5}$) at the birth address was associated with increased asthma incidence at age 14–16 years (36). Further evidence comes from a meta-analyses of birth cohort studies showing that increased childhood exposure to $PM_{2.5}$ and black carbon was associated with increased risk of asthma at age 12 years (37). The most dangerous environmental exposure in children derives from Environmental Tobacco Smoke (ETS), which is universally recognized as a major risk factor for asthma. Exposure to prenatal and early postnatal passive smoke may have adverse effect on both the immune system and the structural and functional development of the lung; this may explain the subsequent increased risk of incident asthma (38). Exposure to ETS at school age is associated with an increased risk of severity and exacerbations and may be considered a risk factor for asthma persistence in later life (39). In recent years increasing interest raised the novel concept of Third-Hand Smoke (THS), the combination of tobacco smoke pollutants which remain in an indoor environment after tobacco has been smoked. Since infants and children are prone to the risks related to THS exposure, investigations are warranted to study the health effects of THS relevant to different exposure pathways and profiles occurring also in pre-natal life (40). Lastly, a new threat to the respiratory health of children and adolescents has been raised from the spread of electronic cigarettes, the most commonly used tobacco product among adolescents (41). Recent studies have shown an association with asthma symptoms in adolescents (42, 43). Further research on the health effects of electronic cigarettes is advised.

THE GLOBAL BURDEN OF DISEASE

Lifelong Outcomes

Asthma can appear at any stage throughout life, but it generally develops in childhood (44). Data from the Melbourne Asthma Study reported that 47% of individuals with persistent asthma, and even 75% of subjects classified with severe asthma, at age 6 still had asthma symptoms at age 50 years (45). Noteworthy, children with severe asthma were those at increased risk of developing Chronic Obstructive Pulmonary Disease (COPD) (45–47). Therefore, asthma can be considered a lifelong disease with a major burden especially in subjects suffering from severe asthma.

Morbidity

In 1990, the Global Burden of Disease Study (GBD) proposed the "Disability-adjusted life years" (DALYs) as a measure of disease burden. DALYs quantify how many years of life are lost due to death and/or non-fatal illness or impairment. This health gap measure can be considered as the sum of two components: years of life lost plus years lived with disability (YLDs) (48). The latter measure is calculated as the prevalence of each disease sequela multiplied by the disability weight for that sequela. Asthma was the 14th highest ranked cause of global YLDs at all ages, but specific data for children were not available (49). In the GBD 2015, it accounted for 1.1% of the overall global estimate of DALYs/100,000 for all causes. Overall, asthma represents the second most important respiratory disease after COPD when considering the burden of disease as measured by both YLDs and DALYs.

Mortality

Mortality for asthma is relatively low at all ages. In Europe, asthma is responsible for 0.4% of all deaths (43,000 persons), with wide differences among countries (50). In the GDB 2015, a decrease of 26.7% was observed in comparison with 1990. The decrease in age-standardized death rates was 58.8% between 1990 and 2015. The greatest decrease was observed in HICs, reflecting a better access to health services as well as better treatment options following international guidance (1). Asthma mortality in children is low and is significantly associated with symptoms prevalence and hospital admissions (51). Hence, when comparing childhood asthma mortality between countries, any reduction in prevalence has to be taken into account. Over recent years, asthma mortality in children decreased across Europe, with little difference between countries. This would be attributable to a better control of symptoms due to improvements in treatment of asthma attacks together with the more widespread use of inhaled corticosteroids which have been shown to reduce mortality at all ages (52). Noteworthy, data from the National Review of Asthma Deaths Confidential Enquiry Report showed that in United Kingdome 80% of asthma deaths occurred in people with poor adherence to treatment and in those who had taken more bronchodilators (53).

SOCIO-ECONOMIC COST OF CHILDHOOD ASTHMA

Asthma is a chronic condition that can assume different severity degrees throughout patient's life, with significant social impact and economic burden. In fact, this disease can be associated with limitations on physical and social aspects of daily life of children and their caregivers, especially when symptoms are not controlled (3). Overall, global asthma-related costs are high and significantly vary across countries, depending on several factors, such as the type of health system, financial resources on Public Health and methods of data collection (54).

Usually, asthma-related costs are classified into direct, indirect and intangible costs (**Figure 2**). Direct costs generally account for 50–80% of the total costs and include: disease management (e.g., outpatient visits, visits to emergency services, hospital admission, medications), complementary investigations or treatment and other costs (e.g., assistance in home care, transportation to medical visits) (54, 55). In children and adolescents with asthma the number of outpatient visits as well as the number of visits to emergency services is higher than in non-asthmatics, increasing according to the disease severity degree (56). Asthma is one of the main causes of hospitalization in children which are usually at least twice than in adults. Hospitalizations are particularly common in children aged < 5 years with a prevalence that has been increased during the last two decades, mostly in LMICs (57). Medications account for variable costs, which differ across countries depending on health system and public or private insurance coverage (58). Greater use of asthma drugs, particularly

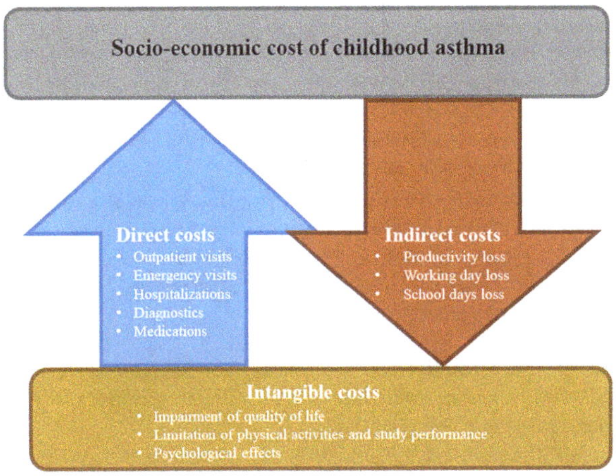

FIGURE 2 | Socio-economic cost of childhood asthma: direct, indirect, and intangible costs.

inhaled steroids, occurred in recent years globally increased costs related to asthma medications (54).

Indirect costs include work-related losses and early mortality. Although loss of working days is not directly applicable in children, absenteeism from school is a comparable consequence. In childhood asthma indirect costs are usually higher than in older patients: a child with an exacerbation of asthma loses on average 3–5 days school days and at least one of her/his caregivers loses the same working time (59).

Intangible costs are unquantifiable, since they are related to impairment of quality of life, limitation of physical activities, and study performance, with consequent psychological effects such as depression and anxiety. Nonetheless, the social burden of asthma is considerable, not only for the child but also for parents. Therefore, when assessing quality of life in asthmatic children, it is important also to assess the quality of life of the caregivers (52).

CONCLUSIONS

During last decades, asthma prevalence has been increasing worldwide. As a chronic condition that usually starts in early childhood, it imposes a high lifetime burden on individuals, their caregivers and the community. Despite significant progress in health care reached in last decades, there are still consistent disparities between countries. Children from LMICs particularly suffer a disproportionately higher burden in terms of morbidity and mortality (54). The implementation of strategies aimed at early detect asthma thus providing access to the proper treatment has been shown to effectively reduce the burden of the disease (50). The Global Asthma Network (GAN) was established in 2002 as a collaboration between individuals from ISAAC and the International Union Against Tubercolosis and Lung Disease in order to globally improve asthma care through enhanced surveillance, research collaboration, funding and capacity building, access to medical care and quality-assured essential medicines, and education of health professionals and public (60). A survey undertaken by GAN in 120 countries during 2013–2014 showed that only about one in four countries had a national asthma strategy, with a lower proportion in LCMIs than in HICs. In countries with a high prevalence of current wheeze, adopting an asthma strategy was significantly more common than what occurred in low prevalence countries. This may be due to lack of interest or to difficulties in engaging in world-wide epidemiological studies. However, extension of asthma strategies in all countries is strongly recommended, since such an approach could have a big impact on the burden of the disease, by decreasing severity and improving symptoms control (61). In this perspective, asthma, as other non-communicable chronic respiratory diseases, must be included in the agenda of each national authority. It is therefore important that monitoring of prevalence and severity continue globally. Further studies focusing on estimates of asthma costs are warranted, especially in LMICs. Moreover, standard methods of data collection are desirable in order to obtain comparable information from different countries (2). Finally, future asthma research should integrate both pediatric and adult populations in longitudinal studies, with the aim of better understand the role of risk and protective factors on disease onset and severity throughout life (1, 62, 63).

AUTHOR CONTRIBUTIONS

GF and SL provided substantial contributions to the conception or design of the work, revised the manuscript for important intellectual content, approved the final version, and agreed to be accountable for all aspects of the work.

REFERENCES

1. Soriano JB, Abajobir AA, Abate KH, Abera SF, Agrawal A, Ahmed MB, et al. Global, regional, and national deaths, prevalence, disability-adjusted life years, and years lived with disability for chronic obstructive pulmonary disease and asthma, 1990–2015: a systematic analysis for the Global Burden of Disease Study 2015. *Lancet Respir Med.* (2017) 5:691–706. doi: 10.1016/S2213-2600(17)30293-X
2. Asher I, Pearce N. Global burden of asthma among children. *Int J Tuberc Lung Dis.* (2014) 18:1269–78. doi: 10.5588/ijtld.14.0170
3. Global Initiative for Asthma. Global Strategy for Asthma Management and Prevention (2018). Available online at: www.ginasthma.org
4. Douwes J, Pearce N. Epidemiology of respiratory allergies and asthma. In: Ahrens W, Pigeot I, editors. *Handbook of Epidemiology.* New York, NY: Springer (2014). p. 2263–319.
5. Asher M, Keil U, Anderson H, Beasley R, Crane J, Martinez F, et al. International study of asthma and allergies in childhood (ISAAC): rationale and methods. *Eur Respir J.* (1995) 8:483–91. doi: 10.1183/09031936.95.08030483
6. Asher MI, Montefort S, Björkstén B, Lai CK, Strachan DP, Weiland SK, et al. Worldwide time trends in the prevalence of symptoms of asthma, allergic rhinoconjunctivitis, and eczema in childhood: ISAAC phases one and three repeat multicountry cross-sectional surveys. *Lancet* (2006) 368:733–43. doi: 10.1016/S0140-6736(06)69283-0
7. Sestini P, De Sario M, Bugiani M, Bisanti L, Giannella G, Kaisermann D, et al. Frequency of asthma and allergies in Italian children and adolescents: results from SIDRIA-2. *Epidemiol Prev.* (2005) 29:24–31.
8. Ciccone G, Camarlengo A, Bugiani M, Dalmasso P, Faggiano F, Volante T, et al. Asthma and respiratory symptoms in 6-7 yr old Italian children: gender, latitude, urbanization and socioeconomic factors. *Eur Respir J.* (1997) 10:1780–6.
9. Uphoff EP, Bird PK, Antó JM, Basterrechea M, von Berg A, Bergström A, et al. Variations in the prevalence of childhood asthma and wheeze in MeDALL cohorts in Europe. *ERJ Open Res.* (2017) 3:00150–2016. doi: 10.1183/23120541.00150-2016
10. Ellwood P, Asher MI, Billo NE, Bissell K, Chiang C-Y, Ellwood EM, et al. The global asthma network rationale and methods for Phase I global surveillance: prevalence, severity, management and risk factors. *Eur Respir J.* (2017) 49:1601605. doi: 10.1183/13993003.01605-2016
11. Lai C, Beasley R, Crane J, Foliaki S, Shah J, Weiland S. Global variation in the prevalence and severity of asthma symptoms: phase three of the International Study of Asthma and Allergies in Childhood (ISAAC). *Thorax* (2009) 64:476–83. doi: 10.1136/thx.2008.106609
12. Pearce N, Aït-Khaled N, Beasley R, Mallol J, Keil U, Mitchell E, et al. Worldwide trends in the prevalence of asthma symptoms: phase III of the International Study of Asthma and Allergies in Childhood (ISAAC). *Thorax* (2007) 62:758–66.

13. Cruz ÁA, Stelmach R, Ponte EV. Asthma prevalence and severity in low-resource communities. *Curr Opin Allergy Clin Immunol.* (2017) 17:188–93. doi: 10.1097/ACI.0000000000000360
14. Galassi C, De Sario M, Biggeri A, Bisanti L, Chellini E, Ciccone G, et al. Changes in prevalence of asthma and allergies among children and adolescents in Italy: 1994–2002. *Pediatrics* (2006) 117:34–42. doi: 10.1542/peds.2004-2709
15. Migliore E, Pearce N, Bugiani M, Galletti G, Biggeri A, Bisanti L, et al. Prevalence of respiratory symptoms in migrant children to Italy: the results of SIDRIA-2 study. *Allergy* (2007) 62:293–300. doi: 10.1111/j.1398-9995.2007.01238.x
16. Nieuwenhuis MA, Siedlinski M, Berge M, Granell R, Li X, Niens M, et al. Combining genomewide association study and lung eQTL analysis provides evidence for novel genes associated with asthma. *Allergy* (2016) 71:1712–20. doi: 10.1111/all.12990
17. Sarnowski C, Sugier P-E, Granell R, Jarvis D, Dizier M-H, Ege M, et al. Identification of a new locus at 16q12 associated with time to asthma onset. *J Allergy Clin Immunol.* (2016) 138:1071–80. doi: 10.1016/j.jaci.2016.03.018
18. Schieck M, Schouten JP, Michel S, Suttner K, Toncheva AA, Gaertner VD, et al. Doublesex and mab-3 related transcription factor 1 (DMRT1) is a sex-specific genetic determinant of childhood-onset asthma and is expressed in testis and macrophages. *J Allergy Clin Immunol.* (2016) 138:421–31. doi: 10.1016/j.jaci.2015.12.1305
19. McGeachie MJ, Yates KP, Zhou X, Guo F, Sternberg AL, Van Natta ML, et al. Genetics and genomics of longitudinal lung function patterns in individuals with asthma. *Am J Respir Crit Care Med.* (2016) 194:1465–74. doi: 10.1164/rccm.201602-0250OC
20. Yang IV, Lozupone CA, Schwartz DA. The environment, epigenome, and asthma. *J Allergy Clin Immunol.* (2017) 140:14–23. doi: 10.1016/j.jaci.2017.05.011
21. Somineni HK, Zhang X, Myers JMB, Kovacic MB, Ulm A, Jurcak N, et al. Ten-eleven translocation 1 (TET1) methylation is associated with childhood asthma and traffic-related air pollution. *J Allergy Clin Immunol.* (2016) 137:797–805. doi: 10.1016/j.jaci.2015.10.021
22. Simpson A, Tan VY, Winn J, Svensen M, Bishop CM, Heckerman DE, et al. Beyond atopy: multiple patterns of sensitization in relation to asthma in a birth cohort study. *Am J Respir Crit Care Med.* (2010) 181:1200–6. doi: 10.1164/rccm.200907-1101OC
23. Stoltz DJ, Jackson DJ, Evans MD, Gangnon RE, Tisler CJ, Gern JE, et al. Specific patterns of allergic sensitization in early childhood and asthma & rhinitis risk. *Clin Exp Allergy* (2013) 43:233–41. doi: 10.1111/cea.12050
24. Burbank AJ, Sood AK, Kesic MJ, Peden DB, Hernandez ML. Environmental determinants of allergy and asthma in early life. *J Allergy Clin Immunol.* (2017) 140:1–12. doi: 10.1016/j.jaci.2017.05.010
25. Rubner FJ, Jackson DJ, Evans MD, Gangnon RE, Tisler CJ, Pappas TE, et al. Early life rhinovirus wheezing, allergic sensitization, and asthma risk at adolescence. *J Allergy Clin Immunol.* (2017) 139:501–7. doi: 10.1016/j.jaci.2016.03.049
26. Fishbein AB, Fuleihan RL. The hygiene hypothesis revisited: does exposure to infectious agents protect us from allergy? *Curr Opin Pediatr.* (2012) 24:98–102. doi: 10.1097/MOP.0b013e32834ee57c
27. Bacharier LB, Cohen R, Schweiger T, Yin-DeClue H, Christie C, Zheng J, et al. Determinants of asthma after severe respiratory syncytial virus bronchiolitis. *J Allergy Clin Immunol.* (2012) 130:91–100. doi: 10.1016/j.jaci.2012.02.010
28. Jackson DJ, Gangnon RE, Evans MD, Roberg KA, Anderson EL, Pappas TE, et al. Wheezing rhinovirus illnesses in early life predict asthma development in high-risk children. *Am J Respir Crit Care Med.* (2008) 178:667–72. doi: 10.1164/rccm.200802-309OC
29. Lemanske RF, Jackson DJ, Gangnon RE, Evans MD, Li Z, Shult PA, et al. Rhinovirus illnesses during infancy predict subsequent childhood wheezing. *J Allergy Clin Immunol.* (2005) 116:571–7. doi: 10.1016/j.jaci.2005.06.024
30. Hansbro PM, Starkey MR, Mattes J, Horvat JC. Pulmonary immunity during respiratory infections in early life and the development of severe asthma. *Ann Am Thorac Soc.* (2014) 11:S297–302. doi: 10.1513/AnnalsATS.201402-086AW
31. Darveaux JI, Lemanske RF. Infection-related asthma. *J Allergy Clin Immunol Pract.* (2014) 2:658–63. doi: 10.1016/j.jaip.2014.09.011
32. Tatum AJ, Shapiro GG. The effects of outdoor air pollution and tobacco smoke on asthma. *Immunol Allergy Clin.* (2005) 25:15–30. doi: 10.1016/j.iac.2004.09.003
33. Rancière F, Bougas N, Viola M, Momas I. Early exposure to traffic-related air pollution, respiratory symptoms at 4 years of age, and potential effect modification by parental allergy, stressful family events, and sex: a prospective follow-up study of the PARIS Birth Cohort. *Environ Health Perspect.* (2017) 125:737–45. doi: 10.1289/EHP239
34. Gehring U, Wijga AH, Brauer M, Fischer P, de Jongste JC, Kerkhof M, et al. Traffic-related air pollution and the development of asthma and allergies during the first 8 years of life. *Am J Respir Crit Care Med.* (2010) 181:596–603. doi: 10.1164/rccm.200906-0858OC
35. Mölter A, Simpson A, Berdel D, Brunekreef B, Custovic A, Cyrys J, et al. A multicentre study of air pollution exposure and childhood asthma prevalence: the ESCAPE project. *Eur Respir J.* (2014) 45:610–24. doi: 10.1183/09031936.00083614
36. Gehring U, Wijga AH, Hoek G, Bellander T, Berdel D, Brüske I, et al. Exposure to air pollution and development of asthma and rhinoconjunctivitis throughout childhood and adolescence: a population-based birth cohort study. *Lancet Respir Med.* (2015) 3:933–42. doi: 10.1016/S2213-2600(15)00426-9
37. Bowatte G, Lodge C, Lowe AJ, Erbas B, Perret J, Abramson MJ, et al. The influence of childhood traffic-related air pollution exposure on asthma, allergy and sensitization: a systematic review and a meta-analysis of birth cohort studies. *Allergy* (2015) 70:245–56. doi: 10.1111/all.12561
38. Ferrante G, Antona R, Malizia V, Montalbano L, Corsello G, La Grutta S. Smoke exposure as a risk factor for asthma in childhood: a review of current evidence. *Allergy Asthma Proc.* (2014) 35:454–61. doi: 10.2500/aap.2014.35.3789
39. La Grutta S, Indinnimeo L, di Coste A, Ferrante G, Landi M, Pelosi U, et al. Environmental risk factors and lung diseases in children: from guidelines to health effects. *Early Hum Dev.* (2013) 89:S59–62. doi: 10.1016/j.earlhumdev.2013.07.025
40. Ferrante G, Simoni M, Cibella F, Ferrara F, Liotta G, Malizia V, et al. Third-hand smoke exposure and health hazards in children. *Monaldi Arch Chest Dis.* (2013) 79:38–43. doi: 10.4081/monaldi.2013.108
41. Ferkol TW, Farber HJ, La Grutta S, Leone FT, Marshall HM, Neptune E, et al. Electronic cigarette use in youths: a position statement of the Forum of International Respiratory Societies. *Eur Respir J.* (2018) 51:1800278. doi: 10.1183/13993003.00278-2018
42. Kim SY, Sim S, Choi HG. Active, passive, and electronic cigarette smoking is associated with asthma in adolescents. *Sci Rep.* (2017) 7:17789. doi: 10.1038/s41598-017-17958-y
43. Schweitzer RJ, Wills TA, Tam E, Pagano I, Choi K. E-cigarette use and asthma in a multiethnic sample of adolescents. *Prev Med.* (2017) 105:226–31. doi: 10.1016/j.ypmed.2017.09.023
44. To T, Wang C, Guan J, McLimont S, Gershon AS. What is the lifetime risk of physician-diagnosed asthma in Ontario, Canada? *Am J Respir Crit Care Med.* (2010) 181:337–43. doi: 10.1164/rccm.200907-1035OC
45. Tai A, Tran H, Roberts M, Clarke N, Gibson A-M, Vidmar S, et al. Outcomes of childhood asthma to the age of 50 years. *J Allergy Clin Immunol.* (2014) 133:1572–8. doi: 10.1016/j.jaci.2013.12.1033
46. Bateman ED, Reddel HK, van Zyl-Smit RN, Agusti A. The asthma–COPD overlap syndrome: towards a revised taxonomy of chronic airways diseases? *Lancet Respir Med.* (2015) 3:719–28. doi: 10.1016/S2213-2600(15)00254-4
47. Bui DS, Lodge CJ, Burgess JA, Lowe AJ, Perret J, Bui MQ, et al. Childhood predictors of lung function trajectories and future COPD risk: a prospective cohort study from the first to the sixth decade of life. *Lancet Respir Med.* (2018) doi: 10.1016/S2213-2600(18)30100-0. [Epub ahead of print].
48. Murray CJ. *Summary Measures of Population Health: Concepts, Ethics, Measurement and Applications.* Geneva: World Health Organization (2002).
49. Vos T, Flaxman AD, Naghavi M, Lozano R, Michaud C, Ezzati M, et al. Years lived with disability (YLDs) for 1160 sequelae of 289 diseases and injuries 1990–2010: a systematic analysis for the Global Burden of Disease Study 2010. *Lancet* (2012) 380:2163–96. doi: 10.1016/S0140-6736(12)61729-2
50. Global Asthma Report 2014. Available at: http://globalasthmareport.org/
51. Anderson H, Gupta R, Kapetanakis V, Asher M, Clayton T, Robertson C, et al. International correlations between indicators of prevalence, hospital

admissions and mortality for asthma in children. *Int J Epidemiol.* (2008) 37:573–82. doi: 10.1093/ije/dyn039

52. Gibson G, Loddenkemper R, Sibille Y, Lundbäck B. *The European Lung White Book: Respiratory Health and Disease in Europe.* Sheffield, UK: European Respiratory Society (2013).
53. Levy M, Andrews R, Buckingham R, Evans H, Francis C, Houston R, et al. *Why asthma still kills: the National Review of Asthma Deaths (NRAD).* Royal College of Physcians (2014).
54. Nunes C, Pereira AM, Morais-Almeida M. Asthma costs and social impact. *Asthma Res Pract.* (2017) 3:1. doi: 10.1186/s40733-016-0029-3
55. Ferreira de Magalhães M, Amaral R, Pereira AM, Sá-Sousa A, Azevedo I, Azevedo LF, et al. Cost of asthma in children: a nationwide, population-based, cost-of-illness study. *Pediatr Allergy Immunol.* (2017) 28:683–91. doi: 10.1111/pai.12772
56. Nunes C, Ladeira S. Asthma, from childhood to adulthood: a prospective 20-year longitudinal study of a cohort of asthmatics. *J Investig Allergol Clin Immunol.* (2002) 12:242–9. doi: 10.1053/rmed.19 99.076
57. Akdis CA, Agache I. *Global Atlas of Asthma.* Zurich: European Academy of Allergy and Clinical Immunology. (2013).
58. Sullivan PW, Ghushchyan V, Navaratnam P, Friedman HS, Kavati A, Ortiz B, et al. National prevalence of poor asthma control and associated outcomes among school-aged children in the United States. *J Allergy Clin Immunol Pract.* (2018) 6:536–44. doi: 10.1016/j.jaip.2017.06.039
59. Braman SS. The global burden of asthma. *Chest* (2006) 130:4S–12S. doi: 10.1378/chest.130.1_suppl.4S
60. Selroos O, Kupczyk M, Kuna P, Lacwik P, Bousquet J, Brennan D, et al. National and regional asthma programmes in Europe. *Eur Respir Rev.* (2015) 24:474–83. doi: 10.1183/16000617.00008114
61. Asher I, Haahtela T, Selroos O, Ellwood P, Ellwood E, Group GANS, others. Global Asthma Network survey suggests more national asthma strategies could reduce burden of asthma. *Allergol Immunopathol.* (2017) 45:105–14. doi: 10.1016/j.aller.2016.10.013
62. Genuneit J, Seibold A, Apfelbacher C, Konstantinou G, Koplin J, La Grutta S, et al. "Overview of systematic reviews in allergy epidemiology (OSRAE)" of the EAACI interest group on epidemiology. overview of systematic reviews in allergy epidemiology. *Allergy* (2017) 72:849–56. doi: 10.1111/all.13123
63. Genuneit J, Seibold AM, Apfelbacher CJ, Konstantinou GN, Koplin JJ, Grutta S, et al. The state of asthma epidemiology: an overview of systematic reviews and their quality. *Clin Transl Allergy* (2017) 7:12. doi: 10.1186/s13601-017-0146-y

6

Epidemiology of Asthma in Children and Adults

Shyamali C. Dharmage[1], *Jennifer L. Perret*[1,2*] *and Adnan Custovic*[3]

[1] *Allergy and Lung Health Unit, School of Population and Global Health, University of Melbourne, Melbourne, VIC, Australia,* [2] *Institute for Breathing and Sleep, Melbourne, VIC, Australia,* [3] *Department of Paediatrics, Imperial College London, London, United Kingdom*

***Correspondence:**
Jennifer L. Perret
jennifer.perret@unimelb.edu.au

Asthma is a globally significant non-communicable disease with major public health consequences for both children and adults, including high morbidity, and mortality in severe cases. We have summarized the evidence on asthma trends, environmental determinants, and long-term impacts while comparing these epidemiological features across childhood asthma and adult asthma. While asthma incidence and prevalence are higher in children, morbidity, and mortality are higher in adults. Childhood asthma is more common in boys while adult asthma is more common in women, and the reversal of this sex difference in prevalence occurs around puberty suggesting sex hormones may play a role in the etiology of asthma. The global epidemic of asthma that has been observed in both children and adults is still continuing, especially in low to middle income countries, although it has subsided in some developed countries. As a heterogeneous disease, distinct asthma phenotypes, and endotypes need to be adequately characterized to develop more accurate and meaningful definitions for use in research and clinical settings. This may be facilitated by new clustering techniques such as latent class analysis, and computational phenotyping methods are being developed to retrieve information from electronic health records using natural language processing (NLP) algorithms to assist in the early diagnosis of asthma. While some important environmental determinants that trigger asthma are well-established, more work is needed to define the role of environmental exposures in the development of asthma in both children and adults. There is increasing evidence that investigation into possible gene-by-environment and environment-by-environment interactions may help to better uncover the determinants of asthma. Therefore, there is an urgent need to further investigate the interrelationship between environmental and genetic determinants to identify high risk groups and key modifiable exposures. For children, asthma may impair airway development and reduce maximally attained lung function, and these lung function deficits may persist into adulthood without additional progressive loss. Adult asthma may accelerate lung function decline and increase the risk of fixed airflow obstruction, with the effect of early onset asthma being greater than late onset asthma. Therefore, in managing asthma, our focus going forward should be firmly on improving not only short-term symptoms, but also the long-term respiratory and other health outcomes.

Keywords: asthma epidemiology, incidence, prevalence, risk factors, lifecourse

KEY POINTS

- Asthma is a major non-communicable disease affecting both children and adults, with high morbidity and relatively low mortality compared with other chronic diseases.
- The global epidemic of asthma that has been observed in both children and adults is still continuing especially in low to middle income countries, although some evidence suggests it has subsided in some high-income countries.
- Asthma is a heterogeneous disease and distinct asthma phenotypes and endotypes need to be adequately characterized. This may be facilitated by cluster and latent class analysis if clusters/classes are associated with clinically important asthma outcomes.
- Computational phenotyping methods to retrieve information from electronic health records using natural language processing (NLP) algorithms are innovative and may assist in the early diagnosis of asthma and in epidemiological research
- While some environmental triggers are well-established, investigation into possible gene-by-environment and environment-by-environment interactions may help to better uncover the determinants of asthma.
- Work-related asthma from occupational sensitizers (asthmagens) and/or irritants is common and is an important consideration for individuals who present with asthma symptoms during their productive working years
- For children, asthma may impair airway development and reduce maximally attained lung function, and these lung function deficits may track (or persist) into adulthood without additional progressive loss.
- Adult asthma may accelerate lung function decline and increase the risk of fixed airflow obstruction, especially for smokers with asthma
- People with asthma are more susceptible to infections and non-communicable chronic co-morbidities which are associated with worse asthma outcomes
- Defining asthma remains an ongoing challenge and innovative methods are needed to identify, diagnose, and accurately classify asthma at an early stage to most effectively implement optimal management and reduce the health burden attributable to asthma

INTRODUCTION

Asthma is one of the most common major non-communicable diseases and for many, has a substantial impact on quality of life. Globally, asthma is ranked 16th among the leading causes of years lived with disability and 28th among the leading causes of burden of disease, as measured by disability-adjusted life years. Around 300 million people have asthma worldwide, and it is likely that by 2025 a further 100 million may be affected (1). There is a large geographical variation in asthma prevalence, severity, and mortality. While asthma prevalence is higher in high income countries, most asthma-related mortality occurs in low-middle income countries (2). Despite the advances in asthma treatment in recent decades, there are still gains to be made in terms of improving patient education, employing new diagnostic approaches, and implementing personalized case management.

Patterns in asthma incidence and prevalence differ between children and adults. It is well-known that asthma often begins in childhood but can occur at any time throughout life, with some developing asthma for the first time as adults. While asthma incidence and prevalence are higher in children, asthma-related healthcare use, and mortality are higher in adults. Interestingly, incidence and prevalence of asthma differs by sex across the lifespan. Pre-pubertal boys have a higher asthma incidence, prevalence, and hospitalization rate than girls of the same age, but this trend reverses during adolescence (3). Females continue to have a higher burden of asthma than males well into the 5th decade of life. However, the female-male gap in asthma burden narrows around the 5th decade. Some even suggest that the sex differential in asthma incidence may reverse again, following a sharp increase in asthma incidence in males around the 4th decade of life (3). The sex reversal in asthma burden around major reproductive events suggests that sex hormones may play a role in the etiology of asthma.

The current evidence suggests that asthma is a complex multifactorial disorder and its etiology is increasingly attributed to interactions between genetic susceptibility, host factors, and environmental exposures. These include environmental factors (air pollution, pollens, mold and other aeroallergens, and weather), host factors (obesity, nutritional factors, infections, allergic sensitization), and genetic factors (asthma susceptibility loci on genes). Although underlying mechanisms of asthma are not yet fully understood, they may include airway inflammation, control of airway tone and reactivity (4). It is also now recognized that asthma may not be a single disease but a group of heterogeneous phenotypes with different etiologies and prognoses (5). While phenotyping individuals with asthma has been used to help guide clinical management, defining the entity of "asthma" has been a major challenge encountered in research, especially in epidemiological research, where in-depth data collection needs to be balanced with the large number of study participants necessary for adequate power.

This is not an exhaustive or systematic review on all the complexities of asthma epidemiology but aims to provide an epidemiological perspective by comparing and contrasting trends, and discussing the current debate on definitions, environmental risk factors, and long-term consequences of childhood and adult asthma. The roles of genetic factors and gene-environment interactions in the etiology of asthma are described in another article in this series and are therefore not addressed here. Similarly, an article published alongside this article will be covering asthma categories, phenotypes and endotypes, although these topics have been introduced in the present review.

GLOBAL EPIDEMIC OF ASTHMA PREVALENCE—SUBSIDING IN SOME PARTS OF THE WORLD

During the second half of the Twentieth century, notably since the 1960s, a sharp increase in asthma prevalence was observed in a number of developed countries. This observation was a result of repeated cross-sectional surveys of prevalence of asthma, mainly in children but also in adults. As a result of this observation, in the 1990s, a series of epidemiological studies were established across the world to estimate global asthma prevalence and incidence, and identify risk factors associated with these outcomes. These include large multinational studies in children [such as the International Study of Asthma and Allergies in Childhood (ISAAC; http://isaac.auckland.ac.nz/) (6–8)] and in adults [such as the European Community Respiratory Health Survey (ECRHS; http://www.ecrhs.org/) (9)]. These studies confirmed that asthma is one of the most common chronic diseases across the globe in all age groups and there is substantial variation in asthma prevalence worldwide. It is now acknowledged that the prevalence of both childhood and adult asthma may have peaked in some areas, predominantly in high-income countries, whereas an increase may be continuing in low and mid-income countries (10). It is important to note that a reduction in the prevalence of current asthma is determined by improved asthma control and/or reduced asthma incidence at a population level. Thus, a reduction in prevalence of current asthma may well-reflect improved asthma control through increased medication use from more widespread prescribing habits and better compliance. Documenting reductions in asthma incidence is complicated as parallel cohort studies with specific age windows are needed to establish patterns with the comparison group ideally from the same geographical region. These challenges might in part explain why studies from Australia and UK have not consistently shown reductions in asthma prevalence and why temporal trends in European and Asian countries between the 1970s and mid-2000s have been conflicting (4).

Although greater awareness, recognition, and/or diagnostic shifts have been suggested as contributory factors to the steep rise in asthma prevalence observed over the last four decades of the Twentieth century, repeated cross-sectional surveys using objective measures, such as bronchial hyperreactivity, have confirmed that these factors are unlikely to fully explain this epidemic (4). Though the specific elements driving this rise in prevalence have not been established, it is now clear that the reasons almost certainly are linked to changing environmental factors, acting through gene-by-environmental interactions. Given the rapidity with which the prevalence has risen, this argues against alterations to the population's genetic makeup alone.

The increase in asthma prevalence has been paralleled by a similar increase in other allergies such allergic rhinitis and eczema (11). Multiple hypotheses have been proposed to explain this epidemic, and these have been investigated but are still debated in the field. In the late 1980s, it was thought that increased exposure to indoor allergens such as house dust mite, cat, and fungi due to modernization of housing with tighter insulation and the use of plush furniture and carpets may have contributed to increases in asthma and allergies. Also, in 1989, Strachan proposed the "hygiene hypothesis," suggesting that decreased exposure to unhygienic environments in early life may have led to the increased prevalence of these conditions (12). In 2003, Rook et al. proposed a lack of exposure to non-pathogenic microbes and commensal organisms as an alternative explanation for the increased prevalence of asthma and allergic diseases (13). This led to the "microbial diversity" hypothesis that suggests that environments rich in microbial diversity in the gut mucosa and respiratory tract are the key factors in priming and regulating the immune system.

Asthma mortality and hospitalization rates with acute severe asthma attacks also increased in all age groups during the period from 1960 to 1985, with the highest rates of increase in young pre-school children (14). Following this period, during the 1990s and early 2000s, a decreasing trend in severity has been observed. However, despite novel treatments and improved inhalers for the administration of topical therapies, no further improvements in either mortality or hospitalization rates have been observed in the last decade, either in children or in adults (15).

Given that some childhood asthma persists into adulthood, it is possible that the "asthma epidemic" in children during the 1980–90s has subsequently translated into an increased adult prevalence. However, establishing this trend is challenging due to increased trends also affecting adult asthma, variable asthma definitions, heterogeneity of asthma phenotypes, and limited sequential studies within distinct geographical regions.

EPIDEMIOLOGICAL DEFINITIONS OF ASTHMA—PART OF THE CHALLENGE

Definitions are key to our understanding of the epidemiology, pathophysiology and etiology of asthma, and ascertaining similarities or differences between childhood and adult asthma. Yet variation in asthma severity, age-of-asthma onset, allergic vs. non-allergic phenotypes and type of airway inflammation add complexity to the standard definitions used in large population-based studies (16).

Despite attempts to reach a consensus definition for epidemiological studies, as many as 60 different definitions of "childhood asthma" have been used across 122 published studies (17). Although some of these definitions may appear almost identical, the multiplicity in the way the primary outcome is defined can have a substantial impact on the estimated prevalence and risk factors. As an example, the above study has shown that the agreement between four seemingly very similar and commonly used definitions was overall relatively low (61%), and well-over a third of children in a study could move from being considered "asthma cases" to "controls" depending on the definition used (17). These differences need to be considered when interpreting results of meta-analyses of asthma epidemiology.

Some epidemiological definitions are more sensitive while others are more specific, with both scenarios leading to misclassification of asthma status. For example, current asthma defined by "wheezy breathing in the last 12 months in the absence of a cold" is a more sensitive definition than using "doctor-diagnosed asthma" as they do not rely on the individual to seek health advice (18), while the latter is a more specific definition. As such, survey definitions that adopt wheezy breathing effectively estimate a greater asthma prevalence than clinical definitions which may also incorporate objective measures such as the co-presence of bronchial hyperreactivity (19).

Furthermore, it is important to consider the age of the participants. Particularly for early childhood cohort studies, it can be difficult to distinguish between transient wheeze precipitated by viral infections and the onset of true asthma in young children, although in many cases, recurrent wheezing episodes during the first few years of life can represent the early stages of asthma. For adults, prospectively collected data on childhood asthma status can minimize the risk of recall bias, otherwise retrospective recall typically misclassifies relapsed childhood asthma as late-onset asthma and preferentially favors those who have more severe childhood disease (20). For older people at risk of co-morbidity, an asthma diagnosis may be difficult to differentiate from other diseases causing breathlessness, especially chronic obstructive pulmonary disease (COPD), and heart failure.

A consolidated definition of asthma may not be desirable given the emerging consensus in the research community that "asthma" is an umbrella term for several diseases with similar clinical manifestations but different underlying pathophysiological mechanisms (5), often referred to as "asthma endotypes" (21, 22). In this context, symptoms associated with asthma (such as wheeze or cough) and objective measures (such as lung function and biomarkers in blood, exhaled breath, sputum, and/or urine) should be viewed as observable traits (or "phenotypes") (23, 24). However, it is important to note that different mechanisms may give rise to similar or almost identical observable traits, while the same underlying mechanism may also result in distinct phenotypes in different patients (25).

To date, the framework of asthma endotypes remains a theoretical concept (23), but this framework may also help in developing accurate asthma definitions to facilitate further discovery of their underlying mechanisms (23). With increasing interest in endotypes, there have even been calls to abolish the term "asthma" altogether. However, the term "asthma" provides a practical and functional framework for clinicians to manage patients and for scientists to search for mechanisms; and before abolishing it, we first need to propose more useful and meaningful terminology, which will only come through a more thorough understanding of asthma endotypes.

To further this concept, asthma heterogeneity that features multiple different subtypes has major implications for future studies. However, phenotyping asthma from questionnaire data alone seems increasingly insufficient. While previous cluster analyses have been used to identify patient clusters based on asthma symptoms and airway eosinophilia (16), newer statistical techniques such as latent class analyses (LCA) also have the potential to effectively deal with asthma heterogeneity. Essentially, LCA methods are able to identify novel and statistically distinct classes among individuals in a relatively unbiased way, and are based on measured variables that relate to asthma symptoms (26) and/or biomarkers such as bronchial hyperresponsiveness and atopy (27, 28). A notable example that extended the knowledge of the observed wheezing phenotypes in childhood from the TAHS cohort (29) identified a new phenotype known as "intermediate onset wheezers" (30). This class was subsequently found to have persistent deficits in post-bronchodilator FEV_1 in adolescence (31). Thus, while LCA can readily document asthma heterogeneity, it is of most value if associations are shown between the LCA classifications and clinically important asthma outcomes. To assist in the early identification and diagnosis of asthma, there are currently available innovative computational phenotyping methods that leverage complex electronic health record data that have been validated in different practice settings (32, 33). Using natural language processing (NLP) algorithms, asthma is identified via automated chart review based on predetermined asthma criteria (PAC) via a two-step process: (1) finding asthma-related concepts in text that match specified criteria, then (2) assigning an asthma status classification to individual records (34). While this artificial intelligence algorithm is being developed to improve overall asthma care as a population management tool, it can potentially retrieve information for large-scale, multi-center population studies which has previously been an underutilized data source for asthma research.

SEVERE ASTHMA IN ADULTS AND CHILDREN

Severe asthma represents a small subgroup of individuals who have a disproportionately high health burden. The European Respiratory Society (ERS)/American Thoracic Society (ATS) Task Force defines severe asthma as "asthma which requires treatment with high dose of inhaled corticosteroids (ICS) plus a second controller (and/or systemic corticosteroids) to prevent it from becoming "uncontrolled," or which remains "uncontrolled" despite this therapy" (35). This definition applies to both children and adults with asthma, and it is highly likely that the condition we refer to as "severe asthma" is the extreme end of the spectrum for several different asthma endotypes.

There is considerable variation in the prevalence estimates of severe asthma. For example, in has been reported that 4.2% of Swedish adult asthmatic patients in primary care settings have severe disease (36). Surveys in Denmark described a higher proportion of ~8% of severe asthmatics (37), while some studies report that as high as 20% or even more than 30% of asthmatic patients have at least some features of severe disease (38, 39). The proportion of severe asthmatics appears lower in childhood asthma compared to adult asthma (40). For example, in a birth cohort in Sweden, only seven of 329 12-year old asthmatic children had severe asthma as defined by the World Health Organization (WHO) (41), suggesting a prevalence of 0.23% in the general population and 2.1% among children with asthma (42). Among 616 children in a Norwegian birth cohort, 67 had asthma, of whom only three were defined as having a severe disease, with an estimated population prevalence of severe asthma at age 10 years of 0.5, and 4.5% among asthmatic children (43). A study conducted within a birth cohort in Manchester (UK), identified a latent class of persistent troublesome wheezers, comprising children with high number of acute asthma attacks, hospital admissions, and unscheduled healthcare visits, which accounted for ~10% of children with doctor-diagnosed asthma, and 3.2% of the general population (44). These children exhibited numerous features associated with severe asthma including diminished lung function, high FeNO and hyperreactive airways

(44), with a significant loss of lung function between preschool and mid-school age (45). However, when "severe asthma" was defined using ERS/ATS (35) or WHO (41) criteria, only a small number of children were classified as having severe asthma, suggesting that we need to look beyond the amount of medication and disease control when defining severe disease (46).

In the absence of linking data with national pharmaceutical schemes, capturing detailed information on medication use is challenging in epidemiological studies, although such information is critical when defining severe asthma. For example, in children the "maximum treatment" used to define severe asthma includes high doses of ICS or oral corticosteroids, often in combination with add-on therapy with long-acting β-2 agonists (LABA) and/or leukotriene-receptor antagonists (LTRA) (47–49). The limitation of the use of "maximum treatment" is that there may be different reasons for poor asthma control among patients on "maximum treatment," such as the wrong diagnosis (46), non-adherence with medication (50), or therapy-resistant disease (48).

To provide a more useful clinical and research framework for the investigation of severe childhood asthma, Bush et al. have proposed the term "Problematic severe asthma" (PSA) for children who require specialist referral because of the apparent poor response to maximum asthma treatment (48, 49). Once other potential causes of asthma-like symptoms are excluded and asthma diagnosis is confirmed, children with PSA can be broadly divided into three distinct (but occasionally overlapping) groups: Difficult-to-treat (or difficult) asthma (DA); Asthma with co-morbidities ("Asthma plus"); and Severe therapy-resistant asthma (STRA) (49). The main characteristics of DA are that principal factors which contribute to troublesome symptoms are potentially modifiable. These include poor adherence with medication (51), ongoing exposure to adverse environmental factors such as allergens (52–54), tobacco smoke (55), and air pollution (56–58), and psychosocial factors (59–61). If these modifiable factors are addressed, this should result in better asthma control, including improvement in symptoms, and reduction in severe asthma attacks (62, 63). Children with troublesome asthma and comorbid conditions such as food allergy (64), allergic rhinitis (65), and/or obesity (66) are considered to have "Asthma plus" (i.e., asthma + comorbidities). Treatment of these disorders co-occurring with asthma may improve asthma control (65), although there is a paucity of evidence to support this from well-designed randomized intervention trials (67). However, despite interventions and treatments aimed at addressing modifiable factors and comorbidities, some children with DA and Asthma plus may not improve [e.g., because of the continued poor adherence with medications (50, 68), or ongoing high exposure to allergens (69–71)], in which case they should be considered as having refractory DA or refractory Asthma plus (46, 72).

Although there is considerable within-group heterogeneity in each of the above categories, and strict differentiation may be challenging and on occasion not possible, the concepts which distinguish PSA, DA, and STRA are useful in both a research and clinical context (73), and can also be used in adult severe asthma (74).

A number of studies have described differences between childhood and adult severe asthma based on symptom patterns. Severe asthma is predominantly persistent in adults, but much more variable with rapidly evolving severe attacks in children, often remaining symptom-free between the attacks (75, 76). However, we would argue that these differences may have been over-emphasized. It is possible that severe asthmatics who are currently seen in adult clinics reflect the patterns seen in pediatric clinics 10–20 years ago, and that the pattern of severe disease currently seen in pediatric severe asthma clinics may be foreshadowing the severe adult asthma in years to come. It is possible that the differences observed in cross-sectional studies carried out contemporaneously in children and adults can in part be explained by a cohort effect.

Impaired innate anti-viral immunity with diminished interferon induction to rhinovirus has been reported in both children and adults with severe asthma (77–79). A recent study has identified different patterns of cytokine responses by blood mononuclear cells after stimulation with rhinovirus-16 between children with early-onset troublesome asthma compared to those with late-onset mild allergic asthma (80). The synergism between allergic sensitization, high allergen exposure, and viral infection (mostly rhinovirus) has been shown to increase the risk of hospitalization, both in children (52) and in adults (81) with asthma.

One factor strongly associated with severe asthma in children and adolescents is allergic sensitization (82–87). Several studies in recent years have suggested that there may be different classes of sensitization and that some of these sensitization subtypes are more pathologic than others (85, 88, 89). Further studies using component-resolved diagnostics rather than standard skin and blood tests to whole allergen extracts have identified different cross-sectional and longitudinal patterns of component-specific IgE responses associated with different risk of asthma presence, persistence and severity in children (90–93). If the above notion is correct, this may be an indicator of adult severe asthma research and practice in years to come.

ENVIRONMENTAL EXPOSURES ASSOCIATED WITH ASTHMA IN CHILDREN AND ADULTS

Childhood asthma and adult onset asthma are known to share many of the same causes and triggers. While there is stronger evidence on the role of environmental factors as triggers than causes, there is increasing evidence for interactions among and between environmental and other intrinsic factors, such as genetics and atopy, to potentially cause asthma. The vast majority of childhood onset asthma manifests as an allergic phenotype, while there is a predominance of the non-allergic phenotype in adult onset asthma. However, both allergic and non-allergic asthma can exhibit individual responses to both allergic and non-allergic airborne triggers such as animal hair and dander, pollen, and mold (fungal) spores, food allergens, tobacco smoke, or other pollutant exposures (**Table 1**). Other than this table that provides key references to the main environmental exposures associated with asthma across the lifespan, the typical non-allergic, food and animal triggers of asthma are not described further in this chapter. Subsequent text has focused on the relationships between outdoor, indoor and workplace air pollutants and allergens and asthma, followed by a section on lifestyle factors such as obesity, diet, and breastfeeding.

Parental and Personal Smoking

In utero maternal smoking and parental smoking in early life has been shown to be temporally associated with increased asthma in young children (116). Recent evidence from multi-generational studies suggest that grandmaternal smoking while the mother is *in utero* and paternal smoking during his adolescence can independently increase the risk of subsequent offspring childhood asthma. These findings suggest that tobacco smoking may cause heritable modifications of the epigenome, which increase the risk of asthma in future generations (128).

Smoking also seems to interact with sex. Female smokers had a higher prevalence of asthma than female non-smokers, but this difference was less frequent for males, suggesting that females may be more susceptible. Many studies have found that personal smoking predisposes an individual to increased risk of incident or new-onset asthma, although smoking-onset in adolescence, or adulthood typically occurs after early-onset asthma (119). As non-atopic asthma becomes increasingly common compared with atopic asthma in adults, this is most likely because this phenotype frequently coincides with a substantial history of cigarette smoking and its potential to predispose to chronic airflow limitation (119, 120, 129). Smokers with asthma form a distinct group that are more likely to have suboptimal asthma control (119) and develop asthma-COPD overlap syndrome (ACOS) in later life, characterized by incompletely reversed airflow obstruction following an inhaled bronchodilator (130).

From an epidemiological viewpoint, smoking is common in people with asthma, with around one-quarter of adults from 70 countries receiving recent asthma treatment also reporting to be current smokers (2). Some evidence suggests that people with asthma may be more likely to smoke, and this was seen especially in adolescents who have more severe disease (130).

Outdoor Air Pollutants

Outdoor air pollution almost certainly has a major global impact on asthma for children and adults, especially in China and India (121). Worldwide, in 2015, 9–23 million and 5–10 million annual asthma emergency room visits have been attributed to the outdoor air pollutants ozone and particulate matter with an aerodynamic diameter $<2.5\ \mu m$ ($PM_{2.5}$), respectively.(Exposure to PM_1 has been found to increase the risk of asthma and asthma-related symptoms, especially among boys, and those with allergic predisposition (122). Residential markers of traffic-related air pollution, including nitrogen dioxide (NO_2) exposure and distance to major roads, have been associated with increased risk for new-onset asthma, persistence of asthma and current asthma in a middle-aged, asthma-enriched, population-based cohort (125). In a natural experiment of 60 young to middle-aged adults with mild-to-moderate asthma, when compared with walking in the less polluted Hyde Park in London, walking along Oxford Street was associated with reductions in lung function, neutrophilic inflammation and airway acidification (126). These changes were greater for individuals with moderate asthma compared with mild disease at baseline.

Outdoor Allergens

Exposure to ambient grass pollen is an important trigger for childhood asthma exacerbations requiring emergency department attendance and this has been recently confirmed by a systemic review (99). There is also scant evidence on the role of early life exposure to pollen in the development of childhood asthma (131). However, less evidence is available on the role of pollen in adult asthma (132), except in "Thunderstorm asthma" which is related to a combination of factors as described below.

In relation to other outdoor allergens, increasing evidence indicates that asthmatic children are susceptible to exacerbations that lead to hospitalization when exposed to outdoor fungal spores (104). Furthermore, high concentrations of outdoor fungal/mold exposure on peak days have been linked to asthma exacerbation and mortality in adults (103, 133, 134). IgE sensitization to fungal species is associated with increased asthma severity, neutrophilic inflammation, and reduced lung function consistent with ACOS (105).

Thunderstorm Asthma

Thunderstorm asthma is defined as epidemics that occur during or shortly after a thunderstorm, where individuals affected would experience asthma-related symptoms such as breathlessness, wheezing and coughing. "Thunderstorm asthma" (106, 107) is the outcome of a complex interaction between multiple factors but not necessarily any one of them individually. Under certain weather conditions such as a thunderstorm, pollen grains may swell and burst to form fine respirable particles that are sufficiently small to enter the lower respiratory tract and precipitate severe asthma in those susceptible. This can occur in sensitized individuals who may or may not have a prior history of asthma or asthma symptoms, but who often have a history of allergic rhinitis. Fungal spore allergens may also be involved (133, 134).

On the 21st of November 2016, Melbourne, Australia, experienced a thunderstorm asthma health emergency (106, 107) that exceeded all previously reported thunderstorm asthma events [mainly in the UK and Australia (135, 136)]. In addition to a 4.3-fold increase in emergency attendances for acute respiratory distress symptoms after adjustment for temporal trends (107), nine deaths over the subsequent 10-day period were attributed to asthma as the primary cause (137). This mortality statistic was 50% more than expected based on the average for the same period over the previous 3 years (137), with a total of 10 deaths (immediate and delayed) attributed to the specific epidemic.

Indoor Environment

Indoor pollutants such as products of combustion, including PM and NO_2, and airborne allergens have been the subject of intense scrutiny as determinants of asthma given that most of our time is spent indoors.

TABLE 1 | Environmental exposures associated with asthma spanning childhood to adulthood.

Environmental exposure	Feature	Children	Adolescents	Adults
ALLERGIC				
Airborne triggers - House dust mite (HDM) - Animal hair and dander - Pollen exposure - Mold (fungal) spores - Thunderstorm asthma	HDM aeroallergen is a perennial asthma trigger linked to asthma incidence in high-risk children	(94–96)	(94)	(94)
	Association between pet allergen exposure and asthma is conflicting and non-conclusive	(94, 97, 98)	(98)	(98)
	Grass pollen triggers asthma exacerbations requiring emergency department attendances	(99)	(99)	
	Indoor fungal spore exposure can worsen asthma control; decreased visible indoor mold reduces symptoms but not PEFM variability	(100, 101)	(100, 101)	(100, 101)
	High outdoor Alternaria exposure may contribute to severe asthma/ respiratory arrest (ages 11–25)	(102)	(103)	(103)
	Fungal spores, especially Cladosporium are associated with asthma hospitalization (ages 2–17)	(104)	(104)	
	IgE sensitization to mycoses linked to neutrophilic airway inflammation and lower lung function			(105)
	Thunderstorm asthma can be triggered by outdoor pollen, and possibly fungal, spores	(106, 107)	(106, 107)	(106, 107)
Food allergens ($n = 170$), e.g.,	In asthma, c/w non-atopy, odds for current asthma increased 3.8-fold if food allergy was likely	(108)	(108)	(108)
- Egg white - Peanut	Food allergy is an uncommon trigger in asthma, but may present as life-threatening asthma, especially to peanut and other tree nut allergens	(109, 110)		
- Tree nuts - Shellfish - Cows milk	Co-existing, poorly-controlled asthma is a risk factor for severe or fatal food-induced anaphylaxis	(110, 111)		
Occupational sensitizing agents (with latency)	Extensive lists of occupational asthmagens known to cause new-onset occupational asthma and/or exacerbate pre-existing asthma[†] - Sensitizing HMW agents (e.g., plant allergens like flour, flowers, latex; animal allergens by animal handlers and lab workers; biological enzymes; fungi-yeasts) - Sensitizing LMW agents (e.g., chemicals like isocyanates, reactive dyes, industrial cleaning/sterilizing agents; metals; pharmaceuticals like antibiotics, opiates; solder flux; wood dusts)		(112–115)	(112–115)
NON-ALLERGIC				
Non-allergic triggers - Respiratory viral infections - Cold air - Humidity - Exercise	Typically trigger variations in asthma symptoms and airflow limitation, and their presence increases the probability that the individual has asthma	(94)	(94)	(94)
Tobacco smoke exposure - Parental smoking	Parental smoking linked to increased incidence of childhood asthma and wheeze	(116)		
- Second-hand smoke exposure	Incident asthma from regular smoking from late childhood; may be greater for those non-allergic compared with allergic, and for those exposed to maternal smoking *in utero*	(117, 118)	(117, 118)	
- Personal smoking	Personal smoking may worsen asthma control/ exacerbations		(119)	(119)
	Personal smoking predisposes to post-BD airflow obstruction and asthma-COPD overlap			(120)
Traffic-related air pollution (TrAP)	Air pollutants (O_3, $PM_{2.5}$) linked to new asthma cases and increased ED admissions globally	(121)	(121)	(121)
- Car exhaust fumes	Long-term exposure to PM_1 may worsen asthma, especially for young males with childhood allergy	(122)	(122)	
	Pollution-related decline in FEV_1 growth was similar between those with and without asthma	(123, 124)	(123, 124)	
	Residential TrAP may contribute to new-onset and persistence of asthma in middle-aged adults			(125)
	Natural experiment of diesel exhaust exposure and adverse short-term changes in spirometry			(126)
Household air pollution (HAP)	Non-polluting home heating improved asthma symptoms, days off school, and healthcare utilization	(127)		
Occupational agents (no latency)	Airway irritants (e.g., chlorine, ammonia) - Irritant occupational asthma - Work exacerbated (pre-existing) asthma		(113, 114)	(113, 114)

BD, bronchodilator; COPD, chronic obstructive pulmonary disease; HMW, high molecular weight; FEV_1, forced expiratory volume in 1 second; LMW, low molecular weight; O_3, ozone; PM, particulate matter.

[†]A web-based list of asthmagens can be found at www.occupationalasthma.com.

There is substantial evidence to suggest that indoor allergens generated by house dust mite, mold and cat are triggers for both childhood and adult asthma, especially in those sensitized (100–102). However, their role in the etiology of asthma is not clear. On the other hand, primary prevention trials on reduction of allergen exposure in early life have failed to detect any benefits. Some observational studies have even reported exposure to allergens in infancy may help develop tolerance and reduce the risk of asthma. However, the evidence is not consistent. Interestingly, there is increasing evidence on this tolerance hypothesis in the etiology of food allergy in which a clinical trial has shown that early consumption of peanuts can reduce the development of peanut allergy (138, 139). These findings suggest that it may be worth exploring this notion of early exposure to allergens leading to development of tolerance, which in turn may reduce the risk of developing asthma.

Occupational Exposures

Occupational exposures to asthmagens or inciting sensitizing agents are common and often under-recognized causes of work-related asthma (WRA). WRA includes two distinct subtypes: work-aggravated/exacerbated asthma (WEA) occurring in individuals with pre-existing asthma, and occupational asthma (OA) occurring in individuals without previous asthma. OA is typically subclassified into immunoglobulin (Ig)-E-mediated or sensitizer-induced OA (90%) and irritant-induced occupational asthma (10%) (140). A diagnosis of WRA requires the objective diagnosis of asthma with symptoms temporally related to the individual's place of employment (141). Over 250 agents may potentially cause sensitization and possibly occupational asthma (OA), and comprehensive lists are available (**Table 1**) (112–115). Briefly, the two main classes of sensitizing agents, namely high molecular weight (HMW) and low molecular weight (LMW) agents can cause sensitizer-induced asthma which is usually after a latency period and this may contrast the frequent rapid action of irritant agent exposure. A web-based list of agents can be found at www.occupationalasthma.com.

Differentiating sensitizer-induced OA from WEA can be a major challenge for managing clinicians. The time-to-diagnosis of sensitizer-induced OA varies but is usually made between 2 and 4 years following the onset of work-related symptoms, and this timeframe is substantially shorter for the diagnosis of WEA as these individuals are usually medically managed for pre-existing asthma (142). Among compensation claims, confirmed OA diagnoses most have a causative sensitizing agent identified (143).

Despite challenges in estimating the true incidence of OA, around 10–20% of all adult-onset asthma is thought to be caused by respiratory sensitizers and/or irritants in the occupational setting. Of note, this figure can vary widely (from 4 to 58%) (144) and is largely derived from populations in high income countries (144–146). To contrast, work-related exacerbations can occur frequently in 20–25% of working adults who have pre-existing asthma (147), although objective evidence of poorer asthma control is often difficult to demonstrate (140). While past under-recognition and/or under-reporting of OA might have obscured changing trends over recent decades, the health care industry has successfully reduced the risk of latex-induced allergy and OA by substituting natural rubber latex (NRL) gloves for powder-free, protein-poor NRL gloves. This successful approach for exposure minimization highlights the benefit of identifying those at risk from occupationally-related asthma and minimizing potentially harmful exposures.

Lifestyle Factors

Although already mentioned as an "asthma-plus" co-morbidity, the prevalence of obesity in countries in which a Westernized diet predominates is now of epidemic proportions. These dietary patterns feature a high calorie intake which is high in saturated fat and refined sugars and associated with a high glycaemic index, as well as low nutritional value in terms of dietary fiber and vitamins. While this "obesogenic diet" may lack antioxidant and anti-inflammatory properties (148), a meta-analysis has found being overweight and obese to be associated with a dose-response increase in incident asthma in adults (149). While this review did not find significant sex-related differences, female obesity has been associated with a pauci-eosinophil and non-atopic asthma endotype that is symptom-predominant and less steroid-responsive in previous cluster and LCA (16, 28). For all individuals with otherwise poorly controlled asthma, the behavior of avoiding strenuous exercise might confuse severe disease with well-controlled asthma, and this in turn can lead to poorer fitness levels and a propensity to weight gain (94). This is of particular importance to children with asthma, at a time when lifestyle patterns are being especially shaped by external factors.

The role of infant breastfeeding in the prevention of asthma is debated, however this has been largely clarified by findings from the TAHS cohort. This longitudinal study of participants who were followed between childhood and middle-age showed that breast feeding reduced the risk of childhood asthma and conversely increased the risk of adult asthma, but for only those with a familial predisposition (150). In 2015, a systematic review summarized the overall estimate for a longer compared with shorter duration of breastfeeding to be modestly protective for asthma in later childhood-adolescence [odds ratio 0.90 (95%CI 0.84–0.97), $I^2 = 63\%$] (151). While the effect was stronger when restricted to studies from lower-to-middle income countries, no association was seen when restricting the meta-analysis to only cohort studies. The overall conclusion was that the evidence was of low quality. The authors primarily hypothesized that breastfeeding-related reductions in childhood wheeze might relate to the known beneficial immunological factors which could reduce childhood viral infections that predispose to asthma.

IMPACT OF CHILDHOOD AND ADULT ASTHMA ON LUNG FUNCTION TRAJECTORIES AND COPD

Childhood Asthma and Lung Function

Studies that have investigated the impact of childhood asthma on lung function from childhood to adolescence have found that different asthma phenotypes differentially impact long-term lung function outcomes. This is particularly relevant to longitudinal asthma phenotypes, which earlier studies attempted to identify by manually classifying the change of symptoms, but more recent studies have identified distinct longitudinal phenotypes using advanced statistical techniques such as Latent Class Analysis (LCA) as mentioned above. Overall, the use of LCA has led to the identification of more asthma phenotypes and therefore has helped to better disentangle the long-term effects of childhood asthma. The majority of studies have shown that persistent wheeze is related to reduced lung function development throughout adolescence (31, 45, 152, 153), while some suggest the effects of persistent wheeze and relapsed wheeze on lung function are established from mid-childhood, without further decline in tracking of FEV_1 over time (154, 155). It has also been reported that childhood asthma associated with allergic comorbidities, such as eczema and allergic rhinitis, has persistent lung function impairment from birth to adolescence as compared to asthma without such comorbidities (156). These findings have led to the hypothesis that asthma with atopic dermatitis and allergic rhinitis may represent a specific phenotype originating *in utero* (156).

Several longitudinal studies have investigated the long-term impacts of childhood asthma on lung function decline and COPD. Childhood asthma has been associated with adult lung function deficits and increased risk of COPD (157–159). While a number of studies have reported that childhood asthma itself has no impact on adult lung function decline (154, 157, 158, 160), a study that collected childhood asthma status retrospectively has reported that it is associated with greater lung function decline, which may be related to recall bias (161). More recent findings suggest that childhood asthma is related to longitudinal lung function trajectories that are "below normal" within both the general population (162) and asthmatics (163).

Overall, current evidence suggests that many children with childhood asthma/wheeze, especially early persistent asthma/wheeze, may have reduced airway and lung development and not reach their peak lung function potential as influenced by pre-determined lung function trajectories. These lung function deficits may track (or persist) into adulthood without additional progressive loss. However, it is not clear whether childhood asthma can directly affect the rate of lung function decline unless it continues as adult asthma.

Adult Asthma and Lung Function

While asthma in adults is often the persistence or relapse of asthma from childhood, "true" adult onset asthma is a distinct phenotype most often related to environmental risk factors such as smoking (164). The impact of adult asthma on lung function outcomes appears to vary by phenotype including age-at-onset. It has been shown that both early and late onset adult current asthma were associated with a reduction in lung function and an increased risk of fixed airflow obstruction at 45 years, with the effect of early onset asthma being greater than late onset asthma (165–167). These findings differ from the above mentioned systematic review and meta-analysis which found greater levels of fixed airflow obstruction for those with late-onset adult asthma, which most likely relates to inaccurate retrospective recall of childhood asthma by adults (164).

Further evidence from longitudinal studies suggests that adults with asthma have greater lung function decline than those without asthma (168–170). While both early and late onset adult asthma seem to be associated with faster lung function decline, the decline associated with early onset adult asthma is greater than that with late onset adult asthma (167).

An important question is whether we can disentangle the components of lung function deficits in adults with asthma over the life course. Lung function deficits in those with early onset adult asthma may result from both the tracking of reduced lung function from childhood and additional loss from a greater rate of decline in adulthood (167, 171). It has been suggested that adults who developed new-onset asthma had reduced lung function at baseline (172, 173), but it is unknown whether lower lung function before early adulthood, in the absence of childhood asthma, predisposes to "true" adult onset asthma. However, asthma/wheeze status in early life is often forgotten by adults leading to misclassification of "true" adult-onset asthma (20). On the other hand, lung function deficits in adult-onset asthma after peak lung function has been attained are also likely to be due to faster lung function decline.

OTHER HEALTH IMPACTS OF CHILDHOOD AND ADULT ASTHMA

Another major impact of asthma is through its associated additional morbidities, including a predisposition to serious infections such as bacterial pneumonia from a higher nasopharyngeal carriage of *Streptococcus pneumoniae* (174). Although not well-understood, asthma-related chronic airway inflammation with damaged airway mucosa and immunomodulating treatments such as inhaled corticosteroids have been implicated, and lower antibody levels in response to the Pneumococcal vaccine have also been observed (174). In addition to a 2.4-fold increased risk for invasive pneumococcal disease (175), susceptibility to respiratory and non-respiratory infections (such as Herpes zoster and *E. coli* bacteraemia) in never smokers with asthma has been compared with the relative risk of diabetes (176). This susceptibility to infection supports the hypothesis of weaker T_H1 immune responses associated with T_H2-related disease. However, recommendations for Pneumococcal immunization are inconsistent (94) suggesting more evidence is needed to gain consensus of its benefits (177, 178).

Adult asthma is also associated with a number of chronic conditions. The associations between childhood asthma and allergies such as eczema and food allergy are very well-established. Adult asthma is known to be commonly associated with diabetes, osteoporosis, metabolic syndrome, cardiovascular diseases, and issues with mental illness such as anxiety and depression while there are a number of other morbidities that have been linked (179). When a chronic condition is present in people with asthma, that is known as asthma co-morbidity. Almost two-thirds (62.6%) of patients with asthma have at least one comorbid condition with 16% having four co-morbidities (180). This prevalence of these morbidities in asthmatics is too high to be simply due to the chance development of chronic conditions while aging but these associations do not imply causality. The etiology of asthma co-morbidities may be linked to asthma itself, other morbidities, shared mechanisms, shared environmental, and/or shared genetic risk factors. Regardless of the etiology, it is well-known that asthma comorbidities are associated with worse outcomes for the patients and the healthcare systems (181), and managing asthma comorbidities has been associated with significant improvement in its prognosis. Revising guidelines on to handle comorbidities may lead to a more targeted treatment for comorbidities and more patient-centered asthma management, which in turn lead to better outcomes.

SUMMARY

The evidence on the trends and environmental determinants for childhood and adult asthma are similar, although the evidence is stronger for childhood asthma, which is partly related to the stronger attention that childhood asthma has received from the research community. The global epidemic of asthma is continuing, especially in low to middle income countries, although it has subsided in some high income countries. Epidemiological research has helped to uncover some important environmental determinants that trigger asthma, but the role of environmental factors in the etiology of asthma remains largely unknown. Research into interactions between potential determinants may help tease out the etiology. Therefore, there is an urgent need to further investigate the complex mechanisms driving the interrelationship between environmental and genetic determinants to identify high risk groups and key modifiable exposures. Given the long term impact of both childhood and adult asthma, we would argue that our focus going forward to reduce the health burden of asthma should be firmly on improving not only short-term symptoms, but also the long-term respiratory and other health outcomes (182).

AUTHOR CONTRIBUTIONS

The authors alone are responsible for the content and writing of the article. AC, SD, and JP wrote sections of the initial draft of the manuscript which was then critically revised for flow and important content areas by SD and JP. All authors approved the final version of the manuscript.

REFERENCES

1. Network GA. *The Global Asthma Report*, Auckland, New Zealand. (2018).
2. To T, Stanojevic S, Moores G, Gershon AS, Bateman ED, Cruz AA, et al. Global asthma prevalence in adults: findings from the cross-sectional world health survey. *BMC Public Health.* (2012) 12:5. doi: 10.1186/1471-2458-12-204
3. Fuhlbrigge AL, Jackson B, Wright R. Gender and asthma. *Immunol Allergy Clin North Am.* (2002) 22:10. doi: 10.1016/S0889-8561(02)00022-X
4. Eder W, Ege MJ, von Mutius E. The asthma epidemic. *N Engl J Med.* (2006) 355:2226–35. doi: 10.1056/NEJMra054308
5. Pavord ID, Beasley R, Agusti A, Anderson GP, Bel E, Brusselle G, et al. After asthma: redefining airways diseases. *Lancet.* (2018) 391:350–400. doi: 10.1016/S0140-6736(17)30879-6
6. Ellwood P, Asher MI, Beasley R, Clayton TO, Stewart AW, Committee IS. The international study of asthma and allergies in childhood (ISAAC): phase three rationale and methods. *Int J Tubercul Lung Dis.* (2005) 9:10–6.
7. Weiland SK, Bjorksten B, Brunekreef B, Cookson WO, von Mutius E, Strachan DP, et al. Phase II of the international study of asthma and allergies in childhood (ISAAC II): rationale and methods. *Eur Respirat J.* (2004) 24:406–12. doi: 10.1183/09031936.04.00090303
8. Asher MI, Keil U, Anderson HR, Beasley R, Crane J, Martinez F, et al. International Study of Asthma and Allergies in Childhood (ISAAC): rationale and methods. *Eur Respirat J.* (1995) 8:483–91. doi: 10.1183/09031936.95.0803 0483
9. Variations in the prevalence of respiratory symptoms, self-reported asthma attacks, and use of asthma medication in the European Community Respiratory Health Survey (ECRHS). *Eur Respir J.* (1996) 9:687–95. doi: 10.1183/09031936.96.09040687
10. Asher MI, Montefort S, Bjorksten B, Lai CK, Strachan DP, Weiland SK, et al. Worldwide time trends in the prevalence of symptoms of asthma, allergic rhinoconjunctivitis, and eczema in childhood: ISAAC Phases One and Three repeat multicountry cross-sectional surveys. *Lancet.* (2006) 368:733–43. doi: 10.1016/S0140-6736(06)69283-0
11. Addo-Yobo EO, Woodcock A, Allotey A, Baffoe-Bonnie B, Strachan D, Custovic A. Exercise-induced bronchospasm and atopy in Ghana: two surveys ten years apart. *PLoS Med.* (2007) 4:e70. doi: 10.1371/journal.pmed.0040070
12. Strachan DP. Hay fever, hygiene, and household size. *BMJ.* (1989) 299:2. doi: 10.1136/bmj.299.6710.1259
13. Rook GA, Martinelli R, Brunet LR. Innate immune responses to mycobacteria and the downregulation of atopic responses. *Curr Opin Allergy Clin Immunol.* (2003) 3:5. doi: 10.1097/00130832-200310000-00003
14. Mitchell EA. International trends in hospital admission rates for asthma. *Arch Dis Childhood.* (1985) 60:376–8. doi: 10.1136/adc.60.4.376
15. Ebmeier S, Thayabaran D, Braithwaite I, Benamara C, Weatherall M, Beasley R. Trends in international asthma mortality: analysis of data from the WHO Mortality Database from 46 countries (1993–2012). *Lancet.* (2017) 390:935–45. doi: 10.1016/S0140-6736(17)31448-4
16. Haldar P, Pavord ID, Shaw DE, Berry MA, Thomas M, Brightling CE, et al. Cluster analysis and clinical asthma phenotypes. *Am J Respir Crit Care Med.* (2008) 178:218–24. doi: 10.1164/rccm.200711-1754OC
17. Van Wonderen KE, Van Der Mark LB, Mohrs J, Bindels PJ, Van Aalderen WM, Ter Riet G. Different definitions in childhood asthma: how dependable is the dependent variable? *Eur Respir J.* (2010) 36:48–56. doi: 10.1183/09031936.00154409
18. Jenkins MA, Clarke JR, Carlin JB, Robertson CF, Hopper JL, Dalton MF, et al. Validation of questionnaire and bronchial hyperresponsiveness against respiratory physician assessment in the diagnosis of asthma. *Int J Epidemiol.* (1996) 25:609–16. doi: 10.1093/ije/25.3.609
19. Peat JK. Epidemiology and the Changing Prevalence of Asthma. In: Walls RS, Jenkins CR, editors. *Understanding Asthma A Management Companion.* Sydney, NSW: MacLennan and Petty Pty Limited. (2000). p. 11–19.
20. Burgess JA, Walters EH, Byrnes GB, Wharton C, Jenkins MA, Abramson MJ, et al. Who remembers whether they had asthma as children? *J Asthma.* (2006) 43:727–30. doi: 10.1080/02770900601028587
21. Anderson GP. Endotyping asthma: new insights into key pathogenic mechanisms in a complex, heterogeneous disease. *Lancet.* (2008) 372:1107–19. doi: 10.1016/S0140-6736(08)61452-X
22. Lotvall J, Akdis CA, Bacharier LB, Bjermer L, Casale TB, Custovic A, et al. Asthma endotypes: a new approach to classification of disease entities within the asthma syndrome. *J Allergy Clin Immunol.* (2011) 127:355–60. doi: 10.1016/j.jaci.2010.11.037

23. Custovic A, Ainsworth J, Arshad H, Bishop C, Buchan I, Cullinan P, et al. The Study Team for Early Life Asthma Research (STELAR) consortium 'Asthma e-lab': team science bringing data, methods and investigators together. *Thorax.* (2015) 70:799–801. doi: 10.1136/thoraxjnl-2015-206781
24. Belgrave DC, Custovic A, Simpson A. Characterizing wheeze phenotypes to identify endotypes of childhood asthma, and the implications for future management. *Exp Rev Clin Immunol.* (2013) 9:921–36. doi: 10.1586/1744666X.2013.836450
25. Belgrave D, Henderson J, Simpson A, Buchan I, Bishop C, Custovic A. Disaggregating asthma: big investigation versus big data. *J Allergy Clin Immunol.* (2017) 139:400–7. doi: 10.1016/j.jaci.2016.11.003
26. Makikyro EM, Jaakkola MS, Jaakkola JJ. Subtypes of asthma based on asthma control and severity: a latent class analysis. *Resp Res.* (2017) 18:24. doi: 10.1186/s12931-017-0508-y
27. Weinmayr G, Keller F, Kleiner A, du Prel JB, Garcia-Marcos L, Batlles-Garrido J, et al. Asthma phenotypes identified by latent class analysis in the ISAAC phase II Spain study. *Clin Exp Allergy.* (2013) 43:223–32. doi: 10.1111/cea.12035
28. Jeong A, Imboden M, Hansen S, Zemp E, Bridevaux PO, Lovison G, et al. Heterogeneity of obesity-asthma association disentangled by latent class analysis, the SAPALDIA cohort. *Respir Med.* (2017) 125:25–32. doi: 10.1016/j.rmed.2017.02.014
29. Martinez FD, Wright AL, Taussig LM, Holberg CJ, Halonen M, Morgan WJ. Asthma and wheezing in the first six years of life. The Group Health Medical Associates. *N Engl J Med.* (1995) 332:133–8. doi: 10.1056/NEJM199501193320301
30. Lodge CJ, Zaloumis S, Lowe AJ, Gurrin LC, Matheson MC, Axelrad C, et al. Early-life risk factors for childhood wheeze phenotypes in a high-risk birth cohort. *J Pediatr.* (2014) 164:289–94 e1–2. doi: 10.1016/j.jpeds.2013.09.056
31. Lodge CJ, Lowe AJ, Allen KJ, Zaloumis S, Gurrin LC, Matheson MC, et al. Childhood wheeze phenotypes show less than expected growth in FEV1 across adolescence. *Am J Respir Crit Care Med.* (2014) 189:1351–8. doi: 10.1164/rccm.201308-1487OC
32. Wi CI, Sohn S, Ali M, Krusemark E, Ryu E, Liu H, et al. Natural language processing for asthma ascertainment in different practice settings. *J Allergy Clin Immunol Pract.* (2018) 6:126–31. doi: 10.1016/j.jaip.2017.04.041
33. Wi CI, Sohn S, Rolfes MC, Seabright A, Ryu E, Voge G, et al. Application of a natural language processing algorithm to asthma ascertainment. an automated chart review. *Am J Respir Crit Care Med.* (2017) 196:430–7. doi: 10.1164/rccm.201610-2006OC
34. Sohn S, Wang Y, Wi CI, Krusemark EA, Ryu E, Ali MH, et al. Clinical documentation variations and NLP system portability: a case study in asthma birth cohorts across institutions. *J Am Med Inform Assoc.* (2018) 25:353–9. doi: 10.1093/jamia/ocx138
35. Chung KF, Wenzel SE, Brozek JL, Bush A, Castro M, Sterk PJ, et al. International ERS/ATS guidelines on definition, evaluation and treatment of severe asthma. *Eur Resp J.* (2014) 43:343–73. doi: 10.1183/09031936.00202013
36. Larsson K, Stallberg B, Lisspers K, Telg G, Johansson G, Thuresson M, et al. Prevalence and management of severe asthma in primary care: an observational cohort study in Sweden (PACEHR). *Respir Res.* (2018) 19:12. doi: 10.1186/s12931-018-0719-x
37. von Bulow A, Kriegbaum M, Backer V, Porsbjerg C. The prevalence of severe asthma and low asthma control among Danish adults. *J Allergy Clin Immunol Pract.* (2014) 2:759–67. doi: 10.1016/j.jaip.2014.05.005
38. Bleecker ER. *The Epidemiology of Severe Asthma: The TENOR Study and SARP (NIH).* Available online at: http://wwwworldallergyorg/educational_programs/world_allergy_forum/barcelona2008/bleeckerphp
39. Mincheva R, Ekerljung L, Bossios A, Lundback B, Lotvall J. High prevalence of severe asthma in a large random population study. *J Allergy Clin Immunol.* (2018) 141:2256–64.e2. doi: 10.1016/j.jaci.2017.07.047
40. Rusconi F, Fernandes RM, Pijnenburg MWH, Grigg J, Collaboration SCR. European Lung Foundation severe asthma patient advisory g. The Severe Paediatric Asthma Collaborative in Europe (SPACE) ERS Clinical Research Collaboration: enhancing participation of children with asthma in therapeutic trials of new biologics and receptor blockers. *Eur Resp J.* (2018) 52:1801665. doi: 10.1183/13993003.01665-2018
41. Bousquet J, Mantzouranis E, Cruz AA, Ait-Khaled N, Baena-Cagnani CE, Bleecker ER, et al. Uniform definition of asthma severity, control, and exacerbations: document presented for the World Health Organization Consultation on Severe Asthma. *J Allergy Clin Immunol.* (2010) 126:926–38. doi: 10.1016/j.jaci.2010.07.019
42. Nordlund B, Melen E, Schultz ES, Gronlund H, Hedlin G, Kull I. Prevalence of severe childhood asthma according to the WHO. *Respir Med.* (2014) 108:1234–7. doi: 10.1016/j.rmed.2014.05.015
43. Lang A, Carlsen KH, Haaland G, Devulapalli CS, Munthe-Kaas M, Mowinckel P, et al. Severe asthma in childhood: assessed in 10 year olds in a birth cohort study. *Allergy.* (2008) 63:1054–60. doi: 10.1111/j.1398-9995.2008.01672.x
44. Belgrave DCM, Simpson A, Semic-Jusufagic A, Murray CS, Buchan I, Pickles A, et al. Joint modeling of parentally reported and physician-confirmed wheeze identifies children with persistent troublesome wheezing. *J Allergy Clin Immunol.* (2013) 132:575–83.e12. doi: 10.1016/j.jaci.2013.05.041
45. Belgrave DC, Buchan I, Bishop C, Lowe L, Simpson A, Custovic A. Trajectories of lung function during childhood. *Am J Respir Crit Care Med.* (2014) 189:1101–9. doi: 10.1164/rccm.201309-1700OC
46. Bush A, Saglani S, Fleming L. Severe asthma: looking beyond the amount of medication. *Lancet Respir Med.* (2017) 5:844–6. doi: 10.1016/S2213-2600(17)30379-X
47. Fitzpatrick AM. Severe asthma in children: lessons learned and future directions. *J Allergy Clin Immunol Pract.* (2016) 4:11–9. quiz 20–1. doi: 10.1016/j.jaip.2015.10.008
48. Bush A, Saglani S. Management of severe asthma in children. *Lancet.* (2010) 376:814–25. doi: 10.1016/S0140-6736(10)61054-9
49. Bush A, Hedlin G, Carlsen KH, de Benedictis F, Lodrup-Carlsen K, Wilson N. Severe childhood asthma: a common international approach? *Lancet.* (2008) 372:1019–21. doi: 10.1016/S0140-6736(08)61422-1
50. Jochmann A, Artusio L, Jamalzadeh A, Nagakumar P, Delgado-Eckert E, Saglani S, et al. Electronic monitoring of adherence to inhaled corticosteroids: an essential tool in identifying severe asthma in children. *Eur Resp J.* (2017) 50:1700910. doi: 10.1183/13993003.00910-2017
51. McDonald VM, Yorke J. Adherence in severe asthma: time to get it right. *Eur Resp J.* (2017) 50:1702191. doi: 10.1183/13993003.02191-2017
52. Murray CS, Poletti G, Kebadze T, Morris J, Woodcock A, Johnston SL, et al. Study of modifiable risk factors for asthma exacerbations: virus infection and allergen exposure increase the risk of asthma hospital admissions in children. *Thorax.* (2006) 61:376–82. doi: 10.1136/thx.2005.042523
53. Tunnicliffe WS, Fletcher TJ, Hammond K, Roberts K, Custovic A, Simpson A, et al. Sensitivity and exposure to indoor allergens in adults with differing asthma severity. *Eur Resp J.* (1999) 13:654–9. doi: 10.1183/09031936.99.13365499
54. Lowe LA, Woodcock A, Murray CS, Morris J, Simpson A, Custovic A. Lung function at age 3 years: effect of pet ownership and exposure to indoor allergens. *Arch Pediatr Adolesc Med.* (2004) 158:996–1001. doi: 10.1001/archpedi.158.10.996
55. Puranik S, Forno E, Bush A, Celedon JC. Predicting severe asthma exacerbations in children. *Am J Respir Crit Care Med.* (2017) 195:854–9. doi: 10.1164/rccm.201606-1213PP
56. Gehring U, Gruzieva O, Agius RM, Beelen R, Custovic A, Cyrys J, et al. Air pollution exposure and lung function in children: the ESCAPE project. *Environ Health Perspect.* (2013) 121:1357–64. doi: 10.1289/ehp.1306770
57. Molter A, Simpson A, Berdel D, Brunekreef B, Custovic A, Cyrys J, et al. A multicentre study of air pollution exposure and childhood asthma prevalence: the ESCAPE project. *Eur Resp J.* (2015) 45:610–24. doi: 10.1183/09031936.00083614
58. Taggart SC, Custovic A, Francis HC, Faragher EB, Yates CJ, Higgins BG, et al. Asthmatic bronchial hyperresponsiveness varies with ambient levels of summertime air pollution. *Eur Resp J.* (1996) 9:1146–54. doi: 10.1183/09031936.96.09061146
59. Osman LM. Psychological factors in asthma control and attack risk. *Thorax.* (2002) 57:190–1. doi: 10.1136/thorax.57.3.190
60. Calam R, Gregg L, Simpson A, Simpson B, Woodcock A, Custovic A. Behavior problems antecede the development of wheeze in childhood: a birth cohort study. *Am J Respir Crit Care Med.* (2005) 171:323–7. doi: 10.1164/rccm.200406-791OC

61. Calam R, Gregg L, Simpson B, Morris J, Woodcock A, Custovic A. Childhood asthma, behavior problems, and family functioning. *J Allergy Clin Immunol.* (2003) 112:499–504. doi: 10.1016/S0091-6749(03)00008-3
62. Saglani S, Fleming L. How to manage a child with difficult asthma? *Exp Rev Respir Med.* (2016) 10:873–9. doi: 10.1080/17476348.2016.1191355
63. Yorke J, Fleming SL, Shuldham C. A systematic review of psychological interventions for children with asthma. *Pediatr Pulmonol.* (2007) 42:114–24. doi: 10.1002/ppul.20464
64. Roberts G. Asthma comorbidities and making progress with food allergy. *Clin Exp Allergy.* (2017) 47:1230–1. doi: 10.1111/cea.13028
65. Deliu M, Belgrave D, Simpson A, Murray CS, Kerry G, Custovic A. Impact of rhinitis on asthma severity in school-age children. *Allergy.* (2014) 69:1515–21. doi: 10.1111/all.12467
66. Wang R, Custovic A, Simpson A, Belgrave DC, Lowe LA, Murray CS. Differing associations of BMI and body fat with asthma and lung function in children. *Pediatr Pulmonol.* (2014) 49:1049–57. doi: 10.1002/ppul.22927
67. Porsbjerg C, Menzies-Gow A. Co-morbidities in severe asthma: clinical impact and management. *Respirology.* (2017) 22:651–61. doi: 10.1111/resp.13026
68. Chan AH, Stewart AW, Harrison J, Camargo CA Jr., Black PN, Mitchell EA. The effect of an electronic monitoring device with audiovisual reminder function on adherence to inhaled corticosteroids and school attendance in children with asthma: a randomised controlled trial. *Lancet Respir Med.* (2015) 3:210–9. doi: 10.1016/S2213-2600(15)00008-9
69. Langley SJ, Goldthorpe S, Craven M, Morris J, Woodcock A, Custovic A. Exposure and sensitization to indoor allergens: association with lung function, bronchial reactivity, and exhaled nitric oxide measures in asthma. *J Allergy Clin Immunol.* (2003) 112:362–8. doi: 10.1067/mai.2003.1654
70. Langley SJ, Goldthorpe S, Craven M, Woodcock A, Custovic A. Relationship between exposure to domestic allergens and bronchial hyperresponsiveness in non-sensitised, atopic asthmatic subjects. *Thorax.* (2005) 60:17–21. doi: 10.1136/thx.2004.027839
71. Langley SJ, Goldthorpe S, Custovic A, Woodcock A. Relationship among pulmonary function, bronchial reactivity, and exhaled nitric oxide in a large group of asthmatic patients. *Ann Allergy Asthma Immunol.* (2003) 91:398–404. doi: 10.1016/S1081-1206(10)61688-2
72. Bush A, Fleming L, Saglani S. Severe asthma in children. *Respirology.* (2017) 22:886–97. doi: 10.1111/resp.13085
73. Pike KC, Levy ML, Moreiras J, Fleming L. Managing problematic severe asthma: beyond the guidelines. *Arch Dis Childhood.* (2018) 103:392–7. doi: 10.1136/archdischild-2016-311368
74. von Bulow A, Backer V, Bodtger U, Soes-Petersen NU, Vest S, Steffensen I, et al. Differentiation of adult severe asthma from difficult-to-treat asthma - Outcomes of a systematic assessment protocol. *Respir Med.* (2018) 145:41–7. doi: 10.1016/j.rmed.2018.10.020
75. Guilbert TW, Bacharier LB, Fitzpatrick AM. Severe asthma in children. *J Allergy Clin Immunol Pract.* (2014) 2:489–500. doi: 10.1016/j.jaip.2014.06.022
76. Ramratnam SK, Bacharier LB, Guilbert TW. Severe asthma in children. *J Allergy Clin Immunol Pract.* (2017) 5:889–98. doi: 10.1016/j.jaip.2017.04.031
77. Jackson DJ, Johnston SL. The role of viruses in acute exacerbations of asthma. *J Allergy Clin Immunol.* (2010) 125:1178–87. quiz 88–9. doi: 10.1016/j.jaci.2010.04.021
78. Kim CK, Callaway Z, Gern JE. Viral Infections and associated factors that promote acute exacerbations of asthma. *Allergy Asthma Immunol Res.* (2018) 10:12–7. doi: 10.4168/aair.2018.10.1.12
79. Edwards MR, Regamey N, Vareille M, Kieninger E, Gupta A, Shoemark A, et al. Impaired innate interferon induction in severe therapy resistant atopic asthmatic children. *Mucosal Immunol.* (2013) 6:797–806. doi: 10.1038/mi.2012.118
80. Custovic A, Belgrave D, Lin L, Bakhsoliani E, Telcian AG, Solari R, et al. Cytokine Responses to rhinovirus and development of asthma, allergic sensitization and respiratory infections during childhood. *Am J Respir Crit Care Med.* (2018) 197, 1265–74. doi: 10.1164/rccm.201708-1762OC
81. Green RM, Custovic A, Sanderson G, Hunter J, Johnston SL, Woodcock A. Synergism between allergens and viruses and risk of hospital admission with asthma: case-control study. *BMJ.* (2002) 324:763. doi: 10.1136/bmj.324.7340.763
82. Fitzpatrick AM, Gaston BM, Erzurum SC, Teague WG, National Institutes of Health/National Heart L, Blood Institute Severe Asthma Research P. Features of severe asthma in school-age children: Atopy and increased exhaled nitric oxide. *J Allergy Clin Immunol.* (2006) 118:1218–25. doi: 10.1016/j.jaci.2006.08.019
83. Frith J, Fleming L, Bossley C, Ullmann N, Bush A. The complexities of defining atopy in severe childhood asthma. *Clin Exp Allergy.* (2011) 41:948–53. doi: 10.1111/j.1365-2222.2011.03729.x
84. Just J, Gouvis-Echraghi R, Rouve S, Wanin S, Moreau D, Annesi-Maesano I. Two novel, severe asthma phenotypes identified during childhood using a clustering approach. *Eur Resp J.* (2012) 40:55–60. doi: 10.1183/09031936.00123411
85. Holt PG, Strickland D, Bosco A, Belgrave D, Hales B, Simpson A, et al. Distinguishing benign from pathologic TH2 immunity in atopic children. *J Allergy Clin Immunol.* (2016) 137:379–87. doi: 10.1016/j.jaci.2015.08.044
86. Konradsen JR, Nordlund B, Onell A, Borres MP, Gronlund H, Hedlin G. Severe childhood asthma and allergy to furry animals: refined assessment using molecular-based allergy diagnostics. *Pediatr Allergy Immunol.* (2014) 25:187–92. doi: 10.1111/pai.12198
87. Sylvestre L, Jegu J, Metz-Favre C, Barnig C, Qi S, de Blay F. Component-based allergen-microarray: Der p 2 and Der f 2 Dust mite sensitization is more common in patients with severe asthma. *J Investig Allergol Clin Immunol.* (2016) 26:141–3. doi: 10.18176/jiaci.0035
88. Simpson A, Tan VY, Winn J, Svensen M, Bishop CM, Heckerman DE, et al. Beyond atopy: multiple patterns of sensitization in relation to asthma in a birth cohort study. *Am J Respir Crit Care Med.* (2010) 181:1200–6. doi: 10.1164/rccm.200907-1101OC
89. Lazic N, Roberts G, Custovic A, Belgrave D, Bishop CM, Winn J, et al. Multiple atopy phenotypes and their associations with asthma: similar findings from two birth cohorts. *Allergy.* (2013) 68:764–70. doi: 10.1111/all.12134
90. Simpson A, Lazic N, Belgrave DCM, Johnson P, Bishop C, Mills C, et al. Patterns of IgE responses to multiple allergen components and clinical symptoms at age 11 years. *J Allerg Clin Immunol.* (2015) 136:1224–31. doi: 10.1016/j.jaci.2015.03.027
91. Custovic A, Sonntag H-J, Buchan IE, Belgrave D, Simpson A, Prosperi MCF. Evolution pathways of IgE responses to grass and mite allergens throughout childhood. Journal of Allergy and Clinical Immunology. (2015) 136:1645–52.e8. doi: 10.1016/j.jaci.2015.03.041
92. Howard R, Belgrave D, Papastamoulis P, Simpson A, Rattray M, Custovic A. Evolution of IgE responses to multiple allergen components throughout childhood. *J Allergy Clin Immunol.* (2018) 142:1322–30. doi: 10.1016/j.jaci.2017.11.064
93. Fontanella S, Frainay C, Murray CS, Simpson A, Custovic A. Machine learning to identify pairwise interactions between specific IgE antibodies and their association with asthma: a cross-sectional analysis within a population-based birth cohort. *PLoS Med.* (2018) 15:e1002691. doi: 10.1371/journal.pmed.1002691
94. Global Initiative for Asthma. *Global Strategy for Asthma Management and Prevention 2018.* Available online at: www.ginasthma.org Accessed 30.03.2018
95. Celedon JC, Milton DK, Ramsey CD, Litonjua AA, Ryan L, Platts-Mills TA, et al. Exposure to dust mite allergen and endotoxin in early life and asthma and atopy in childhood. *J Allergy Clin Immunol.* (2007) 120:144–9. doi: 10.1016/j.jaci.2007.03.037
96. Lodge CJ, Lowe AJ, Gurrin LC, Hill DJ, Hosking CS, Khalafzai RU, et al. House dust mite sensitization in toddlers predicts current wheeze at age 12 years. *J Allergy Clin Immunol.* (2011) 128:782–8.e9. doi: 10.1016/j.jaci.2011.06.038
97. Lodrup Carlsen KC, Roll S, Carlsen KH, Mowinckel P, Wijga AH, Brunekreef B, et al. Does pet ownership in infancy lead to asthma or allergy at school age? Pooled analysis of individual participant data from 11 European birth cohorts. *PLoS ONE.* (2012) 7:e43214. doi: 10.1371/journal.pone.0043214
98. Takkouche B, Gonzalez-Barcala FJ, Etminan M, Fitzgerald M. Exposure to furry pets and the risk of asthma and allergic rhinitis: a meta-analysis. *Allergy.* (2008) 63:857–64. doi: 10.1111/j.1398-9995.2008.01732.x
99. Erbas B, Jazayeri M, Lambert KA, Katelaris CH, Prendergast LA, Tham R, et al. Outdoor pollen is a trigger of child and adolescent asthma emergency

department presentations: a systematic review and meta-analysis. *Allergy.* (2018) 73:1632–41. doi: 10.1111/all.13407
100. Salo PM, Arbes SJ Jr., Sever M, Jaramillo R, Cohn RD, London SJ, et al. Exposure to Alternaria alternata in US homes is associated with asthma symptoms. *J Allergy Clin Immunol.* (2006) 118:892–8. doi: 10.1016/j.jaci.2006.07.037
101. Burr ML, Matthews IP, Arthur RA, Watson HL, Gregory CJ, Dunstan FD, et al. Effects on patients with asthma of eradicating visible indoor mould: a randomised controlled trial. *Thorax.* (2007) 62:767–72. doi: 10.1136/thx.2006.070847
102. Downs SH, Mitakakis TZ, Marks GB, Car NG, Belousova EG, Leuppi JD, et al. Clinical importance of alternaria exposure in children. *Am J Respir Crit Care Med.* (2001) 164:455–9. doi: 10.1164/ajrccm.164.3.2008042
103. O'Hollaren MT, Yunginger JW, Offord KP, Somers MJ, O'Connell EJ, Ballard DJ, et al. Exposure to an aeroallergen as a possible precipitating factor in respiratory arrest in young patients with asthma. *N Engl J Med.* (1991) 324:359–63. doi: 10.1056/NEJM199102073240602
104. Tham R, Vicendese D, Dharmage SC, Hyndman RJ, Newbigin E, Lewis E, et al. Associations between outdoor fungal spores and childhood and adolescent asthma hospitalizations. *J Allergy Clin Immunol.* (2017) 139:1140–7.e4. doi: 10.1016/j.jaci.2016.06.046
105. Fairs A, Agbetile J, Hargadon B, Bourne M, Monteiro WR, Brightling CE, et al. IgE sensitization to Aspergillus fumigatus is associated with reduced lung function in asthma. *Am J Respir Crit Care Med.* (2010) 182:1362–8. doi: 10.1164/rccm.201001-0087OC
106. Thien F, Beggs PJ, Csutoros D, Darvall J, Hew M, Davies JM, et al. The Melbourne epidemic thunderstorm asthma event 2016: an investigation of environmental triggers, effect on health services, and patient risk factors. *Lancet Planet Health.* (2018) 2:e255–e63. doi: 10.1016/S2542-5196(18)30120-7
107. Andrew E, Nehme Z, Bernard S, Abramson MJ, Newbigin E, Piper B, et al. Stormy weather: a retrospective analysis of demand for emergency medical services during epidemic thunderstorm asthma. *BMJ.* (2017) 359:j5636. doi: 10.1136/bmj.j5636
108. Liu AH, Jaramillo R, Sicherer SH, Wood RA, Bock SA, Burks AW, et al. National prevalence and risk factors for food allergy and relationship to asthma: results from the National Health and Nutrition Examination Survey 2005–2006. *J Allergy Clin Immunol.* (2010) 126:798–806.e13. doi: 10.1016/j.jaci.2010.07.026
109. Burks AW, Tang M, Sicherer S, Muraro A, Eigenmann PA, Ebisawa M, et al. ICON: food allergy. *J Allergy Clin Immunol.* (2012) 129:906–20. doi: 10.1016/j.jaci.2012.02.001
110. Bock SA, Munoz-Furlong A, Sampson HA. Further fatalities caused by anaphylactic reactions to food, 2001–2006. *J Allergy Clin Immunol.* (2007) 119:1016–8. doi: 10.1016/j.jaci.2006.12.622
111. Pumphrey RS, Gowland MH. Further fatal allergic reactions to food in the United Kingdom, 1999–2006. *J Allergy Clin Immunol.* (2007) 119:1018–9. doi: 10.1016/j.jaci.2007.01.021
112. Crewe J, Carey R, Glass D, Peters S, Abramson MJ, Benke G, et al. A comprehensive list of asthmagens to inform health interventions in the Australian workplace. *Aust N Z J Public Health.* (2016) 40:170–3. doi: 10.1111/1753-6405.12479
113. Tarlo SM, Lemiere C. Occupational asthma. *N Engl J Med.* (2014) 370:640–9. doi: 10.1056/NEJMra1301758
114. Malo JL, Chan-Yeung M. Agents causing occupational asthma. *J Allergy Clin Immunol.* (2009) 123:545–50. doi: 10.1016/j.jaci.2008.09.010
115. Baur X, Bakehe P. Allergens causing occupational asthma: an evidence-based evaluation of the literature. *Int Arch Occup Environ Health.* (2014) 87:339–63. doi: 10.1007/s00420-013-0866-9
116. Burke H, Leonardi-Bee J, Hashim A, Pine-Abata H, Chen Y, Cook DG, et al. Prenatal and passive smoke exposure and incidence of asthma and wheeze: systematic review and meta-analysis. *Pediatrics.* (2012) 129:735–44. doi: 10.1542/peds.2011-2196
117. Gilliland FD, Islam T, Berhane K, Gauderman WJ, McConnell R, Avol E, et al. Regular smoking and asthma incidence in adolescents. *Am J Respir Crit Care Med.* (2006) 174:1094–100. doi: 10.1164/rccm.200605-722OC
118. Genuneit J, Weinmayr G, Radon K, Dressel H, Windstetter D, Rzehak P, et al. Smoking and the incidence of asthma during adolescence: results of a large cohort study in Germany. *Thorax.* (2006) 61:572–8. doi: 10.1136/thx.2005.051227
119. McLeish AC, Zvolensky MJ. Asthma and cigarette smoking: a review of the empirical literature. J Asthma (2010) 47:16. doi: 10.3109/02770900903556413
120. Perret JL, Bonevski B, McDonald CF, Abramson MJ. Smoking cessation strategies for patients with asthma: improving patient outcomes. *J Asthma Allergy.* (2016) 9:117–28. doi: 10.2147/JAA.S85615
121. Anenberg SC, Henze DK, Tinney V, Kinney PL, Raich W, Fann N, et al. Estimates of the global burden of ambient [Formula: see text], Ozone, and [Formula: see text] on asthma incidence and emergency room visits. *Environ Health Perspect.* (2018) 126:107004. doi: 10.1289/EHP3766
122. Yang M, Chu C, Bloom MS, Li S, Chen G, Heinrich J, et al. Is smaller worse? New insights about associations of PM1 and respiratory health in children and adolescents. *Environ Int.* (2018) 120:516–24. doi: 10.1016/j.envint.2018.08.027
123. Gauderman WJ, Gilliland GF, Vora H, Avol E, Stram D, McConnell R, et al. Association between air pollution and lung function growth in southern California children: results from a second cohort. *Am J Respir Crit Care Med.* (2002) 166:76–84. doi: 10.1164/rccm.2111021
124. Gauderman WJ, McConnell R, Gilliland F, London S, Thomas D, Avol E, et al. Association between air pollution and lung function growth in southern California children. *Am J Respir Crit Care Med.* (2000) 162(4 Pt 1):1383–90. doi: 10.1164/ajrccm.162.4.9909096
125. Bowatte G, Erbas B, Lodge CJ, Knibbs LD, Gurrin LC, Marks GB, et al. Traffic-related air pollution exposure over a 5-year period is associated with increased risk of asthma and poor lung function in middle age. *Eur Respir J.* (2017) 50:1602357. doi: 10.1183/13993003.02357-2016
126. McCreanor J, Cullinan P, Nieuwenhuijsen MJ, Stewart-Evans J, Malliarou E, Jarup L, et al. Respiratory effects of exposure to diesel traffic in persons with asthma. *N Engl J Med.* (2007) 357:2348–58. doi: 10.1056/NEJMoa071535
127. Howden-Chapman P, Pierse N, Nicholls S, Gillespie-Bennett J, Viggers H, Cunningham M, et al. Effects of improved home heating on asthma in community dwelling children: randomised controlled trial. *BMJ.* (2008) 337:a1411. doi: 10.1136/bmj.a1411
128. Accordini S, Calciano L, Johannessen A, Portas L, Benediktsdottir B, Bertelsen RJ, et al. A three-generation study on the association of tobacco smoking with asthma. *Int J Epidemiol.* (2018) 47:1106–17. doi: 10.1093/ije/dyy031
129. Zbikowski SM, Klesges RC, Robinson LA, Alfano CM. Risk factors for smoking among adolescents with asthma. *J Adolesc Health.* (2002) 30:279–87. doi: 10.1016/S1054-139X(01)00394-9
130. Diagnosis of Diseases of Chronic Airflow Limitation: Asthma, COPD and Asthma-COPD Overlap Syndrome (ACOS). *Based on the Global Strategy for Asthma Management and Prevention and the Global Strategy for the Diagnosis, Management and Prevention of Chronic Obstructive Pulmonary Disease.* Available online at: https://goldcopd.org/asthma-copd-asthma-copd-overlap-syndrome/ (accessed 11 August, 2018).
131. Erbas B, Lowe AJ, Lodge CJ, Matheson MC, Hosking CS, Hill DJ, et al. Persistent pollen exposure during infancy is associated with increased risk of subsequent childhood asthma and hayfever. *Clin Exp Allergy.* (2013) 43:337–43. doi: 10.1111/cea.12071
132. Guilbert A, Cox B, Bruffaerts N, Hoebeke L, Packeu A, Hendrickx M, et al. Relationships between aeroallergen levels and hospital admissions for asthma in the Brussels-Capital Region: a daily time series analysis. *Environ Health.* (2018) 17:35. doi: 10.1186/s12940-018-0378-x
133. Packe GE, Ayres JG. Asthma outbreak during a thunderstorm. *Lancet.* (1985) 2:199–204. doi: 10.1016/S0140-6736(85)91510-7
134. Alderman PM, Sloan JP, Basran GS. Asthma and thunderstorms. *Arch Emerg Med.* (1986) 3:260–2. doi: 10.1136/emj.3.4.260
135. Elliot AJ, Hughes HE, Hughes TC, Locker TE, Brown R, Sarran C, et al. The impact of thunderstorm asthma on emergency department attendances across London during July 2013. *Emerg Med J.* (2014) 31:675–8. doi: 10.1136/emermed-2013-203122
136. Davidson AC, Emberlin J, Cook AD, Venables KM. A major outbreak of asthma associated with a thunderstorm: experience of accident and emergency departments and patients' characteristics. Thames Regions

Accident and Emergency Trainees Association. *BMJ.* (1996) 312:601–4. doi: 10.1136/bmj.312.7031.601

137. Tan HT, Ellis JA, Koplin JJ, Matheson MC, Gurrin LC, Lowe AJ, et al. Filaggrin loss-of-function mutations do not predict food allergy over and above the risk of food sensitization among infants. *J Allergy Clin Immunol.* (2012) 130:1211–3 e3. doi: 10.1016/j.jaci.2012.07.022
138. Du Toit G, Roberts G, Sayre PH, Bahnson HT, Radulovic S, Santos AF, et al. Randomized trial of peanut consumption in infants at risk for peanut allergy. *N Engl J Med.* (2015) 372:803–13. doi: 10.1056/NEJMoa1414850
139. Gruchalla RS, Sampson HA. Preventing peanut allergy through early consumption–ready for prime time? *N Engl J Med.* (2015) 372:875–7. doi: 10.1056/NEJMe1500186
140. Vandenplas O, Suojalehto H, Cullinan P. Diagnosing occupational asthma. *Clin Exp Allergy.* (2017) 47:6–18. doi: 10.1111/cea.12858
141. Beach J, Russell K, Blitz S, Hooton N, Spooner C, Lemiere C, et al. A systematic review of the diagnosis of occupational asthma. *Chest.* (2007) 131:569–78. doi: 10.1378/chest.06-0492
142. Santos MS, Jung H, Peyrovi J, Lou W, Liss GM, Tarlo SM. Occupational asthma and work-exacerbated asthma: factors associated with time to diagnostic steps. *Chest.* (2007) 131:1768–75. doi: 10.1378/chest.06-2487
143. Tarlo SM, Liss G, Corey P, Broder I. A workers' compensation claim population for occupational asthma. Comparison of subgroups. *Chest.* (1995) 107:634–41. doi: 10.1378/chest.107.3.634
144. Balmes J, Becklake M, Blanc P, Henneberger P, Kreiss K, Mapp C, et al. American thoracic society statement: occupational contribution to the burden of airway disease. *Am J Respir Crit Care Med.* (2003) 167:787–97. doi: 10.1164/rccm.167.5.787
145. Blanc PD, Toren K. How much adult asthma can be attributed to occupational factors? *Am J Med.* (1999) 107:580–7. doi: 10.1016/S0002-9343(99)00307-1
146. Toren K, Blanc PD. Asthma caused by occupational exposures is common - a systematic analysis of estimates of the population-attributable fraction. *BMC Pulm Med.* (2009) 9:7. doi: 10.1186/1471-2466-9-7
147. Henneberger PK, Redlich CA, Callahan DB, Harber P, Lemiere C, Martin J, et al. An official american thoracic society statement: work-exacerbated asthma. *Am J Respir Crit Care Med.* (2011) 184:368–78. doi: 10.1164/rccm.812011ST
148. Wood LG. Diet, Obesity, and Asthma. *Anna Am Thor Soc.* (2017) 14(Supplement_5):S332–S8. doi: 10.1513/AnnalsATS.201702-124AW
149. Beuther DA, Sutherland ER. Overweight, obesity, and incident asthma: a meta-analysis of prospective epidemiologic studies. *Am J Respir Crit Care Med.* (2007) 175:661–6. doi: 10.1164/rccm.200611-1717OC
150. Matheson MC, Erbas B, Balasuriya A, Jenkins MA, Wharton CL, Tang ML, et al. Breast-feeding and atopic disease: a cohort study from childhood to middle age. *J Allergy Clin Immunol.* (2007) 120:1051–7. doi: 10.1016/j.jaci.2007.06.030
151. Lodge CJ, Tan DJ, Lau MX, Dai X, Tham R, Lowe AJ, et al. Breastfeeding and asthma and allergies: a systematic review and meta-analysis. *Acta Paediatr.* (2015) 104:38–53. doi: 10.1111/apa.13132
152. Hallberg J, Thunqvist P, Schultz ES, Kull I, Bottai M, Merritt AS, et al. Asthma phenotypes and lung function up to 16 years of age-the BAMSE cohort. *Allergy.* (2015) 70:667–73. doi: 10.1111/all.12598
153. Strunk RC, Weiss ST, Yates KP, Tonascia J, Zeiger RS, Szefler SJ. Mild to moderate asthma affects lung growth in children and adolescents. *J Allergy Clin Immunol.* (2006) 118:1040–7. doi: 10.1016/j.jaci.2006.07.053
154. Sears MR, Greene JM, Willan AR, Wiecek EM, Taylor DR, Flannery EM, et al. A longitudinal, population-based, cohort study of childhood asthma followed to adulthood. *N Engl J Med.* (2003) 349:1414–22. doi: 10.1056/NEJMoa022363
155. Morgan WJ, Stern DA, Sherrill DL, Guerra S, Holberg CJ, Guilbert TW, et al. Outcome of asthma and wheezing in the first 6 years of life: follow-up through adolescence. *Am J Respir Crit Care Med.* (2005) 172:1253–8. doi: 10.1164/rccm.200504-525OC
156. Lødrup Carlsen KC, Mowinckel P, Hovland V, Håland G, Riiser A, Carlsen K-H. Asthma and lower airway disease: lung function trajectories from birth through puberty reflect asthma phenotypes with allergic comorbidity. *J Allergy Clin Immunol.* (2014) 134:917–23. doi: 10.1016/j.jaci.2014.05.020
157. Phelan PD, Robertson CF, Olinsky A. The melbourne asthma study: 1964–1999. *J Allergy Clin Immunol.* (2002) 109:189–94. doi: 10.1067/mai.2002.120951
158. Tagiyeva N, Devereux G, Fielding S, Turner S, Douglas G. Outcomes of childhood asthma and wheezy bronchitis. A 50-year cohort study. *Am J Respir Crit Care Med.* (2016) 193:23–30. doi: 10.1164/rccm.201505-0870OC
159. Bui DS, Walters HE, Burgess JA, Perret JL, Bui MQ, Bowatte G, et al. Childhood respiratory risk factor profiles and middle-age lung function: a prospective cohort study from the first to sixth decade. *Ann Am Thor Soc.* (2018) 15:1057–66. doi: 10.1513/AnnalsATS.201806-374OC
160. Marossy AE, Strachan DP, Rudnicka AR, Anderson HR. Childhood chest illness and the rate of decline of adult lung function between ages 35 and 45 years. *Am J Respir Crit Care Med.* (2007) 175:355–9. doi: 10.1164/rccm.200607-1023OC
161. Svanes C, Sunyer J, Plana E, Dharmage S, Heinrich J, Jarvis D, et al. Early life origins of chronic obstructive pulmonary disease. *Thorax.* (2010) 65:14–20. doi: 10.1136/thx.2008.112136
162. Bui DS, Lodge CJ, Burgess JA, Lowe AJ, Perret J, Bui MQ, et al. Childhood predictors of lung function trajectories and future COPD risk: a prospective cohort study from the first to the sixth decade of life. *Lancet Respir Med.* (2018) 6:535–44. doi: 10.1016/S2213-2600(18)30100-0
163. McGeachie MJ, Yates KP, Zhou X, Guo F, Sternberg AL, Van Natta ML, et al. Patterns of growth and decline in lung function in persistent childhood asthma. *N Engl J Med.* (2016) 374:1842–52. doi: 10.1056/NEJMoa1513737
164. Tan DJ, Walters EH, Perret JL, Lodge CJ, Lowe AJ, Matheson MC, et al. Age-of-asthma onset as a determinant of different asthma phenotypes in adults: a systematic review and meta-analysis of the literature. *Exp Rev Resp Med.* (2015) 9:109–23. doi: 10.1586/17476348.2015.1000311
165. Perret JL, Dharmage SC, Matheson MC, Johns DP, Gurrin LC, Burgess JA, et al. The interplay between the effects of lifetime asthma, smoking, and atopy on fixed airflow obstruction in middle age. *Am J Respir Crit Care Med.* (2013) 187:42–8. doi: 10.1164/rccm.201205-0788OC
166. Tan DJ, Walters EH, Perret JL, Burgess JA, Johns DP, Lowe AJ, et al. Clinical and functional differences between early-onset and late-onset adult asthma: a population-based tasmanian longitudinal health study. *Thorax.* (2016) 71:981–7. doi: 10.1136/thoraxjnl-2015-208183
167. Aanerud M, Carsin AE, Sunyer J, Dratva J, Gislason T, Jarvis D, et al. Interaction between asthma and smoking increases the risk of adult airway obstruction. *Eur Respir J.* (2015) 45:635–43. doi: 10.1183/09031936.00055514
168. Lange P, Parner J, Vestbo J, Schnohr P, Jensen G. A 15-year follow-up study of ventilatory function in adults with asthma. *N Engl J Med.* (1998) 339:1194–200. doi: 10.1056/NEJM199810223391703
169. James AL, Palmer LJ, Kicic E, Maxwell PS, Lagan SE, Ryan GF, et al. Decline in lung function in the Busselton Health Study: the effects of asthma and cigarette smoking. *Am J Respir Crit Care Med.* (2005) 171:109–14. doi: 10.1164/rccm.200402-230OC
170. Peat JK, Woolcock AJ, Cullen K. Rate of decline of lung function in subjects with asthma. *Eur J Resp Dis.* (1987) 70:171–9.
171. Tai A, Tran H, Roberts M, Clarke N, Gibson AM, Vidmar S, et al. Outcomes of childhood asthma to the age of 50 years. *J Allergy Clin Immunol.* (2014) 133:1572–8.e3. doi: 10.1016/j.jaci.2013.12.1033
172. Porsbjerg C, Lange P, Ulrik CS. Lung function impairment increases with age of diagnosis in adult onset asthma. *Respir Med.* (2015) 109:821–7. doi: 10.1016/j.rmed.2015.04.012
173. Anto JM, Sunyer J, Basagana X, Garcia-Esteban R, Cerveri I, de Marco R, et al. Risk factors of new-onset asthma in adults: a population-based international cohort study. *Allergy.* (2010) 65:1021–30. doi: 10.1111/j.1398-9995.2009.02301.x
174. Zaidi SR, Blakey JD. Why are people with asthma susceptible to pneumonia? A review of factors related to upper airway bacteria. *Respirology.* (2019) 24:423–30. doi: 10.1111/resp.13528
175. Talbot TR, Hartert TV, Mitchel E, Halasa NB, Arbogast PG, Poehling KA, et al. Asthma as a risk factor for invasive pneumococcal disease. *N Engl J Med.* (2005) 352:2082–90. doi: 10.1056/NEJMoa044113
176. Helby J, Nordestgaard BG, Benfield T, Bojesen SE. Asthma, other atopic conditions and risk of infections in 105 519 general population never and ever smokers. *J Int Med.* (2017) 282:254–67. doi: 10.1111/joim.12635

177. Juhn YJ. Risks for infection in patients with asthma (or other atopic conditions): is asthma more than a chronic airway disease? *J Allergy Clin Immunol.* (2014) 134:247–57. quiz 58–9. doi: 10.1016/j.jaci.2014.04.024
178. Klemets P, Lyytikainen O, Ruutu P, Ollgren J, Kaijalainen T, Leinonen M, et al. Risk of invasive pneumococcal infections among working age adults with asthma. *Thorax.* (2010) 65:698–702. doi: 10.1136/thx.2009.132670
179. Kankaanranta H, Kauppi P, Tuomisto LE, Ilmarinen P. Emerging comorbidities in adult asthma: risks, clinical associations, and mechanisms. *Mediat Inflamm.* (2016) 2016:3690628. doi: 10.1155/2016/3690628
180. Weatherburn CJ, Guthrie B, Mercer SW, Morales DR. Comorbidities in adults with asthma: population-based cross-sectional analysis of 1.4 million adults in Scotland. *Clin Exp Allergy.* (2017) 47:1246–52. doi: 10.1111/cea.12971
181. Gershon AS, Guan J, Wang C, Victor JC, To T. Describing and quantifying asthma comorbidity [corrected]: a population study. *PLoS ONE.* (2012) 7:e34967. doi: 10.1371/journal.pone.0034967
182. Szefler SJ. Asthma across the lifespan: time for a paradigm shift. *J Allergy Clin Immunol.* (2018) 142:773–80. doi: 10.1016/j.jaci.2018.03.010

7

Immunotherapy and Asthma in Children

Maria A. Tosca[1], Amelia Licari[2], Roberta Olcese[1], Gianluigi Marseglia[2], Oliviero Sacco[3] and Giorgio Ciprandi[4]*

[1] Department of Pediatrics, Allergy Center, Istituto Giannina Gaslini (IRCCS), Genoa, Italy, [2] Department of Pediatrics, Ospedale San Matteo (IRCCS), Pediatrics Clinic, University of Pavia, Pavia, Italy, [3] Pediatric Pulmonology and Endoscopy, Istituto Giannina Gaslini (IRCCS), Genoa, Italy, [4] Allergy Clinic, Ospedale San Martino (IRCCS), Genoa, Italy

***Correspondence:**
Maria A. Tosca
mariangelatosca@gaslini.org

Allergen immunotherapy (AIT) is still the only disease-modifying treatment strategy for IgE-mediated allergic diseases, with consolidated evidence both in adults and children. AIT is effective in determining clinical improvement of allergic rhinitis and asthma, such as reduced symptoms, medication use, and improvement of quality of life, with a long-lasting effect after cessation of treatment. Results from recent clinical studies have implemented the evidence of effectiveness and safety of allergen immunotherapy for the treatment of allergic asthma, so that the current asthma guidelines now recommend sublingual immunotherapy as an add-on therapy for asthma in adults and adolescents with house dust mite allergy, allergic rhinitis, and exacerbations despite low-to-moderate dose ICS, with forced expiratory volume in 1 second more than 70% predicted. AIT may also reduce the risk of progression from allergic rhinitis to asthma in children and prevent the onset of new sensitizations, thus representing a potentially preventive method of treatment. The aim of this review is to present an updated overview of the clinical indications of AIT, with particular reference to pediatric asthma, of the mechanisms of clinical and immunological tolerance to allergens, and of the potential biomarkers predicting clinical response.

Keywords: allergen immunotherapy, subcutaneous immunotherapy, sublingual immunotherapy, allergic rhinitis, asthma

INTRODUCTION

Allergen immunotherapy (AIT) is the administration of the causal allergen to control allergic inflammation and symptoms. AIT has been used for over a century and it is actually considered the only disease-modifying treatment strategy for IgE-mediated allergic diseases, as causing a persistent immunological and clinical tolerance toward the causal allergen (1).

Both subcutaneous AIT (SCIT) and sublingual (SLIT) are used and accepted as effective treatments for adults and children with allergic rhinitis (AR) with or without asthma (2, 3). Historically, SCIT was early proposed as the first route of AIT administration, since first report (4). However, despite its proven effectiveness, the use of SCIT is still limited by the need for frequent injections by a doctor over a minimum of 3 years, and, mostly important, the potential occurrence of systemic severe reactions. Consequently, SCIT should be administered in a medical setting by clinicians able to manage anaphylaxis (1). Furthermore, the risk of systemic reactions to SCIT is greater in subjects with uncontrolled asthma and with accelerated dosing schedules (5). Given these disadvantages, SLIT may represent a viable alternative to SCIT, mainly in children, allowing safe self-administration at home (6–8). So, route selection vaccine is based on availability or approval, cost, and the patient's age or the physician's or patient's preference (9).

SCIT or SLIT products cannot be actually compared due to their heterogeneous composition and allergen concentration (10). Existing studies suggest that both may induce similar immunologic changes (11). Allergens are used for SCIT as aqueous or physically-adsorbed (depot) extracts, as well as chemically modified allergens (allergoids) as depot formulations. Allergens for SLIT are used as drops or tablets. Waiting for a harmonized and international AIT products regulation, they are still available most commonly either by being distributed as "named patient products" (NPP), prepared simply in compliance with Good Manufacturing Practice, and by obtaining a formal marketing authorization (12). SLIT tablets for grass pollen and house dust mite (HDM) have been recently registered for use in children, adolescents, and adults (13, 14).

Through complex molecular and cellular mechanisms inducing immune tolerance, effective AIT may modify the natural course of allergic disease, both preventing the onset of new sensitizations and the clinical disease progression (from rhinitis to asthma). AIT may also control allergic symptoms that are unresponsive to avoidance strategies and medications, reduce medication use, and improve quality of life, with a long-lasting effect after cessation (15, 16). Results from recent trials have implemented the evidence of effectiveness and safety of AIT for the treatment of allergic asthma, so that updated asthma guidelines now recommend SLIT as an add-on therapy for asthma in adults and adolescents with HDM allergy, under certain conditions (3).

The aim of this review is to present an updated overview of the clinical indications of AIT, with particular reference to pediatric asthma, of the mechanisms of clinical and immunological tolerance to allergens, and of the potential biomarkers predicting clinical response. A literature search was performed through Medline via Pubmed to identify all relevant articles published in English, on the basis of the following three search terms: "allergen immunotherapy", "children," and "asthma." From the articles retrieved in the first round of search, additional references were identified by a manual search among the cited references.

OVERVIEW OF THE MECHANISMS OF ALLERGEN IMMUNOTHERAPY

AIT targets the upper and lower respiratory allergic symptoms by modulating the IgE-mediated response consequent to allergen exposure. Through multiple mechanisms involving both innate and adaptive immunity, AIT regulates T- and B-cells, changing antibody isotypes, decreases mediator release, and migration of inflammatory cells to tissues (17–19).

A key mechanism in inducing immunologic tolerance is the upregulation of allergen-specific T-regulatory (Treg) cells and B-regulatory (Breg) cells, which primarily down-regulate the Th_2 response (19) (**Table 1**). Regulatory cells inhibit the activation of allergen-specific Th_2 lymphocytes, suppress allergic inflammation, and ultimately shift toward a Type 1-mediated immune response, releasing cytokines, interleukin (IL)-10 and transforming growth factor-β (TGF-β) (20).

TABLE 1 | Mechanisms of immunologic tolerance mediated by T and B regulatory cells during allergen immunotherapy.

Treg-mediated mechanisms
Release regulatory cytokines (IL-10, TGF-β, and IL-35)
Induce tolerogenic DCs subsets
Reduced number of ILC2
Suppress activation of allergen-specific Th_2 lymphocytes
Downregulate the expression of FCεRI receptors on mast cells,
Decrease allergen-specific IgE synthesis
Promote B-cell production of IgG_4 antibody
Breg-mediated mechanisms
Release regulatory cytokines (IL-10, TGF-β)
Induce the synthesis of IgG4 blocking antibodies
Inhibit activation and proliferation of effector T lymphocytes
Suppress Th_2-dependent inflammation
Promote T-cell expression of Foxp3 and generation of functional Treg cells

Breg, B regulatory; DCs, dendritic cells; FCεRI, high-affinity receptor for the Fc region of IgE; Foxp3, forkhead box P3; IgE, immunoglobulin E; IgG_4, immunoglobulin G subtype 4; IL, interleukin; ILC2, innate lymphoid cells type 2; TGF, transforming growth factor; Th_2, T helper type 2; Treg, T regulatory.

After high-dose allergen administration by AIT, dendritic cells (DCs) produce IL-12, IL-27, and IL-10, generating and activating distinct phenotypes of Tregs: natural (nTreg) and inducible (iTreg) cells (17, 19). Both nTreg and iTreg cells suppress allergic response through direct and indirect mechanisms: release regulatory cytokines (IL-10, TGF-β, and IL-35), directly induce tolerogenic DCs subsets, suppress activation of allergen-specific Th_2 lymphocytes, downregulate the expression of FCεRI receptors on mast cells, decrease allergen-specific IgE synthesis, and promote B-cell production of IgG4 in an allergen-independent manner (17, 19). IL-10 directly inhibits T-cell-associated cytokines, including IL-4 and IL-5, reduces proinflammatory cytokine from mast cells and eosinophils, decreases allergen-specific IgE production, and increases IgA and IgG_4 levels (19). Competitively binding to the same site epitopes recognized by IgE, IgG_4 exert a sort of "immunologic blockade" inhibiting mast cell and basophil degranulation. In addition, IgG_4 has been proposed to co-stimulate the inhibitory IgG receptor FcγRIIb, which can negatively regulate FcεRI signaling and in turn inhibit effector cell activation. IgG_4 also inhibit IgE-mediated facilitation of allergen presentation to T lymphocytes (20). TGF-β suppresses both activity and proliferation of Th_2 cells and innate lymphoid cells type 2 (ILC2), thus inhibiting Th_2-cytokines (IL-4, IL-5, IL-9, and IL-13), and consequently decreasing the activation of eosinophils, basophils, mast cells and IgE-secreting B lymphocytes (17, 19).

Bregs play a key role in inducing immune tolerance to allergens, directly promoting the synthesis of allergen-specific IgG_4, inhibiting activation and proliferation of effector T lymphocytes, suppressing Th_2-dependent inflammation, increasing Treg cells (21). Overall, AIT is able to restore the impaired allergen tolerance.

CLINICAL INDICATIONS OF AIT IN CHILDREN WITH RESPIRATORY ALLERGY

AIT should be considered in patients who have AR with or without conjunctivitis, and/or asthma with documented sensitization consisting with symptoms after sensitizing-allergen exposure (22). Candidates for AIT are patients with uncontrolled symptoms by medications and/or environmental prevention or experiencing drug adverse effects or wishing reduction of long-term treatment (22).

The evidence of efficacy and safety of AIT in AR and/or asthma have been documented both in adults and children (6, 23, 24).

Allergic Rhinitis

AIT is the established treatment of choice for AR patients experiencing failed allergen avoidance and/or medical therapy (2, 25). European Academy of Allergy and Clinical Immunology (EAACI) 2018 guidelines recommend AIT in AR patients, with or without conjunctivitis, with evident sensitization to one or more clinically relevant allergens and moderate-to-severe symptoms despite regular and/or avoidance strategies (6, 26). This statement is based on a body of international trials evidence providing a comprehensive assessment of AIT in AR: both SCIT and SLIT are effective for seasonal and perennial AR in achieving short-term improvements in symptom, medication use, and combined symptom and medication scores (27, 28). The evidence of longer-term effectiveness is documented for grass AIT, especially for tablets (26). Thus, standardized and validated AIT products should be used when available, and a product-specific evaluation of evidence is actually recommended before initiating treatment with a specific product (6, 26).

With particular reference to children, AIT should be considered similarly to adults (26). Although major gaps still exist for the pediatric age (29), it can be actually recommended: (i) continuous, pre- and pre/co-seasonal SCIT for children with seasonal AR; (ii) continuous SCIT for perennial AR (weak recommendation due to the lack of exclusive pediatric data); (iii) pre-co-seasonal and continuous SLIT for seasonal AR (both tablet and drop); (iv) poor evidence for perennial AR, although the effectiveness of SLIT tablet approach has been demonstrated in the short term in mixed adult/adolescent studies (26). It is also recommended a minimum of 3-year course to achieve long-term efficacy (6).

Asthma

Asthma is a common chronic disease affecting all age groups, with up to 20% of children aged 6–7 years experiencing severe wheezing episodes within a year (30). The actual asthma management is control-based: therapeutic strategies are based on a stepwise approach and adjusted in a continuous cycle involving assessment, treatment and review (3, 31–33). However, standard pharmacotherapy does not affect the underlying pathogenetic immune response, as it is withdrawn symptoms and inflammation occur again.

SLIT is actually recommended as add-on treatment option in adult HDM-sensitized asthmatics with concomitant AR who have exacerbations despite inhaled corticosteroids (ICS] treatment, with forced expiratory volume in 1 s (FEV_1) more than 70% predicted, as stated in the latest Global Initiative for Asthma Report (GINA) update (3). Asthma must be mild-to-moderate and allergic, and well or "partially" controlled by standard pharmacotherapy; asthma control has to be maintained throughout AIT course (34). Conversely, AIT is still restricted in patients with uncontrolled asthma, as it represents a significant risk factor for serious and even fatal adverse reactions (5). Coupling anti-IgE biological therapy (omalizumab) with AIT has been proposed as a suitable option to increase SCIT effectiveness and safety (35–38).

This significant change in the GINA strategy draws upon recent Phase III clinical trial evaluating the treatment of asthma with the standardized quality (SQ) HDM SLIT-tablet in adults: the addition of HDM SLIT to maintenance therapies reduced ICS or the time to first exacerbation upon ICS reduction, suggesting that SQ HDM SLIT-tablet may improve overall asthma control (39). While these data require further studies to confirm long-term efficacy and safety of this product in adults, less information is available for adolescents (40, 41) and studies are in progress in children (42). HDM sensitization in early childhood represents an important risk factor for the development of asthma (43) and is linked to the impairment of lung function in school-age asthmatic children (43, 44) and asthma persistence into adulthood (45). So, other single HDM SLIT preparations have been tested in children and adolescents with allergic asthma. Among others, SLIT with the 300 index of reactivity (IR)-standardized HDM extract, in children aged 6–18 years with AR with or without allergic asthma, improved rhinitis and/or asthma symptoms scores, together with a reduction of rescue medications (46).

Meta-analyses confirmed the effectiveness and the safety profile of AIT in allergic asthma for adults and children (27, 47–51), mainly concerning SLIT in children (22, 52–54). Consistent reduction in combined AR and asthma symptom and medication scores have been demonstrated in pediatric patients with asthma and comorbid AR treated with SLIT (48, 53, 55). These clinical effects have been also demonstrated to be persistent after AIT discontinuation up to 5 years (56). SCIT has demonstrated effectiveness in controlling asthma and reducing medication use (49, 50, 57). Meta-analyses of randomized clinical trials using SCIT in asthma have demonstrated a significant reduction in symptoms, medication use, and AHR both in children and adults, while the effect on lung function showed conflicting results (49, 50). Studies conducted in children showed similar results (58–61). SCIT may have a long-term impact on childhood asthma, as demonstrated in a prospective study using HDM SCIT: after 3 years of SCIT discontinuation, a global remission of asthma (in particular reduced doses of ICS, lower asthma symptom scores, higher quality of life scores, less AHR, and higher FEV_1) was reported in treated patients compared to controls (62). In another retrospective study, asthmatics allergic to either HDM or grass pollen, treated with SCIT in childhood, were re-evaluated 9 years after the discontinuation, showing a three-time lower risk of frequent asthma symptoms than controls, but without any difference in lung function or medication use (63).

Overall, both SCIT and SLIT appear to be effective for the treatment of AR and asthma in children (64, 65). Of particular interest for the pediatric population, it is the AIT ability (both SCIT and SLIT) to reduce ICS doses together with the impact on asthma control. These promising results highlight the immunomodulating pivotal role of AIT in controlling and inducing remission of disease activity. Furthermore, the persistence of these clinical effects after discontinuation separates AIT uniquely from other anti-allergic therapies.

Prevention of Allergy Progression and Asthma Onset

Over the last decade, the disease-modifying properties of AIT have been largely investigated, mainly focusing on the prevention of allergic sensitization and asthma onset.

Developing new sensitizations is characteristic of the natural history of allergy. A preventive effect of AIT on the onset of new sensitizations has been reported (1, 66) and demonstrated in asthmatic children mono-sensitized to HDM (67, 68). However, a recent systematic review and meta-analysis on this topic reported a low level of evidence related to the heterogeneity and the high risk of bias of the included studies (69, 70). A recent EAACI-funded meta-analysis highlighted a reduced risk of developing new sensitizations at least over the short period, but none on the long-term (71).

Children with AR have an increased risk of developing asthma later on in life when compared to those without AR, especially those with AHR (72). Few but significant studies investigated disease modification in children, mainly concerning AIT (73–77). The prevention of allergy (PAT) study was a large prospective randomized controlled study to evaluate the preventive effect of SCIT in children (aged 6–14 years) with grass and/or birch AR without asthma (73–75). Actively-treated children had a significantly reduced risk of developing asthma and fewer asthma symptoms after 3 year treatment compared to controls (73). This preventive effect persisted at 5 years (74) and 7 years (75) after SCIT discontinuation. The preventive effect of SLIT was evaluated in two open trials conducted on children with AR with or without asthma: a 3-year course of SLIT improved AR symptoms, reduced onset of asthma, and decreased AHR (78, 79). Although promising, these findings had a major limitation as derived from open studies with a limited number of subjects. The results of the grass tablet asthma prevention (GAP) study, the first randomized, double-blind, placebo-controlled trial, have been recently published (77). The GAP study involved 812 children (aged 5–12 years), with grass-pollen AR and without asthma, who received 3-year SQ grass-SLIT-tablet or placebo and were followed for 2 years after discontinuation (77). Treated children significantly reduced the risk of experiencing asthma symptoms or using asthma medication, as well as AR-related symptoms and medications, at the end of the trial, during the 2-year post-treatment follow-up, and during the entire 5-year trial period (77). Taken together, these studies suggest that AIT might reduce the risk of developing asthma symptoms in children, especially in those with AR. EAACI guidelines on the PAT recommend a 3-year course of AIT in children with moderate-to-severe AR and grass/birch pollen allergy, uncontrolled with pharmacotherapy for short-term and possibly long-term prevention of asthma symptoms in addition to improving the control of AR (6, 16).

Finally, the role of AIT in the primary PAT is currently under investigation. In a recent proof of concept study, 111 young children (aged 5–9 months), not sensitized, but at high risk of atopy, were treated with prophylactic HDM SLIT (80). A significant sensitization prevention was demonstrated in the active group; however, no significant preventive effect was observed on HDM sensitization or allergy-related symptoms (80). Further studies are expected to clarify the role of AIT as early-intervention in high-risk children.

PATIENT SELECTION AND BIOMARKERS OF RESPONSE

Since AIT is allergen-specific, a detailed clinical history and appropriate allergy diagnostic tests are essential to properly identify the triggering clinical relevant allergen(s) (2). In case of polysensitized patients, the identification of major allergens should be supported by the use of component-resolved diagnostics (81). Uncontrolled AR symptoms despite antihistamines and/or topical corticosteroids and allergen avoidance measures and/or side-effects of medication, the duration of AR symptoms, as well as the assessment of asthma control, are essential to consider AIT as a therapeutic option (2). Each patient should be evaluated individually by considering the benefits and the risks, and the ability to comply/cooperate with AIT (26). Although some clinical studies have demonstrated efficacy and safety of AIT in preschool children (82, 83), there is no consensus on a specific lower age limit for initiating AIT for respiratory allergy (8). However, this issue still deserves further extensive studies in the perspective of preventive strategies.

Although highly effective, some patients could not respond to AIT treatment. Thus, the identification and validation of potential predictive biomarkers of AIT effectiveness is an active filed of research and could enhance the selection and the clinical management of patients receiving AIT. Biomarkers are quantitative measurement predicting clinical and immunological effects of AIT (84). In particular, ideal biomarkers for AIT should assist in patient selection and identification of responders and predict clinical and immunological response during treatment and after discontinuation of treatment (84). The EAACI Taskforce recently reviewed all candidate biomarkers used in clinical trials of AR patients with or without asthma (18, 84) (**Table 2**). Markers can be cellular (Tregs), humoral (allergen-specific IgG_4 ($sIgG_4$), IgE/IgG_4), molecular (interleukins), or functional (IgE FAB and blocking factor). Although several studies have included biomarkers as secondary outcomes, specifically AIT biomarker studies are still lacking. To date, raised serum allergen-specific IgE (sIgE) are considered the only useful biomarker to select candidates for AIT, in the

TABLE 2 | Potential biomarkers for allergen immunotherapy (AIT).

Categories	Candidate biomarkers	Domain	Advantages	Disadvantages, unmet need	Possible applications
Biomarkers for diagnosis	IgE (sIgE, tIgE, sIgE/tIgE)	Antibodies	Elevated serum IgE levels in the context of a clear history of allergic symptoms is a biomarker for selection of patients for AIT	No clear correlation with clinical outcome Lack of validation in RDBPCT Lack of standardization of assay platform and reference ranges/cut-off values	Prediction of disease severity and/or progression
	CD63, CD203c, DAO, basophil histamine release				
Biomarkers predictive of AIT safety	CD63, CD203c, DAO, basophil histamine release	Basophil activation	Small amount of blood (<2 ml) is required to perform the test	Mechanism of allergen induced basophil hyperresponsiveness during AIT not completely known Limited number of studies Need for standardized assays	Reduced risk of side effects and improvement of patients' compliance to treatment
Biomarkers of AIT efficacy	IgG subclasses ($sIgG_1$, $sIgG_4$, $sIgE/IgG_4$)	Antibodies	$sIgG_4$ is a biomarker of immunologic response of AIT	No clear correlation with clinical outcome Limited data on local antibody levels and activities	Prediction of patients' compliance
	sIgE/total IgE	Antibodies	Potential positive predictive biomarker of response for AIT	Lack of validation in RDBPC	Prediction of clinical response
	IgE FAB, IgE-BF	Serum Inhibitory activity for IgE	Highly reproducible serum-based assay Association with clinical outcome has been reported in some studies	Availability limited to specialized centers or laboratories	
Not yet determined	CCR3, ECP, eotaxin, IFN-γ, IL-2, IL-2R, IL-4/5/6, IL-8/9/10, IL-13/18, MCP-1, TARC, transthyretin	Cytokines and chemokines	May be useful to further explore mechanisms of AIT	No correlation with clinical outcome	Not known
	DCs, Breg, Treg	Cellular biomarkers	Early biomarkers of immunologic response	Not routinely performed, limited applications in clinical practice No clear correlation with clinical outcome	Prediction of immunological response
	SPT, Id, In, chamber studies	*In vivo* biomarkers	Provocation tests used as surrogate biomarkers of clinical response to AIT Provocation methods are recommended as primary endpoints in proof-of-concept and dose-finding trials of AIT	Standardization and validation differ from the various challenge protocols Comparison between provocation test results and symptoms after natural exposure are currently lacking	Prediction of clinical response

Adapted from Shamji et al. (84). BF, binding factor; Breg, B regulatory cell; CCR, chemokine receptor; CD, cluster of differentiation; DAO, diamine oxidase; DC, dendritic cell; ECP, eosinophil cationic protein; FAB, facilitated antigen binding; Id, intradermal test; IFN, interferon; Ig, immunoglobulin; IL, interleukin; In, intranasal test; MCP, monocyte chemoattractive protein; RDBPCT, Randomized double-blinded placebo-controlled trial; sIg, allergen-specific Ig; SPT, skin prick test; TARC, thymus and activation-regulated chemokine; tIg, total Ig; Treg, T regulatory cell.

context of a clear history of symptoms on exposure to the relevant allergen (84). In particular, preliminary data suggest that higher levels of sIgE in children could be helpful to predict AIT efficacy (85). Furthermore, sIgG4, sIgE/total IgE ratio, and IgE-FAB are in the pipeline as candidate biomarkers for compliance and response to AIT, respectively (84). More research is needed to confirm and interpret the possible association of biomarkers with both clinical response and persistence of clinical benefit after discontinuation of AIT.

CONCLUSIONS

AIT represents a valuable therapeutic option, especially in childhood, to modify the progression of allergic disease. AIT may be particularly useful in children with AR and new-onset asthma because it may modify the long-term prognosis of their airway disease. Both SCIT and SLIT seem to be effective in pediatric allergic asthma, showing a promising steroid-sparing effect of which patients treated with high-dose pharmacotherapy for a long term could benefit most. To date, uncontrolled asthma remains a clear contraindication for AIT treatment; however, coupling novel biological therapies with AIT could represent a novel approach to treat these patients with high risk of adverse reactions. Over the last decade considerable advances in the AIT approach have been also made to move forward this therapeutic field in the context of personalized medicine. The advanced knowledge of the mechanisms of sustaining clinical and immunological tolerance toward allergens, the implementation of vaccination strategies (using recombinant allergen extracts, or modified extracts at increased safety/efficacy, or adjuvants to further stimulate the immune system), the implementation and diffusion of international guidelines, the definition of regulatory aspects such as standardization and registration of AIT products, the standardization of clinical trial outcomes, as well as the planning of future dedicated pediatric studies, will all implement the evidence of efficacy and safety of AIT for allergic children.

AUTHOR CONTRIBUTIONS

All authors made substantial contribution to the conception of the work, reviewed the literature on the subject, and drafted the final version of the manuscript. AL and MT revised it critically for important intellectual content. All authors finally approved the version to be published and agreed to be accountable for all aspects of the work in ensuring that questions related to the accuracy or integrity of any part of the work are appropriately investigated and resolved.

REFERENCES

1. Jutel M, Agache I, Bonini S, Burks AW, Calderon M, Canonica W, et al. International consensus on allergy immunotherapy. *J Allergy Clin Immunol.* (2015) 136:556–68. doi: 10.1016/j.jaci.2015.04.047
2. Brozek JL, Bousquet J, Agache I, Agarwal A, Bachert C, Bosnic-Anticevich S, et al. Allergic rhinitis and its impact on asthma (ARIA) guidelines-2016 revision. *J Allergy Clin Immunol.* (2017) 140:950–58. doi: 10.1016/j.jaci.2017.03.050
3. Global Initiative for Asthma. *GINA Guidelines 2018. Global Strategy for Asthma Management and Prevention* (2018). Available online at: http://www.ginasthma.org/
4. Noon L. Prophylactic inoculation against hayfever. *Lancet* (1911) 1:1572 doi: 10.1016/S0140-6736(00)78276-6
5. Pitsios C, Demoly P, Bilò MB, Gerth van Wijk R, Pfaar O, Sturm GJ, et al. Clinical contraindications to allergen immunotherapy: an EAACI position paper. *Allergy* (2015) 70:897–909. doi: 10.1111/all.12638
6. Muraro A, Roberts G, Halken S, Agache I, Angier E, Fernandez-Rivas M, et al. EAACI guidelines on allergen immunotherapy: executive statement. *Allergy* (2018) 73:739–43. doi: 10.1111/all.13420
7. Rodríguez Del Río P, Vidal C, Just J, Tabar AI, Sanchez-Machin I, Eberle P, et al. The European survey on adverse systemic reactions in allergen immunotherapy (EASSI): a paediatric assessment. *Pediatr Allergy Immunol.* (2017) 28:60–70. doi: 10.1111/pai.12660
8. Pajno GB, Bernardini R, Peroni D, Arasi S, Martelli A, Landi M, et al. Clinical practice recommendations for allergen-specific immunotherapy in children: the Italian consensus report. *Ital J Pediatr.* (2017) 43:13. doi: 10.1186/s13052-016-0315-y
9. Burks AW, Calderon MA, Casale T, Cox L, Demoly P, Jutel M, et al. Update on allergy immunotherapy: american academy of allergy, asthma & immunology/european academy of allergy and clinical immunology/PRACTALL consensus report. *J Allergy Clin Immunol.* (2013) 131:1288.e3–96. doi: 10.1016/j.jaci.2013.01.049
10. Bauer CS, Rank MA. Comparative efficacy and safety of subcutaneous versus sublingual immunotherapy. *J Allergy Clin Immunol.* (2014) 134:765.e2–765. doi: 10.1016/j.jaci.2014.07.024
11. Nelson HS, Makatsori M, Calderon MA. Subcutaneous immunotherapy and sublingual immunotherapy: comparative efficacy, current and potential indications, and warnings – United States Versus Europe. *Immunol Allergy Clin North Am.* (2016) 36:13–24. doi: 10.1016/j.iac.2015.08.005
12. Bonertz A, Roberts GC, Hoefnagel M, Timon M, Slater JE, Rabin RL, et al. Challenges in the implementation of EAACI guidelines on allergen immunotherapy: a global perspective on the regulation of allergen products. *Allergy* (2018) 73:64–76. doi: 10.1111/all.13266
13. EMA. Committee for medicinal products for human use (CHMP). *Guideline on the Clinical Development of Products for Specific Immunotherapy for the Treatment of Allergic Diseases.* London (2011).
14. EMA. Committee for Medicinal Products for human use (CHMP). *Guideline on Allergen Products Standardization and Quality Issues.* London (2014).
15. Jutel M, Agache I, Bonini S, Burks AW, Calderon M, Canonica W, et al. International consensus on allergen immunotherapy II: mechanisms, standardization, and pharmacoeconomics. *J Allergy Clin Immunol.* (2016) 137:358–68. doi: 10.1016/j.jaci.2015.12.1300
16. Halken S, Larenas-Linnemann D, Roberts G, Calderón MA, Angier E, Pfaar O, et al. EAACI guidelines on allergen immunotherapy: prevention of allergy. *Pediatr Allergy Immunol.* (2017) 28:728–45. doi: 10.1111/pai.12807
17. Shamji MH, Durham SR. Mechanisms of allergen immunotherapy for inhaled allergens and predictive biomarkers. *J Allergy Clin Immunol.* (2017) 140:1485–98. doi: 10.1016/j.jaci.2017.10.010
18. Berings M, Karaaslan C, Altunbulakli C, Gevaert P, Akdis M, Bachert C, et al. Advances and highlights in allergen immunotherapy: on the way to sustained clinical and immunologic tolerance. *J Allergy Clin Immunol.* (2017) 140:1250–67. doi: 10.1016/j.jaci.2017.08.025
19. Akdis CA, Akdis M. Mechanisms of allergen-specific immunotherapy and immune tolerance to allergens. *World Allergy Organ J.* (2015) 8:17. doi: 10.1186/s40413-015-0063-2
20. Kappen JH, Durham SR, Veen HI, Shamji MH. Applications and mechanisms of immunotherapy in allergic rhinitis and asthma. *Ther Adv Respir Dis.* (2017) 11:73–86. doi: 10.1177/1753465816669662
21. van de Veen W, Wirz OF, Globinska A, Akdis M. Novel mechanisms in immune tolerance to allergens during natural allergen exposure and allergen-specific immunotherapy. *Curr Opin Immunol.* (2017) 48:74–81. doi: 10.1016/j.coi.2017.08.012
22. Cox L, Nelson H, Lockey R, Calabria C, Chacko T, Finegold I, et al. Allergen immunotherapy: a practice parameter third update. *J Allergy Clin Immunol.* (2011) 127:S1–55. doi: 10.1016/j.jaci.2010.09.034
23. Larenas-Linnemann D, Luna-Pech JA. What you should not miss from the systematic reviews and meta-analyses on allergen-specific immunotherapy in 2017. *Curr Opin Allergy Clin Immunol.* (2018) 18:168–176. doi: 10.1097/ACI.0000000000000439
24. Pfaar O, Alvaro M, Cardona V, Hamelmann E, Mösges R, Kleine-Tebbe J. Clinical trials in allergen immunotherapy: current concepts and future needs. *Allergy* (2018). doi: 10.1111/all.13429. [Epub ahead of print].
25. Wise SK, Lin SY, Toskala E, Orlandi RR, Akdis CA, Alt JA, et al. International consensus statement on allergy and rhinology: allergic rhinitis. *Int Forum Allergy Rhinol.* (2018) 8:108–352. doi: 10.1002/alr.22073
26. Roberts G, Pfaar O, Akdis CA, Ansotegui IJ, Durham SR, Gerth van Wijk R, et al. EAACI guidelines on allergen immunotherapy: allergic rhinoconjunctivitis. *Allergy* (2018) 73:765–98. doi: 10.1111/all.13317
27. Dhami S, Nurmatov U, Arasi S, Khan T, Asaria M, Zaman H, et al. Allergen immunotherapy for allergic rhinoconjunctivitis: a systematic review and meta-analysis. *Allergy* (2017) 72:1597–1631. doi: 10.1111/all.13201
28. Nurmatov U, Dhami S, Arasi S, Roberts G, Pfaar O, Muraro A, et al. Allergen immunotherapy for allergic rhinoconjunctivitis: a systematic

overview of systematic reviews. *Clin Transl Allergy* (2017) 7:24. doi: 10.1186/s13601-017-0159-6

29. Comberiati P, Marseglia GL, Barberi S, Passalacqua G, Peroni DG Allergen-specific immunotherapy for respiratory allergy in children: unmet needs and future goals. *J Allergy Clin Immunol Pract.* (2017) 5:946–50. doi: 10.1016/j.jaip.2017.01.024
30. Lai CK, Beasley R, Crane J, Foliaki S, Shah J, Weiland S, et al. Global variation in the prevalence and severity of asthma symptoms: phase three of the international study of asthma and allergies in childhood (ISAAC). *Thorax* (2009) 64:476–83. doi: 10.1136/thx.2008.106609
31. Taylor DR, Bateman ED, Boulet LP, Boushey HA, Busse WW, Casale TB, et al. A new perspective on concepts of asthma severity and control. *Eur Respir J.* (2008) 32:545–54. doi: 10.1183/09031936.00155307
32. Dinakar C, Chipps BE. Clinical tools to assess asthma control in children. *Pediatrics* (2017) 139:e20163438. doi: 10.1542/peds.2016-3438
33. Licari A, Marseglia GL. Current and future challenges in pediatric severe asthma. *Curr Med Res Opin.* (2018) 34:943–4. doi: 10.1080/03007995.2018.1439463
34. Tsabouri S, Mavroudi A, Feketea G, Guibas GV. Subcutaneous and sublingual immunotherapy in allergic asthma in children. *Front Pediatr.* (2017) 5:82. doi: 10.3389/fped.2017.00082
35. Licari A, Marseglia A, Caimmi S, Castagnoli R, Foiadelli T, Barberi S, et al. Omalizumab in children. *Paediatr Drugs* (2014) 16:491–502. doi: 10.1007/s40272-014-0107-z
36. Ciprandi G, Marseglia GL, Castagnoli R, Valsecchi C, Tagliacarne C, Caimmi S, et al. From IgE to clinical trials of allergic rhinitis. *Expert Rev Clin Immunol.* (2015) 11:1321–33. doi: 10.1586/1744666X.2015.1086645
37. Licari A, Castagnoli R, Bottino C, Marseglia A, Marseglia G, Ciprandi G. Emerging drugs for the treatment of perennial allergic rhinitis. *Expert Opin Emerg Drugs* (2016) 21:57–67. doi: 10.1517/14728214.2016.1139082
38. Licari A, Castagnoli R, Brambilla I, Marseglia A, Tosca MA, Marseglia GL, et al. New approaches for identifying and testing potential new anti-asthma agents. *Expert Opin Drug Discov.* (2018) 13:51–63. doi: 10.1080/17460441.2018.1396315
39. Virchow JC, Backer V, Kuna P, Prieto L, Nolte H, Villesen HH, et al. Efficacy of a house dust mite sublingual allergen immunotherapy tablet in adults with allergic asthma: a randomized clinical trial. *JAMA* (2016) 315:1715–25. doi: 10.1001/jama.2016.3964
40. Mauro M, Boni E, Makri E, Incorvaia C. Pharmacodynamic and pharmacokinetic evaluation of house dust mite sublingually administered immunotherapy tablet in the treatment of asthma. *Expert Opin Drug Metab Toxicol.* (2015) 11:1937–43. doi: 10.1517/17425255.2015.1113255
41. Mosbech H, Deckelmann R, de Blay F, Pastorello EA, Trebas-Pietras E, Andres LP, et al. Standardized quality (SQ) house dust mite sublingual immunotherapy tablet (ALK) reduces inhaled corticosteroid use while maintaining asthma control: a randomized, double-blind, placebo-controlled trial. *J Allergy Clin Immunol.* (2014) 134:568.e7–75. doi: 10.1016/j.jaci.2014.03.019
42. Maloney J, Prenner BM, Bernstein DI, Lu S, Gawchik S, Berman G, et al. Safety of house dust mite sublingual immunotherapy standardized quality tablet in children allergic to house dust mites. *Ann Allergy Asthma Immunol.* (2016) 116:59–65. doi: 10.1016/j.anai.2015.10.024
43. Lodge CJ, Lowe AJ, Gurrin LC, Hill DJ, Hosking CS, Khalafzai RU, et al. House dust mite sensitization in toddlers predicts current wheeze at age 12 years. *J Allergy Clin Immunol.* (2011) 128:782.e9–88. doi: 10.1016/j.jaci.2011.06.038
44. Lau S, Illi S, Sommerfeld C, Niggemann B, Bergmann R, von Mutius E, et al. Early exposure to house-dust mite and cat allergens and development of childhood asthma: a cohort study. *Lancet* (2000) 356:1392–7. doi: 10.1016/S0140-6736(00)02842-7
45. Illi S, von Mutius E, Lau S, Niggemann B, Grüber C, Wahn U, et al. Perennial allergen sensitisation early in life and chronic asthma in children: a birth cohort study. *Lancet* (2006) 368:763–70. doi: 10.1016/S0140-6736(06)69286-6
46. Ferrés J, Justicia JL, García MP, Muñoz-Tudurí M, Alvà V. Efficacy of high-dose sublingual immunotherapy in children allergic to house dust mites in real-life clinical practice. *Allergol Immunopathol.* (2011) 39:122–7. doi: 10.1016/j.aller.2010.01.008
47. Rice JL, Diette GB, Suarez-Cuervo C, Brigham EP, Lin SY, Ramanathan M Jr, et al. Allergen-specific immunotherapy in the treatment of pediatric asthma: a systematic review. *Pediatrics* (2018) 141:e20173833. doi: 10.1542/peds.2017-3833
48. Penagos M, Passalacqua G, Compalati E, Baena-Cagnani CE, Orozco S, Pedroza A, et al. Meta-analysis of the efficacy of sublingual immunotherapy in the treatment of allergic asthma in pediatric patients, 3 to 18 years of age. *Chest* (2008) 133:599–609. doi: 10.1378/chest.06-1425
49. Ross RN, Nelson HS, Finegold I. Effectiveness of specific immunotherapy in the treatment of asthma: a meta-analysis of prospective, randomized, double-blind, placebo-controlled studies. *Clin Ther.* (2000) 22:329–41. doi: 10.1016/S0149-2918(00)80037-5
50. Abramson MJ, Puy RM, Weiner JM. Injection allergen immunotherapy for asthma. *Cochrane Database Syst Rev.* (2010) 8:CD001186. doi: 10.1002/14651858.CD001186.pub2
51. van de Griendt EJ, Tuut MK, de Groot H, Brand PLP. Applicability of evidence from previous systematic reviews on immunotherapy in current practice of childhood asthma treatment: a GRADE (Grading of Recommendations Assessment, Development and Evaluation) systematic review. *BMJ Open* (2017) 7:e016326. doi: 10.1136/bmjopen-2017-016326
52. Compalati E, Braido F, Canonica GW. An update on allergen immunotherapy and asthma. *Curr Opin Pulm Med.* (2014) 20:109–17. doi: 10.1097/MCP.0000000000000016
53. Calamita Z, Saconato H, Pelá AB, Atallah AN. Efficacy of sublingual immunotherapy in asthma: systematic review of randomized-clinical trials using the cochrane collaboration method. *Allergy* (2006) 61:1162–72. doi: 10.1111/j.1398-9995.2006.01205.x
54. Normansell R, Kew KM, Bridgman AL. Sublingual immunotherapy for asthma. *Cochrane Database Syst Rev.* (2015) 8:CD011293. doi: 10.1002/14651858.CD011293.pub2
55. Lin SY, Erekosima N, Kim JM, Ramanathan M, Suarez-Cuervo C, Chelladurai Y, et al. Sublingual immunotherapy for the treatment of allergic rhinoconjunctivitis and asthma: a systematic review. *JAMA* (2013) 309:1278–88. doi: 10.1001/jama.2013.2049
56. Di Rienzo V, Marcucci F, Puccinelli P, Parmiani S, Frati F, Sensi L, et al. Long-lasting effect of sublingual immunotherapy in children with asthma due to house dust mite: a 10-year prospective study. *Clin Exp Allergy* (2003) 33:206–10. doi: 10.1046/j.1365-2222.2003.01587.x
57. Dominguez-Ortega J, Delgado J, Blanco C, Prieto L, Arroabarren E, Cimarra M, et al. Specific allergen immunotherapy for the treatment of allergic asthma: a review of current evidence. *J Investig Allergol Clin Immunol.* (2017) 27(Suppl. 1):1–35. doi: 10.18176/jiaci.0149
58. Roberts G, Hurley C, Turcanu V, Lack G. Grass pollen immunotherapy as an effective therapy for childhood seasonal allergic asthma. *J Allergy Clin Immunol.* (2006) 117:263–8. doi: 10.1016/j.jaci.2005.09.054
59. Eng PA, Reinhold M, Gnehm HP. Long-term efficacy of preseasonal grass pollen immunotherapy in children. *Allergy* (2002) 57:306–12. doi: 10.1034/j.1398-9995.2002.1o3264.x
60. Hedlin G, Wille S, Browaldh L, Hildebrand H, Holmgren D, Lindfors A, et al. Immunotherapy in children with allergic asthma: effect on bronchial hyperreactivity and pharmacotherapy. *J Allergy Clin Immunol.* (1999) 103:609–14. doi: 10.1016/S0091-6749(99)70232-0
61. Zielen S, Kardos P, Madonini E. Steroid-sparing effects with allergen-specific immunotherapy in children with asthma: a randomized controlled trial. *J Allergy Clin Immunol.* (2010) 126:942–9. doi: 10.1016/j.jaci.2010.06.002
62. Stelmach I, Sobocinska A, Majak P, Smejda K, Jerzynska J, Stelmach W. Comparison of the long-term efficacy of 3- and 5-year house dust mite allergen immunotherapy. *Ann Allergy Asthma Immunol.* (2012) 109:274–8. doi: 10.1016/j.anai.2012.07.015
63. Cools M, Van Bever HP, Weyler JJ, Stevens WJ. Long-term effects of specific immunotherapy, administered during childhood, in asthmatic patients allergic to either house-dust mite or to both house-dust mite and grass pollen. *Allergy* (2000) 55:69–73. doi: 10.1034/j.1398-9995.2000.00191.x
64. Asamoah F, Kakourou A, Dhami S, Lau S, Agache I, Muraro A, et al. Allergen immunotherapy for allergic asthma: a systematic overview of systematic reviews. *Clin Transl Allergy* (2017) 7:25. doi: 10.1186/s13601-017-0160-0

65. Kim JM, Lin SY, Suarez-Cuervo C, Chelladurai Y, Ramanathan M, Segal JB, et al. Allergen-specific immunotherapy for pediatric asthma and rhinoconjunctivitis: a systematic review. *Pediatrics* (2013) 131:1155–67. doi: 10.1542/peds.2013-0343
66. Canonica GW, Cox L, Pawankar R, Baena-Cagnani CE, Blaiss M, Bonini S, et al. Sublingual immunotherapy: world allergy organization position paper 2013 update. *World Allergy Organ J.* (2014) 7:6. doi: 10.1186/1939-4551-7-6
67. Pajno GB, Barberio G, De Luca F, Morabito L, Parmiani S. Prevention of new sensitizations in asthmatic children monosensitized to house dust mite by specific immunotherapy. a six-year follow-up study. *Clin Exp Allergy* (2001) 31:1392–7. doi: 10.1046/j.1365-2222.2001.01161.x
68. Inal A, Altintas DU, Yilmaz M, Karakoc GB, Kendirli SG, Sertdemir Y. Prevention of new sensitizations by specific immunotherapy in children with rhinitis and/or asthma monosensitized to house dust mite. *J Investig Allergol Clin Immunol.* (2007) 17:85–91.
69. Di Bona D, Plaia A, Leto-Barone MS, La Piana S, Macchia L, Di Lorenzo G. Efficacy of allergen immunotherapy in reducing the likelihood of developing new allergen sensitizations: a systematic review. *Allergy* (2017) 72:691–704. doi: 10.1111/all.13104
70. Di Lorenzo G, Leto-Barone MS, La Piana S, Plaia A, Di Bona D. The effect of allergen immunotherapy in the onset of new sensitizations: a meta-analysis. *Int Forum Allergy Rhinol.* (2017) 7:660–69. doi: 10.1002/alr.21946
71. Kristiansen M, Dhami S, Netuveli G, Halken S, Muraro A, Roberts G, et al. Allergen immunotherapy for the prevention of allergy: a systematic review and meta-analysis. *Pediatr Allergy Immunol.* (2017) 28:18–29. doi: 10.1111/pai.12661
72. Burgess JA, Walters EH, Byrnes GB, Matheson MC, Jenkins MA, Wharton CL, et al. Childhood allergic rhinitis predicts asthma incidence and persistence to middle age: a longitudinal study. *J Allergy Clin Immunol.* (2007) 120:863–9. doi: 10.1016/j.jaci.2007.07.020
73. Möller C, Dreborg S, Ferdousi HA, Halken S, Høst A, Jacobsen L, et al. Pollen immunotherapy reduces the development of asthma in children with seasonal rhinoconjunctivitis (the PAT-study). *J Allergy Clin Immunol.* (2002) 109:251–6. doi: 10.1067/mai.2002.121317
74. Jacobsen L, Niggemann B, Dreborg S, Ferdousi HA, Halken S, Høst A, et al. Specific immunotherapy has long-term preventive effect of seasonal and perennial asthma: 10-year follow-up on the PAT study. *Allergy* (2007) 62:943–8. doi: 10.1111/j.1398-9995.2007.01451.x
75. Niggemann B, Jacobsen L, Dreborg S, Ferdousi HA, Halken S, Høst A, et al. Five-year follow-up on the PAT study: specific immunotherapy and long-term prevention of asthma in children. *Allergy* (2006) 61:855–9. doi: 10.1111/j.1398-9995.2006.01068.x
76. Valovirta E, Berstad AK, de Blic J, Bufe A, Eng P, Halken S, et al. Design and recruitment for the GAP trial, investigating the preventive effect on asthma development of an SQ-standardized grass allergy immunotherapy tablet in children with grass pollen-induced allergic rhinoconjunctivitis. *Clin Ther.* (2011) 33:1537–46. doi: 10.1016/j.clinthera.2011.09.013
77. Valovirta E, Petersen TH, Piotrowska T, Laursen MK, Andersen JS, Sørensen HF, et al. Results from the 5-year SQ grass sublingual immunotherapy tablet asthma prevention (GAP) trial in children with grass pollen allergy. *J Allergy Clin Immunol.* (2018) 141:529.e13–38. doi: 10.1016/j.jaci.2017.06.014
78. Novembre E, Galli E, Landi F, Caffarelli C, Pifferi M, De Marco E, et al. Coseasonal sublingual immunotherapy reduces the development of asthma in children with allergic rhinoconjunctivitis. *J Allergy Clin Immunol.* (2004) 114:851–7. doi: 10.1016/j.jaci.2004.07.012
79. Marogna M, Tomassetti D, Bernasconi A, Colombo F, Massolo A, Businco AD, et al. Preventive effects of sublingual immunotherapy in childhood: an open randomized controlled study. *Ann Allergy Asthma Immunol.* (2008) 101:206–11. doi: 10.1016/S1081-1206(10)60211-6
80. Zolkipli Z, Roberts G, Cornelius V, Clayton B, Pearson S, Michaelis L, et al. Randomized controlled trial of primary prevention of atopy using house dust mite allergen oral immunotherapy in early childhood. *J Allergy Clin Immunol.* (2015) 136:1541–1547.e11. doi: 10.1016/j.jaci.2015.04.045
81. Melioli G, Passalacqua G, Canonica GW, Baena-Cagnani CE, Matricardi P. Component-resolved diagnosis in pediatric allergic rhinoconjunctivitis and asthma. *Curr Opin Allergy Clin Immunol.* (2013) 13:446–51. doi: 10.1097/ACI.0b013e32836274d8
82. Fiocchi A, Pajno G, La Grutta S, Pezzuto F, Incorvaia C, Sensi L, et al. Safety of sublingual-swallow immunotherapy in children aged 3 to 7 years. *Ann Allergy Asthma Immunol.* (2005) 95:254–8. doi: 10.1016/S1081-1206(10)61222-7
83. Agostinis F, Tellarini L, Canonica GW, Falagiani P, Passalacqua G. Safety of sublingual immunotherapy with a monomeric allergoid in very young children. *Allergy* (2005) 60:133. doi: 10.1111/j.1398-9995.2004.00616.x
84. Shamji MH, Kappen JH, Akdis M, Jensen-Jarolim E, Knol EF, Kleine-Tebbe J, et al. Biomarkers for monitoring clinical efficacy of allergen immunotherapy for allergic rhinoconjunctivitis and allergic asthma: an EAACI position paper. *Allergy* (2017) 72:1156–73. doi: 10.1111/all.13138
85. Tosca MA, Pistorio A, Accogli A, Silvestri M, Rossi GA, Ciprandi G. Egg allergy: the relevance of molecular-based allergy diagnostics. *Clin Exp Allergy* (2014) 44:1094–5. doi: 10.1111/cea.12360

8

Use of Symptoms Scores, Spirometry and Other Pulmonary Function Testing for Asthma Monitoring

Marcella Gallucci [1], Paolo Carbonara [2], Angela Maria Grazia Pacilli [2], Emanuela di Palmo [1], Giampaolo Ricci [1] and Stefano Nava [2]*

[1] *Department of Pediatrics, S. Orsola-Malpighi Hospital, University of Bologna, Bologna, Italy,* [2] *Department of Specialistic, Diagnostic and Experimental Medicine (DIMES), University of Bologna, Alma Mater Studiorum, Bologna, Italy*

***Correspondence:**
Giampaolo Ricci
giampaolo.ricci@unibo.it*

Asthma is a global problem affecting millions of people all over the world. Monitoring of asthma both in children and in adulthood is an indispensable tool for the optimal disease management and for the maintenance of clinical stability. To date, several resources are available to assess the asthma control, first is the monitoring of symptoms, both through periodic follow-up visits and through specific quality of life measures addressed to the patient in first person or to parents. Clinical monitoring is not always sufficient to predict the risk of future exacerbations, which is why further instrumental examinations are available including lung function tests, the assessment of bronchial hyper-reactivity and bronchial inflammation. All these tools may help in quantifying the future risk for each patient and therefore they potentially may change the natural history of asthmatic disease. The monitoring of asthma in children as in adults is certainly linked by many aspects, however the asthmatic child is a future asthmatic adult and it is precisely during childhood and adolescence that we should implement all the efforts and strategies to prevent the progression of the disease and the subsequent impairment of lung function. For these reasons, asthma monitoring plays a crucial role and must be particularly close and careful. In this paper, we evaluate several tools currently available for asthma monitoring, focusing on current recommendations emerging from various guidelines and especially on the differences between the monitoring in pediatric age and adulthood.

Keywords: asthma, guidelines, asthma monitoring, lung function tests, children, adults

INTRODUCTION

Asthma is one of the most widespread diseases in the world and affects about 300 million patients (1). Despite the high prevalence of asthma in industrialized countries, overall asthma control is still not completely satisfactory. In Europe, only 15% of patients under steroid treatment achieve adequate disease control (2, 3). These findings highlight the importance of optimizing the asthma management in order to improve disease control. Asthma monitoring is an essential step of disease management, which cannot disregard the understanding of the asthma pathogenesis. The main goals of an effective management is the achievement of an optimal control and the prevention of serious exacerbations and impairment of lung function. Achieving control is ensured by monitoring.

The tools for monitoring asthma include the assessment of frequency and severity of symptoms (patient/parents reported or through specific scores) and the use of objective measurements such as spirometry, airway hyper-responsiveness and inflammatory markers.

During the pediatric age, the asthma monitoring must take into account that children are "growing subjects" with the need for continuous treatment adjustments related to the different stages of development not only physical but also psycho-relational. Moreover, healthcare providers do not face a patient but a family unit that must take care of the problem, with all the implications related to school and sports activities.

All guidelines recommend periodic follow-up visits, the interval between visits depends on initial assessment and treatment. Despite the availability of several asthma guidelines, detailed recommendations on asthma monitoring in children and young people (aged 5–16) are poorly defined.

The 2007 American National Asthma Education and Prevention Program (NAEPP) guidelines focuses their attention on the concepts of "impairment and risk" to determine the levels of asthma control and severity, assessed through symptom frequency and measures of lung function among children 5–11 years of age (4). NAEPP guidelines introduced a categorization of asthmatic patients defining them as having "persistent asthma" if they have experienced two or more exacerbations treated with oral corticosteroids (OCS) in the previous 6 months, with a consequent increased future risk. More recently, GINA guidelines state that a previous severe exacerbation in the last 12 months, a history of access into an intensive care or intubation are major independent risk factors for exacerbations (4, 5).

Others factors that increase the future risk in children and adults include the following: socioeconomic or psychological problems, comorbidities such as obesity, chronic rhino-sinusitis, food allergy, exposure to smoke or allergens, low FEV1, higher bronchodilator reversibility, high SABA use, inadequate treatment, sputum or blood eosinophilia and elevated FeNO (5).

The latter two performed before and after the preventive therapy are useful in the assessment of response to medical treatments.

Therefore, the need to quantify the "future risk" for each patient, led the scientific community to search for specific indicators of future exacerbations, such as biomarkers, individual characteristics and genetic factors. These indicators could play a crucial role in asthma monitoring, although some methods are not yet standardized or used in clinical practice.

Scottish Intercollegiate Guidelines Network (SIGN) recommends the monitoring of asthma in children mainly through the assessment of symptoms, number of exacerbations, school absences, evaluation of therapy adherence and inhaler technique, measurement of height, and weight at least annually (6).

Abbreviations: NAEPP, American National Asthma Education and Prevention Program; BDR, bronchodilator reversibility; BHR, bronchial hyper-responsiveness; GINA, Global Initiative for Asthma; FeNO, fractional exhaled nitric oxide; IOS, impulse oscillometry; FOT, technique of forced oscillations; COPD, Chronic Obstructive Pulmonary Disease.

A close monitoring of asthma should include also an early detection of the impairment in lung function as well as the presence of bronchial hyper-responsiveness and bronchial inflammation. These findings are even more relevant in patients at risk, especially in those at high risk of exacerbations or with poor/inadequate disease control (7).

Ideally, a successful management should minimize both daily symptoms and risk factors for exacerbations/complications.

As recommended by the most recent published guidelines (GINA, NICE, SIGN/BTS) the follow up of asthmatic patients should be centered on continuing patients self-monitoring and periodical ambulatory visits for the assessments of the clinical status and lung function parameters (5, 6, 8).

The frequency of follow-up visits depends on asthma severity and the need of treatment adjustments. According to GINA recommendations, the lung function should be recorded at diagnosis, 3–6 months after starting treatment and "periodically" thereafter.

Among pediatric population, an adequate parents training can have a role in reducing the frequency of follow-up visits (9–11).

The main purpose of this article is to compare recommendations of various guidelines about asthma monitoring but also highlighting the differences between recommendations for pediatric and adult patients. In particular, we focus our attention on the availability of clinical tools for assessment of frequency and severity of symptoms, the use of lung function tests and inflammatory markers and the early detection of comorbidities and risk factors for severe asthma.

Monitoring asthma also means investigating the causes of poor medication adherence as well as comprising practical difficulties in using inhaler devices and understanding therapeutic plans especially in adult patients with comorbidities. The lack of awareness and detailed information regarding the importance of treatment adherence, avoidance of triggers, proper inhaler technique significantly contributes to the poor disease control.

Many tools are currently available for clinical and instrumental asthma monitoring, some of these can be performed by patients or caregivers (e.g., PEF), others (such as FeNO, spirometry, or asthma scores) can be made by general practitioners and/or by pulmonologists while some other (such as sputum analysis and oscillometry) only by pulmonologists.

In this paper, we will analyze each of these tools by evaluating different applications in the disease monitoring and comparing different guidelines.

CLINICAL TOOLS

Asthma Control Scores

The clinical history is crucial to assess the asthma control and should include simple key questions and specific asthma scores to collected information about exacerbations, limitations of daily activities, nocturnal awakenings and reliever medication use.

For young children, asthma control should be determined with help from the child's parent through.

TABLE 1 | Main Asthma control scores in children and adults.

	Children	Adults	Normal value/Note
Asthma Control Questionnaire (ACQ) (7 questions) (9)	Validated in adults and children older than 5 years		Well controlled ≤0.75, Inadequately controlled ≥1.5 Minimal important difference 0.5
ACQ shortened (5 five question symptoms only)	Validated in adults and children older than 5 years		More accurate for subjects with normal or near-normal FEV1
Asthma Control Test (ACT) (5 questions) (6)	Validated in children aged for 4–11 year olds	Validated in adults	Reasonably well controlled 20–24; under control 25
Mini Asthma Quality of Life Questionnaire (AQLQ) (32 questions) (10)	–	Validated in adults	Symptoms assessed over the preceding 2 weeks
Pediatric Asthma Quality of Life Questionnaire (PAQLQ) (23 questions) (12, 13)	Validated for age range 7–17 years	–	Higher scores indicate better quality of life
Royal College of Physicians (RCP) (3 questions) (11)	Not validated in children	Not well validated in adults	Probably useful in day-to-day clinical practice
Asthma Therapy Assessment Questionnaire (ATAQ) (20-item) (14)	Mainly used in research	Not used in adults	Include 4 different domains on symptom control, behavior and attitude barriers, self-efficacy barriers, and communication gaps

Both in adult and children, GINA guidelines distinguishes between controlled, partly controlled and poorly controlled asthma based on level of symptoms during the past 4 weeks (5).

This categorization take into account the presence of daily symptoms (>2 per week), any night awakenings, reliever needed (>2 per week) and any activity limitation due to asthma, therefore, controlled asthma is defined by minimal daily symptoms and need of short acting bronchodilator, no nocturnal symptoms and no limitation of activities.

Further and more specific tools to assess the asthma control include quality-of-life measures such as questionnaires applicable in both adults and children (**Table 1**).

The Asthma Control Test (ACT) and the Asthma Control Questionnaire (ACQ) are recommended by all Guidelines and have been studied and extensively validated for both adults and children (the childhood ACT for children 4–11 years of age and the ACQ for children older than 5 years).

ACT includes 5 questions, 3 related to symptoms, 1 related to medication use, and 1 about overall control during the past 4 weeks with separate sections for parent and child; a score ≤ 19 indicate a poor symptoms control (15–17).

The C-ACT include seven items and it is divided into two parts. The first part is addressed to the child and consists of four questions on perception of asthma control, limitation of activities, coughing and awakenings at night. The second one is completed by parents and consists of three questions (daytime complaints, daytime wheezing and awakenings at night) with six response options. The score ranges from 0 (poorest asthma control) to 27 (optimal asthma control). ACT and ACQ are useful to assess the response to longer-term treatment.

The ACQ includes 7 questions, 5 related to symptoms, 1 on rescue treatment use and 1 on FEV1 finding; the control is assessed over the preceding week. For children with normal FEV1 a version of five-point questionnaire is preferable (12).

Other available scores include the Mini Asthma Quality of Life Questionnaire, validated for adults (its counterparts for patients 7–17 years of age is the Pediatric Quality of life Questionnaire) and the Royal College of Physicians 3 Questions (13, 14). The first values the control over the preceding 2 weeks and could be used to assess response to longer-term treatment trials. The latter although not well validated in both adults and children, could be used in day-to-day clinical practice thanks to his simplicity.

In the pediatric setting, GINA guidelines also include the Test for Respiratory and Asthma Control in Kids (TRACK) and the Composite Asthma Severity Index (CASI) both including the assessment of exacerbations. The TRACK is the first validated questionnaire designed to assess asthma control exclusively in young children (<4 years). This score may be more sensible in children since it reflects the changes in asthma control over a short follow up period and take into account the assessment of exacerbations (18, 19). Nevertheless, children may experience more exacerbations during one season vs. another while most of the clinical scores investigate trends over the last month, so they may not be totally indicative of asthma control in children with seasonal wheezing (20).

SIGN guidelines also recommend the use of the Pediatric Asthma Quality of life Questionnaire (PAQLQ) to assess health-related QoL in children with asthma and including 23 questions that investigate 4 domains (symptoms, activity limitations, emotional function, and environmental stimuli), validated for the age range 7–17 years (21, 22).

A further questionnaire is the Asthma Therapy Assessment Questionnaire (ATAQ), a 20-item parent-completed questionnaire, developed to assist clinicians to identify children at risk for adverse outcomes of asthma and including 4 different domains on symptom control, behavior and attitude barriers, self-efficacy barriers, and communication gaps (23).

TABLE 2 | Positive test threshold of objective tests in children (aged 5 years and over) and adults.

	NICE (8)		GINA (5)		SIGN (6)	
	Children	**Adults**	**Children**	**Adults**	**Children**	**Adults**
Obstructive spirometry	FEV1/FVC ratio <70% (or below the lower limit of normal if this value is available)		FEV1/FVC ratio <0.90	FEV1/FVC ratio <0.75–0.80	FEV1/FVC ratio <70%	
Bronchodilator reversibility test	Improvement in FEV1 of 12% or more	Improvement in FEV1 of 12% or more and increase in volume of 200 ml or more	Improvement in FEV1 of 12% or more	Improvement in FEV1 of 12% or more and increase in volume of 200 ml or more	Improvement in FEV1 of 12% or more	Improvement in FEV1 of 12% or more and increase in volume of 200 ml or more**
Peak expiratory flow variability	Variability over 20%		>13%*	>10%*	Variability over 20%***	
FeNO	35 ppb or more	40 ppb or more	FENO >50 ppb has been associated with a good short-term response to ICS		35 ppb or more	40 ppb or more
CHALLENGE TEST						
Methacholine and histamine (both non-specific direct broncho-provocation tests)	n/a	PC20°: 8 mg/ml or less	n/a	Fall in FEV1 of 20% or more with standard dose from baseline	n/a	C20 8 mg/ml or less°
Mannitol	n/i	n/i	n/a	Fall in FEV1 of 15% or more from baseline, with standard dose	Fall in FEV1 15% or more at cumulative dose of 635 mg	
Exercise challenge	n/i	n/i	Fall in FEV1 of >12% predicted , or PEF >15%	Fall in FEV1 of >10% and >200 ml from baseline	n/i	n/i

*Comparison between the different guidelines. n/a, not applicable; n/i, not included. *Calculated from twice-daily readings (best of each time): (HighestPEF-LowestPEF)/mean of the day's highest and lowest PEF, and averaged over 1–2 weeks. **School children using a threshold of 9% change. ***Monitor peak flows for 2–4 weeks. °PC20: provocative concentration of methacholine causing a 20% fall in FEV1.*

A new score defined Severe Asthma questionnaire (SAQ) is being validated in adults; it can be used to detect the impact of both asthma symptoms and treatment on quality of life (24).

Usually, in daily practice, the possibility of using asthma control questionnaires and above all quality of life measures is significantly higher in the pediatric clinical routine.

Certainly, in the pediatric age the supervision of parents ensures a further control and makes these scores more reliable than those compiled by asthmatic patients. Moreover, in the adulthood comorbidities play an important role in the care management, often with reduced time to apply these clinical tools by healthcare professionals.

Concluding, we believe that asthma control scores are simple and useful monitoring tools, but the most of these refer to a short previous period and are often influenced by the subjective (or caregivers') symptom perception, for this reason they should be combined, when possible, with more objective tests such as pulmonary function tests or a careful clinical follow-up.

Patients and Parents Self-Monitoring

Patients as well as parents should be encouraged to keep track of symptoms consequently healthcare practitioners should adequately train them on this issue.

As recognized by several guidelines, many patients can benefit from a written action plan in which, according to the disease control, the patient is instructed to recognize the need for action (e.g., to step up therapy or seek medical advice) (5, 25).

A detailed education program for both adults and pediatric patients should cover: training on treatment adherence and correct use of medication, recognition and avoidance of triggers and risk factors for exacerbations or worsening of symptoms (such as exposure to allergens, influenza virus or rhinoviruses, smoke both active and passive or other environmental factors, including workplace related factors) (25, 26).

Among adults, educational programs have been repeatedly proven effective in improving symptoms control, quality of life and treatment compliance therefore they potentially can prevent or reduce severe exacerbations conducive to urgent visits and hospital admissions (4, 5).

A recent prospective randomized controlled trial including 160 adults with asthma showed that a single 10 min, educational session provided by a respiratory specialist, could substantially improve asthma control determined by the ACT score after 3 months. The educational program included basic information about asthma treatment and instructions on inhalation technique for about 10 min (27).

More recently, new tools for the self-assessment of asthma control are available such as applications for smartphones, often produced by respiratory societies, which can often be obtained for free (28, 29).

These applications enable patients to enter in their profile daily data such as symptoms and their frequency, ACT, PEF values etc. The app can therefore calculate the level of asthma control. Some apps have up to date pollen maps and calendars, or have personalized acoustic memos to remind patients to take the inhaled therapy (30).

Vasbinder et al. in their randomized controlled trial e-MATIC (e-Monitoring of Asthma Therapy to Improve Compliance in children), proposed the use of the "real-time medication monitoring (RTMM)" for improving adherence to inhaled corticosteroids. The study failed to prove a significant improvement in asthma control, quality of life or asthma exacerbations with high costs in the intervention group, although RTMM with tailored SMS reminders improved adherence to ICS (31).

Nevertheless, e- devices may be precious tools for monitoring, especially in adolescence. Teenagers, in particular, may experience age-related difficulties as they accept responsibility for self-management from their parents; the negative impacts of asthma are largely preventable if adolescents engage in self-management behaviors, including symptom prevention as treatment adherence and trigger avoidance or symptom monitoring. It has been proved that the use of "asthma apps" can positively influence adolescents' self-management behaviors through increased self-observation, self-judgment and increased self-efficacy (32).

The availability of these new promising resources certainly opens up new possibilities in the management and monitoring of asthma, even though a recent Cochrane meta-analysis (including 21 studies in adults and children), concluded that tele-healthcare for asthma did not seems to improve QoL or reduce exacerbation rate in children (33). Therefore, further evidences and studies will be needed to routinely recommend the use of these tools in the clinical practice.

LUNG FUNCTION TESTS AND INFLAMMATORY MARKERS

Spirometry

The functional hallmark of asthma is a reversible airway obstruction and its detection is often required for the diagnosis of the disease. The severity of obstruction is a known risk factor for exacerbations, therefore functional monitoring is essential in order to achieve optimal control.

Moreover, severity of obstruction does not always correlate with symptoms: a significant bronchial obstruction may be present also in asymptomatic children and adults. It has been shown that children with chronic obstruction are less likely to perceive the symptom of dyspnea than children with an acute obstruction (34). For this reason, children with poor perception of chronic obstruction are at risk of developing severe exacerbations, associated with poor lung function. Therefore, a regular assessment of lung function is crucial.

The spirometry is the main test for detecting and measuring airway obstruction in children over 5 years old and adults and it has some precision for predicting future attacks.

Reference values of the lung function tests suggested by several guidelines are reported in **Table 2.**

The presence of expiratory airflow limitation should be valued at diagnosis or at the beginning of treatment (in order to evaluate increase in treatment dose), after 3–6 months of controller therapy and then periodically depending on clinical course, although SIGN and GINA guidelines do not indicate clear recommendations on monitoring FEV1 in children (5, 6).

NICE guidelines specify to perform a spirometry for monitoring asthma at each visit or at least after 3 or 6 months from the beginning of therapy and then every 1–2 years (8).

Spirometer parameters should be adjusted according to sex, age, and ethnicity. According to GINA guidelines, the FEV/FVC ratio cut-off of normality is 0.90 in children and 0.75–0.80 in adults (5). Different guidelines often diverge in the choice of this cut-off (according to NICE guidelines, it is 0.70 in both pediatric and adult age) (8) (**Table 2**).

In general, a fixed threshold might lead to an overestimation of obstruction in elderly patients and an underestimation in young ones (35).

In **Table 3** we reported the main lung function tests used in our clinical setting in monitoring asthma.

FEV1 is the most widely used functional index in the asthma follow up; in particular, among asthmatic children a FEV1 <60% is a risk factor for exacerbations and its decrease is associated with increasing asthma severity (36). Children with FEV1 <60% of the predicted seem to have a double risk of asthma exacerbations in the following year compared to those with FEV1> 80% (4, 37).

In order to compare spirometry findings in children, Global Lung Initiative recommend that the spirometry values should be expressed in z score, even though these recommendation is poorly applied worldwide (5).

Adults with an accelerated FEV_1 decline (>30 ml/year) may be either steroid-resistant/difficult-to-treat asthmatics or not adequately treated principally due to under-perception or poorly adherence to maintenance therapy (38).

Some authors have argued that other indices, such as FVC, should be also considered, as some patients with severe obstruction respond to bronchodilators with a significant increase in FVC but not FEV1 (39).

In order to compare spirometry findings in children, Global Lung Initiative recommend that the spirometry values should be expressed in z score, even though these recommendation is poorly applied worldwide (8).

It is well known that the confirmation of the diagnosis requires a positive reversibility test (according to GINA guidelines improvement in FEV1 ≥12 in children, ≥12% together with an increase in volume ≥200 ml in adults). American Thoracic Society recommendations define a significant bronchodilator response (BDR) as an increase in FEV1 ≥12% and/or 200 ml in both adults and children (40).

TABLE 3 | Main lung function tests used in our clinical setting in monitoring asthma.

	Children >5 years	Adults	Normal value	Note
Spirometry	Values widely available, usually within normal range in adults and children with asthma		FEV1/FVC >0.90 in children >0.75–0.80 in adults	Less applicable in acute severe asthma
Positive bronchodilator (BD) reversibility test from baseline suggestive for asthma	++	++	Children FEV1 <10% Adults FEV1<12% and <200 mL	In children sometimes also suggestive also FEV1 >10% In adults more robust FEV1>15% and >400 mL
Peak expiratory flow (PEF) average diurnal variability over 2 weeks	Not routinely used	+	<8% with twice daily readings	Confirmed airflow limitation by variability
AIRWAY RESPONSIVENESS				
Exercise test	Used preferentially for diagnosis and not to monitor disease		Children <12-% adults <10%	Not applicable in patients with impaired lung function (i.e., FEV1/FVC <0.7 and FEV1<70% predicted)
Exhaled nitric oxide (FENO)	Used only in specific protocols for diagnosis and monitoring		<25 ppb at exhaled flow of 50 ml/sec	>50 ppb highly predictive of eosinophilic airway inflammation and positive response to corticosteroid therapy
Eosinophil differential count in induced sputum	–	+	Normal range <2%	Close relationship between raised sputum eosinophil count and corticosteroid responsiveness

+, dubious role in asthma monitoring; ++, potentially useful in asthma monitoring.

Some studies showed that in children, this cut-off may be too high and then less sensitive to assess airway obstruction, suggesting that a lower cut-off (8%) should be used to improve the diagnosis of asthma (41).

The assessment of bronchodilator reversibility (BDR) can be useful not only to confirm the diagnosis but also in the asthma monitoring. In severe pediatric asthma, the spirometry should be always performed with a bronchodilator test to detect airway obstruction and its reversibility since it has been shown that these children have an increased bronchodilator response that may be associated with higher risk of impairment of lung function (42, 43). A persistent BDR may also be associated with poor therapy compliance or wrong inhaler technique and seems to correlate to some indices of airway inflammation, such as the exhaled nitric oxide fraction (FeNO), therefore it might be predictive for a positive response to inhaled corticosteroids (ICSs) (44).

Regarding the most appropriate setting to perform lung function tests, although spirometry performed in the primary care setting may be a useful tool in asthma monitoring, concerns have been raised about the quality and standardization of this procedure compared to hospital-based or laboratory spirometry. The spirometry provides objective data of lung function, but the outcome is often dependent on the operator. Therefore, in our opinion, expert personnel that spurs the patient to an optimal execution should perform it.

Peak Expiratory Flow

Home monitoring of peak expiratory flow (PEF) may be use as an additional functional test in the monitoring of asthma. There is still lack of evidence that PEF monitoring over time might result in better disease control. PEF measurement can be used to document the variability of bronchial obstruction in asthma even if PEF is not related to FEV1 values and may underestimate the degree of airflow limitation and air trapping. Moreover, PEF values vary depending on the meter used therefore it is advisable to compare its measurement with the best personal value (obtained during the disease control phase or during maximum treatment) using the same meter. PEF "personal best" has proved to be useful in improving the progression of asthma, but the patient needs to be adequately trained since measures are effort dependent (45, 46).

According with most of the guidelines, PEF measurement should not be routinely used to monitor asthma in children, unlike in adults where it is recommended for subjects with severe asthma or with poor perception of airflow limitation (5, 6, 8). Certainly, PEF measurements do not give information about the obstruction characteristics (obstructive or restrictive) or site. Nevertheless, NICE guidelines recommend a monitoring of peak flow variability for 2–4 weeks in children and young people (aged 5–16) if there is "diagnostic uncertainty after initial assessment with a normal or obstructive spirometry, irreversible airways obstruction (negative BDR) and a FeNO level of 35 ppb or more" (8). NICE guideline also recommend considering a value of more than 20% variability as a positive test. Even GINA guidelines in the diagnostic assessment of asthma include the use of diurnal PEF variability calculated from twice daily over 2 weeks; for children diurnal variability >13% is considered excessive [unlike in adult where the cut-off of PEF variability is >10% (5)] (**Table 2**).

The ease of execution even in pediatric age and the possibility of being performed at home and during acute phase make this test easy to handle and reproducible, even though its monitoring does not improve asthma control in addition to clinical scores in adults and children (6, 47). For this reason, PEF assessment is not recommended in pediatric age in asthma monitoring.

Impulse Oscillometry, Forced Oscillations Technique, and Expiratory Flow Limitation

During childhood, impulse oscillometry (IOS) and the technique of forced oscillations (FOT) may be used as an alternative technique to assess lung function, since measurements are made from tidal breathing and younger children are able to comply compared to spirometry. IOS measures respiratory resistance and reactance by analyzing responses to pressure waves of different frequency. The assessment of airflow resistance can be an indirect indicator of airway caliber, while spirometry mainly reflects airflow characteristics. IOS is easily performed during tidal breathing therefore it only need a partial collaboration of small patients, even though it is not available in all centers and in some cases, it is difficult to interpret. ERS/ATS guidelines give practice information about the test modality and its analysis (48).

Several studies showed a significant association between findings of the IOS and those of spirometry. In asthma, IOS has been used to assess the bronchodilator response and the therapeutic response to different treatments. In studies utilizing both IOS and spirometry, the first one has proved to be more useful than spirometry in early detection of asthmatic children from normal cohorts (49).

Many evidence showed that peripheral airways (PAW) in children as in adults are the initial site of inflammation and obstruction in asthmatic disease (50).

IOS can evaluate peripheral airways more accurately than spirometry identifying a PAW impairment before symptoms and spirometric abnormalities occur. For these reasons, it could be used to guide an early therapeutic approach to prevent clinical symptoms and further lung damage (51).

In adulthood, excluding patients with severe chronic asthma and marked airway obstruction, an expiratory flow limitation (ELF) at rest is seldom observed, unless under severe and prolonged bronchoconstriction.

One way to value EFL is by the forced oscillation technique (FOT) through the application of negative pressure at the mouth during tidal expiration (NEP).

When the oscillatory pressure applied at the mouth does not reach alveoli during expiration due to a flow-limiting segment in the bronchial tree, the reactance signal, instead of reflecting the mechanical properties of the lung parenchyma and airways, is influenced only by those of the airways and becomes much more negative with a clear distinction between inspiration and expiration.

This application of the FOT is useful to identify flow limitation during tidal breathing, but the closure of intrathoracic airways eventually occurring at end expiratory lung volume (EELV) must be considered as an important limiting factor of this technique, since the distortion of the reactance signal is similar (52, 53).

In addition, when EFL originates in the peripheral airways, it is mainly due to the viscous, density-independent, flow-limiting mechanism, while the speed wave, density-dependent, flow-limiting mechanism is substantially involved when the EFL originates in the central airways.

Despite several potential applications of FOT and oscillometry, larger longitudinal studies will be needed to confirm the usefulness of these techniques as routinely monitoring tools in asthma.

Blood and Sputum Eosinophils

As indicated in the recent ERS/ATS guidelines, the assessment of asthma phenotype (eosinophilic or non-eosinophilic) may play a crucial role in the management of patients with severe disease (54). The ideal tool for this purpose is represented by the cell count on BAL during bronchoscopy. The invasive nature of the procedure has obviously limited the number of subjects studied, therefore the scientific community has sought surrogates that allowed the identification of different asthma phenotypes such as eosinophils count in induced sputum and the peripheral eosinophilia.

Based on the sputum analysis, patients with asthma can be grouped in four different inflammatory phenotypes: eosinophilic asthma, neutrophilic asthma, mixed granulocytic asthma, and paucigranulocytic asthma. Eosinophilic asthma defined as a sputum eosinophil count of 2–3% or higher, represents almost half of the asthmatic population (55).

Several studies have found higher levels of sputum eosinophils in uncontrolled asthmatics, therefore sputum analysis may be a useful method of objectively monitoring asthma (56). Moreover, the short-term response to inhaled corticosteroids depends on the amount of eosinophils present in the sputum therefore this technique may be a guide for modulating steroid therapy (57).

A recent study by Fleming et al. included 55 children with severe asthma and showed that incorporating the control of sputum eosinophils into the management algorithm reduce exacerbations in the short term even though did not significantly reduce overall exacerbations or improve asthma control (58).

It is difficult for children to collect sputum because they tend to swallow more than expectorate.

Among pediatric patients with bronchial hyperactivity, induced sputum, through stimulation with hypertonic saline, may allow to understand the type of inflammation, the presence of cells and lower respiratory tract mediators (59–61).

Several studies have evaluated the safety of sputum induced in asthmatic children aged 6 to 16, demonstrating how moderate bronchospasm occurs in 10% of children and resolves with the administration of the bronchodilator (62, 63).

In clinical practice, the use of these tools for the diagnosis and monitoring of asthma certainly has limitations, however among pulmonologists and also in our center these may be a precious help for the assessment of the type of inflammation, the diagnostic confirmation and the adjustment of the preventive therapy.

In asthma, blood eosinophil are considered a good surrogate marker for sputum eosinophil count (over 2–3% with a cut-off of 220 cells per mm^3 or 3% among adults). High eosinophil count in peripheral blood is a recognized risk factor for disease severity and for future exacerbations (58, 64). During childhood, the asthma predictive index (API) also include blood eosinophils within minor criteria as predictor of future recurrent wheezing (65, 66).

Nadif et al. showed that patients with high blood eosinophilia (>250 cells per mm^3) had lower FEV1 values and worse asthma control than those with eosinophils in normal range (67).

For these reasons, the bronchial and peripheral eosinophilia could be considered a potentially useful biomarker for the selection of patients who will respond to anti IL5 therapy, a monoclonal antibody used in patient older than 12 years with refractory eosinophilic asthma.

Fractional Exhaled Nitric Oxide (FeNO)

As already mentioned, the detection of different asthma phenotypes guided the scientific community searching for specific biomarkers that could guide and improve the disease monitoring and the therapeutic approach. The monitoring of asthma should also include the determination of minimally invasive inflammatory markers.

Fractional exhaled nitric oxide (FeNO) measurement correlates with eosinophilic airway inflammation and therefore with the most common asthma endotype, independently of gender, and age. FeNO levels are higher in asthmatic children compared to non-asthmatic children and in one study values rose further during exacerbations and rapid decline after oral steroid treatment (68–70). British guidelines recognize that a FeNO <20 ppb in children under 12 years may have a role in identifying patients who can step down corticosteroid treatment (5). This relationship is lost in adults smokers (superior cut off in children >35 ppb, in adults >50 ppb) (6) (**Table 3**).

Agency for Healthcare Research and Quality (AHRQ), recently conducted a systematic review (including 175 studies) about the role of FeNO in the diagnosis, treatment and monitoring of asthma. Both in adults and in children FeNO results can predict which patients will respond to inhaled corticosteroid therapy, therefore the use of this marker in long-term managing of treatments can reduce the frequency of exacerbations. Moreover, the review showed that FeNO diagnostic accuracy was modestly better in steroid-naïve asthmatics, children and non-smokers than the overall population. Nevertheless, regarding the asthma monitoring in preschooler children authors concluded that there is insufficient evidence supporting the use of FeNO in this category for predicting a future diagnosis of asthma (69).

Two recent Cochrane reviews, including both pediatric and adulthood studies, showed that tailoring asthma medications based on FeNO levels decreased the frequency of asthma exacerbations but did not impact on day-to-day clinical symptoms or inhaled corticosteroid dose (71–73).

In conclusion, FeNO role in asthma management has not been concretely proven due to incomplete evidence therefore it is not routinely recommended in all patients, at least in monitoring, even though it may be useful in subjects who respond poorly to inhaled corticosteroids (73).

Nevertheless, the use of biomarkers as tools for phenotyping asthma and personalizing therapy is certainly attractive but it has not yet entered clinical practice.

AIRWAY HYPERRESPONSIVENESS

Bronchial Provocation Tests

A hallmark feature of asthma is increased responsiveness of the airways to inhaled stimuli. The assessment of bronchial responsiveness through provocation tests can be useful for both research purposes and clinical practice. Bronchial provocation tests include the direct inhalation of different substances such as methacholine, histamine, mannitol, inhalation of allergens or the use of "stimuli" such as exercise, inhalation of cold air and hyperventilation with dry air (74).

Monitoring of bronchial hyper-responsiveness (BHR) is not routinely recommended in current guidelines, since its role is more typically confined to the diagnostic process.

However, some data seem to indicate a potential usefulness of BHR among asthmatic adults, as an indicator of exacerbation risk and inhaled corticosteroid response (75, 76).

Bronchial provocations tests are not usually performed in asthmatic children and several papers support this recommendation including one clinical trial (77). Nevertheless, BHR assessments could have a role in asthma monitoring among children with exercise limitations or with reduced perception of symptoms (78).

Within the pediatric population, the exercise test may be a precious tool for the evaluation of indirect BHR (79). A reduction in post-exercise FEV1 compared to the baseline is considered a sign of bronchial obstruction induced by exercise. GINA guidelines recognize that the exercise challenge may provide information about airway hyper-responsiveness but "only undertake a challenge if it is otherwise difficult to assess asthma control." A positive exercise challenge for children is considered for a fall in FEV1 >12% of predicted or PEF >15% (for adult a fall in FEV1 >10% and >200 ml from baseline).

NICE guideline clearly recommend of "do not use challenge testing to monitor asthma control," while SIGN group state that "regular monitoring of airway responsiveness not proven to improve asthma control in children" (6, 8) (**Table 2**).

COMORBIDITIES AND RISK FACTORS

Both for adults and children, the detection of potentially modifiable risk factors for exacerbations may be useful in asthma monitoring and includes the exposure to specific allergens, smoking, high SABA use, poor adherence to therapy and incorrect inhaler technique. As already mentioned, GINA guidelines state that a previous sever exacerbation in last 12 months and a history of access into an intensive care or intubation are major independent risk factors for exacerbations (5).

Moreover, the asthma monitoring cannot be separated from an early identification and management of associated comorbidities (**Table 4**).

This term defines factors and/or pathological conditions, which can coexist with asthma, contribute to its severity and to poor control.

Comorbidities are obviously more frequent in adults and may significantly complicate the management of asthma throughout

TABLE 4 | Principal asthma comorbidities.

	Children	Adults	Note
Anxiety and depressive disorders	++	+	Especially during adolescence
Gastro-esophageal reflux disease	+	++	More common in adults, although empiric treatment of asymptomatic GERD in asthmatics does not seem useful (68)
Obesity	++	+++	Asthma is more difficult to control in obese patients
Food allergy/anaphylaxis	+	+	Food allergy is a rare trigger but the association with asthma is a risk factor for anaphylaxis
Allergic rhinitis/Sinusitis	+	++	Often coexist
Nasal polyps	−	++	Exacerbated by aspirin or NSAIDs
Pregnancy	−	+	Change asthma control
Perimenstrual asthma	±	++	Possible role during adolescence
Respiratory infections	+++	++	Often exacerbation factors
Tobacco smoking and environmental exposure	++	+++	Chronic mechanism
Cardiovascular diseases	−	+++	Frequent in elderly
Chronic pulmonary diseases	−	+++	Frequent in elderly

−, not relevant; ±, some relevance; ++, relevant; +++, very relevant.

all its stages, from diagnosis to treatment. All guidelines present this point as relevant in the workup of asthma. The most frequent comorbidities among adult population include upper airway diseases (rhinitis, chronic rhinosinusitis), obesity, COPD, gastro-esophageal reflux disease (GERD), bronchiectasis; in elderly patients, heart failure is very common.

From an epidemiological point of view, rhinitis, and rhinosinusitis are the most frequent comorbidities of asthma for all ages and the former seems to be associated with an increased risk of exacerbations (80). The presence of GERD is associated with worse asthma symptoms and poorer quality of life while obesity can worsen asthma by compromising lung function, inducing corticosteroid insensitivity and systemic inflammation (81–83).

All these conditions often exacerbate or simulate symptoms of asthma causing a poor response to treatment. For these reasons, it is essential to assess and carefully monitor these comorbidities also by implementing integrated care pathways.

Other conditions that may present with elevated blood eosinophilia and a clinical picture mimicking a severe refractory asthma, such as chronic eosinophilic pneumonia, Churg-Strauss syndrome, allergic bronchopulmonary aspergillosis (ABPA), should be taken into account during asthma monitoring (84).

Finally, a subset of adult patients (usually over 40 years of age) present a combination of both asthma and COPD features which is known as Asthma-COPD overlap syndrome (ACOS), likely resulting from different phenotypes of airway disease. They are often smokers, but may have allergies and a family or personal history of asthma with a not completely reversible airway obstruction (5).

Additional diagnostic findings include eosinophilic airway inflammation, a good response to corticosteroid therapy, and high concentrations of exhaled nitric oxide, which should be assessed in the monitoring of these patients (85). Since ACOS outcome is generally worse than asthma with higher treatment needs, the management should be especially careful therefore it might be advisable to refer these patients to specialized center.

ASTHMA ACTION PLAN

The asthma action plan helps asthmatic adults and/or caregivers recognize worsening asthma and gives clear instructions on what to do in response. Each asthmatic patient is different, so each action plan will be too.

An accurate action plan should cover every of these points:

- What medicines to take and when
- A list of potential triggers
- Early symptoms of flare-ups and what to do if they happen
- Know how to manage a full-blown flare-up
- When to get emergency care

The asthma action plan should be based on symptoms trend or peak expiratory flow (PEF) measurements and is individualized according to the pattern of the patient's disease. In children, symptom-based plans are preferred.

Inclusion of PEF measurements in the asthma action plan can be beneficial for adults with more severe or difficult-to-control asthma and those with poor symptoms perception. When PEF is used, the asthma action plan should be based on personal best rather than on predicted values.

Regular review of the asthma action plan is an important part of asthma monitoring since the level of asthma severity and control may change over time (86, 87).

CONCLUSION

An ideal asthma monitoring should provide a personalized approach for each asthmatic patient.

The personalized asthma care should use specific monitoring tools for different patients, preferably with different fields. This assumption therefore represent a fundamental part of comprehensive asthma management.

In light of reported evidences, it may be noted that some advice in monitoring of asthma may apply to both adults and children.

1. The categorization of asthma based on disease severity, which is crucial for the therapeutic planning, require an accurate combination and evaluation of the clinical and functional status.
2. The assessment of risk factors for exacerbations and for severe asthma should be carefully investigated.
3. Moreover, the estimation of future risk allows identifying patients who require a closed follow-up in order to prevent

acute exacerbations and to detect an early impairment of lung function.

4. The use of a written and simple action plan (clear indications on which drugs to take every day, how to spot if asthma's getting worse, and what to do if you have an asthma attack) for both adults and children is advisable and it should be reviewed during each control.
5. At each visit, the patient's adherence to the treatment and correct use of inhaler devices should be assessed and reviewed. For patients who monitor their PEF at home, is advisable to review periodically the correct use of the instrument.
6. Pediatricians should always remember that a careful monitoring of growth and possible side effects of therapy is essential among asthmatic children.
7. Self-management tests associated with monitoring tools for the assessment of pulmonary function and measures of airways inflammation must be appropriate for pediatric age.

Ideally, the follow-up of asthmatic patients should have as its objective a responsible self-monitoring associated with a periodic outpatient check of the clinical status and lung function findings.

As healthcare professionals, we should arouse awareness and self-management. Particularly among adolescents, we should implement a shared decision-making and find ways to connect with them effectively.

The use of new technologies in monitoring asthma is inevitable and may help us to provide great opportunities to monitor patients remotely and to improve the communication.

AUTHOR CONTRIBUTIONS

MG and PC performed the literature review. AP, SN, and EdP contributed to data collection and interpretation of the literature data. GR coordinated the writing group. All authors critically reviewed the manuscript, read and approved the final version.

REFERENCES

1. Bahadori K, Doyle-Waters MM, Marra C, Lynd L, Alasaly K, Swiston J, et al. Economic burden of asthma: a systematic review. *BMC Pulm Med.* (2009) 9:24. doi: 10.1186/1471-2466-9-24
2. Cazzoletti L, Marcon A, Janson C, Corsico A, Jarvis D, Pin I, et al. Therapy and health economics group of the European community respiratory health survey. Asthma control in Europe: a real-world evaluation based on an international population-based study. *J Allergy Clin Immunol.* (2007) 120:1360–7. doi: 10.1016/j.jaci.2007.09.019
3. Demoly P, Paggiaro P, Plaza V, Bolge SC, Kannan H, Sohier B, et al. Prevalence of asthma control among adults in France, Germany, Italy, Spain and the UK. *Eur Respir Rev.* (2009) 18:105–12. doi: 10.1183/09059180.00001209
4. National Asthma Education and Prevention Program. Expert Panel Report 3 (EPR-3): guidelines for the diagnosis and management of asthma-summary Report 2007. *J Allergy Clin Immunol.* (2007) 120(Suppl. 5):S94–138. doi: 10.1016/j.jaci.2007.09.029
5. Global Initiative for Asthma. *GINA Report: Global Strategy for Asthma Management and Prevention.* (2017). Available online at: https://ginasthma.org/gina-reports/
6. British Thoracic Society/Scottish Intercollegiate Guideline Network. *British Guideline on the Management of Asthma.* (2016). Available online at:https://www.brit-thoracic.org.uk/document-library/clinical-information/asthma/btssign-asthma-guideline-2016/
7. Sears MR, Greene JM, Willan AR, Wiecek EM, Taylor DR, Flannery EM, et al. A longitudinal, population-based, cohort study of childhood asthma followed to adulthood. *N Engl J Med.* (2003) 349:1414–22. doi: 10.1056/NEJMoa022363
8. National Institute for Health and Care Excellence. *Asthma: Diagnosis, Monitoring and Chronic Asthma Management.* (2017). Available online at https://www.nice.org.uk/guidance/ng80
9. Holt EW, Cook EF, Covar RA, Spahn J, Fuhlbrigge AL. Identifying the components of asthma health status in children with mild to moderate asthma. *J Allergy Clin Immunol.* (2008) 121:1175–80. doi: 10.1016/j.jaci.2008.02.015
10. Global Initiative for Asthma. *GINA Report: Global Strategy for Asthma Management and Prevention.* (2018). Available online at: https://ginasthma.org/gina-reports/
11. Klok T, de Groot EP, Brouwer AFJ, Brand PLP. Follow-up of children with asthma. *Eur Respir Monogr.* (2012) 56:210–23. doi: 10.1183/1025448x.10018110
12. Liu AH, Zeiger R, Sorkness C, Mahr T, Ostrom N, Burgess S, et al. Development and cross sectional validation of the Childhood Asthma Control Test. *J Allergy Clin Immunol.* (2007) 119:817–25. doi: 10.1016/j.jaci.2006.12.662
13. Juniper EF, Guyatt GH, Cox FM, Ferrie PJ, King DR. Development and validation of the Mini Asthma Quality of Life Questionnaire. *Eur Respir J.* (1999) 14:32–8. doi: 10.1034/j.1399-3003.1999.14a08.x
14. Thomas M, Gruffydd-Jones K, Stonham C, Ward S, Macfarlane TV. Assessing asthma control in routine clinical practice: use of the Royal College of Physicians '3 questions'. *Prim Care Respir J.* (2009) 18:83–8. doi: 10.3132/pcrj.2008.00045
15. Nathan RA, Sorkness CA, Kosinski M, Schatz M, Li JT, Marcus P, et al. Development of the asthma control test: a survey for assessing asthma control. *J Allergy Clin Immunol.* (2004) 113:59–65. doi: 10.1016/j.jaci.2003.09.008
16. Schatz M, Kosinski M, Yarlas AS, Hanlon J, Watson ME, Jhingran P. The minimally important difference of the Asthma Control Test. *J Allergy Clin Immunol.* (2009) 124:719–23.e1. doi: 10.1016/j.jaci.2009.06.053
17. Juniper EF, Gruffydd-Jones K, Ward S, Svensson K. Asthma Control Questionnaire in children: validation, measurement properties, interpretation. *Eur Respir J.* (2010) 36:1410–6. doi: 10.1183/09031936.00117509
18. Zeiger RS, Mellon M, Chipps B, Murphy KR, Schatz M, Kosinski M, et al. Test for Respiratory and Asthma Control in Kids (TRACK): clinically meaningful changes in score. *J Allergy Clin Immunol.* (2011) 128:983–8. doi: 10.1016/j.jaci.2011.08.010
19. Wildfire JJ, Gergen PJ, Sorkness CA, Mitchell HE, Calatroni A, Kattan M, et al. Development and validation of the Composite Asthma Severity Index-an outcome measure for use in children andadolescents. *J Allergy Clin Immunol.* (2012) 129:694–701. doi: 10.1016/j.jaci.2011.12.962
20. Covar RA, SzeflerSJ, Zeiger RS, Sorkness CA, Moss M, Mauger DT, et al. Factors associated with asthma exacerbations duringa long-term clinical trial of controller medications in children. *J Allergy Clin Immunol.* (2008) 122:741–7. doi: 10.1016/j.jaci.2008.08.021
21. Juniper EF, Guyatt GH, Feeny DH, Ferrie PJ, Griffith LE, Townsend M. Measuring quality of life in children with asthma. *Qual Life Res.* (1996) 5:35–46. doi: 10.1007/BF00435967
22. Juniper EF, Guyatt GH, Feeny DH, Ferrie PJ, Griffith LE, Townsend M. Measuring quality of life in the parents of children with asthma. *Qual Life Res.* (1996) 5:27–34. doi: 10.1007/BF00435966

23. Skinner EA, Diette GB, Algatt-Bergstrom PJ, Nguyen TT, Clark RD, Markson LE, et al. The Asthma Therapy Assessment Questionnaire (ATAQ) for children and adolescents. *Dis Manag.* (2004) 7:305–13. doi: 10.1089/dis.2004.7.305
24. Hyland ME, Jones RC, Lanario JW, Masoli M. The construction and validation of the Severe Asthma Questionnaire. *Eur Respir J.* (2018) 52:1800618. doi: 10.1183/13993003.00618-2018
25. Banasiak NC. Childhood asthma practice guideline part three: update of the 2007 National Guidelines for the Diagnosis and Treatment of Asthma. The National Asthma Education and Prevention Program. *J Pediatr Health Care.* (2009) 23:59–61. doi: 10.1016/j.pedhc.2008.10.004
26. Vasileiou E, Sheikh A, Butler C, El Ferkh K, von Wissmann B, McMenamin J, et al. Effectiveness of influenza vaccines in asthma: a systematic review and meta-analysis. *Clin Infect Dis.* (2017) 65:1388–95. doi: 10.1093/cid/cix524
27. Schuermans D, Hanon S, Wauters I, Verbanck S, Vandevoorde J, Vanderhelst E. Impact of a single 10 min education session on asthma control as measured by ACT. *Respir Med.* (2018) 143:14–7. doi: 10.1016/j.rmed.2018.08.003
28. McKay FH, Cheng C, Wright A, Shill J, Stephens H, Uccellini M. Evaluating mobile phone applications for health behaviour change: a systematic review. *J Telemed Telecare.* (2018) 24:22–30. doi: 10.1177/1357633X16673538
29. Hui CY, Walton R, McKinstry B, Jackson T, Parker R, Pinnock H. The use of mobile applications to support self-management for people with asthma: a systematic review of controlled studies to identify features associated with clinical effectiveness and adherence. *J Am Med Inform Assoc.* (2017) 24:619–32. doi: 10.1093/jamia/ocw143
30. Triveldi D. Cochrane review summary: smartphone and tablet self-management apps for asthma. *Prim Health Care Res Dev.* (2015) 16:111–3. doi: 10.1017/S1463423615000018
31. Vasbinder EC, Goossens LM, Rutten-van Mölken MP, de Winter BC, van Dijk L, Vulto AG, et al. e-Monitoring of Asthma Therapy to Improve Compliance in children (e-MATIC): a randomised controlled trial. *Eur Respir J.* (2016) 48:758–67. doi: 10.1183/13993003.01698-2015
32. Pinnock H, Parke HL, Panagioti M, Daines L, Pearce G, Epiphaniou E, et al. PRISMS and RECURSIVE groups. Systematic meta-review of supported self-management for asthma: a healthcare perspective. *BMC Med.* (2017) 15:64. doi: 10.1186/s12916-017-0823-7
33. McLean S, Chandler D, Nurmatov U, Liu J, Pagliari C, Car J, et al. Telehealthcare for asthma: a Cochrane review. *CMAJ.* (2011) 183:E733–42. doi: 10.1503/cmaj.101146
34. Rietveld S, Everaerd W. Perceptions of asthma by adolescents at home. *Chest.* (2000) 117: 434–9. doi: 10.1378/chest.117.2.434
35. Swanney MP, Ruppel G, Enright PL, Pedersen OF, Crapo RO, Miller MR, et al. Using the lower limit of normal for the FEV1/FVC ratio reduces the misclassification of airway obstruction. *Thorax.* (2008) 63:1046–51. doi: 10.1136/thx.2008.098483
36. Moeller A, Carlsen KH, Sly PD, Baraldi E, Piacentini G, Pavord I, et al. ERS Task Force Monitoring Asthma in Children. Monitoring asthma in childhood: lung function, bronchial responsiveness and inflammation. *Eur Respir Rev.* (2015) 24:204–15. doi: 10.1183/16000617.00003914
37. National Asthma Education and Prevention Program. National Asthma Education and Prevention Program. Expert panel report: guidelines for the diagnosis and management of asthma update on selected topics – 2002. *J Allergy Clin Immunol.* (2002) 110(Suppl.):S141–219.
38. Sposato B. Could FEV1 decline have a role in daily clinical practice for asthma monitoring? *Curr Med Res Opin.* (2013) 29:1371–81. doi: 10.1185/03007995.2013.821057
39. Chhabra SK, Bhatnagar S. Comparison of bronchodilator responsiveness in asthma and chronic obstructive pulmonary disease. *Indian J Chest Dis Allied Sci.* (2002) 44:91–7.
40. Reddel HK, Taylor DR, Bateman ED, Boulet LP, Boushey HA, Busse WW, et al. An official American Thoracic Society/European Respiratory Societystatement: asthma control and exacerbations: standardizing endpoints for clinical asthma trials and clinical practice. *Am J Respir Crit Care Med.* (2009) 180:59–99. doi: 10.1164/rccm.200801-060ST
41. Tse SM, Gold DR, Sordillo JE, Hoffman EB, GillmanMW, Rifas-Shiman SL, et al. Diagnostic accuracy of the bronchodilator response in children. *J Allergy Clin Immunol.* (2013) 132:554–9.e5. doi: 10.1016/j.jaci.2013.03.031
42. Teague WG, Phillips BR, Fahy JV, Wenzel SE, Fitzpatrick AM, Moore WC, et al. Baseline features of the Severe Asthma Research Program (SARP III) cohort: differences with age. *J Allergy Clin Immunol Pract.* (2018) 6:545–54.e4. doi: 10.1016/j.jaip.2017.05.032
43. Liu AH. Biomarkers and childhood asthma: improving control today and tomorrow. *Allergy Asthma Proc.* (2005) 26:249–54.
44. Tantisira KG, Fuhlbrigge AL, Tonascia J, Van Natta M, Zeiger RS, Strunk RC, et al. Bronchodilation and bronchoconstriction: predictors of future lung function in childhood asthma. *J Allergy Clin Immunol.* (2006) 117:1264–71. doi: 10.1016/j.jaci.2006.01.050
45. Scichilone N, Contoli M, Paleari D, Pirina P, Rossi A, Sanguinetti CM, et al. Assessing and accessing the small airways; implications for asthma management. *Pulmonary Pharmacol Therap.* (2013) 26:172–9. doi: 10.1016/j.pupt.2012.10.001
46. Reddel HK, Vincent SD, Civitico J. The need for standardization of Peak Flow charts. *Thorax.* (2005) 60:164–7. doi: 10.1136/thx.2004.030437
47. Beydon N, Davis SD, Lombardi E, Allen JL, Arets HG, Aurora P, et al. An official American Thoracic Society/European Respiratory Society statement: pulmonary function testing in preschool children. *Am J Respir Crit Care Med.* (2007) 175:1304–45. doi: 10.1164/rccm.200605-642ST
48. Bickel S, Popler J, Lesnick B, Eid N. Impulse oscillometry: interpretation and practical applications. *Chest.* (2014) 146:841–7. doi: 10.1378/chest.13-1875
49. Komarow HD, Skinner J, Young N, Gaskins D, Nelson C, Gergen PJ, et al. Study on the use of impulse oscillometry in the evaluation of children with asthma: analysis of lung parameters, order effect, and utility compared with spirometry. *Pediatr Pulmonol.* (2012) 47:18–26. doi: 10.1002/ppul.21507
50. Shi Y, Aledia AS, Galant SP, George SC. Peripheral airway impairment measured by oscillometry predicts loss of asthma control in children. *J Allergy Clin Immunol.* (2013) 131:718–23. doi: 10.1016/j.jaci.2012.09.022
51. Galant SP, Komarow HD, Shin HW, Siddiqui S, Lipworth BJ. The case for impulse oscillometry in the management of asthma in children and adults. *Ann Allergy Asthma Immunol.* (2017) 118:664–71. doi: 10.1016/j.anai.2017.04.009
52. Boczkowski J, Murciano D, Pichot MH, Ferretti A, Pariente R, Milic-Emili J. Expiratory flow limitation in stable asthmatic patients during resting breathing. *Am J Respir Crit Care Med.* (1997) 156(3 Pt 1):752–7. doi: 10.1164/ajrccm.156.3.9609083
53. Tantucci C, Ellaffi M, Duguet A, Zelter M, Similowski T, Derenne JP, et al. Dynamic hyperinflation and flow limitation during methacholine-induced bronchoconstriction in asthma. *Eur Respir J.* (1999) 14:295–301. doi: 10.1183/09031936.99.142
54. Chung KF, Wenzel SE, Brozek JL, Bush A, Castro M, et al. International ERS/ATS guidelines on definition, evaluation and treatment of severe asthma. *Eur Respir J.* (2014) 43:343–73. doi: 10.1183/09031936.00202013
55. Green RH, Brightling CE, McKenna S, Hargadon B, Parker D, Bradding P, et al. Asthma exacerbations and sputum eosinophil counts: a randomized controlled trial. *Lancet.* (2002) 360:1715–21. doi: 10.1016/S0140-6736(02)11679-5
56. Romagnoli M, Vachier I, Tarodo de la Fuente P, Meziane H, Chavis C, Bousquet J, et al. Eosinophilic inflammation in sputum of poorly controlled asthmatics. *Eur Respir J.* (2002) 20:1370–7. doi: 10.1183/09031936.02.00029202
57. Petsky HL, Li A, Chang AB. Tailored interventions based on sputum eosinophils versus clinical symptoms for asthma in children and adults. *Cochrane Database Syst Rev.* (2017) 8:CD005603. doi: 10.1002/14651858.CD005603.pub3
58. Fleming L, Wilson N, Regamey N, Bush A. Use of sputum eosinophil counts to guide management in children with severe asthma. *Thorax.* (2012) 67:193–8. doi: 10.1136/thx.2010.156836
59. Gogate S, Katial R. Pediatric biomarkers in asthma: exhaled nitric oxide, sputum eosinophils and leukotriene E4. *Curr Opin Allergy Clin Immunol.* (2008) 8:154–7. doi: 10.1097/ACI.0b013e3282f60f61
60. Hargreave FE, Nair P. Point: Is measuring sputum eosinophils useful in the management of severe asthma? Yes. *Chest.* (2011) 139:1270–2. doi: 10.1378/chest.11-0618
61. Chen DH, Zhong GY, Luo W, Chen QL, Sun BQ, Chen RC, et al. Reference values of induced sputum cytology in healthy children in guangzhou,

southern china. *Pediatrics.* (2013) 131:e518–24. doi: 10.1542/peds.2012-0946

62. Lex C, Payne DN, Zacharasiewicz A, Li AM, Wilson NM, Hansel TT, et al. Sputum induction in children with difficult asthma: safety, feasibility, and inflammatory cell pattern. *Pediatr Pulmonol.* (2005) 39:318–24. doi: 10.1002/ppul.20159
63. Covar RA, Spahn JD, Martin RJ, Silkoff PE, Sundstrom DA, Murphy J, et al. Safety and application of induced sputum analysis in childhood asthma. *J Allergy Clin Immunol.* (2004) 114:575–82. doi: 10.1016/j.jaci.2004.06.036
64. Carr TF, Berdnikovs S, Simon HU, Bochner BS, Rosenwasse LJ. Eosinophilic bioactivities in severe asthma. *World Allergy Organ J.* (2016) 9:21. doi: 10.1186/s40413-016-0112-5
65. Zeiger RS, Schatz M, Li Q, Chen W, Khatry DB, Gossage D, et al. High blood eosinophil count is a risk factor for future asthma exacerbations in adult persistent asthma. *J Allergy Clin Immunol Pract.* (2014) 2:741–50. doi: 10.1016/j.jaip.2014.06.005
66. Amin P, Levin L, Epstein T, Ryan P, LeMasters G, Khurana Hershey G, et al. Optimum predictors of childhood asthma: persistent wheeze or the Asthma Predictive Index? *J Allergy Clin Immunol Pract.* (2014) 2:709–15. doi: 10.1016/j.jaip.2014.08.009
67. Nadif R, Siroux V, Oryszczyn MP, Ravault C, Pison C, Pin I, et al. Heterogeneity of asthma according to blood inflammatory patterns. *Thorax.* (2009) 64:374–80. doi: 10.1136/thx.2008.103069
68. Busse W, Chupp G, Nagase H, Albers FC, Doyle S, Shen Q, et al. Anti-IL-5 treatments in patients with severe asthma by blood eosinophil thresholds: indirect treatment comparison. *J Allergy Clin Immunol.* (2018) 143:190–200.e20. doi: 10.1016/j.jaci.2018.08.031
69. Wang Z, Pianosi P, Keogh K, Zaiem F, Alsawas M, Alahdab F, et al. *The Clinical Utility of Fractional Exhaled Nitric Oxide (FeNO) in Asthma Management.* Rockville, MD: Agency for Healthcare Research and Quality (US) (2017). doi: 10.23970/AHRQEPCCER197
70. Harnan SE, Tappenden P, Essat M, Gomersall T, Minton J, Wong R, et al. Measurement of exhaled nitric oxide concentration in asthma: a systematic review and economic evaluation of NIOX MINO, NIOX VERO and NObreath. *Health Technol Assess.* (2015) 19:1–330. doi: 10.3310/hta19820
71. Petsky HL, Kew KM, Chang AB. Exhaled nitric oxide levels to guide treatment for children with asthma. *Cochrane Database Syst Rev.* (2016) 11:CD011439. doi: 10.1002/14651858.CD011439.pub2
72. Petsky HL, Kew KM, Turner C, Chang AB. Exhaled nitric oxide levels to guide treatment for adults with asthma. *Cochrane Database Syst Rev.* (2016) 9:CD011440. doi: 10.1002/14651858.CD011440.pub2
73. Caudri D, Wijga AH, Hoekstra MO, Kerkhof M, Koppelman GH, Bruekreef B, et al. Prediction of asthma in symptomatic preschool children using exhaled nitric oxide, Rint and specific IgE. *Thorax.* (2010) 65:801–7. doi: 10.1136/thx.2009.126912
74. Lehtimaki L, Csonka P, Makinen E, Isojarvi J, Hovi SL, Ahovuo-Saloranta A. Predictive value of exhaled nitric oxide in the management of asthma: a systematic review. *Eur Respir J.* (2016) 48:706–14. doi: 10.1183/13993003.00699-2016
75. Cockcroft DW, Davis BE. Diagnostic and therapeutic value of airway challenges in asthma. *Curr Allergy Asthma Rep.* (2009) 9:247–53. doi: 10.1007/s11882-009-0036-z
76. Cockcroft DW. Direct challenge tests: airway hyperresponsiveness in asthma: its measurement and clinical significance. *Chest.* (2010) 138(Suppl. 2):18–24S. doi: 10.1378/chest.10-0088
77. Nuijsink M, Hop WC, Sterk PJ, Duiverman EJ, de Jongste JC. Long-term asthma treatment guided by airway hyperresponsiveness in children: a randomized controlled trial. *Eur Respir J.* (2007) 30:457–66. doi: 10.1183/09031936.00111806
78. Galera R, Casitas R, Martínez-Cerón E, Romero D, García-Río F. Does airway hyperresponsiveness monitoring lead to improved asthma control? *Clin Exp Allergy.* (2015) 45:1396–405. doi: 10.1111/cea.12539
79. Riiser A, Hovland V, Carlsen KH, Mowinckel P, Lødrup Carlsen KC. Does bronchial hyperresponsiveness in childhood predict active asthma in adolescence? *Am J Respir Crit Care Med.* (2012) 186:493–500 doi: 10.1164/rccm.201112-2235OC
80. Chiang WC, Chen YM, Tan HK, Balakrishnan A, Liew WK, Lim HH, et al. Allergic rhinitis and non-allergic rhinitis in children in the tropics: prevalence and risk associations. *Pediatric Pulmonol.* (2012) 47:1026–33. doi: 10.1002/ppul.22554
81. McCallister JW, Parsons JP, Mastronarde JG. The relationship between gastroesophageal reflux and asthma: an update. *Ther Adv Respir Dis.* (2011) 5:143–50. doi: 10.1177/1753465810384606
82. Tay TR, Hew M. Comorbid "treatable traits" in difficult asthma: current evidence and clinical evaluation. *Allergy.* (2018) 73:1369–82. doi: 10.1111/all.13370
83. Scott HA, Gibson PG, Garg ML, Wood LG. Airway inflammation is augmented by obesity and fatty acids in asthma. *Eur Respir J.* (2011) 38:594–602. doi: 10.1183/09031936.00139810
84. Cottin V. Eosinophilic lung diseases. *Clin Chest Med.* (2016) 37:535–56. doi: 10.1016/j.ccm.2016.04.015
85. Sorino C, Scichilone N, D'Amato M, Patella V, DI Marco F. Asthma-COPD overlap syndrome: recent advances in diagnostic criteria and prognostic significance. *Minerva Med.* (2017) 108(3 Suppl. 1):1–5. doi: 10.23736/S0026-4806.17.05321-6
86. Gibson PG, Powell H. Written action plans for asthma: an evidence-based review of the key components. *Thorax.* (2004) 59:94–9. doi: 10.1136/thorax.2003.011858
87. Gibson PG, Coughlan J, Wilson AJ, Abramson M, Bauman A, Hensley MJ, et al. Self-management education and regular practitioner review for adults with asthma. *Cochrane Database Syst Rev.* (2000) 2:CD001117. doi: 10.1002/14651858.CD001117

9

Classification of Pediatric Asthma: From Phenotype Discovery to Clinical Practice

Ceyda Oksel[1†], *Sadia Haider*[1†], *Sara Fontanella*[1], *Clement Frainay*[2,3] *and Adnan Custovic*[1*]

[1] Section of Paediatrics, Department of Medicine, Imperial College London, London, United Kingdom, [2] Department of Epidemiology and Biostatistics, Faculty of Medicine, School of Public Health, Imperial College London, London, United Kingdom, [3] INRA, UMR1331, Toxalim, Research Centre in Food Toxicology, Toulouse, France

***Correspondence:**
Adnan Custovic
a.custovic@imperial.ac.uk

† These authors have contributed equally to this work

Advances in big data analytics have created an opportunity for a step change in unraveling mechanisms underlying the development of complex diseases such as asthma, providing valuable insights that drive better diagnostic decision-making in clinical practice, and opening up paths to individualized treatment plans. However, translating findings from data-driven analyses into meaningful insights and actionable solutions requires approaches and tools which move beyond mining and patterning longitudinal data. The purpose of this review is to summarize recent advances in phenotyping of asthma, to discuss key hurdles currently hampering the translation of phenotypic variation into mechanistic insights and clinical setting, and to suggest potential solutions that may address these limitations and accelerate moving discoveries into practice. In order to advance the field of phenotypic discovery, greater focus should be placed on investigating the extent of within-phenotype variation. We advocate a more cautious modeling approach by "supervising" the findings to delineate more precisely the characteristics of the individual trajectories assigned to each phenotype. Furthermore, it is important to employ different methods within a study to compare the stability of derived phenotypes, and to assess the immutability of individual assignments to phenotypes. If we are to make a step change toward precision (stratified or personalized) medicine and capitalize on the available big data assets, we have to develop genuine cross-disciplinary collaborations, wherein data scientists who turn data into information using algorithms and machine learning, team up with medical professionals who provide deep insights on specific subjects from a clinical perspective.

Keywords: asthma, phenotypes, disease progression, machine learning, longitudinal data, big data

INTRODUCTION

Asthma is a term describing a heterogeneous medical condition characterized by variable symptom expression, airway inflammation and therapeutic responses, making the clinical diagnosis challenging and long-term prognosis uncertain (1). Identifying genetic risk factors, environmental associates and pathophysiological mechanisms of asthma is further complicated by the fact that there is no uniform definition of this condition (2–4). In research settings, different studies use different definitions, which may lead to the under- or over-estimation of cases, and any signal in genetic of environmental association studies may be diluted as a consequence of the heterogeneity of the primary outcome measure (5). For example, Van Wonderen et al. reviewed 122 published articles and reported a staggering 60 different definitions of childhood asthma used in cohort studies (4). After selecting four common definitions used in the literature and applying them to a single cohort, the authors found that prevalence estimates varied from 15.1 to 51.1% (4). For the clinical setting, the UK National Institute of Health and Care Excellence (NICE) guidance recommends algorithm for diagnosing childhood asthma which is based on sequential assessment of four objective tests of lung function/airway inflammation (spirometry, bronchodilator reversibility, fractional exhaled nitric oxide, and peak flow variability; https://www.nice.org.uk/guidance). However, a recent study has found a poor agreement between the proposed algorithm and a strict epidemiological definition of asthma (physician diagnosis, current symptoms, and regular use of inhaled corticosteroids) in a birth cohort study (6). The authors suggested that the proposed NICE guidance on asthma diagnosis in children should not be implemented, emphasizing the uncertainties of how to accurately diagnose asthma, and which objective tests are useful (6).

There is increasing recognition that asthma is not a single disease, but a collective noun used to describe a set of clinical symptoms and features which may arise through different pathophysiological mechanisms (7, 8). While the subtypes of asthma sharing similar observable characteristics are often labeled as "phenotypes," "asthma endotypes" are defined on the basis of pathophysiological mechanisms associated with discrete subtypes. There is a general consensus in the medical community that different endotypes of asthma do exist, however, there is no consensus as to what these endotypes are, or how to define them (9). One approach to endotype discovery capitalizes on the advances in computer sciences and software engineering and uses unbiased, data-driven approaches in an attempt to uncover different "phenotypes" of asthma, with the assumption that patterns of clinical symptoms are a reflection of specific underlying pathophysiological mechanisms (9). It is important to emphasize that disease subtypes discovered using data-driven approaches are not observed, but latent (i.e., hidden) by nature, and ideally should not be referred to as "phenotypes" (i.e., observable characteristics). However, as the term "phenotype" has been used in this context for more than a decade (10), we will maintain this nomenclature in this review. A thorough review of the implementation of data-driven methods for phenotype discovery in pediatric asthma has been conducted recently, with a particular focus on childhood wheezing illness and different "wheezing phenotypes" at a population level (11, 12). We will expand the discussion beyond the existing approaches to understanding phenotypic complexity in asthma, and highlight the role of clinical context and clinical experience in linking latent "phenotypes" to underlying biological mechanisms and tailored treatment approaches. We start by highlighting the heterogeneity of asthma and its phenotypic expression, and then discuss potential solutions to maximize the gain from different sources of data, and their clinical utility in asthma research.

DISENTANGLING ASTHMA HETEROGENEITY: FROM SUBJECTIVE TO DATA-DRIVEN APPROACHES

The idea of characterizing asthma subtypes based on the temporal pattern of symptoms through the life-course is not new (13), but has gained momentum in recent years with emerging of data-driven analytic approaches. Over the past two decades, subtyping approaches have progressed from subjective sub-typing to statistical classification techniques. **Table 1** summarizes different approaches for discovering pediatric asthma phenotypes. In subjective sub-typing, phenotypes are identified using predefined or hypothesized criteria based on investigators' insights about clinical features, symptoms, age of onset, and progression rate (14, 23). The main limitation of this approach is that less obvious or rare patterns may be missed. A risk of artificially limiting the set of inputs or imposing a structure on the data is that it may limit the predictive ability of a model by missing associations which do, in fact, exist (9). In contrast, data-driven classification relies on techniques and algorithms that mine the large data sets to uncover the underlying structures and patterns "hidden" in the data. Statistical methods such as cluster analysis and latent class analysis (LCA) (11, 24–26), principal component analysis (20, 27), and exploratory factor analysis (21), have been widely applied to discover homogeneous subtypes of asthma. These procedures ranged from univariate approaches (a single symptom measured over time) to more sophisticated, multivariate approaches that simultaneously model several variables, including symptoms and other clinical and environmental characteristics. By incorporating the longitudinal structure of data, the latter has enabled investigators to capture the multidimensionality of the disease and to characterize phenotypic heterogeneity across the life-course (28).

Nowadays, big data set containing many thousands of variables (such as clinical variables, objective tests, various biomarkers, genome-wide genotyping, proteomics etc.), are extensively used in medical research. In particular, the concept of "big" is difficult to pin down and relative to each field. Big data in healthcare refers to the large volumes of data accumulated from numerous sources, patients and populations that can no longer be easily handled by traditional statistical analysis methods due to its complexity. One of the advantages of big data in medicine is its capacity to examine heterogeneity between diverse populations, build better predictive models around individual patients and deliver more personalized and effective care. As an example, big data could be used to develop analytical tools that can help identify at-risk asthma patients before an attack occurs[1], to identify patients with exacerbations and inadequately controlled asthma (29) and to understand how variations in environmental factors influence childhood asthma hospitalization (30).

In the context of "big data analytics," it is not possible to define *a priori* all possible causal and associational mechanisms (9). By allowing algorithms to model a large number of potential associations in an unsupervised way, patterns can be identified

[1]http://www.propellerhealth.com

TABLE 1 | Different approaches for phenotypic discovery with the associated advantages and disadvantages.

References	Age (years)	Sample size	Methodology	Strengths	Limitations
(13)	1–6	54	Subjective sub-typing	- Phenotypes are observable expressions - Choice of cutoff guided by investigator expertise - Simple	- Predefined or hypothesized criteria needed - Rare patterns may be missed - Risk of over- or under- fitting as there are no objective statistical criteria for judging fit - Subjective cut-offs need to be recalibrated when new data becomes available - Un-validated cut-offs pose challenge for comparing findings across studies
(14)	1–6	826			
(15)	1–6	6265	Latent class analysis	- Probabilistic class allocation. - No prior knowledge is needed. - Hidden patterns may be uncovered that could not be a priori. - Hypothesis generating - Objective statistical criteria for judging whether phenotypes represent true variation	- Discovered sub-types are latent and retrospective by nature - Within-class heterogeneity arising from individuals whose patterns do not exemplify any phenotype - Meaningful clinical interpretation required to explain the patterns - Number of derived phenotypes may be related to the frequency and timing of data collection - Unclear to what extent established phenotype labels convey temporal patterns
(10)	1–7	689			
(16)	1–9	953			
(17)	1–8	5760			
	1–8	2810			
(18)	1–8	1184			
(19)	8–12	3890			
(20)	3–5	946	Principal component analysis	- Accounts for - coexisting symptoms - Reduces the variable dimensions in complex diseases	- Difficult clinical interpretation - Not useful for categorical and longitudinal data unless properly specified
(21)	7–35	925	Exploratory factor analysis		
(22)	6–18	613	Hierarchical clustering	- No a priori info about the number of classes required	- Risk of misclassifying distinct phenotypes that are present at low frequency

that could not have been predicted in advance, even by experts in the field. As such, data is allowed to speak for itself, often without relying on any prior knowledge. However, a danger of this approach is that it may become divorced from rigorous scientific scrutiny and meaningful clinical interpretation (9), since big data can only explain part of the picture (31). In the absence of guidance about the clinical plausibility of findings, there is a risk of identifying false positive associations as the number of relationships being tested increases (32). To be genuinely successful, the "data-driven" approach should encompass making decisions based on both data analysis and interpretation (**Figure 1**), which can only be achieved through a true synergy between the expertise in data science and clinical domain (22).

LATENT VARIABLE MODELING PARADIGMS FOR "PHENOTYPE" IDENTIFICATION

One way to address the complexity of asthma is to derive asthma phenotypes that differentiate groups of patients presenting with similar combinations of symptoms, and to understand how biological factors shape each of these disease "phenotypes" (5). One such approach is latent class trajectory modeling, a class of probabilistic models in which repeated measurements of observable symptoms are modeled to identify homogeneous sub-populations within the larger heterogeneous population. Over the last few decades, latent modeling approaches [reviewed in (9, 11, 12)] have been extensively used to identify longitudinal trajectories of childhood wheeze (10, 17, 33, 34), atopy (34–37), and asthma (11, 12, 19), and to evaluate their associations with early life risk factors. For example, recent studies which used data from several population-based birth cohort studies have described four discrete trajectories of lung function from early childhood to young adulthood (38, 39), providing evidence that early life influences might be crucial not only for childhood asthma, but also for the pathogenesis of COPD in adulthood (28).

However, despite the increasing utilization of (and reliance on) latent class methods to stratify asthma and allergic diseases, there is a striking lack of enquiry into the extent of between-individual variation within the supposedly homogeneous "phenotypes." Latent class methods use posterior probabilities which provide researchers with an objective basis for assigning individuals to classes (phenotypes) that best typify their pattern of symptom development. As these probabilities collectively measure specific individual's likelihood of belonging to each of the classes discovered by a model, a class (or "phenotype") membership is not fixed, and all individuals are assigned a non-zero probability of belonging to each class. It is a common practice to then assign individuals to one of the latent classes according to the maximum posterior probability for an individual belonging to a particular class. Once classified in such way, the individuals are often considered as members of a single class, despite occasionally a considerable variations in posterior probabilities and marginal class assignments.

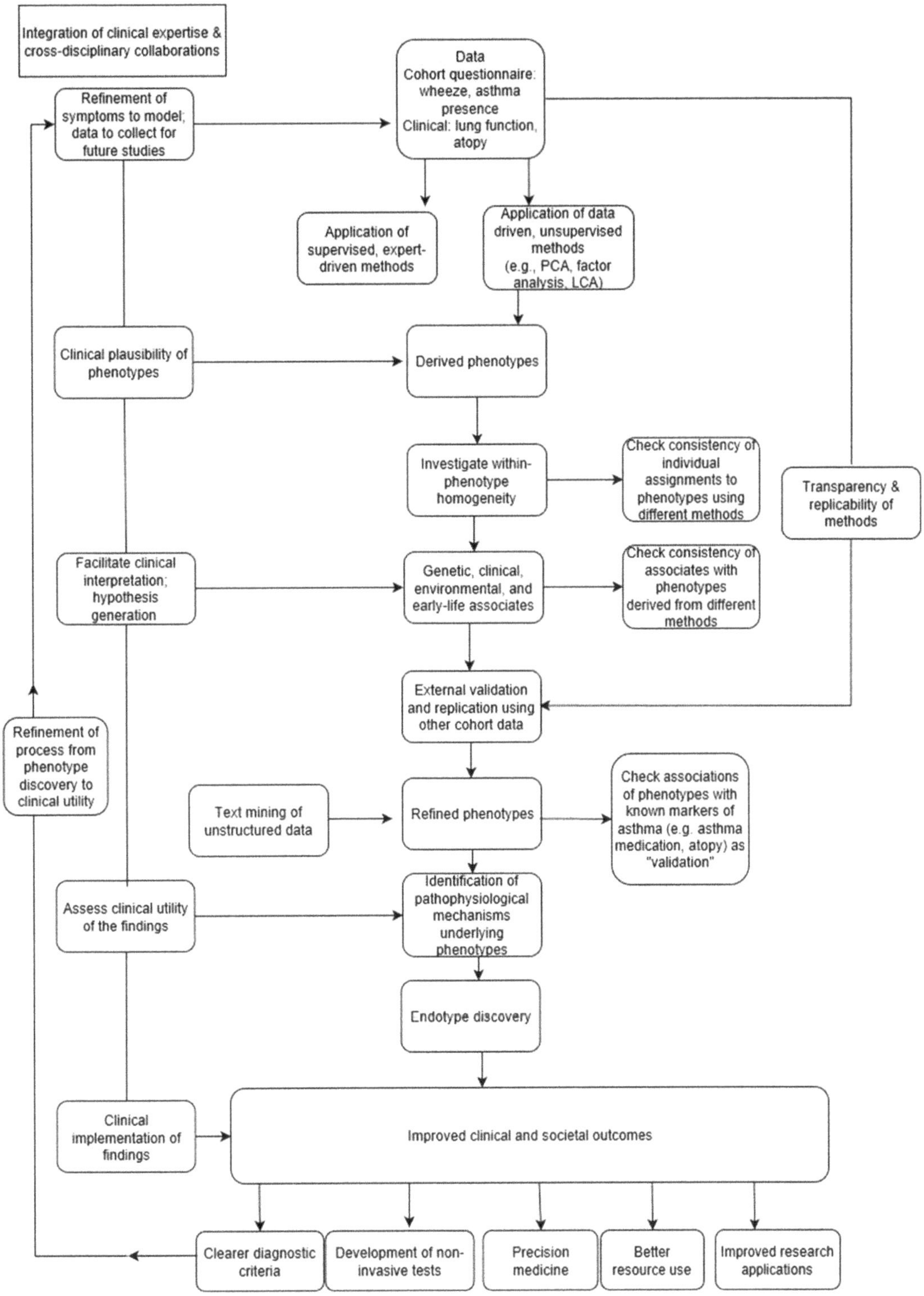

FIGURE 1 | From phenotype discovery to clinical utility.

However, in some cases, there may be subjects who have low posterior probabilities for all classes, and/or whose patterns do not exemplify any phenotype. As an example, an individual may have a 0.5 probability of belonging to "phenotype 1," 0.30 probability of belonging to "phenotype 2," and 0.20 probability of being in "phenotype 3," yet such classification would assign a person into "phenotype 1," ignoring the underlying uncertainty in class assignment. An implication of this is that the latent classes may not, in fact, reflect homogeneous patterns. If we are to understand pathophysiological processes underpinning different phenotypes, then each phenotype should include only individuals whose patterns fit well within the assigned class with a high probability (close to 1), and with a very low probability of belonging to other classes.

Furthermore, it is unclear to what extent the phenotypic nomenclature adequately conveys the temporal characteristics of individuals assigned to the classes, for example, whether "persistent" wheeze means long and/or uninterrupted spells of wheeze, and/or whether "early transient" means absolutely no recurrence of wheeze later in life. Also, one has to be careful not to assume that a persistence of symptoms (such as wheeze) necessarily reflects a persistence of the same pathophysiological process. For example, children with "persistent wheeze" may develop symptoms in early life due to impaired anti-virus responses (40), while the cause of the wheezing later in the school age may be related to other mechanisms such as IgE-mediated sensitisation (41). We would also like to highlight that phenotypes derived from different birth cohort studies often share the same nomenclature (such as "transient early," "late-onset" and "persistent"), but phenotypes with the same assignment often differ substantially in terms of their age of onset, temporal trajectory and distributions within a population. Although common labels are frequently ascribed to latent classes (phenotypes) across studies, it has not been established whether individuals with similar longitudinal profiles are classified to the "same" phenotype in different cohorts sharing similar time points (or even within the same cohort). Moreover, classifications derived from latent class methods appear to be based on a combination of the timing of onset of symptoms and their frequency, but there has been a lack of research into whether there are different levels of disease "severity" within each phenotype, and how would the addition of information on severity impact classification.

A recent review of childhood wheeze phenotypes discovered using data-driven methods found a lack of consistent associations with risk factors and associates across different studies (18). We propose that within-class heterogeneity may be a in part responsible for these discrepancies, and may mask potentially important and consistent associations. Given that the optimal solution for the number of phenotypes may be an artifact of the underlying assumptions of the methods employed, idiosyncrasies particular to a cohort, and within-class heterogeneity, we encourage researchers to investigate the characteristics of the individual trajectories assigned to the phenotypes, and in doing so, question whether the model assumptions are appropriate for the data at hand. In order to reduce misclassification and derive more holistic phenotypes which reflect a" real life" and clinical practice, we would also suggest that rather than focusing on a single symptom (e.g., wheeze), we should employ methods that can incorporate a more comprehensive set of symptoms and/or comorbidities (for example, rhinitis, atopic dermatitis) (42). Thus, in order to achieve more consistency in phenotype discovery (in particular with respect to the role of different risk factors), it may be necessary to move beyond LCA and employ other methods for phenotype discovery.

ADVANCING PHENOTYPE DISCOVERY: THE CASE FOR A MORE REFINED APPROACH

As outlined above, the identification of asthma phenotypes and their underlying distinct pathophysiological mechanisms is crucial for the development of targeted therapeutic strategies (1, 5, 8, 9). In order to achieve this goal, it is imperative that researchers derive asthma phenotypes that are truly homogenous. Whilst data-driven approaches have provided a framework for unearthing a structure within large datasets, there is a risk of assuming that the results represent the "truth," in particular when this assumption is based on a reliance on objective statistical criteria, such as the Bayesian information criterion (BIC), Akaike information criterion (AIC), etc. For the clinical community, the proliferation of machine learning techniques and their associated language inventory of "new" terms [hidden Markov models (34), random forest (42), Bayesian networks (42), latent variable modeling (42), clustering (22), etc.,] are complex to comprehend, even by the statistically literate. Rigorous scientific assessment, reproducibility and transparency of models are increasingly challenging with the availability of diverse programming languages (R, Python, Stata, MATLAB, Infer.Net, MPlus, etc.,). The density of code underlying some algorithms makes it difficult to replicate and validate models (43). Although performance measures to compare the predictive adequacy of various machine learning techniques (area under the curve [AUC], sensitivity, specificity, positive and negative predictive values [PPV and NPV respectively], etc.,) are routinely published, studies rarely demonstrate how numeric improvements in prediction translate into better outcomes for patients. Hence, there is a pressing need for big data research to include data's relationship to improved outcomes at its core. In addition, steps need to be taken to improve the statistical literacy of healthcare professionals through greater education to bridge the divide with the big data "industry." It is essential that clinicians embrace new findings and engage in debates surrounding big data and healthcare.

Birth cohorts have been instrumental in shedding light on asthma heterogeneity, but they alone cannot address all important questions, particularly in relation to severe disease, and the pathophysiological mechanisms underlying different phenotypes. Patient cohorts contain data which complement the information from birth cohorts, and bringing together these data assets may be essential to disaggregate asthma. Such a multi-cohort approach would enhance the credibility, reproducibility and generalizability of phenotyping results, while maximizing the benefits of accumulated and readily available evidence, but methodological challenge of how best to co-analyse the data from different contexts remains unanswered.

THE CLINICAL UTILITY OF DATA-DRIVEN PHENOTYPES

To date, numerous asthma classifications have been proposed based on observable clinical characteristics, disease severity, triggers, age of onset and inflammatory markers. For example, various atopic phenotypes (pollen sensitization with severe exacerbations, multiple allergies with severe asthma, house dust mite, multiple early/late, and late mixed inhalant) were defined based on asthma severity and allergic sensitization in pediatric populations from the TAP (44), MAAS (45), and CAPS (37) cohorts. Similarly, several inflammatory phenotypes (46) such as eosinophilic asthma, neutrophilic asthma, pauci-granulocytic asthma (24, 47–50), and Th2-high asthma (51), and trigger-induced asthma phenotypes such as cigarette smoke-induced asthma (52), air pollution-induced asthma (53), and exercise-induced asthma (54) have been identified in different populations. Although the long-term goal of the phenotype-driven approach is to broaden the personalized management of asthma, translation into clinically actionable endotypes is not readily apparent. This may, in part, be due to the limited ability to identify causative pathophysiological mechanisms of distinct subgroups of childhood asthma. The clinical utility of phenotype classification and their use in everyday clinical practice requires an improved understanding of pathophysiological mechanisms that underlie each asthma subgroup.

One way of bridging the findings from data-driven analytics into day-to-day clinical practice is by linking identified phenotypes to a specific underlying pathology, and tailoring treatment choices based on pathophysiologic mechanisms. Recent advances in molecular techniques offer promising opportunities to link phenotypes with underlying pathological mechanisms. For example, by employing machine learning, a recent study has described an architecture of multiple cytokine responses by human blood mononuclear cells to rhinovirus stimulation comprising six response profiles, and observed major differences in trajectories of asthma, allergic sensitization and lower respiratory tract infections during childhood between these profiles, suggesting that impaired anti-virus immunity may contribute to the development of a specific phenotype of troublesome childhood asthma (41). In another study, Bønnelykke et al (45). identified a novel gene (*CDHR3*) that was associated with a specific phenotype of early onset asthma with severe exacerbations. In subsequent studies, the risk variant in *CDHR3* has been reported to facilitate rhinovirus-C binding and replication (55), suggesting that the *CDHR3* may pose a risk to early-onset asthma with severe exacerbations and hospitalisations through an interaction with RV-C infection (56). Collectively, these findings highlight how the use of umbrella term "asthma" masks the complexity of disease heterogenity, and that the derivation of more precise and internally-homogenous phenotypes may be useful for providing more accurate assessment of underlying pathophysiology. Several recent studies which used machine learning-based methodologies applied to a large amount of data generated by multiplex arrays measuring IgE to more than 100 individual allergenic proteins suggest that it may be possible to develop better diagnostic algorithms to help practicing physicians differentiate between benign and clinically important allergic sensitisation to help asthma diagnosis (57–59).

In short term, the continued validation and replication of asthma phenotypes in different populations, and the integration of novel approaches such as whole genome sequencing and omics profiling to tease out pathological mechanisms underlying different phenotypes are needed to help deliver personalized medicine in clinical practice. In the longer-term, findings from large-scale data have the potential for the development of non-invasive and quick diagnostic assessments for use in clinics (57, 60).

FUTURE POTENTIAL FOR REFINING PHENOTYPES: INTEGRATING TEXT MINING APPROACHES INTO ASTHMA RESEARCH

The exponential growth in the amount of data which is being generated in healthcare setting often makes it difficult to extract knowledge and value from a vast amount of unstructured data, or to understand whether these insights are relevant to the clinical setting (9). To date, over 119,200 scientific articles are indexed in the PubMed database under the "asthma" label, with a publication rate of more than 3,000 asthma-related papers each year (https://www.ncbi.nlm.nih.gov/pubmed/). Methodologies such as text mining are usually seen as a specialization of the broader data-mining field, with the ultimate aim of extracting useful information from unstructured data and unlocking full insight contained in huge volumes of data. They commonly rely on Natural Language Processing (NLP) methods, a key component of many Artificial Intelligence systems, dedicated to the automatic treatment of written, typed or spoken resources. The biomedical field has extended NLP solutions to biological and medical domain (also known as bioNLP) (61, 62), and demonstrated its potential use for performing extraction of asthma candidate genes (63, 64), biological and clinical concepts (65), protein-protein interactions (66), and gene-disease associations (67). Earlier applications of bioNLP in asthma research were limited to text-searching from clinical notes to characterize patients with asthma exacerbation (68), and asthma as a principal diagnosis (69). More recent studies have extended their use to include classification components of NLP which help to classify asthma status at a patient level (70).

The application of NLP to clinical problems holds out great promise of extracting biomedical relations from scientific literature and clinical narratives, and unlocking clinical information from various medical documents such as consultation notes, patient narratives or medical admission and discharge records. However, such clinical information is commonly omitted in phenotyping studies, mostly due to the unstructured nature of the data. While the integration of bioNLP methodologies with machine learning tools may help tackle the inconsistency in asthma ascertainment over many studies, one of the key limitation of bio-text mining approaches is that they still require manual curation and shared annotated datasets which are currently very limited in asthma research (71). The collaborative efforts of biomedical community toward shared objectives and tasks (72), may help overcome the current limits in BioNLP, unlock its full potential for deciphering complex disease, and provide solutions to medical problems that are too complex for a single discipline or method to resolve.

CONCLUSION

Despite a significant contribution of recent phenotyping studies to our understanding of asthma heterogeneity, the translation of findings to clinical practice is hampered by a number of methodological challenges. The promise of data-driven "revolution" to support clinical decision making will not be fulfilled by technological and methodological advances alone, but by a fundamental change in medical culture, and the advancement of a team science approach (5). If we are to make a step change toward personalized medicine and capitalize on the available big data assets, we have to develop genuine cross-disciplinary collaborations, wherein data scientists who turn data into information using algorithms and machine learning, team up with medical professionals who provide deep insights on specific subjects from a clinical perspective, and prioritize which problems to solve. This may facilitate more meaningful and robust disease classification through, for example, a more informed choice of prognostic indicators, and inform the clinical decision-making process. Bringing together diverse disciplines and skill sets is a challenge for medical science in general, and complex heterogeneous long-term conditions such as asthma may offer an example ofs how targeting a particular health problem by looking at it from multiple perspectives can achieve insights that translate to patient benefit through the delivery of personalized medicine.

AUTHOR CONTRIBUTIONS

AC, CO, and SH conceived the idea; SF and CF provided input on the methodology; All authors wrote the report.

REFERENCES

1. Pavord ID, Beasley R, Agusti A, Anderson GP, Bel E, Brusselle G, et al. After asthma: redefining airways diseases. *Lancet* (2018) 391:350–400. doi: 10.1016/S0140-6736(17)30879-6
2. Luo G, Nkoy FL, Stone BL, Schmick D, Johnson MD. A systematic review of predictive models for asthma development in children. *BMC Med Inform Decis Mak.* (2015) 15:99. doi: 10.1186/s12911-015-0224-9
3. Rodriguez-Martinez CE, Sossa-Briceno MP, Castro-Rodriguez JA. Factors predicting persistence of early wheezing through childhood and adolescence: a systematic review of the literature. *J Asthma Allergy* (2017) 10:83–98. doi: 10.2147/JAA.S128319
4. Van Wonderen KE, Van Der Mark LB, Mohrs J, Bindels PJ, Van Aalderen WM, Ter Riet G. Different definitions in childhood asthma: how dependable is the dependent variable? *Eur Respir J.* (2010) 36:48–56. doi: 10.1183/09031936.00154409
5. Custovic A, Ainsworth J, Arshad H, Bishop C, Buchan I, Cullinan P, et al. The Study Team for Early Life Asthma Research (STELAR) consortium 'Asthma e-lab': team science bringing data, methods and investigators together. *Thorax* (2015) 70:799–801. doi: 10.1136/thoraxjnl-2015-206781
6. Murray C, Foden P, Lowe L, Durrington H, Custovic A, Simpson A. Diagnosis of asthma in symptomatic children based on measures of lung function: an analysis of data from a population-based birth cohort study. *Lancet Child Adolesc Health* (2017) 1:114–23. doi: 10.1016/S2352-4642(17)30008-1
7. Anderson GP. Endotyping asthma: new insights into key pathogenic mechanisms in a complex, heterogeneous disease. *Lancet* (2008) 372:1107–19. doi: 10.1016/S0140-6736(08)61452-X
8. Lotvall J, Akdis CA, Bacharier LB, Bjermer L, Casale TB, Custovic A, et al. Asthma endotypes: a new approach to classification of disease entities within the asthma syndrome. *J Allergy Clin Immunol.* (2011) 127:355–60. doi: 10.1016/j.jaci.2010.11.037
9. Belgrave D, Henderson J, Simpson A, Buchan I, Bishop C, Custovic A. Disaggregating asthma: big investigation versus big data. *J Allergy Clin Immunol.* (2017) 139:400–7. doi: 10.1016/j.jaci.2016.11.003
10. Henderson J, Granell R, Heron J, Sherriff A, Simpson A, Woodcock A, et al. Associations of wheezing phenotypes in the first 6 years of life with atopy, lung function and airway responsiveness in mid-childhood. *Thorax* (2008) 63:974–80. doi: 10.1136/thx.2007.093187
11. Deliu M, Belgrave D, Sperrin M, Buchan I, Custovic A. Asthma phenotypes in childhood. *Expert Rev Clin Immunol.* (2017) 13:705–13. doi: 10.1080/1744666X.2017.1257940
12. Howard R, Rattray M, Prosperi M, Custovic A. Distinguishing asthma phenotypes using machine learning approaches. *Curr Allergy Asthma Rep.* (2015) 15:1–10. doi: 10.1007/s11882-015-0542-0
13. Wilson NM. Wheezy bronchitis revisited. *Arch Dis Child.* (1989) 64:1194–9. doi: 10.1136/adc.64.8.1194
14. Martinez FD, Wright AL, Taussig LM, Holberg CJ, Halonen M, Morgan WJ. Asthma and wheezing in the first six years of life. *N Engl J Med.* (1995) 332:133–8. doi: 10.1056/NEJM199501193320301
15. Depner M, Fuchs O, Genuneit J, Karvonen AM, Hyvärinen A, Kaulek V, et al. Clinical and epidemiologic phenotypes of childhood asthma. *Am J Respir Crit Care Med.* (2014) 189:129–38. doi: 10.1164/rccm.201307-1198OC
16. Chen Q, Just AC, Miller RL, Perzanowski MS, Goldstein IF, Perera FP, et al. Using latent class growth analysis to identify childhood wheeze phenotypes in an urban birth cohort. *Ann Allergy Asthma Immunol.* (2012) 108:311–5. e1. doi: 10.1016/j.anai.2012.02.016
17. Savenije OE, Granell R, Caudri D, Koppelman GH, Smit HA, Wijga A, et al. Comparison of childhood wheezing phenotypes in 2 birth cohorts: ALSPAC and PIAMA. *J Allergy Clin Immunol.* (2011) 127:1505–12. e14. doi: 10.1016/j.jaci.2011.02.002
18. Belgrave DC, Custovic A, Simpson A. Characterizing wheeze phenotypes to identify endotypes of childhood asthma, and the implications for future management. *Expert Rev Clin Immunol.* (2013) 9:921–36. doi: 10.1586/1744666X.2013.836450
19. Weinmayr G, Keller F, Kleiner A, du Prel J, Garcia-Marcos L, Batllés-Garrido J, et al. Asthma phenotypes identified by latent class analysis in the ISAAC phase II Spain study. *Clin Exp Allergy* (2013) 43:223–32. doi: 10.1111/cea.12035
20. Smith JA, Drake R, Simpson A, Woodcock A, Pickles A, Custovic A. Dimensions of respiratory symptoms in preschool children. *Am J Respir Crit Care Med.* (2008) 177:1358–63. doi: 10.1164/rccm.200709-1419OC
21. Pillai SG, Tang Y, Van Den Oord E, Klotsman M, Barnes K, Carlsen K, et al. Factor analysis in the Genetics of Asthma International Network family study identifies five major quantitative asthma phenotypes. *Clin Exp Allergy* (2008) 38:421–9. doi: 10.1111/j.1365-2222.2007.02918.x
22. Deliu M, Yavuz TS, Sperrin M, Belgrave D, Sahiner UM, Sackesen C, et al. Features of asthma which provide meaningful insights for understanding the disease heterogeneity. *Clin Exp Allergy* (2018) 48:39–47. doi: 10.1111/cea.13014
23. Jankovic J, McDermott M, Carter J, Gauthier S, Goetz C, Golbe L, et al. Variable expression of Parkinson's disease. *Neurology (*1990) 40:1529. doi: 10.1212/WNL.40.10.1529
24. Haldar P, Pavord ID, Shaw DE, Berry MA, Thomas M, Brightling CE, et al. Cluster analysis and clinical asthma phenotypes. *Am J Respir Crit Care Med.* (2008) 178:218–24. doi: 10.1164/rccm.200711-1754OC
25. Erro R, Vitale C, Amboni M, Picillo M, Moccia M, Longo K, et al. The heterogeneity of early Parkinson's disease: a cluster analysis on newly diagnosed untreated patients. *PLoS ONE* (2013) 8:e70244. doi: 10.1371/journal.pone.0070244
26. Veltman EM, Lamers F, Comijs HC, de Waal MWM, Stek ML, van der Mast RC, et al. Depressive subtypes in an elderly cohort identified using latent class analysis. *J Affect Disord.* (2017) 218:123–30. doi: 10.1016/j.jad.2017.04.059

27. Hilvering B, Vijverberg S, Houben L, Schweizer R, Lammers J-W, Koenderman L. The identification of asthma phenotypes by categorical PCA: combinatorial analysis of clinical parameters and dysfunctional blood eosinophils. *Eur Respir J.* (2014) 44:P3006.
28. Bui DS, Lodge CJ, Burgess JA, Lowe AJ, Perret J, Bui MQ, et al. Childhood predictors of lung function trajectories and future COPD risk: a prospective cohort study from the first to the sixth decade of life. *Lancet Respir Med.* (2018) 6:535–44. doi: 10.1016/S2213-2600(18)30100-0
29. Teach SJ, Gill MA, Togias A, Sorkness CA, Arbes Jr SJ, Calatroni A, et al. Preseasonal treatment with either omalizumab or an inhaled corticosteroid boost to prevent fall asthma exacerbations. *J Allergy Clin Immunol.* (2015) 136:1476–85. doi: 10.1016/j.jaci.2015.09.008
30. Kuo CY, Pan RH, Chan CK, Wu CY, Phan DV, Chan CL. Application of a time-stratified case-crossover design to explore the effects of air pollution and season on childhood asthma hospitalization in cities of differing urban patterns: big data analytics of government open data. *Int J Environ Res Public Health* (2018) 15:647. doi: 10.3390/ijerph15040647
31. Neff G. Why Big Data Won't Cure Us. *Big Data* (2013) 1:117–23. doi: 10.1089/big.2013.0029
32. Rumsfeld JS, Joynt KE, Maddox TM. Big data analytics to improve cardiovascular care: promise and challenges. *Nat Rev Cardiol.* (2016) 13:350–9. doi: 10.1038/nrcardio.2016.42
33. Granell R, Henderson AJ, Sterne JA. Associations of wheezing phenotypes with late asthma outcomes in the Avon Longitudinal Study of Parents and Children: a population-based birth cohort. *J Allergy Clin Immunol.* (2016) 138:1060–70. e11. doi: 10.1016/j.jaci.2016.01.046
34. Lazic N, Roberts G, Custovic A, Belgrave D, Bishop C, Winn J, et al. Multiple atopy phenotypes and their associations with asthma: similar findings from two birth cohorts. *Allergy* (2013) 68:764–70. doi: 10.1111/all.12134
35. Lee E, Lee SH, Kim YH, Cho HJ, Yoon J, Yang SI, et al. Association of atopy phenotypes with new development of asthma and bronchial hyperresponsiveness in school-aged children. *Ann Allergy Asthma Immunol.* (2017) 118:542–50. e1. doi: 10.1016/j.anai.2017.02.008
36. Havstad S, Johnson CC, Kim H, Levin AM, Zoratti EM, Joseph CL, et al. Atopic phenotypes identified with latent class analyses at age 2 years. *J Allergy Clin Immunol.* (2014) 134:722–7. e2. doi: 10.1016/j.jaci.2014.01.022
37. Garden F, Simpson J, Marks G. Atopy phenotypes in the Childhood Asthma Prevention Study (CAPS) cohort and the relationship with allergic disease. *Clin Exp Allergy* (2013) 43:633–41. doi: 10.1111/cea.12095
38. Belgrave DCM, Granell R, Turner SW, Curtin JA, Buchan IE, Le Souef PN, et al. Lung function trajectories from pre-school age to adulthood and their associations with early life factors: a retrospective analysis of three population-based birth cohort studies. *Lancet Respir Med.* (2018) 6:526–34. doi: 10.1016/S2213-2600(18)30099-7
39. Berry CE, Billheimer D, Jenkins IC, Lu ZJ, Stern DA, Gerald LB, et al. A distinct low lung function trajectory from childhood to the fourth decade of life. *Am J Respir Crit Care Med.* (2016) 194:607–12. doi: 10.1164/rccm.201604-0753OC
40. Semic-Jusufagic A, Belgrave D, Pickles A, Telcian AG, Bakhsoliani E, Sykes A, et al. Assessing the association of early life antibiotic prescription with asthma exacerbations, impaired antiviral immunity, and genetic variants in 17q21: a population-based birth cohort study. *Lancet Respir Med.* (2014) 2:621–30. doi: 10.1016/S2213-2600(14)70096-7
41. Custovic A, Belgrave D, Lin L, Bakhsoliani E, Telcian AG, Solari R, et al. Cytokine responses to rhinovirus and development of asthma, allergic sensitization and respiratory infections during childhood. *Am J Respir Crit Care Med.* (2018). doi: 10.1164/rccm.201708-1762OC
42. Prosperi MC, Belgrave D, Buchan I, Simpson A, Custovic A. Challenges in interpreting allergen microarrays in relation to clinical symptoms: a machine learning approach. *Pediatr Allergy Immunol.* (2014) 25:71–9. doi: 10.1111/pai.12139
43. Groeneveld PW, Rumsfeld JS. Can big data fulfill its promise? *Circ Cardiovasc Qual Outcomes* (2016) 9:679–82. doi: 10.1161/CIRCOUTCOMES.116.003097
44. Just J, Saint-Pierre P, Gouvis-Echraghi R, Laoudi Y, Roufai L, Momas I, et al. Childhood allergic asthma is not a single phenotype. *J Pediatr.* (2014) 164:815–20. doi: 10.1016/j.jpeds.2013.11.037
45. Bønnelykke K, Sleiman P, Nielsen K, Kreiner-Møller E, Mercader JM, Belgrave D, et al. A genome-wide association study identifies CDHR3 as a susceptibility locus for early childhood asthma with severe exacerbations. *Nat Genet.* (2014) 46:51–5. doi: 10.1038/ng.2830
46. Fahy JV. Eosinophilic and neutrophilic inflammation in asthma: insights from clinical studies. *Proc Am Thorac Soc.* (2009) 6:256–9. doi: 10.1513/pats.200808-087RM
47. Wenzel SE, Schwartz LB, Langmack EL, Halliday JL, Trudeau JB, Gibbs RL, et al. Evidence that severe asthma can be divided pathologically into two inflammatory subtypes with distinct physiologic and clinical characteristics. *Am J Respir Crit Care Med.* (1999) 160:1001–8. doi: 10.1164/ajrccm.160.3.9812110
48. Moore WC, Meyers DA, Wenzel SE, Teague WG, Li H, Li X, et al. Identification of asthma phenotypes using cluster analysis in the Severe Asthma Research Program. *Am J Respir Crit Care Med.* (2010) 181:315–23. doi: 10.1164/rccm.200906-0896OC
49. Moore WC, Hastie AT, Li X, Li H, Busse WW, Jarjour NN, et al. Sputum neutrophil counts are associated with more severe asthma phenotypes using cluster analysis. *J Allergy Clin Immunol.* (2014) 133:1557–63. e5. doi: 10.1016/j.jaci.2013.10.011
50. Simpson JL, Scott R, Boyle MJ, Gibson PG. Inflammatory subtypes in asthma: assessment and identification using induced sputum. *Respirology* (2006) 11:54–61. doi: 10.1111/j.1440-1843.2006.00784.x
51. Woodruff PG, Modrek B, Choy DF, Jia G, Abbas AR, Ellwanger A, et al. T-helper type 2–driven inflammation defines major subphenotypes of asthma. *Am J Respir Crit Care Med.* (2009) 180:388–95. doi: 10.1164/rccm.200903-0392OC
52. Henneberger PK, Redlich CA, Callahan DB, Harber P, Lemiere C, Martin J, et al. An official American Thoracic Society statement: work-exacerbated asthma. *Am J Respir Crit Care Med.* (2011) 184:368–78. doi: 10.1164/rccm.812011ST
53. Guarnieri M, Balmes JR. Outdoor air pollution and asthma. *Lancet* (2014) 383:1581–92. doi: 10.1016/S0140-6736(14)60617-6
54. Hallstrand TS, Moody MW, Aitken ML, Henderson WR. Airway immunopathology of asthma with exercise-induced bronchoconstriction. *J Allergy Clin Immunol.* (2005) 116:586-93. doi: 10.1016/j.jaci.2005.04.035
55. Bochkov YA, Watters K, Ashraf S, Griggs TF, Devries MK, Jackson DJ, et al. Cadherin-related family member 3, a childhood asthma susceptibility gene product, mediates rhinovirus C binding and replication. *Proc Natl Acad Sci USA.* (2015) 112:5485–90. doi: 10.1073/pnas.1421178112
56. Bønnelykke K, Ober C. Leveraging gene-environment interactions and endotypes for asthma gene discovery. *J Allergy Clin Immunol.* (2016) 137:667–79. doi: 10.1016/j.jaci.2016.01.006
57. Simpson A, Lazic N, Belgrave DCM, Johnson P, Bishop C, Mills C, et al. Patterns of IgE responses to multiple allergen components and clinical symptoms at age 11 years. *J Allergy Clin Immunol.* (2015) 136:1224–31. doi: 10.1016/j.jaci.2015.03.027
58. Custovic A, Sonntag H-J, Buchan IE, Belgrave D, Simpson A, Prosperi MCF. Evolution pathways of IgE responses to grass and mite allergens throughout childhood. *J Allergy Clin Immunol.* (2015) 136:1645–52.e8. doi: 10.1016/j.jaci.2015.03.041
59. Howard R, Belgrave D, Papastamoulis P, Simpson A, Rattray M, Custovic A. Evolution of IgE responses to multiple allergen components throughout childhood. *J Allergy Clin Immunol.* (in press). doi: 10.1016/j.jaci.2017.11.064
60. Holt PG, Strickland D, Bosco A, Belgrave D, Hales B, Simpson A, et al. Distinguishing benign from pathologic TH2 immunity in atopic children. *J Allergy Clin Immunol.* (2016) 137:379–87. doi: 10.1016/j.jaci.2015.08.044
61. Rebholz-Schuhmann D, Oellrich A, Hoehndorf R. Text-mining solutions for biomedical research: enabling integrative biology. *Nat Rev Genet.* (2012) 13:829. doi: 10.1038/nrg3337
62. Gonzalez GH, Tahsin T, Goodale BC, Greene AC, Greene CS. Recent advances and emerging applications in text and data mining for biomedical discovery. *Brief Bioinform.* (2015) 17:33–42. doi: 10.1093/bib/bbv087
63. Perez-Iratxeta C, Wjst M, Bork P, Andrade MA. G2D: a tool for mining genes associated with disease. *BMC Genetics* (2005) 6:45. doi: 10.1186/1471-2156-6-45

64. Tremblay K, Lemire M, Potvin C, Tremblay A, Hunninghake GM, Raby BA, et al. Genes to diseases (G2D) computational method to identify asthma candidate genes. *PLoS ONE* (2008) 3:e2907. doi: 10.1371/journal.pone.0002907
65. Krallinger M, Valencia A. Text-mining and information-retrieval services for molecular biology. *Genome Biol.* (2005) 6:224. doi: 10.1186/gb-2005-6-7-224
66. Ono T, Hishigaki H, Tanigami A, Takagi T. Automated extraction of information on protein–protein interactions from the biological literature. *Bioinformatics* (2001) 17:155–61. doi: 10.1093/bioinformatics/17.2.155
67. Van Driel MA, Bruggeman J, Vriend G, Brunner HG, Leunissen JA. A text-mining analysis of the human phenome. *Eur J Hum Genet.* (2006) 14:535. doi: 10.1038/sj.ejhg.5201585
68. Himes BE, Kohane IS, Ramoni MF, Weiss ST. Characterization of patients who suffer asthma exacerbations using data extracted from electronic medical records. *AMIA Annu Symp Proc.* (2008) 2008:308-12.
69. Zeng QT, Goryachev S, Weiss S, Sordo M, Murphy SN, Lazarus R. Extracting principal diagnosis, co-morbidity and smoking status for asthma research: evaluation of a natural language processing system. *BMC Med Inform Decis Makin.* (2006) 6:30. doi: 10.1186/1472-6947-6-30
70. Wi CI, Sohn S, Rolfes MC, Seabright A, Ryu E, Voge G, et al. Application of a natural language processing algorithm to asthma ascertainment. An automated chart review. *Am J Resp Crit Care Med.* (2017) 196:430–7. doi: 10.1164/rccm.201610-2006OC
71. Chapman WW, Nadkarni PM, Hirschman L, D'avolio LW, Savova GK, Uzuner O. Overcoming barriers to NLP for clinical text: the role of shared tasks and the need for additional creative solutions. *J Am Med Inform Assoc.* (2011):540–3. doi: 10.1136/amiajnl-2011-000465
72. Huang CC, Lu Z. Community challenges in biomedical text mining over 10 years: success, failure and the future. *Brief Bioinform.* (2015) 17:132–44. doi: 10.1093/bib/bbv024

10

Asthma Across Age: Insights from Primary Care

Alan Kaplan[1], Antony Hardjojo[2], Shaylynn Yu[2] and David Price[2,3,4]*

[1] Department of Family and Community Medicine, University of Toronto, Toronto, ON, Canada, [2] Observational and Pragmatic Research Institute, Singapore, Singapore, [3] Division of Applied Health Sciences, Centre of Academic Primary Care, University of Aberdeen, Aberdeen, United Kingdom, [4] Optimum Patient Care, Cambridge, United Kingdom

***Correspondence:**
David Price
dprice@opri.sg

Asthma is a heterogeneous disease comprising of multiple phenotypes and affects patients from childhood up to old age. In this review, we summarize the current knowledge on the similarities and differences in asthma across different age-groups, with emphasis on the perspective from primary care. Despite the similar disease presentation, phenotyping studies showed that there are differences in the distribution of phenotypes of asthma presenting in childhood compared to that in adulthood. Whereas, asthma with early age of onset tends to be of the atopic phenotype, the disease shifts toward the non-atopic phenotypes at later ages. Studies within primary care patients aiming to elucidate risk factors for future asthma exacerbation have shown pediatric and elderly patients to be at higher risk for future asthma attacks compared to other adult patients. Regardless, both pediatric and adult studies demonstrated previous asthma episodes and severity, along with high blood eosinophil to predict subsequent asthma attacks. Differences in childhood and adult asthma are not limited to the underlying phenotypes but also extends to the challenges in the diagnosis, treatment, and management of the disease. Diagnosis of asthma is complicated by age-specific differential diagnoses such as infectious wheezing and nasal obstruction in children, and aging-related problems such as heart disease and obesity in the elderly. There are also age-related issues leading to decreased disease control such as non-adherence, tobacco use, difficulty in using inhalers and corticosteroid-related side effects which hinder asthma control at different patient age-groups. Several clinical guidelines are available to guide the diagnosis and drug prescription of asthma in pediatric patients. However, there are conflicting recommendations for the diagnostic tools and treatment for pediatric patients, posing additional challenges for primary care physicians in working with multiple guidelines. While tools such as spirometry and peak flow variability are often available in primary care, their usage in preschool patients is not consistently recommended. FeNO measurement may be a valuable non-invasive tool which can be adopted by primary physicians to assist asthma diagnosis in preschool-age patients.

Keywords: asthma, guidelines, primary care, children, adult, phenotypes, diagnosis, management

INTRODUCTION

The term "asthma" encompasses1 heterogeneous phenotypes of conditions sharing similar symptoms yet different underlying causes and prognosis (1, 2). Depending on the age of presentation, symptoms of asthma may represent different phenotypes of the disease, each with its own challenges in the diagnosis, management, and treatment. A better understanding of the different subsets of asthma is hoped to assist us to better diagnose, manage, and treat this disorder.

Primary care represents the frontline of patient management and not all patients with asthma require referral to secondary care (3). Thus, this article aims to describe the age-related phenotypes of asthma and the challenges presented by asthma across different age groups, with emphasis on insight from primary care.

ASTHMA ACROSS AGES

Phenotypes of Asthma

The traditional method of asthma phenotyping involves grouping of asthma by characteristics such as the age of onset, trigger, atopic status, and presence of biomarkers, in a so-called "biased" approach to phenotyping (4–6). It is well-known that early-onset asthma represents a distinct phenotype compared to adult-onset asthma. Adult-onset asthma may also be further divided into long-standing asthma, asthma which remitted at childhood and subsequently relapsed, and new onset adult asthma (7).

Cluster analysis presents an unbiased statistical approach to phenotype asthma by grouping them into clusters with maximum similar characteristics within clusters and minimum similarity between clusters (**Table 1**). Haldar et al. conducted a cluster analysis from both patents with milder asthma presenting in primary care, as well as patients with refractory asthma diagnosed in secondary care (2). The study identified 3 and 4 separate clusters of asthma from the respective populations, 2 of which were identified from both populations. Two clusters denoted with early onset were both accompanied with positive atopic status, one of which had minimal signs of eosinophilic inflammation. Clusters of late-onset asthma include a cluster of obesity-related non-eosinophilic asthma predominant in females and a male-predominated cluster predominantly marked by active eosinophilic inflammation but fewer symptoms. Both late-onset clusters also consisted of lower proportion of patients with positive atopic status compared to the early onset clusters.

A cluster analysis which combined severe asthma and non-severe asthma patients recruited into the Severe Asthma Research Program (SARP) identified 5 clusters of asthma (8). Similar to the characteristics of the clusters identified by Haldar et al., clusters associated with early age of onset were also associated with higher atopic status while those with later-onset were less atopic. Another cluster analysis study was conducted on children (6–11 years) and adolescent to adult patients (>11 years) with severe or difficult-to-treat asthma from the TENOR (The Epidemiology and Natural History of Asthma: Outcomes and Treatment Regimens) study (9). Five clusters were identified within both age-groups differentiated by demographics, a topic status, tobacco exposure (in children), and aspirin sensitivity (in adolescent to adults). Interestingly, in contrast to adolescent and adult patients, none of the five children clusters had significantly different asthma outcomes (within the next 12 months) among each other, though this is likely due to the population of the study being limited to severe asthma patients.

Results from both classic "biased" phenotyping studies and cluster analysis studies thus confirmed that early onset asthma is more likely to be atopic in nature, while adult-onset asthma tends to have non-atopic causes, primarily obesity. **Figure 1** illustrates a simple representation of this relationship between the atopic status of asthma and age as previously reviewed by Wenzel et al. (6).

Current asthma guidelines state that more research on the value of asthma phenotyping to guide treatment is required (10, 11).

Severe Asthma Across the Age

An estimated 5–10% of asthma patients suffer from a severe form of asthma (12). Despite the rarity, severe asthma poses high healthcare resource burden (13). The GINA (Global INitiatives for Asthma) guideline defined severe asthma as asthma which requires high dose ICS (inhaled corticosteroid)/LABA to prevent it from being uncontrolled or asthma which remains uncontrolled despite this treatment (10). Regardless, there is currently no universally accepted definition for severe asthma, preventing accurate estimation of its global prevalence, which is further contributed by the absence of a global registry for this subset of asthma until the recent creation of the International Severe Asthma Registry (14).

A recent review by Guilbert et al. highlighted the differences between adult and pediatric severe asthma (15). Compared to the adult counterpart, severe asthma in children had a more rapidly changing phenotype. They were also characterized with higher exhaled nitric oxide, IgE, and eosinophil levels. Despite the differences in pediatric and adult severe asthma, the current treatment guidelines for pediatric severe asthma is currently based on extrapolation from adult studies (15). Thus, there is a need for better guidelines on severe childhood asthma.

RISK PREDICTION OF ASTHMA

Asthma exacerbation is a major cause of quality of life disruption and healthcare resource consumption. Thus, a part of asthma management includes managing the risk for future asthma exacerbations/attacks on top of maintaining symptom control (10, 16). The GINA provides a guideline for assessment of asthma exacerbations in primary care setting (10). The guideline suggests documentation of symptom histories such as the onset, severity, potential risk factors, and current therapy, along with physical examination and objective measurements such as pulse oximetry and peak expiratory flow measurement (for patients > 5 year).

Numerous studies have been conducted to investigate potential risk factors for future asthma exacerbations (**Table 2**). Observational studies using primary care data have identified factors such as previous asthma attacks and medication usage in

TABLE 1 | Clusters of asthma phenotypes.

Population analyzed	Additional patient details	Clusters Identified
Haldar et al. (2)		
1. Primary care (n = 184)	Age range: 18–65 years	1. Early-onset atopic (n = 61) 2. Obese, non-eosinophilic (n = 27) 3. Benign (n = 96)
2. Secondary care (n = 187)	Age range: not specified	1. Early-onset atopic (n = 74) 2. Obese, non-eosinophilic (n = 23) 3. Early symptom predominant (n = 22) 4. Inflammation predominant (n = 68)
Moore et al. SARP study, 2010 (8)		
12–80 years old (n = 726), 304 fulfilled criteria for severe asthma	Primary/secondary: not specified	1. Early-onset atopic, normal lung function and low healthcare utilization (n = 110) 2. Early-onset atopic, higher medication requirement (n = 321) 3. Late-onset, less-atopic, obesity-related, lower lung function, and more daily symptoms and healthcare utilization (n = 59) 4. More severe, long-standing, early-onset, atopic, reversible lung obstruction, high ICS usage (n = 120) 5. More severe, long-standing, late-onset, less-atopic, less-reversible lung obstruction, high ICS usage (n = 116)
Schatz et al. TENOR study, 2014 (9)		
6–11 years old (n = 518)	Patients recruited from "managed care organizations, community physicians or group practices, and academic centers"	1. White race with no tobacco exposure (n = 115) 2. Female cluster (n = 81) 3. Non-atopic (n = 162) 4. Passive smoke exposed (n = 87) 5. Non-white race (n = 73)
≥12 years old (n = 3,612)		1. White female adult onset, low IgE (n = 1262) 2. High atopic cluster (n = 659) 3. Male cluster (n = 664) 4. Non-white cluster (n = 596) 5. Non-white race (n = 431)

ICS, Inhaled corticosteroid.

and biomarkers such as blood eosinophil to predict exacerbations in subsequent years (17, 18).

Knowledge of the risk factors for asthma attacks in children is scarce, and even less is known in preschool asthma, where exacerbation may have viral triggers (19). Swern et al. conducted a *post-hoc* analysis of 2–5years old patients (n = 689) previously enrolled in a randomized control trial (20) The trial included patients with physician-diagnosed asthma defined as ≥3 episodes of asthma symptoms in the past year including but not limited to cough, wheezing and shortness of breath. The study identified a combination of daytime cough, daytime wheeze, and night-time β2-agonist use to be predictive of exacerbation in the following day. However, this study did not report risks for exacerbations further than 3 days after the identification of risk factors.

A very recent study by Bloom et al. reported the exacerbation risks on the general asthma population across different age-groups including patients under 5 years old within the UK's national electronic healthcare records (3). Interestingly, patients ≥55 years and <5 years had the highest rate for exacerbations, in comparison to adolescents (5–17 year) and adults (18–54 years). Regardless of the age groups, higher asthma severity (as defined by the BTS [British Thoracic Society] treatment steps) was a significant predictor for annual exacerbation rate and time to next exacerbation, especially within the <5 years group.

Results on older children and adolescents confirmed the findings of the adult studies, i.e., recent asthma attacks and blood/systemic eosinophilia were consistently reported as predictors for future attacks (17, 18, 21–25). A recent observational study combining data from 2 primary care databases in the UK also reported recent asthma attacks, previous consultation for lower respiratory infections, blood eosinophils > 400/μL, and younger age to be indicative of high-risk for future asthma exacerbation in children 5–12 years of age (23). Another large observational study using general practice data of Dutch children 5–18 years old reported asthma exacerbations and asthma treatment in the preceding year and younger age to be risk factors for severe asthma exacerbations (24). While blood eosinophil level of ≥300 cells/uL was not a risk factor, children with heightened blood eosinophil had shorter time till exacerbation.

Interestingly, in contrast to adult population studies where older age was associated with increased risk (17, 18), studies in children reported younger age to be associated with higher risk for asthma attacks/exacerbations (23, 24). This confirms the observation by Bloom et al that patients at both ends of the age spectrum were at the highest risk for exacerbations (**Figure 2**) (3).

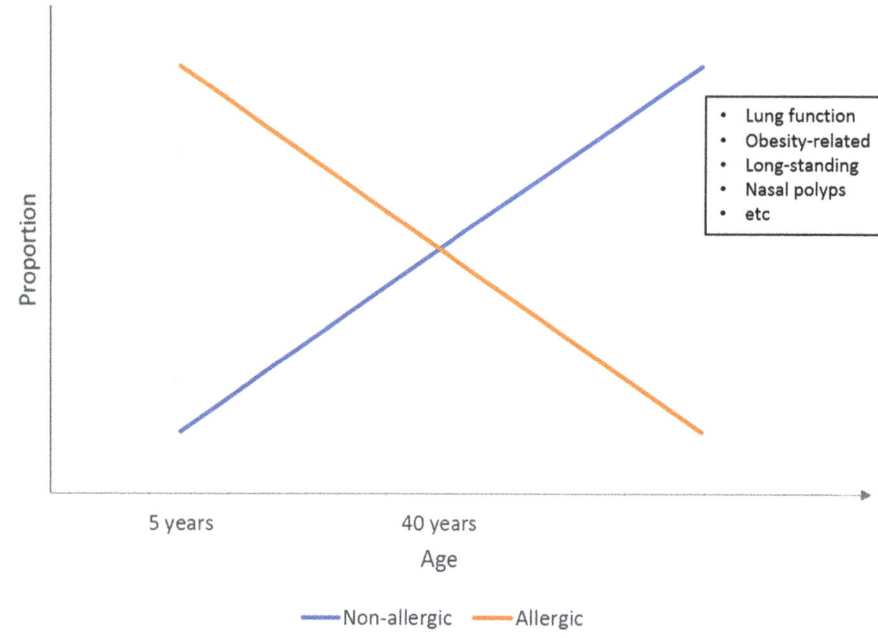

FIGURE 1 | Illustration of the relationship between asthma phenotypes and the age of onset. At younger age, asthma is predominated by the atopic phenotypes, which are gradually phased out by non-atopic phenotypes such as obesity-related asthma at adulthood.

DIAGNOSTIC CHALLENGES ACROSS AGE

There is still a very clear lack of understanding of asthma in children under 5 years, and diagnosis of asthma within the preschool age is challenging due to the lack of proper guideline and definition (26). In this age group, symptoms of wheezing and cough are very common but may be the result of acute respiratory infections instead of asthma (**Figure 3**) (27, 28). The Tucson birth cohort (USA) identified three distinct phenotypes of wheezing in the first 6 years of life: transient early wheezing, late onset wheezing and persistent wheezing (29, 30). The result from subsequent follow-up reported that not all children who wheezed developed asthma in later childhood, although children with atopic wheezing were the most likely (30). Thus, differentiating transient symptoms from symptoms of the more persistent asthma poses a challenge in early age.

The GINA (10) and CTS (Canadian Thoracic Society) (31) guidelines recommend consideration of symptomatology, potential triggers and family history to assist in clinical decision making for this age group of patients. The guidelines additionally recommend observing for signs of airway obstruction and reversibility with inhaled bronchodilators to assist in diagnosis. Similarly, the Australian Asthma Handbook (32) and NICE guideline (33) recommend treating preschool patients with suspected asthma based on clinical observation and conduct objective tests only after 5 years of age.

Objective tools recommended by the clinical guidelines to diagnose asthma across different age groups are summarized in **Table 3**. Lung function tests, primarily spirometry, are recommended to confirm asthma diagnosis in school-aged children and adults within primary care practice (10, 11, 16, 33–35). However, in many countries, spirometry is not available to primary care, and conducting lung function tests on patients <5 years old is challenging due to their inability to produce consistent lung function readings (**Figure 3**) (10, 26, 28, 36). The BTS guideline thus does not recommend lung function measurement to guide asthma management in this age group (16). A joint statement by the American Thoracic Society (ATS) and European Respiratory Society (ERS) suggested taking only one satisfactory measurement, instead of the ideal of at least two separate measurements to accommodate pediatric patients (36). The GEMA emphasizes the need for nursing supervision and suggested measurement of $FEV_{0.5}$ instead of FEV_1 in preschool children 3 years and above (11).

FeNO (Fractional concentration of exhaled Nitric Oxide) is an inflammatory biomarker which may indicate the presence of type 2 asthma (asthma characterized by Type-2 inflammation). The NICE (National Institute for Health and Care Excellence) (33) and GEMA (Spanish Guideline on the Management of Asthma) (11) guideline recommends FeNO measurement for asthma diagnosis. The GINA, on the other hand, do not recommend the usage of FeNO to aid asthma diagnosis in adults, with the argument that FeNO may be elevated in other respiratory conditions, and is not elevated in other asthma phenotypes such as neutrophilic asthma (10). However, the guideline recommends FeNO measurement in preschool-age patients. In agreement with this, a prospective study in a hospital setting reported elevated FeNO level during preschool to be predictive of school-age asthma (37). Additionally, a randomized control trial based on 24 primary care centers and one hospital showed that high

TABLE 2 | Risk prediction of future asthma exacerbations/hospitalization*.

References	Population	Age	Definition of asthma	Outcome	Predictive factors
PEDIATRIC					
Swern et al. (20)	Patient from double-blinded multicenter RCT	2–5 years	Physician-diagnosed asthma: At least 3 episodes of asthma symptoms such as cough, wheeze, shortness of breath	Asthma attacks	• Daytime cough • Daytime wheeze • Night-time β2-agonist
Bloom et al. (3)	Primary care	<5 years and 5–17 years	Patients with read codes for asthma	Annual asthma exacerbation rate and time to first exacerbation	• Higher asthma severity
Haselkorn et al. (21)	Severe asthma children recruited from "Managed care organizations, community physicians or group practices, and academic centers"	6–11 years	Diagnosed with severe asthma or mild/moderate asthma considered to be difficult-to-treat by site specialist.	Future severe exacerbation	• Recent exacerbation • Non-white race (vs. white) • 3-4 allergic triggers • Poor asthma control
Covar et al. (22)	Patient from double-blinded multicenter RCT	6–14 years	Mild-moderate persistent asthma: Diary-reported symptoms or β-agonist use (not including pre-exercise), or mean morning and evening peak flow < 80%.	Asthma exacerbation	• Baseline exacerbation
Turner et al. (19)	Primary care	5–12 years	Read Code for asthma diagnosis.	Asthma attack in 1 year follow-up	• Higher GINA management step • Consultation for LRTI • Blood eosinophil >400/μL • Baseline asthma attacks • Younger age • Lower peak expiratory flow
Engelkes et al. (24)	Primary care	5–18 years	Algorithm-validated from list of patients with ICD code and free-text of asthma	Severe asthma exacerbation	• Younger age • Exacerbations in the previous year • Use of any asthma medication
				Time until next exacerbation	• Younger age • Female gender • Exacerbations in the previous year • Respiratory infection in the previous year • Asthma specialist visit in the previous year • ICS prescription • Blood eosinophil >300/μL • Comorbid eczema
ADULTS					
Bloom et al. (3)	Primary care	18–54 years and ≥55 years	Patients with Read Codes for asthma	Annual asthma exacerbation rate and time to first exacerbation	• Higher asthma severity
Kerkof et al. (25)	Primary care patients with secondary care data linkage	≥5 years	Active asthma defined as having diagnostic Read Codes for asthma, no code for resolved asthma, and at least 2 prescriptions for asthma.	Asthma-related hospital readmission 1 year after discharge	• Blood eosinophil count ≥0.35 × 10^9 cells/L
Blakey et al. (17)	Primary care	12–80 years	Active asthma defined as having diagnostic Read Codes for asthma, no code for resolved asthma, and at least 2 prescriptions for asthma.	Asthma exacerbations in 2 years follow-up period	• Baseline (1 year) asthma exacerbations • Older age, female gender, current smoking, overweight • Co-morbid rhinitis, eczema, GERD, nasal polyps, or anaphylaxis • High blood eosinophil count • Higher daily SABA dose • NSAID, LTRA or LABA prescriptions

(Continued)

TABLE 2 | Continued

References	Population	Age	Definition of asthma	Outcome	Predictive factors
					• More acute OCS course • More asthma-related hospitalization • More primary care visits • Lower PEF%
Price et al. (18)	Primary care	12–80 years	Patients with recorded physician-diagnosis for asthma and no other chronic respiratory diseases.	≥2 severe asthma exacerbations in 1 year follow-up	• Older age, female gender, current smoker, overweight, • Blood eosinophil >400/μL • Co-morbid anxiety, diabetes, eczema, GERD, rhinitis • NSAID prescriptions • Higher asthma treatment step (BTS-SIGN) • General practice consultation for LRTI • Outpatient asthma attendance • Having acute OCS courses • >400 μg/day SABA dose • >800 μg/day ICS dose (FP equivalent)

**Studies which analyzed pediatric and adult patients as a single group are categorized as adult studies. BTS, British Thoracic Society; FP, Fluticasone propionate; GERD, Gastroesophageal reflux disease; GINA, Global Initiatives for Asthma; ICS, Inhaled corticosteroid; LABA, long-acting β-agonists; LRTI, Lower respiratory tract infection; LTRA, Leukotriene receptor antagonists; NSAID, Nonsteroidal anti-inflammatory drugs; OCS, oral corticosteroid; PEF, Peak expiratory flow; SABA, short-acting β-agonist; SIGN, Scottish Intercollegiate Guidelines Network.*

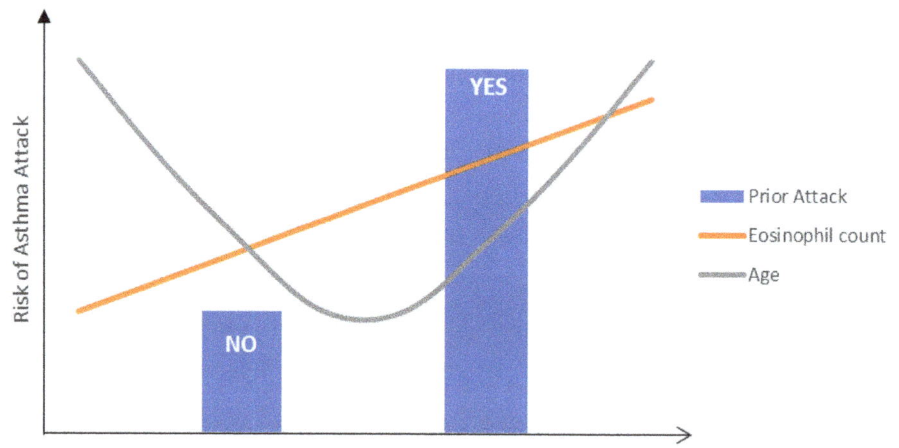

FIGURE 2 | Illustration of the risk factors for future asthma exacerbations.

FeNO level was associated with improved Asthma Control Questionnaire 7 items (ACQ7) score following ICS treatment (38). Therefore, FeNO measurement can be a non-invasive measure conducted in primary care practices to assist asthma diagnosis in preschool children and identifying patients who may benefit from ICS treatment.

Another available tool to assist primary care practitioners to predict whether the presenting wheezing symptoms in preschool children will develop into asthma by school age is the modified version (mAPI) (39) of the Asthma Predictive Index (API) created based on data from the Tucson cohort study (30, 40). The mAPI has been previously shown in an asthma birth cohort study to have high positive predictive capability for asthma at 6, 8, and 11 years based on mAPI score at the first 3 years of life (41).

Older age presents another diagnostic challenge distinct from that in younger patients (**Figure 3**). Symptoms of asthma in old age may be masked by aging-associated changes in pulmonary and other physiological functions (10, 42) and the presence of multiple co-morbid conditions (43). These factors lead to underdiagnosis of asthma within the elderly. The decreased respiratory capacity in the elderly may also make it difficult to conduct lung spirometry, as such the National Institute of Aging recommended alternative techniques which do not require inspiratory efforts such as imaging and forced oscillation (42) The GINA guideline recommends physical examination, such as electrocardiogram and chest x-ray, to aid in the diagnosis of elderly asthma in addition to the routine clinical history taking (10).

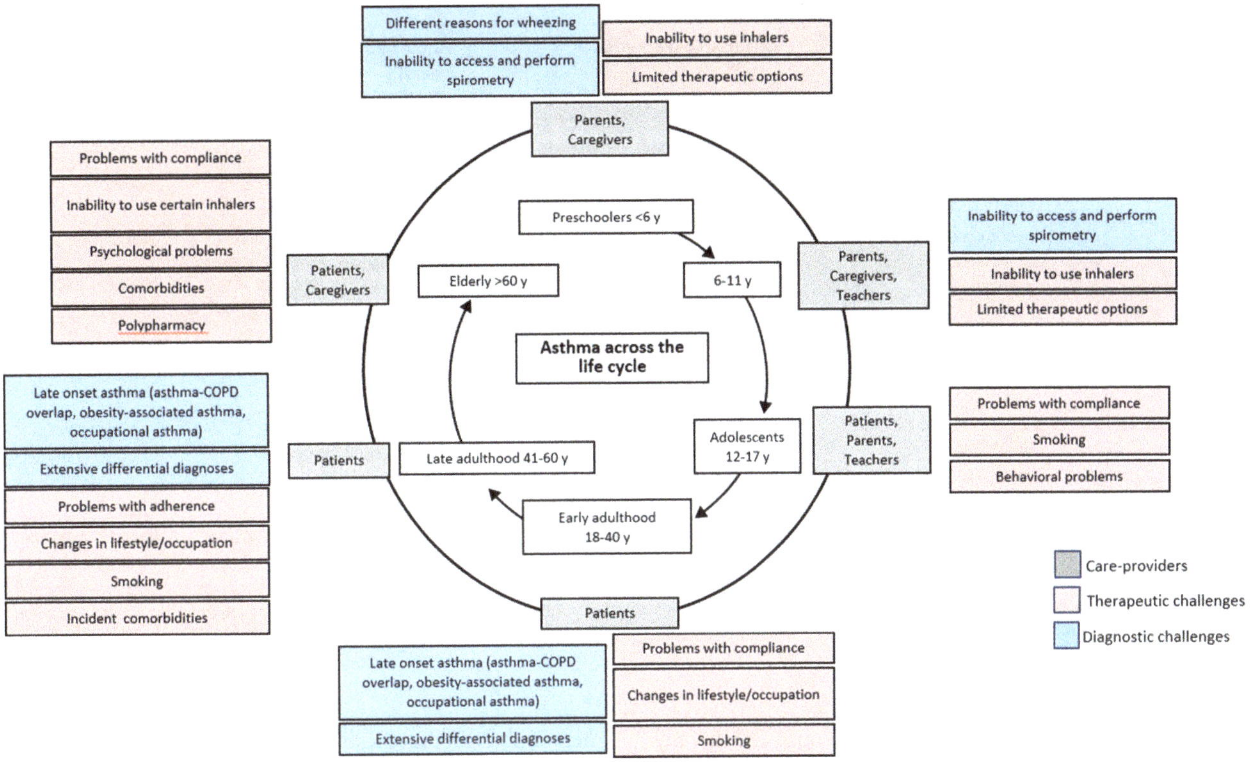

FIGURE 3 | Challenges related to asthma treatment across age. Adapted with permission from: Kaplan A, Covar R, Vanderwalker M. An update on treatment options for children and adults with asthma. Manuscript in Preparation.

Diagnosis of asthma is further complicated by differential diagnosis for symptoms which may mimic asthma. As mentioned above, wheezing and cough in children are likely to be infectious in nature. Non-infectious, non-pulmonary related causes of cough and wheeze, such as gastroesophageal reflux, airway obstruction due to foreign bodies, and congenital heart disease, should also be ruled out before the diagnosis of asthma in children (10). In old age, age-related problems such as heart disease and obesity are the major contributors to differential diagnosis. Chronic obstructive pulmonary disorder (COPD) is also a common cause of misdiagnosis in primary care due to overlapping symptoms with asthma (44). In addition, they may occur concurrently, in a term known as asthma-COPD overlap (ACO). Careful symptom history taking and post-bronchodilator spirometry to test for reversible airway obstruction are recommended to differentiate asthma from COPD and ACOS (10).

THERAPY ISSUES AT DIFFERENT AGES

Differences in Treatment Guidelines

The GINA guideline provides a step-wise management approach for treatment and management of asthma (10). The 2018 updated guideline still recommends as-needed short-acting β-agonists (SABA) for reliever treatment of asthma attacks and ICS as the initial controller medication for asthma, with addition of long-acting β-adrenoceptor agonists (LABA, as combination therapy with ICS), leukotriene receptor antagonists (LTRA) or stepping up of dosage as required for adolescent and adults patients above the age of 12 (10). Recommendations from other guidelines are similar (11, 16, 32–34): initial reliever with SABA, initial preventer treatment of ICS, and when needed, adding LABA in combination with ICS.

Initial treatment option for children 5–12 years follows that of older patients. However, LABA as the initial add-on is not recommended by the GINA (10) for this age group, in contrast to the BTS (16) recommendation. The CTS recommends LABA if stepping up ICS dosage fails to achieve control (34). Alternatively, tiotropium, a long-acting muscarinic antagonist (LAMA), administration by mist inhaler can be prescribed as an add-on in children ≥12 years and adults. LAMA is however not indicated for children <12 years by the GINA (10) and BTS (16) guidelines, though it is indicated for children ≥6 years in the US (45).

The GINA guideline dedicates a section outlining a step-by-step treatment guideline for children 5 years and younger, however, the current guideline is based on more limited evidence (10). Similar to older patients, (SABA) should be given as initial reliever upon presentation of wheezing. When necessary, i.e., symptoms suggestive of asthma or frequent wheezing episode, a

TABLE 3 | Objective tests recommendation in each age-groups and availability in primary care.

	Preschool (<5 years)*	Children (5–12 years)	Adolescent and adults (>12 years)	Availability in primary care
Peak flow variability	Not recommended by BTS	Recommended by GINA, CTS, and NICE; Not recommended by BTS	Recommended by GINA, BTS (in adults), CTS, GEMA and NICE.	Available
Spirometry	Not recommended by GINA† and BTS	Recommended by GINA, BTS, CTS, GEMA, AAH, and NICE	Recommended by GINA, BTS, CTS, GEMA, AAH, and NICE	Available
FeNO	Recommended by GINA, GEMA, and BTS (for 3–4years)	Not recommended by GINA; Recommended by NICE and BTS (for eosinophilic asthma)	Not recommended by GINA; Recommended by NICE, GEMA, and BTS (for eosinophilic asthma)	Not usually available
Bronchial provocation test	Not recommended by GINA	Recommended by GINA, BTS, AAH, and CTS	Recommended by GINA, BTS, CTS, AAH, and NICE (at >17 years)	Available in speciality clinics also
Allergen sensitization	Recommended by GINA and GEMA but not conclusive (doesn't exclude nonatopic asthma)	Recommended by GINA, GEMA, and BTS but not conclusive; Not considered essential by AAH. Not recommended by NICE	Recommended by GINA, GEMA, and BTS but not conclusive Not recommended by NICE	Available through speciality referral
Chest X-ray	Recommended by GINA, BTS, and CTS	Recommended by BTS	Recommended by BTS, and by GINA (in elderly).	Typically available

**NICE guideline does not recommend any objective tests to guide asthma diagnosis in children <5years †According to GINA, children 4–5 years may undergo spirometry with guidance. GINA, Global Initiatives for Asthma; BTS, British Thoracic Society; AAH, Australian Asthma Handbook; NICE, National Institute for Health and Care Excellence; CTS, Canadian Thoracic Society.*

low dose of ICS is recommended as the initial controller therapy. Similarly, GEMA (11) and Australian Asthma handbook (32) recommended initial SABA preventer with addition of low dose ICS when necessary. The BTS (16) guideline recommends SABA for reliever therapy together with low-dose ICS as the preventer, while the CTS guideline for preschool patients (31) recommends daily low-dose ICS as first-line therapy or SABA if symptoms were mild or infrequent. LTRA is recommended as an alternative to ICS by the GINA (10), GEMA (11), Australian Asthma Handbook (32), and BTS (16) but is not recommended for use by the CTS (31). If symptoms remain inadequately controlled with low-dose ICS, the GINA, GEMA and CTS guidelines recommend stepping-up to medium dose ICS, but this is not recommended by the BTS (16).

There is a lack of guideline on the treatment for asthma in elderly patients. Treatment of asthma in the elderly faces additional challenge due to poorer asthma control. However, more studies are required to determine whether this is due to decreased treatment response, difficulty with inhaler technique, or poorer adherence (43).

Challenges in Control

Adherence to inhaled corticosteroid (ICS) treatment is a key factor for reduction of exacerbation and achievement of asthma control. Yet, non-adherence toward ICS is constantly reported to be a very common occurrence, as high as 80% among asthma patients (46, 47). Various factors influencing adherence have been previously described, including educational level and confidence in the treatment (48).

One of the factors influencing adherence includes changes in attitude across ages. Younger children depend on parental intervention for medication, thus it is not surprising that parental concerns on medication to be influential toward adherence in pediatric asthma (49, 50). Improvement of adherence in pediatric patients should focus on parents and caregivers. Interestingly, pediatric asthma therapy adherence has been reported to be inversely correlated with children's age despite the supposedly increased understanding of their condition (50, 51). This could suggest the presence of teenage-related intentional non-adherence, which may be due to several factors such as teenage rebellion, or embarrassment of using prescribed inhaler therapy due to peer pressure (48).

In elderly patients, non-adherence may stem from the patients' struggle due to memory loss coupled with the complexity of the treatment regimen (42). This issue is further exacerbated by the multiple comorbidities in elderly asthma patients which may lead to an increased number of medications, also known as polypharmacy, which subsequently impacts asthma control (52).

Another factor which may negatively impact treatment success is improper inhalation technique, a problem repeatedly reported to commonly occur regardless of the ICS device type (53, 54). The extensive list of possible DPI and MDI device errors and their association with poor asthma outcomes were recently described in a study utilizing primary care records of 7 European countries and Australia (CRITIKAL study) (54). Among the errors reported to be associated with exacerbation is insufficient inspiratory effort for DPI device. This error is well-established to be a major challenge in preschool children and elderly patients (55). An MDI device (28) or soft mist inhaler (56) with properly designed valved holding chamber is more suitable for preschool children.

Smoking has been consistently reported to hinder response to ICS therapy (57, 58), and poor asthma control was associated with smoking status based on an interview of over 10,000 primary care patients aged 12 years and older (59). The BTS guideline recommends higher ICS dose in patients who are current or ex-smokers (16). Smoking remains a global health behavioral problem from teenage to adulthood, with a median reported global prevalence of 10.7% (range 1.7–35.0%) between 2012 and 2015 (60). A recent study on the impact of ICS adherence on asthma exacerbation and control within primary care reported one-third of their patients to be active smokers (47). Tobacco smoking thus represents another "wrench in the gears" in achieving asthma control.

Despite the recommendation for ICS, concerns remain regarding the associated side-effects, which have in turn been reported to negatively impact patient adherence toward ICS treatment (61). ICS is known to be associated with various local side effects such as oral thrush (candidiasis) and hoarseness (62, 63). A previous study reported 63.3% of children under 6 years of age to be affected (64). In addition to local side effects, ICS treatment may also result in growth retardation in children (65). It is therefore recommended to use the lowest ICS dosage for this age group and to monitor for reduced growth velocity (10). The Canadian Society of Allergy and Clinical Immunology (CSACI) also recommended monitoring for adrenal suppression for children and adolescents receiving high dose ICS (66). Another potential systemic side effects of ICS include osteoporosis (which leads to bone fractures), cataracts and diabetes, which pose additional concern on ICS use in older patients (65). Patients administered high dose ICS over a long period (more than 3 months) should thus be monitored for any potential side effect (10, 16).

Issues in Therapy Response

In addition to the challenges in diagnosis, old age poses additional challenges in the treatment of asthma due to decreased response to bronchodilator therapy (3, 67, 68). Knowledge and guidelines on elderly asthma are limited, and clinical trials tend to exclude elderly patients due to the presence of co-morbidities (43). Unlike in preschool children <5 years of age, there is still no dedicated section for elderly patients within the GINA guideline (10). It is also of relevance to understand whether the different phenotypes asthma: early onset atopic and late-onset asthma, would present with different responses to bronchodilator therapy in old age.

Issues Working With Multiple Guidelines

As discussed in the previous section, different guidelines provide different recommendations in terms of prescriptions across patient age groups. The GINA, BTS, NICE, GEMA, and CTS guidelines recommend SABA reliever and ICS preventer as initial treatment for asthma. However, there is less consensus on the subsequent add-on therapy for asthma which remains uncontrolled after the initial therapy in younger age-groups. In children (5–12 by BTS, 6–11 by GINA and CTS), LABA is recommended by the BTS and CTS guidelines as an add-on if symptom control is not achieved with ICS but is not recommended by GINA. Additionally, in the preschool age-group, there are conflicting recommendations regarding the use of LTRA as an alternative to ICS (recommended by GINA, NICE, GEMA, and BTS, but not CTS), and regarding stepping up ICS dosage to achieve control (recommended by GINA, GEMA, and CTS, but not BTS). The NICE guideline, on the other hand, recommended stepping up to a moderate dose of ICS for 8 weeks following initial SABA.

Working with multiple guidelines with different recommendations for asthma management in childhood patients may cause an additional challenge for primary care physicians as highlighted previously by the Primary Care Respiratory Society of UK (69).

Solutions

Despite the utility provided by subjective biomarker measures, they may be unavailable in primary care practices due to the barriers in implementation (70). Data sharing across practices which allow easier physician access to patients' clinical records, including records of past subjective measures, would provide a potential solution to circumvent this challenge. This may also enable a longer observation of patients' medical history to aid in differentiating between asthma, viral wheeze, and COPD in primary care.

To improve cross-sharing of patients' past medical records, there is a need to improve electronic medical records (EMR) systems which are often claims-based and lack uniformity between systems. A potential solution will be the creation of a uniform EMR template which brings together standardized past medical records while enabling patient self-reported information to be provided to primary care practitioners prior to consultation. Creation of a uniform EMR template can be done by utilizing research-based templates such as REDCap (71).

Moving forward, incorporation of clinical decision support systems (CDSS) to EMR systems may aid physicians in making informed clinical decisions despite conflicting treatment guidelines across age-groups (72) and guide the appropriate treatment while warning against the prescription of non-indicated drugs based on the patients' profile (73). Ultimately, a global EMR for primary care, which is capable of conducting machine-learning based on previous data to provide future recommendations, may serve to guide patient management in the lack of guidelines based on strong evidence.

CONCLUSION

Phenotyping studies have shown that depending on the age of onset, symptoms of asthma can represent distinct phenotypes from asthma with later onset. Together with the changing phenotypes across age are the changing challenges for diagnosis, treatment, and control of asthma.

Guidelines for asthma management in young children and the elderly are still based on weaker evidence, despite the higher hurdles in management. Differentiating asthma from other diseases with similar presenting symptoms such as viral wheeze and COPD remains a challenge. Regardless, there are resources such as FeNO measurement and the mAPI (modified Asthma Predictive Index), and spirometry which can assist in the diagnosis of asthma for different age groups within the primary care setting. Future developments in electronic medical record systems to enable cross-sharing of clinical history and implementation of clinical decision support systems (CDSS) can potentially improve patient management across different age-groups.

AUTHOR CONTRIBUTIONS

All authors listed have made a substantial, direct and intellectual contribution to the work, and approved it for publication.

REFERENCES

1. Pavord ID, Beasley R, Agusti A, Anderson GP, Bel E, Brusselle G, et al. After asthma: redefining airways diseases. *Lancet. (London, England).* (2018) 391:350–400. doi: 10.1016/S0140-6736(17)30879-6
2. Haldar P, Pavord ID, Shaw DE, Berry MA, Thomas M, Brightling CE, et al. Cluster analysis and clinical asthma phenotypes. *Am J Respirat Critic Care Med.* (2008) 178:218–24. doi: 10.1164/rccm.200711-1754OC
3. Bloom CI, Nissen F, Douglas IJ, Smeeth L, Cullinan P, Quint JK. Exacerbation risk and characterisation of the UK's asthma population from infants to old age. *Thorax.* (2018) 73:313–20. doi: 10.1136/thoraxjnl-2017-210650
4. Hekking PP, Bel EH. Developing and emerging clinical asthma phenotypes. *J Allergy Clin Immunol Pract.* (2014) 2:671–80. doi: 10.1016/j.jaip.2014.09.007
5. Pavord ID, Korn S, Howarth P, Bleecker ER, Buhl R, Keene ON, et al. Mepolizumab for severe eosinophilic asthma (DREAM): a multicentre, double-blind, placebo-controlled trial. *Lancet. (London, England).* (2012) 380:651–9. doi: 10.1016/S0140-6736(12)60988-X
6. Wenzel SE. Asthma phenotypes: the evolution from clinical to molecular approaches. *Nat Med.* (2012) 18:716–25. doi: 10.1038/nm.2678
7. Fuchs O, Bahmer T, Rabe KF, von Mutius E. Asthma transition from childhood into adulthood. *Lancet Respirat Med.* (2017) 5:224–34. doi: 10.1016/S2213-2600(16)30187-4
8. Moore WC, Meyers DA, Wenzel SE, Teague WG, Li H, Li X, et al. Identification of asthma phenotypes using cluster analysis in the Severe Asthma Research Program. *Am J Respirat Critic Care Med.* (2010) 181:315–23. doi: 10.1164/rccm.200906-0896OC
9. Schatz M, Hsu JW, Zeiger RS, Chen W, Dorenbaum A, Chipps BE, et al. Phenotypes determined by cluster analysis in severe or difficult-to-treat asthma. *J Allergy Clin Immunol.* (2014) 133:1549–56. doi: 10.1016/j.jaci.2013.10.006
10. Global Initiative for Asthma. *Global Strategy for Asthma Management and Prevention.* Updated 2018. Vancouver, USA: GINA; 2018. Available online at: www.ginasthma.org. (accessed July, 25 2018).
11. Plaza Moral V, Alonso Mostaza S, Alvarez Rodriguez C, Gomez-Outes A, Gomez Ruiz F, Lopez Vina A, et al. SPANISH GUIDELINE ON THE MANAGEMENT OF ASTHMA. *J Invest Allergol Clin Immunol.* (2016) 26(Suppl 1):1–92. doi: 10.18176/jiaci.0065.
12. Holgate ST, Polosa R. The mechanisms, diagnosis, and management of severe asthma in adults. *Lancet (London, England).* (2006) 368:780–93. doi: 10.1016/S0140-6736(06)69288-Xr
13. O'Neill S, Sweeney J, Patterson CC, Menzies-Gow A, Niven R, Mansur AH, et al. The cost of treating severe refractory asthma in the UK: an economic analysis from the British thoracic society difficult asthma registry. *Thorax.* (2015) 70:376–8. doi: 10.1136/thoraxjnl-2013-204114
14. Bulathsinhala L, Eleangovan N, Heaney LG, Menzies-Gow A, Gibson PG, Peters M, et al. Development of the international severe asthma registry (ISAR): a modified Delphi study. *J Allergy Clin Immunol Pract.* (2018) 7:578–88.e2. doi: 10.1016/j.jaip.2018.08.016
15. Guilbert TW, Bacharier LB, Fitzpatrick AM. Severe asthma in children. *J Allergy Clin Immunol Pract.* (2014) 2:489–500. doi: 10.1016/j.jaip.2014.06.022
16. British Thoracic Society. *British Guideline on the Management of Asthma: a National Clinical Guideline (SIGN 153).* (2016). Available online at: https://www.sign.ac.uk/assets/sign153.pdf (accessed August 27, 2018).
17. Blakey JD, Price DB, Pizzichini E, Popov TA, Dimitrov BD, Postma DS, et al. Identifying risk of future asthma attacks using UK medical record data: a respiratory effectiveness group initiative. *J Allergy Clin Immunol Pract.* (2017) 5:1015–24 e8. doi: 10.1016/j.jaip.2016.11.007
18. Price D, Wilson AM, Chisholm A, Rigazio A, Burden A, Thomas M, et al. Predicting frequent asthma exacerbations using blood eosinophil count and other patient data routinely available in clinical practice. *J. Asthma Allergy.* (2016) 9:1–12. doi: 10.2147/JAA.S97973
19. Turner S. Predicting and reducing risk of exacerbations in children with asthma in the primary care setting: current perspectives. *Pragmatic Observ Res.* (2016) 7:33–9. doi: 10.2147/POR.S98928
20. Swern AS, Tozzi CA, Knorr B, Bisgaard H. Predicting an asthma exacerbation in children 2 to 5 years of age. *Anna Allergy Asthma Immunol.* (2008) 101:626–30. doi: 10.1016/S1081-1206(10)60226-8
21. Haselkorn T, Zeiger RS, Chipps BE, Mink DR, Szefler SJ, Simons FE, et al. Recent asthma exacerbations predict future exacerbations in children with severe or difficult-to-treat asthma. *J Allergy Clin Immunol.* (2009) 124:921–7. doi: 10.1016/j.jaci.2009.09.006
22. Covar RA, Szefler SJ, Zeiger RS, Sorkness CA, Moss M, Mauger DT, et al. Factors associated with asthma exacerbations during a long-term clinical trial of controller medications in children. *J Allergy Clin Immunol.* (2008) 122:741–7 e4. doi: 10.1016/j.jaci.2008.08.021
23. Turner SW, Murray C, Thomas M, Burden A, Price DB. Applying UK real-world primary care data to predict asthma attacks in 3776 well-characterised children: a retrospective cohort study. *NPJ Prim Care Respir Med.* (2018) 28:28. doi: 10.1038/s41533-018-0095-5
24. Engelkes M, Janssens HM, de Ridder MA, Sturkenboom MC, de Jongste JC, Verhamme KM. Real life data on incidence and risk factors of severe asthma exacerbations in children in primary care. *Respiratory Med.* (2016) 119:48–54. doi: 10.1016/j.rmed.2016.08.016
25. Kerkhof M, Tran TN, van den Berge M, Brusselle GG, Gopalan G, Jones RCM, et al. Association between blood eosinophil count and risk of readmission for patients with asthma: historical cohort study. *PLoS ONE.* (2018) 13:e0201143. doi: 10.1371/journal.pone.0201143
26. Cave AJ, Atkinson LL. Asthma in preschool children: a review of the diagnostic challenges. *J Am Board Fam Med.* (2014) 27:538–48. doi: 10.3122/jabfm.2014.04.130276
27. Ng CW, How CH. Recurrent wheeze and cough in young children: is it asthma? *Singapore Med J.* (2014) 55:236–41. doi: 10.11622/smedj.2014064
28. Pedersen SE, Hurd SS, Lemanske RF, Jr., Becker A, Zar HJ, Sly PD, et al. Global strategy for the diagnosis and management of asthma in children 5 years and younger. *Pediatr Pulmonol.* (2011) 46:1–17. doi: 10.1002/ppul.21321
29. Martinez FD, Wright AL, Taussig LM, Holberg CJ, Halonen M, Morgan WJ. Asthma and wheezing in the first six years of life. the group health medical associates. *N Engl J Med.* (1995) 332:133–8. doi: 10.1056/NEJM199501193320301
30. Taussig LM, Wright AL, Holberg CJ, Halonen M, Morgan WJ, Martinez FD. Tucson children's respiratory study: 1980 to present. *J Allergy Clin Immunol.* (2003) 111:661–75. doi: 10.1067/mai.2003.162
31. Canadian Thoracic Society. *Diagnosis and management of asthma in preschoolers: A Canadian Thoracic Society and Canadian Pediatric Society Position Statement.* Ottowa. (2015). (accessed July 25, 2018).
32. National Asthma Council Australia. *Australian Asthma Handbook*, Version 2.0. National Asthma Council Australia, Melbourne, (2019). Available online at: http://www.asthmahandbook.org.au (accessed March 26, 2019).

33. National Institute for Health and Care Excellence. *Asthma: Diagnosis, Monitoring and Chronic Asthma Management.* (2017). Available online at: http://www.nice.org.uk/guidance/ng80 (accessed September 8, 2018).
34. Canadian Thoracic Society. Guideline Update: Diagnosis and management of asthma in preschoolers, children and adults. Ottowa, ON (2012). (accessed November 13, 2018).
35. Derom E, van Weel C, Liistro G, Buffels J, Schermer T, Lammers E, et al. Primary care spirometry. *Euro Respirat J.* (2008) 31:197–203. doi: 10.1183/09031936.00066607
36. Beydon N, Davis SD, Lombardi E, Allen JL, Arets HG, Aurora P, et al. An official American thoracic society/european respiratory society statement: pulmonary function testing in preschool children. *Am J Respirat Critic Care Med.* (2007) 175:1304–45. doi: 10.1164/rccm.200605-642ST
37. Singer F, Luchsinger I, Inci D, Knauer N, Latzin P, Wildhaber JH, et al. Exhaled nitric oxide in symptomatic children at preschool age predicts later asthma. *Allergy.* (2013) 68:531–8. doi: 10.1111/all.12127
38. Price DB, Buhl R, Chan A, Freeman D, Gardener E, Godley C, et al. Fractional exhaled nitric oxide as a predictor of response to inhaled corticosteroids in patients with non-specific respiratory symptoms and insignificant bronchodilator reversibility: a randomised controlled trial. *Lancet Respirat Med.* (2018) 6:29–39. doi: 10.1016/S2213-2600(17)30424-1
39. Bacharier LB, Guilbert TW. Diagnosis and management of early asthma in preschool-aged children. *J Allergy Clin Immunol.* (2012) 130:287–96. doi: 10.1016/j.jaci.2012.04.025
40. Castro-Rodriguez JA, Holberg CJ, Wright AL, Martinez FD. A clinical index to define risk of asthma in young children with recurrent wheezing. *Am J Respirat Critic Care Med.* (2000) 162(4 Pt 1):1403–6. doi: 10.1164/ajrccm.162.4.9912111
41. Chang TS, Lemanske RF, Jr., Guilbert TW, Gern JE, Coen MH, Evans MD, et al. Evaluation of the modified asthma predictive index in high-risk preschool children. *J Allergy Clin Immunol Pract.* (2013) 1:152–6. doi: 10.1016/j.jaip.2012.10.008
42. Hanania NA, King MJ, Braman SS, Saltoun C, Wise RA, Enright P, et al. Asthma in the elderly: current understanding and future research needs–a report of a national institute on aging (NIA) workshop. *J Allergy Clin Immunol.* (2011) 128(3 Suppl):S4–24. doi: 10.1016/j.jaci.2011.06.048
43. Boulet LP. Asthma in the elderly patient. *Asthma Res Pract.* (2016) 2:3. doi: 10.1186/s40733-015-0015-1
44. Miravitlles M, Andreu I, Romero Y, Sitjar S, Altes A, Anton E. Difficulties in differential diagnosis of COPD and asthma in primary care. *Br J Gen Pract.* (2012) 62:e68–75. doi: 10.3399/bjgp12X625111
45. Boehringer Ingelheim. *Highlights of Prescribing Information.* SPIRIVA® RESPIMAT® (tiotropium bromide) 2017. Available online at: http://docs.boehringer-ingelheim.com/Prescribing%20Information/PIs/Spiriva%20Respimat/spirivarespimat.pdf (accessed November 28, 2017).
46. Dekhuijzen R, Lavorini F, Usmani OS, van Boven JFM. Addressing the impact and unmet needs of nonadherence in asthma and chronic obstructive pulmonary disease: where do we go from here? *J Allergy Clin Immunol Pract.* (2018) 6:785–93. doi: 10.1016/j.jaip.2017.11.027
47. Papi A, Ryan D, Soriano JB, Chrystyn H, Bjermer L, Rodriguez-Roisin R, et al. Relationship of inhaled corticosteroid adherence to asthma exacerbations in patients with moderate-to-severe asthma. *J Allergy Clin Immunol Practice.* (2018) 6:1989–98.e3 doi: 10.1016/j.jaip.2018.03.008
48. Makela MJ, Backer V, Hedegaard M, Larsson K. Adherence to inhaled therapies, health outcomes and costs in patients with asthma and COPD. *Respirat Med.* (2013) 107:1481–90. doi: 10.1016/j.rmed.2013.04.005
49. Koster ES, Raaijmakers JA, Vijverberg SJ, Maitland-van der Zee AH. Inhaled corticosteroid adherence in paediatric patients: the PACMAN cohort study. *Pharmacoepidemiol Drug Saf.* (2011) 20:1064–72. doi: 10.1002/pds.2228
50. van Dellen QM, Stronks K, Bindels PJ, Ory FG, van Aalderen WM. Adherence to inhaled corticosteroids in children with asthma and their parents. *Respirat Med.* (2008) 102:755–63. doi: 10.1016/j.rmed.2007.12.005
51. McQuaid EL. Medication adherence in pediatric asthma: reasoning, responsibility, and behavior. *J Pediatric Psychol.* (2003) 28:323–33. doi: 10.1093/jpepsy/jsg022
52. Wardzynska A, Kubsik B, Kowalski ML. Comorbidities in elderly patients with asthma: association with control of the disease and concomitant treatment. *Geriatr Gerontol Int.* (2015) 15:902–9. doi: 10.1111/ggi.12367
53. Chorao P, Pereira AM, Fonseca JA. Inhaler devices in asthma and COPD–an assessment of inhaler technique and patient preferences. *Respirat Med.* (2014) 108:968–75. doi: 10.1016/j.rmed.2014.04.019
54. Price DB, Roman-Rodriguez M, McQueen RB, Bosnic-Anticevich S, Carter V, Gruffydd-Jones K, et al. Inhaler errors in the CRITIKAL study: type, frequency, and association with asthma outcomes. *J Allergy Clin Immunol Pract.* (2017) 5:1071–81 e9.
55. Haughney J, Price D, Barnes NC, Virchow JC, Roche N, Chrystyn H. Choosing inhaler devices for people with asthma: current knowledge and outstanding research needs. *Respirat Med.* (2010) 104:1237–45. doi: 10.1016/j.rmed.2010.04.012
56. Kamin W, Frank M, Kattenbeck S, Moroni-Zentgraf P, Wachtel H, Zielen S. A handling study to assess use of the respimat ® soft mist inhaler in children under 5 years old. *J Aerosol Med Pulm Drug Deliv.* (2015) 28:372–81. doi: 10.1089/jamp.2014.1159
57. Shimoda T, Obase Y, Kishikawa R, Iwanaga T. Influence of cigarette smoking on airway inflammation and inhaled corticosteroid treatment in patients with asthma. *Allergy Asthma Proc.* (2016) 37:50–8. doi: 10.2500/aap.2016.37.3944
58. Tomlinson JE, McMahon AD, Chaudhuri R, Thompson JM, Wood SF, Thomson NC. Efficacy of low and high dose inhaled corticosteroid in smokers versus non-smokers with mild asthma. *Thorax.* (2005) 60:282–7. doi: 10.1136/thx.2004.033688
59. Chapman KR, Boulet LP, Rea RM, Franssen E. Suboptimal asthma control: prevalence, detection and consequences in general practice. *Euro Respirat J.* (2008) 31:320–5. doi: 10.1183/09031936.00039707
60. Arrazola RA, Ahluwalia IB, Pun E, Garcia de Quevedo I, Babb S, Armour BS. Current tobacco smoking and desire to quit smoking among students aged 13-15 years - global youth tobacco survey, 61 countries, 2012-2015. *MMWR Morbidity Mortal Weekly Rep.* (2017) 66:533–7. doi: 10.15585/mmwr.mm6620a3
61. Cooper V, Metcalf L, Versnel J, Upton J, Walker S, Horne R. Patient-reported side effects, concerns and adherence to corticosteroid treatment for asthma, and comparison with physician estimates of side-effect prevalence: a UK-wide, cross-sectional study. *NPJ Prim Care Respir Med.* (2015) 25:15026. doi: 10.1038/npjpcrm.2015.26
62. Buhl R. Local oropharyngeal side effects of inhaled corticosteroids in patients with asthma. *Allergy.* (2006) 61:518–26. doi: 10.1111/j.1398-9995.2006.01090.x
63. Roland NJ, Bhalla RK, Earis J. The local side effects of inhaled corticosteroids: current understanding and review of the literature. *Chest.* (2004) 126:213–9. doi: 10.1378/chest.126.1.213
64. Dubus JC, Marguet C, Deschildre A, Mely L, Le Roux P, Brouard J, et al. Local side-effects of inhaled corticosteroids in asthmatic children: influence of drug, dose, age, and device. *Allergy.* (2001) 56:944–8. doi: 10.1034/j.1398-9995.2001.00100.x
65. Heffler E, Madeira LNG, Ferrando M, Puggioni F, Racca F, Malvezzi L, et al. Inhaled corticosteroids safety and adverse effects in patients with asthma. *J Allergy Clin Immunol Pract.* (2018) 6:776–81. doi: 10.1016/j.jaip.2018.01.025
66. Issa-El-Khoury K, Kim H, Chan ES, Vander Leek T, Noya F. CSACI position statement: systemic effect of inhaled corticosteroids on adrenal suppression in the management of pediatric asthma. *Allergy Asthma Clin Immunol.* (2015) 11:9. doi: 10.1186/s13223-015-0075-z
67. Banerji A, Clark S, Afilalo M, Blanda MP, Cydulka RK, Camargo CA, Jr. Prospective multicenter study of acute asthma in younger versus older adults presenting to the emergency department. *J Am Geriatr Soc.* (2006) 54:48–55. doi: 10.1111/j.1532-5415.2005.00563.x
68. Dunn RM, Lehman E, Chinchilli VM, Martin RJ, Boushey HA, Israel E, et al. Impact of age and sex on response to asthma therapy. *Am J Respirat Criticl Care Med.* (2015) 192:551–8. doi: 10.1164/rccm.201503-0426OC
69. Keeley D, Baxter N. Conflicting asthma guidelines cause confusion in primary care. *BMJ. (Clinical research ed).* (2018) 360:k29. doi: 10.1136/bmj.k29

70. Walters JA, Hansen E, Mudge P, Johns DP, Walters EH, Wood-Baker R. Barriers to the use of spirometry in general practice. *Australian Family Phys.* (2005) 34:201–3. Available online at: https://eprints.utas.edu.au/1284/
71. Harris PA, Taylor R, Thielke R, Payne J, Gonzalez N, Conde JG. Research electronic data capture (REDCap)–a metadata-driven methodology and workflow process for providing translational research informatics support. *J Biomed Inform.* (2009) 42:377–81. doi: 10.1016/j.jbi.2008.08.010
72. Fathima M, Peiris D, Naik-Panvelkar P, Saini B, Armour CL. Effectiveness of computerized clinical decision support systems for asthma and chronic obstructive pulmonary disease in primary care: a systematic review. *BMC Pulmonary Med.* (2014) 14:189. doi: 10.1186/1471-2466-14-189
73. Ryan D, Blakey J, Chisholm A, Price D, Thomas M, Stallberg B, et al. Use of electronic medical records and biomarkers to manage risk and resource efficiencies. *Eur Clin Respir J.* (2017) 4:1293386. doi: 10.1080/20018525.2017.1293386

11

Measuring Airway Inflammation in Asthmatic Children

Laura Tenero, Marco Zaffanello, Michele Piazza and Giorgio Piacentini*

Department of Surgical Sciences, Dentistry, Gynecology and Pediatrics, University of Verona, Verona, Italy

***Correspondence:**
Laura Tenero
laura.tenero@univr.it

Asthma is the most common chronic respiratory disease in children characterized by airways inflammation, bronchial hyperresponsiveness, recurrent reversible airways obstruction, and respiratory symptoms. The diagnosis of the disease is based on clinical history, airways obstruction at spirometry, and bronchial reversibility. Asthma treatment is aimed to disease control, through the use of controller treatment and monitoring lung function. However, lung function and symptoms not always reflect the underlying airways inflammation and response to the therapy. Objective parameters of asthma inflammation could be important for the clinician in the management of patients with asthma. In the last years, some studies were focused on biomarkers to identify phenotype, inflammation, and pathobiological pathways to help the clinician in the diagnosis and in personalizing the management. Accordingly, clinically feasible tests are represented by the collection of exhaled breath condensate (EBC) and measurement of exhaled nitric oxide (FeNO). Other—methods such as the evaluation of volatile organic compound (VOCs), that reflect airways inflammation and treatment efficacy, are currently used for research purposes For some of these methods, The lack of standardization in pre-collection, collection, post-collection of samples, and interpretation of the results may a problem in clinical practice. Improved these limitations, several biomarkers will be useful to distinguish patients with a different disease condition to personalize the treatment.

Keywords: biomarkers, inflammation, FeNO, exhaled breath condensate, exhaled breath volatile compounds

INTRODUCTION

Asthma is a chronic respiratory disease characterized by inflammation of the airways, bronchial hyperresponsiveness, recurrent reversible airway obstruction, and respiratory symptoms (1). Asthma is the most common chronic respiratory disease in childhood with an incidence between 1 and 18% in people from different countries.

The diagnosis of asthma is based on anamnestic data, clinical evaluation, limitation of the airflow, and bronchial reactivity (1). The goal of asthma treatment is the control of respiratory symptoms with controller daily drugs, reduction of rescue medications needed to maintain a regular daily activity and reaching a normal lung function (1). Though airways inflammation is a pivotal characteristic of the disease, it is not directly related to lung function test or symptoms (2) and with the real response to the therapy (3).

Therefore, objective parameters of airway inflammation should be considered relevant for the treatment choice in asthmatic patients.

The assessment of biomarkers in the exhaled breath of patients with asthma and other lung diseases is a very attractive approach to monitor airways inflammation. Biomarkers are objectively measurable indicators of the biological and pathological processes as well as of the pharmacological responses to the therapeutic intervention (4).

An ideal biomarker should be easy to collect and measure, inexpensive, noninvasive, and feasible in children capable to contribute to the phenotyping of the disease and to the assessment of treatment response (4, 5).

In order to have a clinically useful tool, there are important issues regarding sensibility, reproducibility, and variability of the methods, that need to be evaluated before moving from bench to bedside. In the next future, a number of recently proposed methods are expected to be clinically useful to predict the progression of the disease, to the phenotyping and endotyping of the disease in order to move toward a personalized treatment in asthma (**Figure 1**).

Bronchoscopy with bronchoalveolar lavage (BAL) and endobronchial biopsy are considered the gold standards for assessing airway inflammation and remodeling in asthma but, being invasive methods, they have a limited use in the clinical setting, in particular in pediatric care (2).

In recent years, therefore, researchers have focused their studies to define surrogate biomarkers to be proposed in the assessment of airway inflammation in asthmatic children and are shortly revised in the following sections (4–6) (**Figure 1**).

INDUCED SPUTUM

The method of induced sputum is a relatively noninvasive diagnostic procedure able to harvest cells and mediators from the lower airway (2) which, however, requires a level of expertise in the collection in order to obtain adequate samples and reliable results. Sputum can be induced in children older than 6 years after inhalation of nebulized hypertonic saline solution at increasing concentration (7, 8).

The procedure to collect sputum is standardized by European Respiratory Society Task Force and is applicable to children older than 8 years (9, 10).

However, the practical use of this method is limited due to technical issues which can make the feasibility at clinical setting difficult to perform for regular assessment of airways inflammation in children (11, 12). In particular, hypertonic saline inhalation may cause bronchoconstriction, especially in asthmatic children, for whom pre-medication with β2-agonist may be necessary. Furthermore, the post-collection analysis needs skilled laboratory personnel for mediator assay and cell specimens to be transferred onto slides and properly stained. Trained physicians are also needed in order to have a correct reading of the results from the specimens.

Several studies demonstrated a strong correlation between cellular elements of BAL and cells collected from in the airways through the induced sputum method.

The dominant cell in sputum from normal children is the macrophages, and the normal ratio for eosinophils in sputum from children is 2.5% (7).

Different inflammatory patterns are being identified from sputum of asthmatic children and adults: eosinophilic, neutrophilic, mixed, and paucigranulocytic types (13).

Sputum eosinophilia is a marker of severity of allergic inflammation in asthma and is characterized by elevated numbers of eosinophils, and eosinophil cationic protein concentration, as well as increased nitric oxide and hydrogen peroxide levels in exhaled breath. The patients with an eosinophilic pattern are expected to have a better response to corticosteroids therapy (14).

Also, children with stable asthma show increased number of eosinophils and bronchial epithelial cells in their sputum (15, 16). During asthma exacerbation, eosinophils and mast cells are more represented in the samples obtained from the airways through the method of induced sputum and eosinophil cationic protein concentrations are higher in the fluid phase of the samples. Some patients have sputum neutrophilia with improved levels of interleukin 8 (17). On the other hand, children with asymptomatic airway hyperresponsiveness are expected to have normal cell counts, whereas patients with cystic fibrosis have sputum neutrophilia (15, 18).

EXHALED BREATH CONDENSATE

Exhaled breath condensate (EBC) is a noninvasive method aimed to evaluate volatile markers and inflammatory mediators that may contribute to evaluate asthma pathophysiology.

EBC collects particles from airway lining fluid by the condensation of warm humid breath onto a cold surface in a condensing device.

EBC collection, as described in ATS/ERS guidelines, requires a refrigerated device (19) and patient are requested to breath at tidal volume for 10–15 min. During this time the airways lining fluid undergoes an aerosolization process and the exhaled fraction is condensed in a cooling device (0 to −20°C) (20).

The most frequently evaluated parameters in EBC are pH, exhaled markers of oxidative stress and inflammation.

EBC is composed of water vapor, unstable volatiles such as CO_2 and H_2O_2, inorganic (O_2, N_2), and organic (CO_2) particles, exogenous, and endogenous organic compounds, protein, and cytokines (21). In the respiratory tract, H_2O_2 may be released from inflamed cells—including neutrophils, macrophages, eosinophils, and epithelial cells. Nitrogen redox forms such as nitrite (NO_2 -) and nitrate (NO_3 -) are present in the epithelial lining fluid of the human respiratory tract.

High concentrations of NO_2 and NO_2+NO_3 were showed in patients with asthma, CF and bronchiectasis compared with healthy controls (21).

The pH of EBC is a non-specific marker of airway disease being a median normal pH value of 8.0 in children from 0 to 20 years (22). Some studies showed a lower pH in children with stable asthma than healthy controls and a lower pH value in children with severe than mild asthma (23, 24). In addition, asthmatic patients not adequately treated with ICS have been demonstrated to have a lower pH than those properly treated. Patients with acute exacerbation had a higher pH value after the treatment with budesonide (23, 24).

At present, no association has been reported between asthma symptoms, lung function, FeNO, and airway hyperresponsiveness (25, 26).

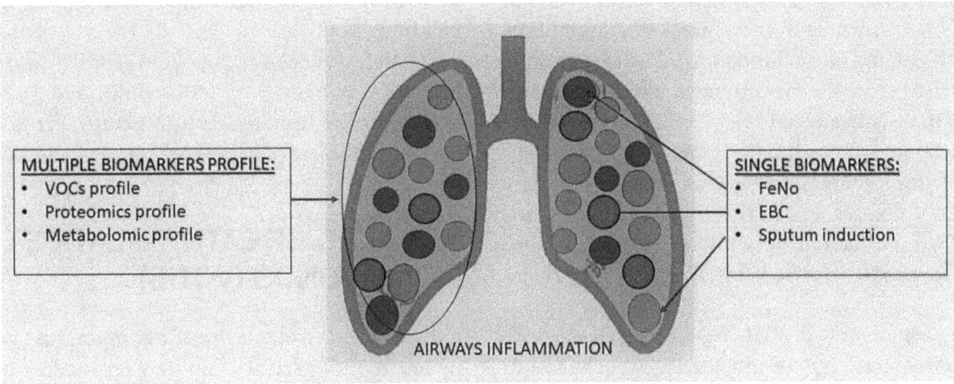

FIGURE 1 | Summary of single and multiple biomarkers detection methods to assess airways inflammation in children.

Biomarkers related to oxidative stress like H_2O_2, 8-isoprostane, asymmetric dimethylarginine (ADMA), aldehydes, and nitrite/nitrate are important to be evaluated in EBC in a number of airway diseases, including asthma.

Asymmetric dimethylarginine (ADMA) is an EBC marker of oxidative stress which can be assessed by the UPLC-MS/MS technique. It is an analog of L-arginine that reduces the synthesis of NO and increases superoxide from inhibition of NOS. A previous study showed that asthmatic children had higher values of ADMA than healthy ones with no difference with ICS treatment (27).

The oxidation of the phospholipid membrane and polyunsaturated fatty acid produces aldehydes and lipid hydroperoxides. One study showed high levels of glutathione in the EBC of asthmatic children with exacerbation and after 5 days of prednisolone therapy, the malondialdehyde level dropped, while glutathione rose (28). Malondialdehyde levels also correlate with air pollution, lung function and inflammatory markers. These results suggest that during exacerbations there is an imbalance between oxidative and antioxidant agents in the airways.

H_2O_2 is released from cells in the airways as superoxide anions, an unstable and reactive particle. In the respiratory system, H_2O_2 can be released from both inflammatory cells—including neutrophils, macrophages, eosinophils—and epithelial cells. In non-asthmatic, non-smoking children, the normal value of this molecule is 0.09 μmol (19). H_2O_2 was higher in asthmatic children during exacerbations and decreased after ICS treatment, supporting the hypothesis that H_2O_2 is a marker of airways inflammation (29, 30). However, other studies failed to demonstrate its ability to predict exacerbations (31, 32).

8-isoprostane, a suitable marker of oxidative stress, is a product of arachidonic acid (33). Children and adults with severe asthma or asthma exacerbation have high levels of this 8-isoprostane (34). The concentrations of 8-isoprostane failed to show any correlation with lung function, FeNO, ICS or leukotriene receptor antagonist therapy (35, 36).

Eicosanoids are another group of markers derived from arachidonic acid that play a role in asthmatic inflammation. The presence of these markers in EBC is confirmed by specific enzyme immunoassay and radioimmunoassays (37).

Asthmatic children have high levels of leukotriene B4 (LTB4), cysteinyl leukotrienes (LTC4, LTD4, and LTE4) in EBC (36, 37). The role of cysteinyl leukotrienes (CysLT) in response to ICS therapy is under debate (38–40). Some authors showed a significant reduction of CysLT after a course of oral corticosteroids and after 6 months of ICS therapy, whereas others did not confirm this result. A significant reduction of CysLTs has been reported after montelukast therapy (41).

Several other markers of inflammation and oxidative stress, such as cytokines and adenosine, have been investigated. Asthmatic children showed high Th2 cytokines and low Th1 cytokines in EBC (42, 43). Moreover, children with asthma had a high IL-4/INFγ ratio related to Th2 inflammation (43). IL-4 was high in asthmatic and atopic children as a predictor of asthma condition, whereas IL-5 could predict exacerbations (32).

FRACTIONAL EXHALED NITRIC OXIDE (FENO)

Nitric oxide in airways is mainly produced by two enzymes: constitutive nitric oxide synthase (cNOS), that produces low quantities of NO, and epithelial inducible NOS (iNOS) that is induced by various inflammatory cytokines (44). FeNO is a marker of eosinophilic airway inflammation, able to evaluate the level of inflammation and the response of anti-inflammatory therapy (45).

FeNO is a noninvasive, repeatable and reproducible method (46) applicable in the pediatric practice. The gold standard technique for cooperative children is the single breath on-line method (47) but also other techniques have been proposed for uncooperative children or in sedated infants (47). Nevertheless, at present, no clear evidence is available regarding the potential clinical application of FeNO measurements in uncooperative children. In this age group, the method deserves additional efforts to standardization because it its potential application to predict asthma (33).

FeNO levels can be influenced by different factors such as patient's age, height, gender, and race, nasal contamination, exhalation flow ambient and air pollution (48). The execution of spirometry or exercise before the measurement, diet or exposure to smoke also need to be considered (48).

The standardization of techniques permits to collect comparable data from different centers in healthy children and subjects with diseases. For this purpose, the first document on FeNO evaluation in children was published in 2002 (47), subsequently revised by ATS/ERS in 2005 (48).

Several studies demonstrated that FeNO correlates with airway hyperresponsiveness, IgE serum levels, bronchodilator response, skin prick tests, asthma symptoms, and lung function (49, 50).

Airway inflammation in allergic asthma results from the activation of Th2-mediated pro-inflammatory cytokine mechanism involving IL-4, IL-5, and IL-13. This mechanism causes the expression of epithelial inducible NO synthase up-regulated via STAT-6, a process which is corticosteroid sensitive (51, 52).

Furthermore, other studies showed that FeNO levels are correlated with serum eosinophilic cation protein, eosinophils in induced sputum, blood eosinophilia, eosinophil infiltration of the airways, and IgE levels in atopic patients (52). High FeNO values characterize Th2-mediated airway inflammation, eosinophilia, and responsiveness to ICS (52).

FeNO is helpful during evaluation of the patients characterizing asthma of the eosinophilic phenotype and predicting asthma exacerbation. In children less than 5-year-old with recurrent coughing and wheezing, increased FeNO levels can predict physician diagnosed asthma at school age (53). Furthermore, increased FeNO levels at the age of 4 years, predict higher risk for wheezing, asthma and need of ICS by school age (54).

The ATS guidelines recommend the use of FeNO for monitoring airway inflammation and for addressing the choice of anti-inflammatory treatment (52, 55, 56). It has been extensively proved a rapid decrease of FeNO values when ICS treatment is started, with a dose-dependent mechanism and a sudden rise when ICS therapy is withdrawn (57). This trend may be helpful in monitoring patient adherence to the therapy (46).

High FeNO values are not always linked to eosinophilic asthma but also to allergic rhinitis, eosinophilic bronchitis and allergen or viral exposure and a correct interpretation is stressed in the ATS/ERS document (55).

In patient treated with omalizumab, FeNO values, blood eosinophils and BMI can predict the response to the therapy (58).

Authors, for a long time, have been very cautious to support the use of FeNO as coadjutant to standard symptom-based management (59, 60).

However, in recent Cochrane review it has been showed that FeNO guided treatment in asthmatic children was associated with a significant reduction in exacerbation as compared with guideline-based treatment (61). On these bases, the most recent GINA document in 2018 included FeNO guided treatment as a proposed for tailoring treatment to be considered in children (1).

Therefore, FeNO can be regarded a useful method to categorize patients with eosinophilic and Th2-mediated asthma evaluating the response to ICS therapy, predicting exacerbations and the compliance to the therapy.

EXHALED BREATH VOLATILE ORGANIC COMPOUNDS (VOCS)

Exhaled breath volatile organic compounds (VOCs) are analyzed by breathomics science and they represent a noninvasive tool to evaluate the lung inflammation. VOCs have a metabolic origin from larger molecules. Airway VOCs originate not only from the upper and lower airways but also from a capillary bed near the alveoli (62). Their concentration in exhaled breath is influenced by blood gas coefficient, cardiac output and alveolar minute volume.

The methodological approach to collect VOCs from exhaled breath requires attention to exclude organic compounds from the ambient air, type of sampling (total vs. alveolar breath), type of collecting materials and other confounding factors (62).

In particular, the collection of airway VOCs needs an inhalation filter to exclude ambient VOCs. The patient is asked to breath into a system which can collect online samples directly via inert tubes into an analyzer or off-line by collecting exhaled air into bags, tubes or syringes. These devices are made of inert materials such as Tedlar bags (63).

Gas chromatography-mass spectrometry (GC-MS) and flame ionization detection (GC-FID) are the most widely used techniques to analyze the samples after collection. These methods can differentiate and quantify VOCs at low concentrations, but they require both qualified technicians and expensive technology (33).

A new non-selective approach to analyze VOCs in exhaled breath is metabolomic profiling that identify and quantify all metabolites in a biological sample without *a priori* hypothesis.

Metabolomic profiles describe the interaction among environmental exposure, medication, nutrition, and toxic substances, genetic expression and microorganisms (33, 62). This method is an interesting approach to patient characterization and personalized medication (33). This approach simultaneously evaluates many metabolites in a sample and generates a profile capable of discriminating between different groups of individuals characterizing the biochemical processes underway in each biological system.

More recently sensor-based device such as the electronic nose, colorimetric sensor array, and gold nanoparticle sensors have been proposed. They adopt specific sensors with optical, chemical or electronic properties that analyze VOCs in the EB (62). Recently, some studies have demonstrated the clinical application of these instruments in respiratory disease (64, 65). VOCs in the EB discriminate between asthma and healthy and between atopic and non-atopic children (64, 65). VOCs profile in exhaled breath was able to discriminate healthy, transient wheezing and asthmatic children starting from the age of 2-3-year-old (66). In the pediatric field, VOCs can also predict asthma exacerbations (67, 68).

Nevertheless, further studies are necessary to evaluate the clinical utility of VOCs in evaluating asthma severity and monitoring asthma symptoms and response to ICS therapy.

CONCLUSIONS

Noninvasive techniques to collect and analyze airways inflammatory biomarkers are helpful in evaluating the airway pathophysiology of asthmatic children.

In clinical practice, FeNO evaluation has been suggested as the only valid and non-invasive technique to test for underlined eosinophilic inflammation, but it would need to be adopted in combination with other useful markers.

The standardization of the new techniques to collect biomarkers in EB and EBC remains problematic. Low reproducibility of exhaled biomarkers and the lack of standardization of the methods of pre-collection, collection, post-collection of the samples, along with the correct interpretation of the results, represent critical issues in clinical practice.

The identification and utilization of ideal and defined biomarkers in asthmatic children remains debated. The reasons for this are the biological aspects of each prospective biomarker, the disease pathobiology, and methods and invasiveness of sample collection. Therefore, the development of novel biomarker with more sensitivity and specificity may lead to prompt diagnosis of severe asthma in future.

AUTHOR CONTRIBUTIONS

MZ, MP, and LT: drafting of the manuscript; GP, MZ, and LT: critical revision.

REFERENCES

1. Global Initiative for Asthma. *Global Strategy for Asthma Management and Prevention*,. Available online at: www.ginasthma.org (2018).
2. Vijverberg SJ, Hilvering B, Raaijmakers JA, Lammers JW, Maitland-van der Zee AH, Koenderman L. Clinical utility of asthma biomarkers: from bench to bedside. *Biologics*.(2013) 7:199–210. doi: 10.2147/BTT.S29976
3. Murugan A, Prys-Picard C, Calhoun WJ. Biomarkers in asthma. *Curr Opin Pulm Med*. (2009) 15:12–8. doi: 10.1097/MCP.0b013e32831de235
4. Kharitonov SA, Barnes PJ. Exhaled markers of inflammation. *Curr Opin Allergy Clin Immunol.* (2001) 1:217–24. doi: 10.1097/00130832-200106000-00004
5. Barnes PJ, Chowdhury B, Kharitonov SA, Magnussen H, Page CP, Postma D, et al. Pulmonary biomarkers in chronic obstructive pulmonary disease. *Am J Respir Crit Care Med.* (2006) 174:6–14. doi: 10.1164/rccm.200510-1659PP
6. Moore WC, Meyers DA, Wenzel SE, Teague WG, Li H, Li X, et al. Identification of asthma phenotypes using cluster analysis in the Severe Asthma Research Program. *Am J Respir Crit Care Med.* (2010) 181:315–23 doi: 10.1164/rccm.200906-0896OC
7. Gibson PG, Henry RL, Thomas P. Noninvasive assessment of airway inflammation in children: induced sputum, exhaled nitric oxide, and breath condensate. *Eur Respir J.* (2000) 16:1008–15.
8. Deykin A, Massaro AF, Drazen JM, Israel E. Exhaled nitric oxide as a diagnostic test for asthma: online versus offline techniques and effect of flow rate. *Am J Respir Crit Care Med.* (2002) 165:1597–601. doi: 10.1164/rccm.2201081
9. Gibson PG, Grootendor DC, Henry RL, Pin I, Rytila PH, Wark P, et al. Sputum induction in children. *Eur Respir J Suppl.* (2002) 37:44s–6s. doi: 10.1183/09031936.02.00004402
10. Robroeks CM, van Berkel JJ, Dallinga JW, Jobsis Q, Zimmermann LJ, Hendriks HJ, et al. Metabolomics of volatile organic compounds in cystic fibrosis patients and controls. *Pediatr Res.* (2010) 68:75–80. doi: 10.1203/PDR.0b013e3181df4ea0
11. Wilson NM, Bridge P, Spanevello A, Silverman M. Induced sputum in children: feasibility, repeatability, and relation of findings to asthma severity. *Thorax* (2000) 55:768–74. doi: 10.1136/thorax.55.9.768
12. Fens N, Zwinderman AH, van der Schee MP, de Nijs SB, Dijkers E, Roldaan AC, et al. Exhaled breath profiling enables discrimination of chronic obstructive pulmonary disease and asthma. *Am J Respir Crit Care Med.* (2009) 180:1076–82. doi: 10.1164/rccm.200906-0939OC
13. Simpson JL, Scott R, Boyle MJ, Gibson PG. Inflammatory subtypes in asthma: assessment and identification using induced sputum. *Respirology* (2006) 11:54–61. doi: 10.1111/j.1440-1843.2006.00784.x
14. Haldar P, Pavord ID, Shaw DE, Berry MA, Thomas M, Brightling CE, et al. Cluster analysis and clinical asthma phenotypes. *Am J Respir Crit Care Med.* (2008) 178:218–24. doi: 10.1164/rccm.200711-1754OC
15. Cai Y, Carty K, Henry RL, Gibson PG. Persistence of sputum eosinophilia in children with controlled asthma when compared with healthy children. *Eur Respir J.* (1998) 11:848–53. doi: 10.1183/09031936.98.11040848
16. Piacentini GL, Vicentini L, Mazzi P, Chilosi M, Martinati L, Boner AL. Mite-antigen avoidance can reduce bronchial epithelial shedding in allergic asthmatic children. *Clin Exp Allergy* (1998) 28:561–7. doi: 10.1046/j.1365-2222.1998.00260.x
17. Norzila MZ, Fakes K, Henry RL, Simpson J, Gibson PG. Interleukin-8 secretion and neutrophil recruitment accompanies induced sputum eosinophil activation in children with acute asthma. *Am J Respir Crit Care Med.* (2000) 161(3 Pt 1):769–74. doi: 10.1164/ajrccm.161.3.9809071
18. Pin I, Radford S, Kolendowicz R, Jennings B, Denburg JA, Hargreave FE, et al. Airway inflammation in symptomatic and asymptomatic children with methacholine hyperresponsiveness. *Eur Respir J.* (1993) 6:1249–56.ho
19. Horvath I, Hunt J, Barnes PJ, Alving K, Antczak A, Baraldi E, et al. Exhaled breath condensate: methodological recommendations and unresolved questions. *Eur Respir J.* (2005) 26:523–48. doi: 10.1183/09031936.05.00029705
20. Baraldi E, Carraro S. Exhaled NO and breath condensate. *Paediatr Respir Rev.* (2006) 7 (Suppl. 1):S20–2. doi: 10.1016/j.prrv.2006.04.017
21. Dent AG, Sutedja TG, Zimmerman PV. Exhaled breath analysis for lung cancer. *J Thorac Dis.* (2013) 5 (Suppl. 5):S540–50. doi: 10.3978/j.issn.2072-1439.2013.08.44
22. Paget-Brown AO, Ngamtrakulpanit L, Smith A, Bunyan D, Hom S, Nguyen A, et al. Normative data for pH of exhaled breath condensate. *Chest* (2006) 129:426–30. doi: 10.1378/chest.129.2.426
23. Carraro S, Folesani G, Corradi M, Zanconato S, Gaston B, Baraldi E. Acid-base equilibrium in exhaled breath condensate of allergic asthmatic children. *Allergy* (2005) 60:476–81. doi: 10.1111/j.1398-9995.2005.00718.x
24. Brunetti L, Francavilla R, Tesse R, Fiermonte P, Fiore FP, Lore M, et al. Exhaled breath condensate cytokines and pH in pediatric asthma and atopic dermatitis. *Allergy Asthma Proc.* (2008) 29:461–7. doi: 10.2500/aap.2008.29.3152
25. Rosias PP, Dompeling E, Dentener MA, Pennings HJ, Hendriks HJ, Van Iersel MP, et al. Childhood asthma: exhaled markers of airway inflammation, asthma control score, and lung function tests. *Pediatr Pulmonol.* (2004) 38:107–14 doi: 10.1002/ppul.20056
26. Ratnawati, Morton J, Henry RL, Thomas PS. Exhaled breath condensate nitrite/nitrate and pH in relation to pediatric asthma control and exhaled nitric oxide. *Pediatr Pulmonol.* (2006) 41:929–36. doi: 10.1002/ppul.20469

27. Carraro S, Giordano G, Piacentini G, Kantar A, Moser S, Cesca L, et al. Asymmetric dimethylarginine in exhaled breath condensate and serum of children with asthma. *Chest* (2013) 144:405–10 doi: 10.1378/chest.12-2379
28. Corradi M, Folesani G, Andreoli R, Manini P, Bodini A, Piacentini G, et al. Aldehydes and glutathione in exhaled breath condensate of children with asthma exacerbation. *Am J Respir Crit Care Med.* (2003) 167:395–9. doi: 10.1164/rccm.200206-507OC
29. Jobsis Q, Raatgeep HC, Hermans PW, de Jongste JC. Hydrogen peroxide in exhaled air is increased in stable asthmatic children. *Eur Respir J.* (1997) 10:519–21.
30. Caffarelli C, Calcinai E, Rinaldi L, Povesi Dascola C, Terracciano L, Corradi M. Hydrogen peroxide in exhaled breath condensate in asthmatic children during acute exacerbation and after treatment. *Respiration* (2012) 84:291–8. doi: 10.1159/000341969
31. Trischler J, Merkel N, Konitzer S, Muller CM, Unverzagt S, Lex C. Fractionated breath condensate sampling: H(2)O(2) concentrations of the alveolar fraction may be related to asthma control in children. *Respir Res.* (2012) 13:14. doi: 10.1186/1465-9921-13-14
32. Robroeks CM, van Vliet D, Jobsis Q, Braekers R, Rijkers GT, Wodzig WK, et al. Prediction of asthma exacerbations in children: results of a one-year prospective study. *Clin Exp Allergy* (2012) 42:792–8. doi: 10.1111/j.1365-2222.2012.03992.x
33. Moschino L, Zanconato S, Bozzetto S, Baraldi E, Carraro S. Childhood asthma biomarkers: present knowledge and future steps. *Paediatr Respir Rev.* (2015) 16:205–12. doi: 10.1016/j.prrv.2015.05.001
34. Baraldi E, Carraro S, Alinovi R, Pesci A, Ghiro L, Bodini A, et al. Cysteinyl leukotrienes and 8-isoprostane in exhaled breath condensate of children with asthma exacerbations. *Thorax* (2003) 58:505–9. doi: 10.1136/thorax.58.6.505
35. Shahid SK, Kharitonov SA, Wilson NM, Bush A, Barnes PJ. Exhaled 8-isoprostane in childhood asthma. *Respir Res.* (2005) 6:79. doi: 10.1186/1465-9921-6-79
36. Loukides S, Kontogianni K, Hillas G, Horvath I. Exhaled breath condensate in asthma: from bench to bedside. *Curr Med Chem.* (2011) 18:1432–43. doi: 10.2174/092986711795328418
37. Thomas PS, Lowe AJ, Samarasinghe P, Lodge CJ, Huang Y, Abramson MJ, et al. Exhaled breath condensate in pediatric asthma: promising new advance or pouring cold water on a lot of hot air? a systematic review. *Pediatr Pulmonol.* (2013) 48:419–42 doi: 10.1002/ppul.22776
38. Csoma Z, Kharitonov SA, Balint B, Bush A, Wilson NM, Barnes PJ. Increased leukotrienes in exhaled breath condensate in childhood asthma. *Am J Respir Crit Care Med.* (2002) 166:1345–9. doi: 10.1164/rccm.200203-233OC
39. Debley JS, Hallstrand TS, Monge T, Ohanian A, Redding GJ, Zimmerman J. Methods to improve measurement of cysteinyl leukotrienes in exhaled breath condensate from subjects with asthma and healthy controls. *J Allergy Clin Immunol.* (2007) 120:1216–7. doi: 10.1016/j.jaci.2007.06.029
40. Steiss JO, Rudloff S, Landmann E, Ruckes-Nilges C, Zimmer KP, Lindemann H. Effect of inhaled corticosteroid treatment on exhaled breath condensate leukotriene E(4) in children with mild asthma. *Allergy Asthma Proc.* (2008) 29:371–5. doi: 10.2500/aap.2008.29.3135
41. Montuschi P, Mondino C, Koch P, Barnes PJ, Ciabattoni G. Effects of a leukotriene receptor antagonist on exhaled leukotriene E4 and prostanoids in children with asthma. *J Allergy Clin Immunol.* (2006) 118:347–53. doi: 10.1016/j.jaci.2006.04.010
42. Karakoc GB, Yukselen A, Yilmaz M, Altintas DU, Kendirli SG. Exhaled breath condensate MMP-9 level and its relationship with asthma severity and interleukin-4/10 levels in children. *Ann Allergy Asthma Immunol.* (2012) 108:300–4. doi: 10.1016/j.anai.2012.02.019
43. Shahid SK, Kharitonov SA, Wilson NM, Bush A, Barnes PJ. Increased interleukin-4 and decreased interferon-gamma in exhaled breath condensate of children with asthma. *Am J Respir Crit Care Med.* (2002) 165:1290–3. doi: 10.1164/rccm.2108082
44. Turner S. Exhaled nitric oxide and the management of childhood asthma–yet another promising biomarker "has been" or a misunderstood gem. *Paediatr Respir Rev.* (2015) 16:88–96. doi: 10.1016/j.prrv.2014.07.005
45. Kharitonov SA, Yates DH, Barnes PJ. Inhaled glucocorticoids decrease nitric oxide in exhaled air of asthmatic patients. *Am J Respir Crit Care Med.* (1996) 153:454–7. doi: 10.1164/ajrccm.153.1.8542158
46. Pijnenburg MW, De Jongste JC. Exhaled nitric oxide in childhood asthma: a review. *Clin Exp Allergy.* (2008) 38:246–59. doi: 10.1111/j.1365-2222.2007.02897.x
47. Baraldi E, de Jongste JC. Measurement of exhaled nitric oxide in children, 2001. *Eur Respir J.* (2002) 20:223–37. doi: 10.1183/09031936.02.00293102
48. ATS/ERS recommendations for standardized procedures for the online and offline measurement of exhaled lower respiratory nitric oxide and nasal nitric oxide, 2005. *Am J Respir Crit Care Med.* (2005) 171:912–30. doi: 10.1164/rccm.200406-710ST
49. Covar RA, Szefler SJ, Martin RJ, Sundstrom DA, Silkoff PE, Murphy J, et al. Relations between exhaled nitric oxide and measures of disease activity among children with mild-to-moderate asthma. *J Pediatr.* (2003) 142:469–75. doi: 10.1067/mpd.2003.187
50. Komakula S, Khatri S, Mermis J, Savill S, Haque S, Rojas M, et al. Body mass index is associated with reduced exhaled nitric oxide and higher exhaled 8-isoprostanes in asthmatics. *Respir Res.* (2007) 8:32. doi: 10.1186/1465-9921-8-32
51. Ludviksdottir D, Diamant Z, Alving K, Bjermer L, Malinovschi A. Clinical aspects of using exhaled NO in asthma diagnosis and management. *Clin Respir J.* (2012) 6:193–207. doi: 10.1111/crj.12001
52. Mahr TA, Malka J, Spahn JD. Inflammometry in pediatric asthma: a review of fractional exhaled nitric oxide in clinical practice. *Allergy Asthma Proc.* (2013) 34:210–9. doi: 10.2500/aap.2013.34.3660
53. Singer F, Luchsinger I, Inci D, Knauer N, Latzin P, Wildhaber JH, Moeller A. Exhaled nitric oxide in symptomatic children at preschool age predicts later asthma. *Allergy* (2013) 68:531–8. doi: 10.1111/all.12127
54. Caudri D, Wijga AH, Hoekstra MO, Kerkhof M, Koppelman GH, Brunekreef B, Smit HA, de Jongste JC. Prediction of asthma in symptomatic preschool children using exhaled nitric oxide, Rint and specific IgE. *Thorax* (2010) 65:801–7. doi: 10.1136/thx.2009.126912
55. Dweik RA, Boggs PB, Erzurum SC, Irvin CG, Leigh MW, Lundberg JO, et al. An official ATS clinical practice guideline: interpretation of exhaled nitric oxide levels (FENO) for clinical applications. *Am J Respir Crit Care Med.* (2011) 184:602–15. doi: 10.1164/rccm.9120-11ST
56. Taylor DR. Advances in the clinical applications of exhaled nitric oxide measurements. *J Breath Res.* (2012) 6:047102. doi: 10.1088/1752-7155/6/4/047102
57. van Rensen EL, Straathof KC, Veselic-Charvat MA, Zwinderman AH, Bel EH, Sterk PJ. Effect of inhaled steroids on airway hyperresponsiveness, sputum eosinophils, and exhaled nitric oxide levels in patients with asthma. *Thorax* (1999) 54:403–8. doi: 10.1136/thx.54.5.403
58. Sorkness CA, Wildfire JJ, Calatroni A, Mitchell HE, Busse WW, O'Connor GT, et al. Reassessment of omalizumab-dosing strategies and pharmacodynamics in inner-city children and adolescents. *J Allergy Clin Immunol Pract.* (2013) 1:163–71. doi: 10.1016/j.jaip.2013.01.011
59. Petsky HL, Cates CJ, Lasserson TJ, Li AM, Turner C, Kynaston JA, et al. A systematic review and meta-analysis: tailoring asthma treatment on eosinophilic markers (exhaled nitric oxide or sputum eosinophils). *Thorax* (2012) 67:199–208. doi: 10.1136/thx.2010.135574
60. Jartti T, Wendelin-Saarenhovi M, Heinonen I, Hartiala J, Vanto T. Childhood asthma management guided by repeated FeNO measurements: a meta-analysis. *Paediatr Respir Rev.* (2012) 13:178–83. doi: 10.1016/j.prrv.2011.11.002
61. Petsky HL1, Kew KM, Chang AB. Exhaled nitric oxide levels to guide treatment for children with asthma. *Cochrane Database Syst Rev.* (2016) 11:CD011439. doi: 10.1002/14651858.CD011439.pub2
62. van Mastrigt E, de Jongste JC, Pijnenburg MW. The analysis of volatile organic compounds in exhaled breath and biomarkers in exhaled breath condensate in children - clinical tools or scientific toys? *Clin Exp Allergy* (2015) 45:1170–88. doi: 10.1111/cea.12454
63. Barker M, Hengst M, Schmid J, Buers HJ, Mittermaier B, Klemp D, et al. Volatile organic compounds in the exhaled breath of young patients with cystic fibrosis. *Eur Respir J.* (2006) 27:929–36. doi: 10.1183/09031936.06.00085105
64. Dallinga JW, Robroeks CM, van Berkel JJ, Moonen EJ, Godschalk RW, Jobsis Q, et al. Volatile organic compounds in exhaled breath as a diagnostic tool for asthma in children. *Clin Exp Allergy* (2010) 40:68–76.

65. Caldeira M, Barros AS, Bilelo MJ, Parada A, Camara JS, Rocha SM. Profiling allergic asthma volatile metabolic patterns using a headspace-solid phase microextraction/gas chromatography based methodology. *J Chromatogr A* (2011) 1218:3771–80. doi: 10.1016/j.chroma.2011.04.026
66. Smolinska A, Klaassen EM, Dallinga JW, van de Kant KD, Jobsis Q, Moonen EJ, et al. Profiling of volatile organic compounds in exhaled breath as a strategy to find early predictive signatures of asthma in children. *PLoS ONE* (2014) 9:e95668. doi: 10.1371/journal.pone.0095668
67. Robroeks CM, van Berkel JJ, Jobsis Q, van Schooten FJ, Dallinga JW, Wouters EF, et al. Exhaled volatile organic compounds predict exacerbations of childhood asthma in a 1-year prospective study. *Eur Respir J.* (2013) 42:98–106. doi: 10.1183/09031936.00010712
68. Raymer JH, Thomas KW, Cooper SD, Whitaker DA, Pellizzari ED. A device for sampling of human alveolar breath for the measurement of expired volatile organic compounds. *J Anal Toxicol.* (1990) 14:337–44.

12

Dysfunctional Breathing in Children and Adults with Asthma

Gary J. Connett and Mike Thomas*

University Hospital Southampton NHS Foundation Trust, Southampton, United Kingdom

***Correspondence:**
Gary J. Connett
gary.connett@uhs.nhs.uk

Asthma occurs across the life course. Its optimal treatment includes the use of personalized management plans that recognize the importance of co-morbidities including so-called "dysfunctional breathing." Such symptoms can arise as a result of induced laryngeal obstruction (ILO) or alterations in the mechanics of normal breathing called breathing pattern disorders. Whilst these two types of breathing abnormalities might be related, studies tend to focus on only one of them and do not consider their relationship. Evidence for these problems amongst childhood asthmatics is largely anecdotal. They seem rare in early childhood. Both types are more frequently recognized in the second decade of life and girls are affected more often. These observations tantalizingly parallel epidemiological studies characterizing the increasing prevalence and severity of asthma that also occurs amongst females after puberty. Exercise ILO is more common amongst adolescents and young adults. It should be properly delineated as it might be causally related to specific treatable factors. More severe ILO occurring at rest and breathing pattern disorders are more likely to be occurring within a psychological paradigm. Dysfunctional breathing is associated with asthma morbidity through a number of potential mechanisms. These include anxiety induced breathing pattern disorders and the enhanced perception of subsequent symptoms, cooling and drying of the airways from hyperventilation induced hyperresponsiveness and a direct effect of emotional stimuli on airways constriction via cholinergic pathways. Hyperventilation is the most common breathing pattern disorder amongst adults. Although not validated for use in asthma, the Nijmegen questionnaire has been used to characterize this problem. Studies show higher scores amongst women, those with poorly controlled asthma and those with psychiatric problems. Evidence that treatment with breathing retraining techniques is effective in a primary care population including all types of asthmatics suggests the problem might be more ubiquitous than just these high-risk groups. Future challenges include the need for studies characterizing all types of dysfunctional breathing in pediatric and adult patient cohorts and clearly defined, age appropriate, interventional studies. Clinicians caring for asthmatics in all age groups need to be aware of these co-morbidities and routinely ask about symptoms that suggest these problems.

Keywords: asthma, dysfunctioal breathing, paradoxical vocal fold motion, hyperventilation, breathing pattern disorders, inducible laryngeal obstruction, exercise inducible laryngeal obstruction, breathing retraining exercises

INTRODUCTION

For most of the time breathing occurs sub-consciously. A network of brain stem neurones at the level of the medulla and pons forms the respiratory center which initiates rhythmic contraction of the respiratory muscles whilst co-ordinating these movements with other activities, such as speaking and swallowing (1). As humans we are able to override this otherwise automatic process, for example by breath holding to dive underwater or to forcefully blow out candles. Breathing can also be impacted upon by emotions. For example, bouts of laughter can harmlessly interrupt normal respiration. However, in some people physiologically inappropriate hyperventilation, in response to feelings of agitation and anxiety, can lead to disabling symptoms and become a chronic problem (2). In others abnormal dysfunctional breathing patterns, such as trying to breath through an obstructed larynx, rapid, shallow breathing, irregular breathing and predominant upper-chest breathing might also lead to troublesome symptoms with or without associated hypocapnia. Identifying such problems as a co-morbidity complicating asthma can be difficult as there is considerable overlap in the types of symptoms that occur and a complex interrelationship (3).

In this article we will review how the asthma phenotype might be impacted upon by dysfunctional breathing problems throughout the life course.

DEFINITIONS AND TERMINOLOGY

Dysfunctional breathing might usefully be regarded as an overarching term that is inclusive of problems that are either thoracic or laryngeal in nature (4). Whilst both types are reported as occurring amongst asthmatics, there are no studies addressing the extent to which they both occur within individual patients. This is despite prevalence studies suggesting that both are common and that therefore there should be considerable overlap. Unfortunately the use of the term dysfunctional can be stigmatizing for patients and especially in children where it might have inappropriate connotations about dysfunctional families and elements of abuse or neglect. To address such issues, breathing pattern disorders is a recently recommended term describing functional abnormalities in the mechanics of the diaphragm and intercostal muscles that result in inefficient breathing. Similarly, a joint task force addressing upper airway problems has recommended the term inducible laryngeal obstruction (ILO) rather than laryngeal dysfunction or paradoxical vocal cord motion to denote extrathoracic airway problems. ILO usefully encompasses obstruction occurring at supraglottic as well as glottic (vocal fold) levels as characterized at laryngoscopy (5).

The most commonly recognized breathing pattern disorder and the first to be described was hyperventilation in adults (6). More recently however, breathing pattern disorders have come to encompass a wider spectrum of breathing abnormalities. These include periodic deep sighing, thoracic dominant breathing, forced abdominal expiration and thoracic-abdominal asynchrony (7, 8). The extent to which these other problems occur amongst asthmatics is unknown.

PATHOPHYSIOLOGY

The pathophysiology of dysfunctional breathing disorders is incompletely understood. It has been suggested that the occurrence of a characteristic complex of symptoms that can include breathlessness, chest tightness, sighing, yawning, chest discomfort, general fatigue, anxiety and abdominal bloating, might usefully be regarded as a learnt conditioned response to some sort of emotional distress that has taken on physical manifestations (9). Those affected often do not recognize that their symptoms are arising in this way and that they might be "catastrophising" their health fearing serious underlying illness. The resulting interference with normal automatic control probably occurs at a sub-conscious level.

Somatisation symptoms typically resemble those of an illness the affected person is aware of, has, or has had in the past. In this context, it is well-recognized that those patients presenting with acute hyperventilation, commonly also have undetected co-existing asthma (10). Amongst known asthmatics however, the situation is far more complex because of the difficulties distinguishing true asthma from asthmatic symptoms induced by dysfunctional breathing. Hyperventilation for example, occurs in the vast majority of acute asthma attacks as demonstrated by low arterial carbon dioxide tensions (11). The mechanism whereby this happens might include stimulation of irritant and stretch receptors, anxiety mediated effects on cholinergic bronchosconstriction (12) and a hyperventilatory response to the perception of increased airways resistance (13). Hyperventilation *per se* might then further worsen true asthma through bronchosconstrictive cooling and airway dehydration.

ILO, the involuntary narrowing of the upper airway during inspiration, is similarly complex and multifactorial. Anxiety and psychological disorders are thought to be major contributory factors in the majority of adults who are affected and particularly when symptoms occur spontaneously at rest (14). Amongst younger asthmatics, exercise induced laryngeal obstruction (EILO) is more common and should usefully be regarded as a separate condition. It can co-exist with exercise-induced asthma and psychological co-morbidities are less predominant than in ILO. Causal factors include the aerodynamic effects of high inspiratory flow rates, neurally mediated laryngeal hyper-reactivity and environmental factors, such as inhaling cold air. Gastro-esophageal reflux has been implicated but this is very common in unaffected individuals of all ages and a causal relationship has not been proven (15). Upper airway symptoms of rhinitis and post-nasal drip might also be a contributory precipitant of upper airway closure but is also unproven (16).

EPIDEMIOLOGY

The findings of the main studies to determine the presence of hyperventilation in asthmatics are summarized in **Table 1**. These studies have used the Nijmegen questionnaire (**Table 2**). This

TABLE 1 | Prevalence studies of dysfunctional breathing identified by Nijmegen scoring in asthmatics.

Study setting	Age	Study size	Age differences; Mean (SD)	Prevalence and sex differences	Comments
UK General Practice (*N* = 7033) (17, 18)	17–65 years	71% of 307 asthmatics provided completed questionnaires	Dysfunctional breathers (DB) were younger: 44.8 years (14.7) vs. 49.0 years (13.8) *P* = 0.05	Overall prevalence; 29%. 35% of females and 20% of males Female:male, 73:27 (*P* = 0.016)	Patients were affected equally across all levels of severity. A follow up study found DB in 9.5% of non-asthmatics (14% of females and 2% males surveyed).
Greece Secondary care mild to moderate asthmatics (19)	20–68 years	162 participants; 94 female, 68 male	Not reported	Overall prevalence; 34% 46.8% of females and 14.7% males Female:male, 81:19	DB was more common in asthmatics that were moderate (72.9%) vs. mild (27.1%) and uncontrolled (81.4%) vs. controlled (18.6%).
Scotland secondary care "problem asthma clinic," 76% of patients on BTS step 4 or 5 (20)	13.5–83 years	102 participants; 72 female, 30 male	Not reported	Overall prevalence 64%	Nijmegen scores were related to poor asthma control but more significantly related to quality of life measures.
Romania secondary care asthma clinics (21)	Mean age 35 years	91 participants; 47 female, 44 male	No significant age difference: 37.9 years in DB vs. 34.4 years	Nijmegen score prevalence: 29.7%, progressive exercise test prevalence: 17.6% 38% of females and 7.3% of males Female:male, 82:18	Severe asthma, lack of control and anxiety all associated with DB
Sweden secondary care clinic (22)	Mean age 47 years	25 participants; 19 female, 6 male	Not reported	Nijmegen score positive: 20%	Patients had well-controlled asthma
Spain secondary care clinic (23)	Mean age 47 years, 15–69 years	157 participants; 96 female, 61 male	DB were older: 49 years (24) vs. 42 years (17) *P* = 0.014	Overall prevalence 36% 47% of females and 19.6% of males Female: male, 79:21	Patients with DB experienced all asthma symptoms more acutely. They had more anxiety but no difference in overall asthma severity
Italy school setting (25)	11–14 years	120 asthmatics identified amongst 760 children (15.8%) 47 female, 73 male	No differences	Overall prevalence 25.8% 36.2% of females and 19.2% of males Female:male, 55:45	Asthma was more common amongst males. Amongst non-asthmatics, DB was found in 2.5% (4.1% of females and 0.9% of males surveyed).
Netherlands secondary care asthma clinic (26)	Mean age 10.4 years	206 consecutive asthmatics seen; 96 female, 144 male	No differences	Overall prevalence 5.3% 12% of females and 2.1% of males Female:male, 73:27	Asthma was more common amongst males. There was a strong dose dependent association between DB and asthma control

TABLE 2 | The Nijmegen Questionnaire, Please circle the number in the column that best represents what you have felt recently*.

	Never	Rarely	Sometimes	Often	Very often
Chest pain	0	1	2	3	4
Feeling tense	0	1	2	3	4
Blurred vision	0	1	2	3	4
Dizzy spells	0	1	2	3	4
Feeling confused	0	1	2	3	4
Faster or deeper breathing	0	1	2	3	4
Short of breath	0	1	2	3	4
Tight feelings in the chest	0	1	2	3	4
Bloated feeling in the stomach	0	1	2	3	4
Tingling fingers	0	1	2	3	4
Unable to breathe deeply	0	1	2	3	4
Stiff fingers or arms	0	1	2	3	4
Tight feelings round mouth	0	1	2	3	4
Cold hands or feet	0	1	2	3	4
Palpitations	0	1	2	3	4
Feelings of anxiety	0	1	2	3	4
Subtotals					
Total					

**A total score of 23 or more has been used to screen for dysfunctional breathing in a UK community setting (17). Cut-off scores to detect "abnormality" will depend on a comparison with normal values in the same setting and culture in which the questionnaire is used.*

was originally developed as a screening tool for symptomatic hyperventilation syndrome and subsequently used as a continuous measure of the benefits of interventions to regulate breathing through capnographic feedback methods (24). Although the questionnaire has not been validated for use in adults with asthma (27) or in children, it does appear to be able to detect a cluster of symptoms that can be characterized as relating to the breathing-related effects of stress and anxiety.

Hyperventilation, as identified with this tool, is recognized as being common and occurs across the whole spectrum of asthma severity. It is more common in those with more severe disease and those with poor control (19, 26). Those studies that have investigated psychological co-morbidities, report that stress and the increased perception of more typical asthma symptoms occur more commonly in hyperventilators (21, 23). Such patients were also more likely to have acute asthma attacks.

All studies report that hyperventilation is more common amongst females vs. males and this sex difference tends to increase through childhood into early adult life. The only study in which asthma was more common amongst boys included a younger age group but, as in all other studies, the percentage of girls with asthma who also had hyperventilation was much higher than boys with asthma and hyperventilation (25).

It is not clear whether hyperventilation is more common in adults. A school study from Italy (25) produced comparable data to that in adult primary care, but a secondary care study from the Netherlands found far less dysfunctional breathing compared with adult data (26). Societal differences in reporting might be an important factor limiting the extent to which the Nijmegen questionnaire identifies abnormalities globally and might also limit the generalisability of such findings (28).

EILO is more common in adolescents and younger adults. It has been described in 26.9% of pediatric referrals to secondary care respiratory services, who were thought to have exercise induced asthma (29). Two population based studies suggest that it can occur in between 5.7 and 7.5% of none asthmatic adolescents (30, 31). Most studies also suggest a female predominance (15).

Adult studies have characterized a very severe phenotype of ILO in which symptoms typically occur without provocation. Amongst a hospital based series of 95 cases, 56% were diagnosed as also having asthma and 28% had suffered episodes needing endotracheal intubation to control symptoms (32). Two studies of adult asthmatics attending secondary care services report prevalences of 19 and 50% (33, 34). The study in which half of the asthmatics had this problem were identified using a novel computerized tomography imaging technique to none invasively assess laryngeal movements.

Poor discrimination between exercise induced inspiratory symptoms and exercise induced bronchoconstriction in adolescents and young adults, might be contributing to the over diagnosis of asthma in these age groups.

DIAGNOSTIC CONSIDERATIONS (SEE TABLE 3)

Symptoms relating to dysfunctional breathing need to be differentiated from symptoms due to other causes. These include undiagnosed respiratory, cardiac or metabolic diseases associated with breathlessness, a lack of physical fitness, panic disorders whereby symptoms are more obviously a part of direct manifestations of anxiety, simply reaching physiological limits when exercising and the less common occurrence of wilfully fabricated or induced illness either by the patient or by proxy during childhood.

Increasing breathing difficulties with prolonged inspiration, throat tightness, stridor and wheeze in the cervical region is highly suggestive of ILO in all age groups. A lack of response to more conventional asthma treatment is also indicative. Clinical clues suggesting the possibility of breathing pattern disorders include chest pain or discomfort with no other obvious cause, very short expiratory breath-holding times (e.g., <20 s), feelings of not being able to take a deep breath, the abrupt onset of breathlessness with no obvious cause and the recognition that getting anxious is a trigger of respiratory symptoms (7).

Lactic acidosis after high doses of beta-2-agonists can of itself cause hyperventilation and further complicate a picture of acute asthma made worse by associated tremor and tachycardia which might compound feelings of anxiety (35).

Unfortunately there is no agreed diagnostic work up for this group of conditions. Screening tools for ILO have been suggested but these have largely been developed to distinguish ILO from asthma rather than recognize the two conditions as co-morbidities (36, 37). The medical history can be usefully

TABLE 3 | Dysfunctional breathing in asthma: adults vs. children.

	Children/young people	Adults
Breathing pattern disorders	Girls more often affected and more common in those with psychological co-morbidity	Present across all asthma types and age groups. Women more often affected and those with more severe asthma and/or poor control and/or psychological co-morbidity.
Exercise inducible laryngeal obstruction	Exercise induced breathlessness poorly responsive to asthma treatment. Adolescents of either sex but more commonly girls who are elite athletes or "A" grade students but usually little in the way of psychological co-morbidity	Young adults predominantly as described in adolescents.
Inducible laryngeal obstruction	Limited evidence, but cases similar to that seen in adults have been described and occurring in increasingly younger age groups.	More common in women. Unprovoked asthma, treatment resistant, acute attacks resulting in escalation to high levels of treatment. High levels of physical and psychological morbidity.

informative about EILO. Although psycho-social stressors are less of a feature amongst young people with this condition compared with those who have unprovoked symptoms, they are typically "A" grade individuals, high performing athletes and commonly striving to fulfill parental or peer group expectations. Symptoms crucially peak during exercise or just after stopping, whereas exercise induced bronchospasm typically comes on 3–15 min after exercise. Whilst abnormal spirometry might be indicative of upper airway problems, it is poorly sensitive and should not be used in isolation for diagnosis (38). Typically there is inspiratory flow limitation, but there might also be a plateau in the expiratory flow rate (39). Laryngoscopy, performed during increasing levels of exercise to provoke symptoms, is regarded as the gold standard test, but diagnostic facilities are not widely available and can be difficult to perform in younger age groups (40).

Getting patients to perform voluntary over breathing challenge tests were recommended as a means of reproducing symptoms to support a diagnosis of hyperventilation (41). Initially, this was thought to occur through induced hypocapnia. However, subsequent studies have suggested that, in the majority of patients, alterations in feelings of anxiety and their central effects on neuro-muscular control of breathing are more important determinants of symptoms than respiratory alkalosis and such tests are no longer in common use (42, 43).

Hyperventilation is commonly screened for in asthma clinics using the Nijmegen questionnaire. The questionnaire matches up fairly well with more sophisticated diagnostic testing, such as graded exercise challenge tests (21). The creators of the questionnaire suggest that when used in clinical practice, it should be in conjunction with more objective measures of assessment (44). However, breathing assessments can be difficult as the use of mouthpieces and breathing circuits can directly alter breathing patterns. New technologies, such as structured light plethysmography, might help to better define breathing patterns in the future (45).

In an out-patient setting, there is usually little to find on clinical examination. If symptoms are present, it might be possible to differentiate upper from lower airway obstruction, but this can be difficult. Observing an abnormal breathing pattern might also be usefully informative, but young children in particular commonly breathe in strange ways when their chest is auscultated. Getting the patient or their family to use a mobile phone to capture episodes of abnormal breathing can sometimes be useful (4, 46).

TREATMENT

An essential pre-requisite to treating dysfunctional breathing is to ensure optimal control of underlying asthma. This can be challenging given how similar respiratory symptoms occur in both problems and the need to contain the over use of medication.

Once problems, such as EILO and hyperventilation are identified, a clear explanation and reassurance about the nature of the problem can sometimes be effective in ameliorating symptoms. In the case of EILO, recordings of the larynx at endoscopy or direct visual feedback at the time of the procedure can be highly effective in explaining the cause of symptoms and the use of measures to overcome them (15). The optimal approach to ongoing treatment of (E)ILO is unclear (47). Many interventions have been suggested, but have only been studied in small, uncontrolled trials (48). The prognosis is also far from clear with conflicting case reports although those who have symptoms with no identifiable physical triggers (ILO) appear to do poorly (49). Most reviewers recommend the input of speech therapy services that have developed an interest and expertise in treating this problem and the use of inspiratory muscle training exercises. One retrospective study including adults and children suggested the benefits of inhaled anticholinergic agents in preventing exercise related problems (50). Laser supraglottoplasty has been used in highly selected cases with favorable results (40).

The intervention most commonly used for breathing pattern disorders is breathing retraining exercises. Pediatric studies are limited to reports of case series (51), but a large adult clinical trial in which asthmatics were taught by a trained physiotherapist or used a self-help online programme, reported significant improvements in quality of life scores compared to placebo (52). A smaller randomized controlled trial also reported positive results (53). A number of adult studies evaluating yoga and including yoga breathing techniques have shown small improvements in quality of life in unselected populations of asthmatics (54).

A pediatric service has reported a case series using individualized field testing protocols to characterize exercise related breathing problem in asthmatics and included the use of laryngoscopy to identify EILO as well as breathing pattern disorders thus facilitating individually tailored care plans (55). A pediatric respiratory physiotherapist led clinic designed to specifically address dysfunctional breathing problems has reported significant improvements in quality of life outcomes in support of this approach to treatment (56).

Whilst there is a good scientific rationale for psychological interventions to treat dysfunctional breathing, it is difficult to carry out well-designed studies in this area and there is little supporting evidence for this approach in any age group (57, 58). Suggestion therapy has been shown to be highly effective in young children with habit cough using a bed sheet as a bandage to strap and heal the chest, but a similar device has not been used for dysfunctional breathing in asthma (59).

Evaluating how psychotherapy might impact on dysfunctional breathing is compounded by the many ways in which environmental stressors might result in airway symptoms and associated confounders, such as poor adherence and poor lifestyle choices. These problems typically increase during adolescence and continue into early adult life. Stress increases the individual sensitivity to changes in airway caliber (60). It has also been shown to induce clinically significant bronchoconstriction in up to 40% of asthmatics under experimental conditions and asthmatics have been shown to develop increased indices of airway inflammation as a direct result of stress inducing challenges (61, 62). Research into psychological interventions in adults with asthma is inconclusive (63), but there are suggestions that interventions, such as cognitive behavioral therapy and mindfulness based stress reduction might improve both anxiety scores and asthma control. There is even less evidence for this type of psychological intervention in children and adolescents and high quality clinical studies with clearly defined outcomes are needed in this area (64).

CONCLUSIONS

The diagnosis and treatment of dysfunctional breathing has mostly evolved through observational experience and a growing realization about the importance of this problem in all age groups. Further studies might usefully identify the extent to which the increasing emergence of this clinical problem is impacting on asthma morbidity and in particular during adolescence and early adult life. Recent epidemiological studies have characterized how asthma becomes more prevalent and severe after puberty and particularly in women (65). These changes parallel the emergence of dysfunctional breathing as an increasing problem in asthmatics.

Further studies are needed to help define the optimal approach to treatment in all age groups and to clearly delineate the long-term outcomes for different types of dysfunctional breathing across the lifecourse. Controlled trials have shown that many adults with asthma can benefit from breathing retraining programmes, most probably as a result of correcting breathing pattern disorders. Similar trials are urgently needed to assess the effectiveness of such interventions in children and adolescents.

AUTHOR CONTRIBUTIONS

All authors listed have made a substantial, direct and intellectual contribution to the work, and approved it for publication.

REFERENCES

1. Russo MA, Santarelli DM, O'Rourke D. The physiological effects of slow breathing in the healthy human. *Breathe* (2017) 13:298–309. doi: 10.1183/20734735.009817
2. Dratcu L. Panic, hyperventilation and perpetuation of anxiety. *Prog Neuropsychopharmacol Biol Psychiatry* (2000) 24:1069–89. doi: 10.1016/S0278-5846(00)00130-5
3. Tay TR, Radhakrishna N, Hore-Lacy F, Smith C, Hoy R, Dabscheck E, et al. Comorbidities in difficult asthma are independent risk factors for frequent exacerbations, poor control and diminished quality of life. *Respirology* (2016) 21:1384–90. doi: 10.1111/resp.12838
4. Depiazzi J, Everard ML. Dysfunctional breathing and reaching one's physiological limit as causes of exercise-induced dyspnoea. *Breathe* (2016) 12:120–9. doi: 10.1183/20734735.007216
5. Christensen PM, Heimdal JH, Christopher KL, Bucca C, Cantarella G, Friedrich G, et al. ERS/ELS/ACCP 2013 inter-national consensus conference nomenclature on inducible laryngeal obstructions. *Eur Respir Rev.* (2015) 24:445–50. doi: 10.1183/16000617.0000 6513
6. Kerr WJ, Dalton JW, Gliebe PA. Some physical phenomena associated with anxiety states and their relation to hyperventilation. *Ann Intern Med.* (1937) 11:961–92.
7. Boulding R, Stacey R, Niven R, Fowler SJ. Dysfunctional breathing: a review of the literature and proposal for classification. *Eur Respir Rev.* (2016) 25:287–94. doi: 10.1183/16000617.0088-2015
8. Courtney R, van Dixhoorn J, Greenwood KM, Anthonissen EL. Medically unexplained dyspnea: partly moderated by dysfunctional (thoracic dominant) breathing pattern. *J Asthma* (2011) 48:259–65. doi: 10.3109/02770903.2011.554942
9. Howell JB. The hyperventilation syndrome: a syndrome under threat? *Thorax* (1997) 52(Suppl. 3):S30–4.
10. Saisch SGN, Wessely S, Gardner WN. Patients with acute hyperventilation presenting to an inner-city emergency department. *Chest* (1996) 110:952–7.
11. McFadden ER, Lyons HA. Arterial-blood gas tension in asthma. *N Engl J Med.* (1968) 278:1027–32. doi: 10.1056/NEJM196805092781901
12. Ritz T, Kullowatz A, Goldman MD, Smith HJ, Kanniess F, Dahme B, et al. Airway response to emotional stimuli in asthma: the role of the cholinergic pathway. *J Appl Physiol. (1985)* (2010) 108:1542–9. doi: 10.1152/japplphysiol.00818.2009
13. Osborne CA, O'Connor BJ, Lewis A, Kanabar V, Gardner WN. Hyperventilation and asymptomatic chronic asthma. *Thorax* (2000) 55:1016–22. doi: 10.1136/thorax.55.12.1016
14. Bardin PG, Low K, Ruane L, Kenneth KL. Controversies and conundrums in vocal cord dysfunction. *Landet Resp Med.* (2017) 5:546–8. doi: 10.1016/S2213-2600(17)30221-7
15. Røksund OD, Heimdal J-H, Clemm H, Vollsæter M, Halvorsen T. Exercise inducible laryngeal obstruction: diagnostics and management. *Paed Resp Rev.* (2017) 21:86–94. doi: 10.1016/j.prrv.2016.07.003
16. Hull JH, Backer V, Gibson PG, Fowler SJ. Laryngeal dysfunction: assessment and management for the clinician. *Am J Respir Crit Care Med.* (2016) 194:1062–72. doi: 10.1164/rccm.201606-1249CI

17. Thomas M, McKinley RK, Freeman E, Foy C. Prevalence of dysfunctional breathing in patients treated for asthma in primary care: cross sectional survey. *BMJ* (2001) 322:1098–100. doi: 10.1136/bmj.322.7294.1098
18. Thomas M, McKinley RK, Freeman E, Foy C, Price D. The prevalence of dysfunctional breathing in adults in the community with and without asthma. *Prim Care Respir J.* (2005) 14:78–82. doi: 10.1016/j.pcrj.2004.10.007
19. Grammatopoulou EP, Skordilis EK, Georgoudis G, Haniotou A, Evangelodimou A, Fildissis G, et al. Hyperventilation in asthma: a validation study of the Nijmegen Questionnaire - NQ. *J Asthma* (2014) 51:839–46. doi: 10.3109/02770903.2014.922190
20. Stanton AE, Vaughn P, Carter R, Bucknall C. An observational investigation of dysfunctional breathing and breathing control therapy in a problem asthma clinic. *J Asthma* (2008) 45:758–65. doi: 10.1080/02770900802252093
21. Agache I, Ciobanu C, Paul G, Rogozea L. Dysfunctional breathing phenotype in adults with asthma–incidence and risk factors. *Clin Transl Allergy* (2012) 2:18. doi: 10.1186/2045-7022-2-18
22. Hagman C, Janson C, Emtner M. A comparison between patients with dysfunctional breathing and patients with asthma. *Clin Respir J.* (2008) 2:86–91. doi: 10.1111/j.1752-699X.2007.00036.x
23. Martínez-Moragón E, Perpiñá M, Belloch A, de Diego A. Prevalence of hyperventilation syndrome in patients treated for asthma in a pulmonology clinic. *Arch Bronconeumol.* (2005) 41:267–71.
24. Doorn PV, Folgering HTM, Colla P. Control of the end-tidal PCO_2 in the hyperventilation syndrome: effects of biofeedback and breathing instructions compared. *Bull Eur Physiopathol Respir.* (1982) 18:829–36.
25. D'Alba I, Carloni I, Ferrante AL, Gesuita R, Palazzi ML, de Benedictis FM. Hyperventilation syndrome in adolescents with and without asthma. *Pediatr Pulmonol.* (2015) 50:1184–90. doi: 10.1002/ppul.23145
26. de Groot EP, Duiverman EJ, Brand PL. Dysfunctional breathing in children with asthma: a rare, but relevant comorbidity. *Eur Respir J.* (2013) 41:1068–73. doi: 10.1183/09031936.00130212
27. Li Ogilvie V, Kersten P. A critical review of the psychometric properties of the Nijmegen questionnaire for hyperventilation syndrome. *N Z J Physiother.* (2015) 43:3–10. doi: 10.15619/NZJP/43.1.01
28. Han JN, Stegen K, Schepers R, Van den Bergh O, Van de Woestijne KP. Subjective symptoms and breathing pattern at rest and following hyperventilation in anxiety and somatoform disorders. *J Psychosom Res.* (1998) 45:519–32.
29. Seear M, Wensley D, West N. How accurate is the diagnosis of exercise induced asthma among Vancouver schoolchildren? *Arch Dis Child.* (2005) 90:898–902. doi: 10.1136/adc.2004.063974
30. Johansson H, Norlander K, Berglund L, Janson C, Malinovschi A, Nordvall L, et al. Prevalence of exercise-induced bronchoconstriction and exercise-induced laryngeal obstruction in a general adolescent population. *Thorax* (2015) 70:57–63. doi: 10.1136/thoraxjnl-2014-205738
31. Christensen PM, Thomsen SF, Rasmussen N, Backer V. Exercise-induced laryngeal obstructions: prevalence and symptoms in the general public. *Head Neck Surg.* (2011) 268:1313–9. doi: 10.1007/s00405-011-1612-0
32. Newman KB, Mason UG, Schmaling KB. Clinical features of vocal cord dysfunction. *Am J Respir Crit Care Med.* (1995) 152(4 Pt 1):1382–6.
33. Yelken K, Yilmaz A, Guven M, Eyibilen A, Aladag I. Paradoxical vocal fold motion dysfunction in asthma patients. *Respirology* (2009) 14:729–33. doi: 10.1111/j.1440-1843.2009.01568.x
34. Low K, Lau KK, Holmes P, Crossett M, Vallance N, Phyland D, et al. Abnormal vocal cord function in difficult-to-treat asthma. *Am J Respir Crit Care Med.* (2011) 184:50–6. doi: 10.1164/rccm.201010-1604OC
35. Tomar RPS, Vasudevan R. Metabolic acidosis due to inhaled salbutamol toxicity: a hazardous side effect complicating management of suspected cases of acute severe asthma. *Med J Armed Forces India* (2012) 68:242–4. doi: 10.1016/j.mjafi.2011.10.002
36. Traister RS, Fajt ML, Landsittel D, Petrov AA. A novel scoring system to distinguish vocal cord dysfunction from asthma. *J Allergy Clin Immunol Pract.* (2014) 2:65–9. doi: 10.1016/j.jaip.2013.09.002
37. Pinto L, Aun M, Cukier-Blaj S, Stelmach R, Cukier A, Kalil J, et al. Vocal cord dysfunction diagnosis may be improved by a screening check list. *Allergol Int.* (2016) 65:180–5. doi: 10.1016/j.alit.2015.11.001
38. Christensen PM, Maltbæk N, Jørgensen IM, Nielsen KG. Can flow-volume loops be used to diagnose exercise-induced laryngeal obstructions? A comparison study examining the accuracy and inter-rater agreement of flow-volume loops as a diagnostic tool. *Prim Care Respir J.* (2013) 22:306–11. doi: 10.4104/pcrj.2013.00067
39. Santiago S, Lopez NA, Almería GE, Villa Asensi JR. Spirometry patterns in vocal cord dysfunction. *An Pediatr (Barc).* (2013) 78:173–7. doi: 10.1016/j.anpedi.2012.07.001
40. Liyanagedara S, McLeod R, Elhassan HA. Exercise induced laryngeal obstruction: a review of diagnosis and management. *Eur Arch Oto-Rhino-Laryngol.* (2017) 274:1781–9. doi: 10.1007/s00405-016-4338-1
41. Lewis RA, Howell JB. Definition of the hyperventilation syndrome. *Bull Eur Physiopathol Respir.* (1986) 22:201–5.
42. Hornsveld HK, Garssen B, Dop MJ, van Spiegel PI, de Haes JC. Double-blind placebo-controlled study of the hyperventilation provocation test and the validity of the hyperventilation syndrome. *Lancet* (1996) 348:154–8.
43. Christensen PM, Rasmussen N. Eucapnic voluntary hyperventilation in diagnosing exercise-induced laryngeal obstructions. *Head Neck Surg.* (2013) 270:3107–13. doi: 10.1007/s00405-013-2571-4
44. Van Dixhoorn J, Folgering H. The Nijmegen questionnaire and dysfunctional breathing. *ERJ Open Res.* (2015) 1:00001-2015. doi: 10.1183/23120541.00001-2015
45. Barker N, Smith L, De Boer W, Everard M. Structured light plethysmography as an assessment tool for dysfunctional breathing in children. *Eur Respir J.* (2014) 44:P4318.
46. de Groot EP. Breathing abnormalities in children with breathlessness. *Paediatr Respir Rev.* (2011) 12:83–7. doi: 10.1016/j.prrv.2010.09.003
47. Weinberger M. Dysfunctional breathing in children and adolescents. *Acta Paediatr.* (2017) 106:1898–9. doi: 10.1111/apa.14006
48. Ibrahim WH, Gheriani HA, Almohamed AA, Raza T. Paradoxical vocal cord motion disorder: past, present and future. *Postgrad Med J.* (2007) 83:164–72. doi: 10.1136/pgmj.2006.052522
49. Hayes JP, Nolan MT, Brennan N, FitzGerald MX. Three cases of paradoxical vocal cord adduction followed up over a 10-year period. *Chest* (1993) 104:678–80.
50. Doshi DR, Weinberger M. Long-term outcome of vocal cord dysfunction. *Ann Allergy Asthma Immunol.* (2006) 96:794–9. doi: 10.1016/S1081-1206(10)61341-5
51. Barker NJ, Jones M, O'Connell NE, Everard ML. Breathing exercises for dysfunctional breathing/hyperventilation syndrome in children. *Cochrane Database Syst Rev.* (2013) CD010376. doi: 10.1002/14651858.CD010376.pub2
52. Bruton A, Lee A, Yardley L, Raftery J, Arden-Close E, Kirby S, et al. Physiotherapy breathing retraining for asthma: a randomised controlled trial. *Lancet Respir Med.* (2018) 6:19–28. doi: 10.1016/S2213-2600(17)30474-5
53. Holloway E, West RJ. Integrated breathing and relaxation training (Papworth Method) for adults with asthma in primary care: a randomised controlled trial. *Thorax* (2007) 62:1039–42. doi: 10.1136/thx.2006.076430
54. Yang ZY, Zhong HB, Mao C, Yuan JQ, Huang YF, Wu XY, et al. Yoga for asthma. *Cochrane Database Syst Rev.* (2016) CD010346. doi: 10.1002/14651858.CD010346.pub2
55. Connett G, Keenan V, Payne S, Evans H. Individualised field testing is a useful tool to evaluate difficult asthma. *Eur Respir J.* (2017) 50:PA4495. doi: 10.1183/1393003.congress-2017.PA4495
56. Barker NJ, Elphick H, Everard ML. The impact of a dedicated physiotherapist clinic for children with dysfunctional breathing. *ERJ Open Res.* (2016) 2:00103-2015. doi: 10.1183/23120541.00103-2015
57. Smith HE, Jones CJ. Psychological interventions in asthma. *Curr Treat Options Allergy* (2015) 2:155. doi: 10.1007/s40521-015-0051-3
58. Yorke J, Fleming SL, Shuldham C. Psychological interventions for children with asthma. *Cochrane Database Syst Rev.* (2005) CD003272. doi: 10.1002/14651858.CD003272.pub2
59. Cohlan SQ, Stone SM. The cough and the bedsheet. *Pediatrics* (1984) 74:11–5.
60. Ritz T. Airway responsiveness to psychological processes in asthma and health. *Front Physiol.* (2012) 3:343. doi: 10.3389/fphys.2012.00343
61. Douwes J, Brooks C, Pearce N. Asthma nervosa: old concept, new insights. *Eur Respir J.* (2011) 37:986–90. doi: 10.1183/09031936.00018511
62. Rosenkranz M, Esnault S, Christian BT, Crisafi G, Gresham LK, Higgins AT, et al. Mind-body interactions in the regulation of airway inflammation in

asthma: a PET study of acute and chronic stress. *Brain Behav Immun.* (2016) 58:18–30. doi: 10.1016/j.bbi.2016.03.024

63. Yorke J, Fleming SL, Shuldham C. Psychological interventions for adults with asthma. *Cochrane Database Syst Rev.* (2006) CD002982. doi: 10.1002/14651858.CD002982.pub3
64. Kew KM, Nashed M, Dulay V, Yorke J. Cognitive behavioural therapy (CBT) for adults and adolescents with asthma. *Cochrane Database Syst Rev.* (2016) CD011818. doi: 10.1002/14651858.CD011818.pub2
65. Zein JG, Erzurum SC. Asthma is different in women. *Curr Allergy Asthma Rep.* (2015) 15:28. doi: 10.1007/s11882-015-0528-y

13

Treating Pediatric Asthma According Guidelines

Riccardina Tesse, Giorgia Borrelli, Giuseppina Mongelli, Violetta Mastrorilli and Fabio Cardinale*

Allergy, Immunology and Pediatric Pulmonology Unit, Ospedale Pediatrico Papa Giovanni XXIII, Bari, Italy

***Correspondence:**
Riccardina Tesse
nucciatesse@googlemail.com

Asthma is a common chronic inflammatory disorder of the lower respiratory airways in childhood. The management of asthma exacerbations and the disease control are major concerns for clinical practice. The Global Strategy for Asthma Management and Prevention, published by GINA, updated in 2017, the British Thoracic Society/Scottish Intercollegiate Guideline Network, revised in 2016, the National Institute for Health and Care Excellence asthma guideline consultation, available in 2017, are widely accepted documents, frequently implemented, with conflicting advices, and different conclusion on asthma definition and treatment. An International Consensus on Pediatric Asthma was carried out in 2012 by a Committee with expertise in the field, to critically review differences on current guidelines. In addition, the specific issue of treating severe and difficult asthma has been recently highlighted throughout the International European Respiratory Society/American Thoracic Society guidelines on severe asthma. The aim of this paper is to describe conventional treatments and some new therapeutic approaches to pediatric asthma according to guidelines, highlighting key aspects, and differences on proposed clinical recommendations for asthma management. Age specific therapy are proposed in steps, according to clinical severity and the level of disease control. If control is not achieved within 3 months, stepping-up should be considered; otherwise, if control is achieved after 3 months, stepping down may be considered. The most used drug classes of asthma medications are beta-2 adrenergic agonists, corticosteroids, and leukotriene modifiers. Intramuscolar triamcinolone has been used for severe asthma treatment. Chromones and xanthines have been extensively used in the past, but they have shown limits related to their efficacy and safety profile. Omalizumab, a monoclonal antibody against IgE, is an immunomodulatory biological agent, used as new drug in patients with confirmed IgE-mediated allergic asthma, only for patient's specific range of total IgE level. There are low evidences in the efficacy of metotrexate, as well as macrolide antibiotics in children with asthma. Antifungal agents are also not recommended in asthmatic patients. Non-pharmacological measures that may improve patient's quality of life should also be attempted. We conclude that treatment decisions on childhood asthma management should be critically made, pondering the differences suggested by agreed international consensus documents.

Keywords: asthma, pharmacology, guidelines, asthma management, children

INTRODUCTION

Asthma is a heterogeneous chronic airway disease very common in childhood, usually characterized by respiratory symptoms including wheeze, breathlessness, chest tightness and cough, together with variable expiratory airflow obstruction (1, 2). There is widespread concern about symptom control in asthmatic patients, as well as risk of adverse outcomes into clinical practice. It is therefore not surprising that several guidelines are available to support health care professionals on asthma management of children and adults.

The Global Strategy for Asthma Management and Prevention (GINA) and the British Thoracic Society (BTS)/Scottish Intercollegiate Guideline Network (SIGN) are widely accepted documents, released in the USA and in Europe, respectively. Since 2002 the GINA Science Committee was established to review published research on asthma. Expert leaders in adult and pediatric asthma research, regularly meet with the American Thoracic Society (ATS) and European Respiratory Society (ERS) international conferences, to critically review asthma-related scientific literature. The major revision of GINA has been updated in 2017, suggesting recent conclusions on asthma definition and treatment (3).

The first BTS guideline dated back to 1990 and the SIGN guidelines to 1996, but in 1999 the two Society jointly produced new asthma guideline, updated annually, until 2016, and made available on websites (4).

Both guidelines are frequently implemented, providing recent updates recommendations for asthma management and prevention, with conflicting advices and different conclusion on asthma definition and treatment (5, 6). In 2015 the United Kingdom (UK) National Institute for Health and Care Excellence (NICE) also released a consultation document for diagnosis and monitoring of asthma, and later, on December 2016, for the management of chronic asthma, including cost benefit analysis that were not considered in the BTS/SIGN guidance (7).

An International Consensus on Pediatric Asthma was carried out in 2012 by a working Committee with expertise in the field (8), to critically review differences on the current abovementioned International guidelines, but also including other reports like the Australian Asthma Management document and the Japanese Guideline for Childhood Asthma (9, 10).

Non pharmacological measures that may improve quality of life and reduce symptoms in asthmatic people should be attempted, particularly in children. They include avoidance of exposure to environmental tobacco smoke or cessation of smoking among adolescents, avoidance of food or drug triggers, in people sensitive to them, avoidance of indoor and/or outdoor pollution and irritants (11, 12). Weight loss in overweight patients should be advised; breathing exercise programmes, following physiotherapist methods should also be encouraged.

However, pharmacotherapy represents the fundament of asthma treatment in adults and children. The international reports define the principles of pharmacological asthma management and indicate age specific treatments in steps, according to clinical severity and the level of disease control, which is determined by the interaction between the patient's genetic background, the ongoing treatment, environment, and psychosocial factors. Asthma severity is assessed retrospectively from the level of treatment required to control symptoms and exacerbations, that may change over months.

Asthma phenotypes have been defined based on specific pathologic features, demographic and clinical patterns or therapy responses and personalized phenotype-guided asthma treatments are under investigation, with the acknowledgment of the patient's adherence to therapy issues (13).

This review gives a practical perspective on the most used drugs and the basic steps of asthma management in children and adolescents, based on current international guidelines recommendations, highlighting the key aspects and differences of these documents.

CATEGORIES OF ASTHMA MEDICATIONS AND STEP-WISE STRATEGIES OF TREATMENT

The pharmacological options for treatment of asthma include, according to their use, reliever medications, which are drugs that allow relief of symptoms within few minutes, during worsening asthma or exacerbations, also used for prevention of exercise-induced bronchoconstriction; controller medications, that are used for maintenance treatment: they control symptoms and reduce airway inflammation and future risks of exacerbations; add-on therapies, proposed for patients with severe persistent asthma symptoms and exacerbations, despite treatment with high dose controller medications.

The most used drug classes of asthma medications are beta-2 adrenergic agonists, corticosteroids, and leukotriene modifiers, usually montelukast.

A stepwise approach for pharmacotherapy management in asthmatic patients has been proposed (**Table 1**). Treatment starts at the step most appropriate to the initial severity of asthma. If control is not achieved within 3 months, stepping-up should be tried, after reconsidering adherence to therapy, environment factors, and associated co-morbidities; otherwise, treatment step down may be attempted once good asthma control and the patient's lowest effective level of treatment has been found and maintained for about 3 months. Each recommendation has been assessed for adults adolescents (over 12 years) and children (5–12 years, and under 5 years) in all guidelines (3, 4).

Medications Used for Rapid Relief of Symptoms

At present, **Step 1** treatment is with as-needed inhaled short-acting beta2-agonists (SABAs) alone, commonly salbutamol. SABAs are used for acute relief of asthma symptoms, mainly in patients with occasional daytime symptoms and with normal lung function. Inhaled anticholinergic agents, usually ipratropium, are second-line relievers (14); they are less effective than SABA, but may have synergistic effects when added to SABA during severe exacerbations in reducing patients hospitalization (3, 4).

TABLE 1 | Stepwise pharmacotherapy management in asthmatic children.

	STEP 1	STEP 2	STEP 3	STEP 4	STEP 5
Reliever therapy	As-needed SABA		As-needed SABA or low dose ICS/ LABA		
Controller therapy		Low dose ICS	Low /medium ICS/LABA	Medium/high ICS/LABA	Add-on treatment (omalizumab)
Other common controller options	Low dose ICS	LTRA	Medium/high dose ICS Low ICS + LTRA	High dose ICS + LTRA	Low dose OCS

SABA, short-acting beta$_2$-agonist; ICS, inhaled corticosteroids; LABA, long-acting beta$_2$-agonist; LTRA, leukotriene receptor antagonists; OCS, oral corticosteroids.

In adults, oral SABA or short-acting theophylline are potential alternatives to SABA, however, they have a slower onset of action than inhaled SABA and a higher risk of side-effects, and they are not recommended in children (15).

Medications Used for Long-Term Asthma Symptoms Control

Inhaled Corticosteroids (ICS)

More frequent symptoms or the presence of any exacerbation risk factors indicate that regular controller treatment is needed. For long term asthma control in children, a maintenance treatment with therapeutic doses of ICS in addition to as-needed SABA, should be considered. Regular low dose ICS improve asthma symptoms and lung function, decrease need for additional medication and hospital admission. In the international reports this combination of drugs is the first option of treatment included into **Step 2** (3, 4). ICS differ in potency and bioavailability; beclomethasone dipropionate (BDP) and budesonide have approximately equivalent effects in clinical practice, although there may be some variations using different delivery devices. Fluticasone propionate and mometasone appear to provide the same clinical activity, compared to BDP and budesonide, at half the dosage. The initial dose of ICS should be appropriate to the severity of disease (**Table 2**). In children and adolescent, the starting ICS dose will usually be less or equal 200 micrograms BDP or equivalent per day, given initially twice daily (except ciclesonide proposed once daily). More than 200–400 μg BDP or equivalent would be considered a pediatric moderate dose, and more than 400 μg a pediatric high dose. The dose of ICS should then be titrate the to the lowest effective dose at which control of asthma is maintained. There is an increasing evidence showing that, at recommended doses, ICS are also safe and effective in young children with asthma (16).

However, long term follow-up studies have demonstrated some effect of the chronic ICS use at intermediate-high doses with growth retardation in pre-pubertal children in the first years of treatment, and the reduction in adult final height (17–19). Poorly-controlled asthma itself may affect patient's growth (20). Therefore, after symptoms control has been achieved, ICS therapy should be gradually tapered to the lowest effective dose.

Clinical adrenal suppression has also been described in a small number of children who had been treated with ICS (21). The duration of ICS treatment that may expose a child at risk of clinical adrenal insufficiency is unknown but is likely to occur at high ICS dose per day (at ≥800 μg BDP per day or equivalent). Tests of adrenal function such as the low-dose adrenocorticotrophic hormone (ACTH) test, may be useful in predicting clinically relevant adrenal insufficiency in a child using high-dose ICS, but it is unknown how frequently would need to be repeated in children.

TABLE 2 | Low, medium, and high inhaled corticosteroids doses in asthmatic children and adolescents.

Inhaled corticosteroid	Total daily dose (mcg)		
	Low	Medium	High
SCHOOL AGED CHILDREN			
Beclometasone dipropionate	100–200	200–400	>400
Budesonide	100–200	200–400	>400
Ciclesonide	80	80–160	>160
Fluticasone propionate	100–200	200–400	>400
Mometasone furoate	110	220–440	>440
Triamcinolone acetonide	400–800	800–1,200	>1,200
ADOLESCENTS			
Beclometasone dipropionate	200–500	500–1,000	>1,000
Budesonide	400–200	400–800	>800
Ciclesonide	80–160	160–320	>320
Fluticasone propionate	100–250	250–500	>500
Mometasone furoate	110–220	220–440	>440
Triamcinolone acetonide	400–1,000	1,000–2,000	>2,000

Moreover, the use of extra-fine (diameter <2 μm) vs. fine particle BDP administered as mono-therapy or in combination with LABA, have shown reduction in exacerbation rates in severe asthmatic patients, in a meta-analysis of observational studies (22). Corticosteroid insensitivity is also another specific issue under investigation: molecular mechanisms including glucocorticoid receptor alteration, have been proposed (23).

For patients with persistent symptoms or recurrent exacerbations despite the use of low dose ICS, may be considered a step up, after checking for medication adherence, inhaler technique, continuous allergen exposure and comorbidities such as rhinosinusitis, gastroesophageal reflux, obesity, and obstructive sleep apnea.

Long-Acting Beta-2 Adrenergic Agonists (LABA)

In adolescents likewise in adults, the combination of ICS and LABA, including salmeterol and formeterol, improves asthma outcomes more than higher doses of ICS, and it should be considered before increasing the dose of 400 μg BDP or equivalent per day and certainly before administering 800 μg of

BDP. A LABA should not be used as monotherapy for asthma but only in fixed-dose combination devices also containing an ICS. Recent studies have shown that the risk of adverse events related to the use of LABA when combined with steroids is similar to the risk of using corticosteroids alone in asthmatic patients (24, 25). However, it is more expensive and does not reduce the risk of further exacerbations compared with ICS alone. In addition to studies reassuring about the use of LABA in adolescent and adults (25), an international trial that followed for 26 weeks 6,208 children, aged 4–11 years, with asthma and an exacerbation in the previous year, has also shown that addition of salmeterol to fixed fluticasone doses is effective and does not lead to increased risk of serious asthma-related adverse outcomes than using the ICS alone (26).

Leukotriene Receptor Antagonists (LTRAs)

LTRAs work by blocking some inflammatory responses, such as tightening of airway muscles and the production of mucus secretion, mediated by leukotriens, which are released during asthmatic reaction by cells involved in the pathogenesis of asthma. In international guidelines LTRA are recommended in monotherapy, as second choice after low dose ICS, for the initial step of chronic asthma treatment. Into the next steps, they are also considered as add-on medications, usually in addition to ICS for improving symptoms and pulmonary function, by an increase in antinflammatory activity (27). They may be considered especially for some patients who experienced side-effects using ICS or children under 5 years old (28), and they are effective especially in exercise-induced asthma (29, 30). A review by Bisgaard et al. on more than 2,700 children and adolescents enrolled in several studies, suggested that the safety profile for montelukast was similar to that of placebo or other usual care therapy, and did not change with long-term use (31).

The options of treatment at **Step 3** differ depending on age group. In young children, a medium dose of ICS plus as-needed SABA is the preferred solution, whereas in adolescents, as well as in adults, the combination of low dose ICS/LABA (BDP/formoterol or budesonide/formoterol) as maintenance treatment with as-needed SABA as reliever, or low dose ICS/LABA (BDP/formoterol) as both maintenance and reliever treatment may be considered. Adding LABA to the same low dose of ICS seem to improve, in this age group, symptoms and lung function and reduce risk of exacerbations, compared with a fixed dose of ICS/LABA as maintenance treatment or a higher dose of ICS, both with as-needed SABA. Another option for adults and adolescents if asthma control remains suboptimal, is to increase ICS to medium dose, but this is less effective than adding a LABA. Other less efficacious options are low dose ICS plus either LTRA or low dose, sustained-release theophylline (3).

For adolescent patients as well as adults, low dose maintenance and reliever ICS/LABA with as-needed SABA, is suggested for **Step 4;** if necessary, in patients with not complete symptoms control, may be considered the use of medium dose ICS. For children <12 years, if asthma control is not achieved using moderate dose ICS, the recommendation is to refer the child for expert assessment. A high dose is recommended only when good asthma control cannot be achieved with medium dose ICS plus LABA and/or a third controller, such as LTRA. However, the increase in ICS dose generally provides little additional benefit, and there is an increased risk of side-effects.

The NICE publication include some conflicting advices on key issues of asthma management in primary care. One controversial difference is about the use of LTRA as first choice add-on therapy for patients whose asthma is not well controlled with low dose ICS. LABA are considered marginally more effective than LTRA, in the analysis by NICE, to justify the additional cost (7). The Primary Care Respiratory Society UK has suggested an initial trial of LTRA as add-on treatment to low dose ICS, but underlie that it should not be changed the treatment of patients already favorably established on a LABA regimen (5).

When patients experience persistent symptoms or exacerbations despite high-dose ICS or ICS/LABA, or other options of Step 4 treatment, there are different pharmacological options that may be considered at **Step 5**, as following listed.

Oral Corticosteroids

Add-on low dose oral corticosteroids ($\leq$7.5 mg/day prednisone equivalent) may be considered, but may be associated with potential side effects especially in long-term treatments. Prednisolone is the most used steroid for maintenance therapy in patients with chronic asthma (32). Blood pressure, urine or blood sugar, cholesterol, bone mineral density, growth (height and weight centile), should be regularly monitored, and cataracts should be screened in patients using steroid tablets.

Omalizumab

Anti-immunoglobulin E (anti-IgE) treatment for patients >12 years of age, with severe allergic asthma, impaired lung function, and proven IgE-mediated sensitivity to inhaled allergens, is also a treatment option. Omalizumab is a humanized monoclonal antibody that interferes with the inflammatory cascade by reducing serum IgE levels and inhibiting IgE binding to receptors. It is given as a subcutaneous injection every 2 or 4 week depending on patient weight and total serum IgE levels. It exhibit a suitable clinical outcome reducing exacerbations, and improving asthma control (33). School-age children and adolescent with moderate-to-severe asthma treated with omalizumab in long-term trials had a significantly reduced number of exacerbation attacks, improved the quality of their life and reduced the need for other standard medications to control asthma (34, 35). Omalizumab is safe and well tolerated but it has the inconvenience of the subcutaneous administration and elevated costs.

Immunotherapy

Studies using both subcutaneous and sublingual allergen immunotherapy (SCIT and SLIT) have demonstrated benefit in reducing asthma symptoms and bronchial hyperreactivity in children who do not completely respond to other preventative strategies including ICS (36). The safety profile of SLIT seems to be better than SCIT. There are, however, few studies of adding immunotherapy to ICS so there is difficulty precisely defining where it should sit in step-wise asthma management.

Mepolizumab

The use of specific anti-IL5 monoclonal antibodies treatment (mepolizumab), based on eosinophilia (>3%) in induced sputum as biomarkers to identify responsive patients is a debated topic. Some trials indicate that anti-eosinophil biologic drug can be effective for treatment of the severe systemic corticosteroid-dependent asthma, with a "eosinophilic" endotype, whose disease is largely dependent on eosinophil pathophisiology, by a beneficial effect on airway remodeling (37).

OTHER PHARMACOLOGICAL OPTIONS

Theophylline and Chromones

Other drug solutions not recommended for routine use are theophylline, the most used methylxanthine, which has low efficacy in asthma bronchoconstriction and common side-effects, especially when administered at higher doses (38), and chromones (nedocromil sodium and sodium cromoglycate) used as mast cell stabilizer, having a suitable safety profile, but low efficacy (39). They are included in guidelines as second-line medications in initial treatment steps and prevention of exercise-induced asthma.

Intramuscolar Triamcinolone

Intramuscolar treatment with triamcinolone has been used for severe asthma treatment. Pediatric studies suggest that it may affect eosinophilic inflammation, improve airway obstruction and prevent exacerbation attacks in children with severe asthma (40, 41), but side effects using it are worse than after treatment with oral corticosteroids (42, 43).

Anticholinergic Agents

The addition of tiotropium bromide, a long-acting inhaled anticholinergic agent, to ICS plus LABA has been shown to improve lung function and asthma symptom control in patients with severe persistent asthma in adults (44). There have been no studies of the use of tiotropium in asthmatic children.

Metotrexate, Antifungal Agents, Macrolides

There are low evidences in the efficacy of metotrexate in children with asthma. A meta-analysis investigating the steroid-sparing effect of oral metotrexate in asthmatics showed a small benefit despite a high recurrence of adverse effect (45).

Antifungal agents are not recommended in asthmatic patients without allergic broncopulmonary aspergillosis (46). Vicencio and coworkers recently documented that a high percentage of children with refractory asthma had fungal sensitization correlated to the severity of their disease. Based to a case report of a positive response to itraconazole treatment of a child with severe asthma, the Authors suggest that antifungal therapy may represent a potential successful treatment in some patients with evidence of fungal sensitization, after eliminating molds in the environment (47, 48).

Macrolides have been also proposed in combination to the treatment regimen of asthmatic children, with the aim of decreasing the need of the patient's daily dosage of corticosteroids, due to its antinflammatory and antimicrobial activity (49). A recent study including 40 school-aged asthmatic children showed that a 3-week course of clarythromicyn given as add-on therapy to regular treatment, was associated with an increased control of symptoms and a decrease in the duration of the asthma exacerbations (50). Since the use of this antibiotic is safe compared to other medications, it may be indicated in severe asthmatic patients who have mainly neutrophilic airway inflammation and show resistance to other therapy. However, in long term treatment the development of macrolide resistance among respiratory pathogens should be considered.

ASTHMA SEVERITY ASSESSMENT

Asthma severity can be assessed when the patient is in a regular control of symptoms with continuous treatment:

- Mild asthma is asthma that is well controlled with Step 1 or Step 2 treatment, i.e., with as-needed reliever medication alone, or with low-dosage controller treatment such as low dose ICS, LTRA, or chromones.
- Moderate asthma is asthma that is well controlled with Step 3 treatment e.g., low dose ICS/LABA.
- Severe asthma is asthma that requires Step 4 or 5 treatment, e.g., high-dose ICS/LABA, to prevent it from becoming "uncontrolled," or asthma that remains "uncontrolled" despite this treatment. The ERS/ATS Task Force on Severe Asthma has published International guidelines providing definition and guidance about the management of patients with uncontrolled asthma (51).

CONCLUSIONS

We conclude that due to heterogeneity of asthma characteristics, treatment decisions should be critically made, pondering the differences highlighted by agreed international consensus documents.

Symptoms control of asthmatic patients should be closely monitored, as well as risk factors and frequency of exacerbations, and the response to any treatment adjustment should be documented and regularly reviewed by specialists. A step up in treatment may be considered if patients do not respond suitably to initial treatment, after checking for comorbidities, or alternative therapy options may be attempted. A follow-up visit within 1 week after an exacerbation attack should be scheduled, and a written asthma action plan should be completed by the patient as part of a personal asthma management education. An occasional short-term step up for weeks in maintenance pharmacological doses may be necessary, for example, during viral infections or seasonal allergen exposure. Sometimes a daily dose adjustment of the maintenance therapy dosage may be needed according to symptoms. Ongoing monitoring adherence to asthma therapy and asthma control by spirometry in children who can perform it, and self-monitoring at home by peak expiratory flow evaluation, together with avoidance of triggers, is also encouraged.

AUTHOR CONTRIBUTIONS

RT designed the review and drafted the manuscript. GB, GM, and VM contributed to data collection and interpretation of the literature data. FC revised the work and provided critical input to the manuscript. All Authors approved the final version of the manuscript as submitted.

REFERENCES

1. Hargreave FE, Nair P. The definition and diagnosis of asthma. *Clin Exp Allergy* (2009) 39:1652–8. doi: 10.1111/j.1365-2222.2009.03321.x
2. Bush A, Fleming L. Diagnosis and management of asthma in children. *BMJ* (2015) 350:h996. doi: 10.1136/bmj.h996
3. Global Initiative for Asthma. *GINA Report: Global Strategy for Asthma Management and Prevention* (2017). Available online at: https://ginasthma.org/gina-reports/
4. British Thoracic Society/Scottish Intercollegiate *Guideline Network, British Guideline on the Management of Asthma* (2016). Available online at: https//www.brit-thoracic.org.uk/document-library/clinical-information/asthma/btssign-asthma-guideline-2016/
5. Primary Care Respiratory Society UK. *Asthma Guidelines Briefing Document* (2017). Available online at: https://pcrs-uk.org/briefing-asthma-guidelines
6. Keeley D, Baxter N. Conflicting asthma guidelines cause confusion in primary care. *BMJ* (2018) 360:k29. doi: 10.1136/bmj.k29
7. National Institute for Health and Care Excellence. *Asthma: Diagnosis, Monitoring and Chronic Asthma Management* (2017) Available online at: https://www.nice.org.uk/guidance/ng80
8. Papadopoulos NG, Arakawa H, Carlsen KH, Custovic A, Gern J, Lemanske R, et al. International consensus on (ICON) pediatric asthma. *Allergy* (2012) 67:976–97. doi: 10.1111/j.1398-9995.2012.02865.x
9. Asthma Management Handbook. *National Asthma Council Australia*. Melbourne, VIC (2006). Available online at: http://www.nationalasthma.org.au/handbook (accessed March 2011).
10. Hamasaki Y, Kohno Y, Ebisawa M, Kondo N, Nishima S, Nishimuta T, et al. Japanese guideline for childhood asthma. *Allergol Int.* (2014) 63:335–56. doi: 10.2332/allergolint.14-RAI-0767
11. Janssens T, Ritz T. Perceived triggers of asthma:key to symptom perception and management. *Clin Exp Allergy* (2013) 43:1000–8. doi: 10.1111/cea.12138
12. Vernon MK, Wiklund I, Bell JA, Dale P, Chapman KR. What do we know about asthma triggers? A review of the literature. *J Asthma* (2012) 49:991–8. doi: 10.3109/02770903.2012.738268
13. Reddy MB, Covar RA. Asthma phenotypes in childhood. *Curr Opin Allergy Clin Immunol.* (2016) 16:127–34. doi: 10.1097/ACI.0000000000000252
14. Rodrigo GJ, Castro-Rodriguez JA. Anticholinergics in the treatment o children and adults with acute asthma: a systematic review with meta-analysis. *Thorax* (2005) 60:740–6. doi: 10.1136/thx.2005.047803
15. Weinberger M, Hendeles L. Theophylline in asthma. *N Engl J Med.* (1996) 334:1380–8. doi: 10.1056/NEJM199605233342107
16. Pedersen S, O'Byrne P. A comparison of the efficacy and safety of inhaled corticosteroids in asthma. *Allergy* (1997) 52:1–34.
17. Guilbert TW, Mauger DT, Allen DB, Zeiger RS, Lemanske RF Jr, Szefer SJ, et al. Growth of preschool children at high risk for asthma 2 years after discontinuation of Futicasone. *J Allergy Clin Immunol.* (2011) 128:956–63.e1-7. doi: 10.1016/j.jaci.2011.06.027
18. Kelly HW, Sternberg AL, Lescher R, Fuhlbrigge AL, Williams P, Zeiger RS, et al. Effect of inhaled glucocorticoids in childhood on adult height. *N Engl J Med.* (2012) 367:904–12. doi: 10.1056/NEJMoa1203229
19. Loke YK, Bianco P, Thavarajah M, Wilson AM. Impact of inhaled corticosteroids on growth in children with asthma: systematic review and meta-analysis. *PLoS ONE* (2015) 10:e0133428. doi: 10.1371/journal.pone.0133428
20. Pedersen SE, Hurd SS, Lemanske RF Jr, Becker A, Zar HJ, Sly PD, et al. Global strategy for the diagnosis and management of asthma in children 5 years and younger. *Pediatr Pulmonol.* (2011) 46:1–17. doi: 10.1002/ppul.21321
21. Ahmet A, Kim H, Spier S. Adrenal suppression: a practical guide to the screening and management of this under-recognized complication of inhaled corticosteroid therapy. *Allergy Asthma Clin Immunol.* (2011) 7:13. doi: 10.1186/1710-1492-7-13
22. Sonnappa S, McQueen B, Postma DS, Martin RJ, Roche N, Grigg J, et al. Extrafine versus fine inhaled corticosteroids in relation to asthma control: a systematic review and meta-analysis of observational real-life studies. *J Allergy Clin Immunol Pract.* (2018) 6:907–15e7. doi: 10.1016/j.jaip.2017.07.032
23. Thomson NC. Addressing corticosteroid insensitivity in adults with asthma. *Expert Rev Respir Med.* (2016) 10:137–56. doi: 10.1586/17476348.2016.1133304
24. Bush A, Frey U. Safety of long-acting beta-agonists in children with asthma. *N Engl J Med.* (2016) 375:889–91. doi: 10.1056/NEJMe1608508
25. Stemptel DA, Raphiou IH, Kral KM, Yeakey AM, Emmett AH, Prazma CM, et al. Serious asthma events with fluticasone plus salmeterol versus fluticasone alone. *N Engl J Med.* (2016) 12:1822–30. doi: 10.1056/NEJMoa1511049
26. Stemptel DA, Szefler SJ, Pedersen S, Zeiger RS, Yeakey AM, Lee LA, et al. Safety of adding salmeterol to fluticasone propionate in children with asthma. *N Engl J Med.* (2016) 375:840–9. doi: 10.1056/NEJMoa1606356
27. Paggiaro P, Bacci E. Montelukast in asthma: a review of its efficacy and place in therapy. *Ther Adv Chronic Dis.* (2011) 2:47–58. doi: 10.1177/2040622310383343
28. Knorr B, Franchi LM, Bisgaard H, Vermeulen JH, LaSouef P, Santanello N, et al. Montelukast, a leukotriene receptor antagonist, for the treatment of persistent asthma in children aged 2 to 5 years. *Pediatrics* (2001) 108:e48. doi: 10.1542/peds.108.3.e48
29. Caggiano S, Cutrera R, Di Marco A, Turchetta A. Exercise-induced bronchospasm and allergy. *Front Pediatr.* (2017) 5:131. doi: 10.3389/fped.2017.00131
30. Weiler JM, Brannan JD, Randolph CC, Hallstrand TS, Parson J, Silvers W, et al. Exercise-induced bronchoconstriction update-2016. *J Allergy Clin Immunol.* (2016) 138:1292–5.e36. doi: 10.1016/jaci.2016.05.029
31. Bisgaard H, Skoner D, Boza ML, Tozzi CA, Newcomb K, Reiss TF, et al. Safety and tolerability of montelukast in placebo-controlled pediatric studies and their open-label extension. *Pediatr Pulmonol.* (2009) 44:568–79. doi: 10.1002/ppul.21018
32. Normansell R, Kew KM, Mansour G. Different oral corticosteroid regimens for acute asthma. *Cochrane Database Syst Rev.* (2016) 5:CD011801. doi:10.1002/14651858. CD011801.pub2
33. Chipps BE, Lanier B, Milgrom H, Deschildre A, Hedlin G, Szefler SJ, et al. Omalizumab in children with uncontrolled allergic asthma: review of clinical trial and real-world experience. *J Allergy Clin Immunol.* (2017) 139:1431–44. doi: 10.1016/j.jaci.2017.03.002
34. Busse WW, Morgan WJ, Gergen P, Mitchell HE, Gern JE, Liu AH, et al. Randomized trial of omalizumab (anti-IgE) for asthma in inner-city children. *N Engl J Med.* (2011) 364:1005–15. doi: 10.1056/NEJMoa1009705
35. Lanier B, Bridges T, Kulus M, Taylor AF, Berhane I, Vidaurre CF. Omalizumab for the treatment of exacerbations in children with inadequately controlled allergic (IgE-mediated) asthma. *J Allergy Clinical Immunol.* (2009) 124:1210–6. doi: 10.1016/j.jaci.2009.09.021
36. Tsabouri S, Mavroudi A, Feketea G, Guibas GV. Subcutaneous and sublingual immunotherapy in allergic asthma in children. *Front Pediatr.* (2017) 5:82. doi: 10.3389/fped.201700082
37. Papathanassiou E, Loukides S, Bakakos P. Severe asthma: anti-IgE or anti-IL-5? *Eur Clin Respir J.* (2016) 3:31813. doi: 10.3402/ecrj.v3.31813
38. Szefer SJ, Nelson HS. Alternative agents for anti-infammatory treatment of asthma. *J Allergy Clin Immunol.* (1998) 102:S23–S35. doi: 10.1016/S0091-6749(98)70003-X
39. Barnes PJ. Drugs for asthma. *Br J Pharmacol.* (2006) 147:S297–S303. doi: 10.1038/sj.bjp.0706437

40. Panickar JR, Bhatnagar N, Grigg J. Exhaled nitric oxide after a single dose of intramuscular triamcinolone in children with difficult to control asthma. *Pediatr Pulmonol.* (2007) 42:573–8. doi: 10.1002/ppul.20583
41. Panickar JR, Kenia P, Silverman M, Grigg J. Intramuscular triamcinolone for difficult asthma. *Pediatr Pulmonol.* (2005) 39:421–5. doi: 10.1002/ppul.20176
42. ten Brinke A, Zwinderman AH, Sterk PJ, Rabe KF, Bel EH. Refractory eosinophilic airway inflammation in severe asthma: effect of parenteral corticosteroids. *Am J Respir Crit Care Med.* (2004) 170:601–5. doi: 10.1164/rccm.200404-440OC
43. Bossley CJ, Saglani S, Kavanagh C, Payne DN, Wilson N, Tsartsali L, et al. Corticosteroid responsiveness and clinical characteristics in childhood difficult asthma *Eur Respir J.* (2009) 34:1052–9. doi: 10.1183/09031936.00186508
44. Kerstjens HA, Engel M, Dahl R, Paggiaro P, Beck E, Vandewalker M, et al. Tiotropium in asthma poorly controlled with standard combination therapy. *N Engl J Med.* (2012) 367:1198–207. doi: 10.1056/NEJMoa1208606
45. Bilocca D, Hargadon B, Pavord ID, Green RH, Brightling CE, Bradding P, et al. The role of oral methotrexate as a steroid sparing agent in refractory eosinophilic asthma. *Chron Respir Dis.* (2018) 15:85–7. doi: 10.1177/1479972317709650
46. Parulekar AD, Diamant Z, Hanania NA. Antifungals in severe asthma. *Curr Opin Pulm Med.* (2015) 2148–54. doi: 10.1097/MCP.0000000000000117
47. Vicencio AG, Santiago MT, Tsirilakis K, Stone A, Worgall S, Foley EA, et al. Fungal sensitization in childhood persistent asthma is associated with disease severity. *Pediatr Pulmonol.* (2014) 49:8–14. doi: 10.1002/ppul.22779
48. Vicencio AG, Muzumdar H, Tsirilakis K, Kessel A, Nandalike K, Goldman DL. Severe asthma with fungal sensitization in a child: response to itraconazole therapy. *Pediatrics* (2010) 125:e1255-8. doi: 10.1542/peds.2009-2443
49. Mikailov A, Kane I, Aronoff SC, Luck R, DelVecchio MT. Utility of adjunctive macrolide therapy in treatment of children with asthma: a systematic review and meta-analysis. *J Asthma Allergy* (2013) 6:23–9. doi: 10.2147/JAA.S38652
50. Koutsoubari I, Papaevangelou V, Kostantinou GN, Makrinioti H, Xepapadaki P, Kafetzis D, et al. Effect of clarithromycin on acute asthma exacerbations in children: an open randomized study. *Pediatr Allergy Immunol.* (2012) 23:385–90. doi: 10.1111/j.1399-3038.2012.01280.x
51. Chung KF, Wenzel SE, Brozek JL, Bush A, Castro M, Sterk PJ, et al. International ERS/ATS guidelines on definition, evaluation and treatment of severe asthma. *Eur Respir J.* (2014) 43:343–73. doi: 10.1183/09031936.00202013

14

Approaches to Asthma Diagnosis in Children and Adults

Sejal Saglani[1,2*] *and Andrew N. Menzie-Gow*[1,3]

[1] *National Heart & Lung Institute, Imperial College London, London, United Kingdom,* [2] *Department of Respiratory Paediatrics, Royal Brompton Hospital, London, United Kingdom,* [3] *Department of Respiratory Medicine, Royal Brompton Hospital, London, United Kingdom*

***Correspondence:**
Sejal Saglani
s.saglani@imperial.ac.uk

Although the hallmark features of asthma include reversible airflow obstruction, airway eosinophilia, and symptoms of recurrent wheeze associated with breathlessness and cough, it is a heterogeneous disease. The extent of the pathophysiological abnormalities are variable between patients. Despite this, until recently, asthma diagnosis had been made very simplistically predominantly from a clinical history and examination, and often a trial of medication such as short acting bronchodilators. The limitations of this approach have become increasingly apparent with evidence of inappropriate over diagnosis, under diagnosis and misdiagnosis. Although there is no gold standard single test to make a diagnosis of asthma, there are several objective tests that can be used to support the diagnosis including physiological measures such as obstructive spirometry associated with bronchodilator reversibility and airway hyperresponsiveness. In addition, non-invasive tests of airway inflammation such as exhaled nitric oxide or peripheral blood eosinophils are important to identify those with an allergic or eosinophilic phenotype. Diagnostic guidelines reflect the importance of using objective tests to support a diagnosis of asthma, however practical application in the clinic may not be straightforward. The focus of this review is to discuss the need to undertake objective tests in all patients to support asthma diagnosis and not just rely on clinical features. The advantages, challenges and limitations of performing tests of lung function and airway inflammation in the clinic, the difficulties related to training and interpretation of results will be explored, and the utility and relevance of diagnostic tests will be compared in adults and children.

Keywords: asthma diagnosis, spirometry, exhaled nitric oxide, guidelines, inflammation, paediatric asthma, lung function, objective tests

INTRODUCTION

The essential components of a detailed history and examination remain central to making a diagnosis of asthma in both children and adults (1). Additional confirmative tests are recommended and will be discussed, but all guidelines emphasize the need to accurately establish the presence of a constellation of symptoms that align with asthma. This fundamental need to accurately identify a collection of symptoms that fit with asthma has recently been agreed by an expert consensus opinion from clinicians, researchers and scientists worldwide (2). It has been suggested that the term "asthma" should only be used as a descriptor that relates to a collection of symptoms. But no associated assumptions should be made about the underlying pathophysiological features driving the symptoms (2). It is suggested that this approach will prevent inappropriate treatments from being used and will encourage increased emphasis on individualized therapy. The focus of this review is to discuss the key features that constitute a diagnosis of asthma and to explore the role of objective confirmatory or supportive tests, highlighting the elements that are common to adult and childhood disease and some components that differ according to the age of the patient. The key components that contribute to a diagnosis of asthma include airway inflammation, hyperresponsiveness, bronchial obstruction, and symptoms. Each of these will be discussed, highlighting the relevance in children and adults and also the role of objective tests and the potential pitfalls that may lead to misdiagnosis.

THE BASICS NEED TO BE CORRECT REGARDLESS OF PATIENT AGE

History and Examination

Asthma is characterized by symptoms including wheeze, cough, breathlessness and chest tightness (3), all of which may fluctuate over time. The symptoms are common to children and adults, and an essential component is to obtain objective confirmation of symptoms either as documented doctor observed symptoms, or by administration of an objective questionnaire. A key issue that often leads to misdiagnosis in children is the mistaken assumption that all noisy breathing equates to wheeze and therefore asthma. Epidemiological data rely heavily on questionnaire reported symptoms, which may not always be accurate and may result in very varied reports of prevalence rates (4). However, for the individual patient, an accurate record of documented wheeze and symptoms consistent with asthma is critical to prevent inappropriate diagnosis, but equally importantly, inappropriate treatment (5, 6).

INCORPORATING OBJECTIVE TESTS TO MAKE A DIAGNOSIS OF ASTHMA: IS IT NECESSARY?

The importance of a correct diagnosis for the individual is obvious, however, equally important is the impact on cost to the health service of avoiding inappropriate prescription of asthma treatments. Application of a secondary screening programme, incorporating objective assessments of lung function and airway hyperresponsiveness, to a population who had a physician diagnosis of asthma, identified 28% of patients with a misdiagnosis (7) of whom 71% were on asthma medication. Moreover, the additional costs of the objective tests were significantly less than the costs of a lifetime of prescription of inappropriate medication. One-third of Canadian adults who had asthma diagnosed in the previous 5 years no longer had current asthma, likely because of an initial misdiagnosis (8). Factors contributing to the misdiagnosis of asthma include failure to confirm reversible airflow obstruction, the relatively poor sensitivity of spirometry alone to absolutely confirm asthma (especially in children), the day to day variability of symptoms and the numerous phenotypes of disease (9). Consequences of misdiagnosis not only include inappropriate treatment, but also lost opportunity and time in making a correct diagnosis to explain the patient's respiratory symptoms. It is important to remember that misdiagnosis incorporates both wrongly labeling another condition as asthma, but equally missing a diagnosis of asthma and failed treatment. Both have significant consequences (9). Given the availability of objective tests that can help to confirm the diagnosis and the potential unwanted effects of inappropriate or wrong diagnosis, many diagnostic algorithms now incorporate the need for objective tests in the diagnosis of asthma.

An important change in the approach to diagnosis has recently been introduced in England, where the National Institute of Health and Care Excellence (NICE), whose purpose is to generate evidence based and cost effective guidelines, has recently been published [https://www.nice.org.uk/guidance/ng80]. It was claimed by NICE that up to 1.2 million of the approximately 4 million people with asthma in the UK were misdiagnosed and therefore being prescribed wrong or inappropriate medication (10). For the first time in England, it has now been recommended that both spirometry and exhaled nitric oxide tests should be used in all patients older than 5 years to help in the confirmation of the diagnosis. This guideline has resulted in much debate and discussion especially because of differences from the British Thoracic Society and Scottish Intercollegiate National Guidance (BTS/SIGN) which have been used by clinicians in the UK for over 2 decades (11). In the context of asthma diagnosis, the big contrast between the two guidelines includes the implementation of objective tests as being absolutely central and essential for making a confirmed diagnosis in adults, and very important, and whenever possible, essential for a diagnosis in children over 5 years in the NICE guidance. Although the BTS/SIGN guidelines recommend the use of lung function tests to support asthma diagnosis, implementation of this to date has been very variable and limited.

TESTS TO ASSESS AIRWAY INFLAMMATION IN ASTHMA DIAGNOSIS

Use of Exhaled Nitric Oxide to Diagnose Asthma—In Adults

The NICE diagnostic algorithm for adults includes the need for an accurate history and physical examination, including wherever possible, objective confirmation of wheeze, however, the critical change at this point is the clear message that a diagnosis cannot be made only on symptoms, without an objective confirmatory test. The first objective test to be used in adults aged 17 years and over is exhaled nitric oxide. If a value of 40 parts per billion (ppb) or higher is measured in a patient with suspected asthma, this is considered a positive result, and is strongly supportive of asthma. However, situations in which exhaled nitric oxide may be low, despite the presence of asthma, are highlighted, the most important for adult patients being cigarette smoking (12).

The upregulation of nitric oxide (NO) by inflammatory cytokines in central and peripheral airways can be monitored in exhaled air. Increased fraction of exhaled NO (FeNO) reflects eosinophilic-mediated inflammatory pathways and likely steroid responsiveness moderately well in asthma (13). As the fundamental pathophysiology underlying asthma incorporates eosinophilic airway inflammation coupled with reversible airflow obstruction, exhaled nitric oxide is considered additive to measures of lung function as an indirect marker of airway inflammation. However, in addition to smoking, other factors, including atopy and current treatment with steroids influence measured exhaled nitric oxide. Therefore, although considered useful to help support a diagnosis of asthma, it is apparent that its clinical utility and accuracy is greatest for steroid naïve and non-smoking patients (14). It is because of the variability of exhaled nitric oxide that it must be remembered that although a high level is supportive of the diagnosis, a level below 40 ppb does not exclude asthma (15).

Use of Exhaled Nitric Oxide to Diagnose Asthma—In Children

Although the NICE guidance includes objective tests for children to help confirm a diagnosis of asthma, in contrast to the adult diagnostic algorithm, exhaled nitric oxide measurement is not a required test for making the diagnosis in those under 17 years. Exhaled nitric oxide measurements are only recommended if there is diagnostic uncertainty after lung function tests and assessments of reversible airflow obstruction have been made [https://pathways.nice.org.uk/pathways/asthma#path=view%3A/pathways/asthma/assessing-and-diagnosing-asthma-in-under-17s.xml&content=view-node%3Anodes-diagnostic-uncertainty]. A systematic review of the utility of exhaled nitric oxide for the diagnosis of asthma in children has shown that the measure may be informative for a diagnosis when used in conjunction with other tests, but importantly, that the cut-off for normal should be lower in children than adults (16). Several factors, of relevance to children have been shown to influence levels of exhaled nitric oxide, including age, height, gender, race and passive smoke exposure (16). Another key issue for children, even if only considering those aged 5 and above, is their technique and ability to perform an adequate maneuver that allows maintenance of a sustained exhalation flow rate and an acceptable recording. With these numerous factors that affect values of exhaled nitric oxide in children, the American Thoracic Society (ATS) guidelines suggest values in children below 20 ppb are very unlikely to be associated with eosinophilic airway inflammation, whilst those above 50 ppb suggest airway eosinophilia and a response to corticosteroids (13). The ATS suggest values between 20 and 35 ppb should be interpreted in light of the clinical context, taking into consideration the various factors that may affect exhaled nitric oxide. Several pediatric studies have used 20 ppb as a cut-off and shown high sensitivity (86%), specificity (89%), positive (92%), and negative (80%) predictive value for asthma in children (17, 18). A significant factor that must be considered for children when interpreting values of exhaled nitric oxide is the influence of atopy. Allergic sensitization alone, without any clinical manifestation of atopic disease or asthma is strongly associated with elevated levels of exhaled nitric oxide (19, 20). Moreover, there is an association between elevated exhaled nitric oxide and current exposure to the allergen that the child is sensitized to and multiple sensitization may result in higher exhaled nitric oxide levels (20, 21). Despite the data from the ATS guidelines suggesting a value >20 ppb may be of clinical relevance in children, the abnormal cut-off level that has been set in the NICE guidelines for children is above 35 ppb for those aged 5–16 years. The test is only recommended in those children with diagnostic uncertainty after initial assessment and those with normal spirometry, or airflow obstruction without evidence of reversibility. On balance, an assessment of exhaled nitric oxide is helpful in supporting a diagnosis of asthma in children aged 5 and above, providing the challenges associated with technical ability to perform the test and the factors that may either elevate or lower the value are considered (**Table 1**). As a result, exhaled nitric oxide is currently predominantly used in specialist centers, where the equipment is used frequently, technical expertise in obtaining measurements is reliable, where children with diagnostic uncertainty are seen, and results are interpreted in the context of the influencing factors.

Sputum Eosinophils

Currently, assessment of airway eosinophils is not a requirement for the diagnosis of mild to moderate asthma. The utility of induced sputum inflammation is predominantly recommended for patients thought to have severe disease (22). In practice, the use of sputum eosinophils to make an asthma diagnosis is challenging because of the time and expertise required for both the induction, processing and analysis of the sample. For this reason, the utility of less invasive biomarkers that may reflect airway eosinophilia are preferred. A meta-analysis of the diagnostic accuracy of minimally invasive biomarkers (exhaled nitric oxide, blood eosinophils, total serum IgE) has shown each of these markers only moderately reflect sputum eosinophils with a sensitivity and specificity of 0.66 and 0.76 for exhaled nitric oxide, 0.71 and 0.77 for blood eosinophils (23). These data highlight that no single biomarker accurately reflects airway eosinophilia and if used alone, there is a substantial risk of both false positive and false negative diagnoses. Overall, it appears that blood eosinophils and exhaled nitric oxide have similar

TABLE 1 | Factors, independent of asthma, influencing exhaled nitric oxide levels.

	Elevated/lower level
Age	Increases with age, lower normal values in children than adults
Height	Increase in taller children
Ethnicity	Higher in Black than Caucasian children
Smoke exposure (passive/active)	Lower with smoke exposure
Allergic sensitization	Higher in atopic patients
Gender	Higher in males
Respiratory infection	Lower with concurrent infection
Technique—maintaining exhalation flow rate	Inaccurate results if flow not maintained
Consumption of nitrite containing foods, caffeine, alcohol	Increased values

accuracy in reflecting sputum eosinophilia, regardless of the asthma phenotype, while serum IgE is less accurate (24). Given the difficulty in obtaining sputum samples and the restriction of its use to specialist respiratory centers, currently an assessment of sputum eosinophils is not routinely undertaken to make a diagnosis of asthma in adults or children.

In adult patients the main use of sputum eosinophils has been to guide management and tailoring of therapy to achieve a reduction in exacerbations, rather than to make the diagnosis of asthma (25). Unfortunately, to date, these results have not been reproduced in children, perhaps because of the longitudinal variability of sputum eosinophils counts within patients over time (26).

Blood Eosinophils

A blood test is easier and can routinely be performed in all clinical settings, thus making the utility of peripheral, rather than airway eosinophils, more attractive to help make a diagnosis of asthma for both adults and children.

In children, several factors need to be considered prior to the interpretation of a blood eosinophil count. Firstly, the cut-off for normal values change with age. The range for blood eosinophils in healthy children aged between 6 months and 13 years is between 500 and 700 cells/mcl (27). Thus, using cut-offs of >300/mcl as suggested in numerous adult studies may be entirely inappropriate. Another factor that must be considered in children is the presence of atopic disease without asthma which may result in elevated blood eosinophils without airway eosinophilia. Therefore, if blood eosinophils are relied upon as a biomarker in a child with eczema and wheeze, disentangling the reason for peripheral eosinophilia is difficult and may lead to a false positive diagnosis (28). Another issue is the impact of steroid treatment on peripheral eosinophil count. If a child is steroid naïve, an elevated blood eosinophil count may truly represent airway eosinophilia, but for children on inhaled corticosteroids, the peripheral eosinophil count may be low or normal, while an airway eosinophilia may persist, this is especially true for children with severe asthma (29). On balance, in school-age children with asthma, given the number of potential caveats that may give a result that does not truly reflect airway eosinophils and without a cut-off for the upper limit of normal yet being established, there is currently no evidence to support the use of blood eosinophils as a diagnostic marker for asthma. The utility of blood eosinophils in preschool children with wheezing to predict asthma development and response to inhaled corticosteroids, has been better evaluated and will be discussed below in the section on preschool wheeze and diagnostic markers. Another caveat to the use of peripheral blood eosinophils in children, is the data showing correlations with airway eosinophils are based on values during stable disease, not during exacerbation. It is unclear whether peripheral blood eosinophils would be helpful in making a diagnosis of asthma during an exacerbation, especially in children, since so many acute attacks are driven by infection, when peripheral or airway inflammation may be predominantly neutrophilic, not eosinophilic.

Unlike the paucity of data supporting the utility of blood eosinophils for a diagnosis of asthma in children, there is significant evidence in adults that blood eosinophils are useful to identify those patients who are more likely to respond to specific therapies such as steroids or the anti-eosinophilic monoclonocal antibodies, Mepolizumab (30) and Benralizumab (31). However, it must be remembered that elevated blood eosinophils only reflect a particular phenotype of asthma, that which is predominantly driven by Th2 mediators and is likely to be steroid responsive. Therefore, an absence of peripheral eosinophilia does not exclude asthma. The need to consider symptom pattern and lung function to help support a diagnosis remains important. The use of blood eosinophils in primary care and even as a point of care test is becoming increasingly feasible, whereby a finger prick point of care device has been shown to have close correlation with differential cell counts obtained from samples by venepuncture (32). However, the most important clinical message when interpreting blood eosinophils for asthma diagnosis, is very high counts (>500 cells/mcl) have a high certainty of an associated airway eosinophilia, but for values <410 cells/mcl the relationship between blood and airway eosinophils becomes less clear and it is important to consider the overall clinical picture and all possible factors that might affect blood eosinophil counts (30).

LUNG FUNCTION TESTS AND ASTHMA DIAGNOSIS

Use of Spirometry to Diagnose Asthma—In Adults

Perhaps the most easily accessible test that can be used to support a diagnosis of asthma is spirometry. The presence of an obstructive picture, with a ratio of FEV_1/FVC <70%, and associated reversibility following administration of bronchodilator is in keeping with asthma. Although it is assumed by most that spirometry is used to help confirm a diagnosis of asthma in adults, its use in primary and secondary care settings is limited. For this reason, the NICE guidelines that have been recently published in England include spirometry as a "must do" objective test for all patients over 5 years old with a suspected diagnosis of asthma (https://www.nice.org.uk/guidance/ng80). If an obstructive spirometry result is present, then it has been recommended that all adults, aged 17 and over, should undergo a bronchodilator reversibility test, and an improvement of ≥12% in FEV_1 and an increase in ≥200 ml is considered a positive test of reversible airflow obstruction. However, one of the key issues about the use of spirometry to help diagnose asthma is the absolute requirement for its correct use and interpretation (15). If this is not done, there is a significant risk of both under and over diagnosis (33). Interpretation of spirometry results varies even between specialist lung function laboratories, with lack of standardization in relation to definitions for the lower limit of normal (34). Another issue that affects the interpretation of spirometry in the context of an asthma diagnosis is that values may be normal when assessed during stable disease in the clinic. The majority of adults seen in primary care have mild disease with well-preserved lung function. Airflow obstruction defined as a ratio of FEV_1/FVC <70% was found in only 21% of adult patients diagnosed with asthma in a primary care setting (35). In the case of normal spirometry results, the NICE guidelines suggest a two to 4 week period of peak flow monitoring and more than 20% variability in results as a positive test supportive of asthma. The American Thoracic Society and the National Asthma Education and Prevention Program, both recommend the use of spirometry for the diagnosis of asthma, these recommendations have been in place since 2007. However, an assessment of the implementation of this recommendation by physicians for patients with newly diagnosed asthma demonstrated that only 47% had spirometry performed within a year of the diagnosis being made (36). Moreover, rates of use of spirometry in primary care were only 23% and 78% of patients were prescribed asthma drugs without previous spirometry (36). Therefore, despite recommendations and guidelines having been introduced for over a decade, implementation and physician practice seems to have remained largely unaffected. This pattern seems consistent across countries, with approximately 50% of patients with a diagnosis of asthma ever having had spirometry in a secondary care or specialist setting, and this value reducing to approximately 25% in primary care (37, 38). Overall, there is agreement among respiratory physicians that spirometry is important in making a diagnosis of asthma in adults. However, in practice, it is difficult to find evidence that the guidelines are being consistently implemented. A combination of physician education to undertake spirometry to the required standards, emphasis of its importance and providing knowledge in interpretation and importantly, resources and incentives to undertake the test from primary through to specialist care, is likely the only way it will be adopted more widely (**Table 2**).

TABLE 2 | Advantages and challenges of the use of spirometry in making a diagnosis of asthma in adults and children.

Advantages	Challenges
Objective evidence of obstructive airways disease	Not reliable if technically inadequate maneuvers performed—skills to undertake procedure and calibrate and maintain equipment needed
Demonstration of variable airflow obstruction if bronchodilator reversibility also applied	Defined and agreed values for lower normal limit needed
Minimizes over diagnosis and misdiagnosis	Normal values do not rule out asthma—tests of airway hyperresponsiveness may be needed
Demonstration of reversible airflow obstruction provides objective evidence of asthma	Requires cooperation, cannot be reliably performed in children under 6 years, except in specialist centers
	Difficulties around agreement of lower normal limit—need to use reference values that allow for ethnicity
	Technical expertise in obtaining a satisfactory result is needed. Often best results obtained with incentive devices, which may not be available in primary care

Use of Spirometry to Diagnose Asthma—In Children

Although confirmation of reversible airflow obstruction is as important for a diagnosis of asthma in children as in adults, the practical application of spirometry in children is even more of a challenge (**Table 2**). This applies to all levels of care from primary to specialist, because of the significant challenges of technical expertise required to undertake reliable and reproducible tests in children and the training and education needed by physicians in the interpretation of the data. These issues are highlighted by American data, which shows that although 52% of physicians who provided primary care to children used spirometry, only 21% used spirometry according to the national guidelines and only 35% of physicians surveyed were comfortable interpreting the test results (39). In addition, 21% of spirometry readings were interpreted incorrectly (40), emphasizing the need for training and quality control prior to use of spirometry for children in primary care. The challenges of using spirometry to diagnose asthma in children and the improvements that can be made following training and education of healthcare staff have been discussed in detail elsewhere (41). Another critical issue for children, even more prevalent than in adults, is that when measured during stable disease, spirometry is frequently normal, even in those with severe disease (42). The significant issues that arise when relying on spirometry in children to make a diagnosis of asthma have been highlighted recently in a study that assessed the usefulness of the recent NICE guidelines in England to accurately make a diagnosis of asthma when applied to a cohort of children being regularly followed. Only two of 89 children aged between 13 and 16 years, who were symptomatic met the definition of asthma when assessed according to the NICE diagnostic algorithm (FEV_1:FVC <70%), but neither met the epidemiological, questionnaire based definition of asthma (43). Although a total of 10 children had FEV_1:FVC <70%, 8 of those did not have symptoms consistent with current asthma (43). The risks of using cut-offs for airway obstruction and lower normal limits extrapolated from adult studies have been highlighted as a significant pitfall for the application of the pediatric NICE guidelines in clinical practice (44).

As asthma is characterized by variable airflow obstruction, a reduced FEV_1/FVC ratio may not be present at all times, therefore, if clinical suspicion remains, spirometry may need to be repeated to demonstrate obstruction. Another way of recording variation in airflow obstruction is to undertake several measurements of peak expiratory flow rate (PEFR) at home for 1–2 weeks. Variation of >13% suggests variable airflow obstruction. However, correct technique must be ensured, and this relies on patient cooperation and adherence in undertaking the measurements (45). Demonstration of improvement in spirometry following bronchodilator may be more sensitive in children than detection of obstruction (46). Demonstration of reversibility after bronchodilator had good specificity for an asthma diagnosis (73%), but using a cut-off of 12% improvement for children carried poor diagnostic sensitivity (35%), while a cut-off of 8% was significantly better (47). Therefore, although demonstration of bronchodilator reversibility is important to help confirm a diagnosis of asthma, but it may not be appropriate to use a strict cut-off for improvement in children.

Reference Values for Spirometry: the Global Lung Function Initiative (GLI)

Global, multi-ethnic all age reference equations are now available and have been endorsed by all major international respiratory societies (48). These are now considered the international gold standard and offer a unified approach to the interpretation and presentation of FEV_1 and other spirometry measures. It is essential that these reference equations are used, but specifically in the context of demonstrating airway obstruction in children, it must be remembered that older reference equations may produce lower predicted values, which result in an over-estimation of lung function when interpreted as %predicted. Therefore, the switch to GLI-2012 will result in lower median FEV_1 %predicted values overall, as well as age-specific and individual patient differences. Data for airway obstruction should be interpreted using the GLI-reference values as recommended by the NICE guidelines.

PERSISTENT AIRFLOW LIMITATION AND ASTHMA DIAGNOSIS

An important sub-group of patients thought to have asthma may have obstructive spirometry, but without evidence of bronchodilator reversibility. These patients have a post-bronchodilator FEV1 and/or an FEV1/FVC less than the lower limits of normal, or persistent airflow limitation (49). Although this is unusual in asthma, it may still be consistent with the diagnosis. A multi-center study of children with persistent airflow limitation on spirometry, showed 93% of all children had a diagnosis of asthma, this was even after other diagnoses and co-morbidities had been excluded (49). Similarly approximately one-third of adults screened in asthma clinics have been shown to have persistent airflow obstruction (50). Those with persistent airflow limitation may have more severe disease, but the most important element prior to labeling these patients as asthma is to refer to a specialist center to ensure other diagnoses have been excluded.

In adults, the most common airway disease associated with fixed airway obstruction is chronic obstructive pulmonary disease (COPD). However, it has now been proposed that there is a gray area of overlap between patients that have asthma (with reversible airflow obstruction) and those with COPD and fixed airflow obstruction. This has led to the diagnostic label asthma-COPD overlap (ACO). Although the term has been proposed as a valid entity, the definition and clinical features of patients that may fit this category have remained uncertain. It appears to be characterized by persistent airflow limitation with several features usually associated with asthma and several features usually associated with COPD. There has been a published consensus definition which includes persistent airflow limitation in symptomatic individuals 40 years of age and older, a well-documented history of asthma in childhood or early adulthood and a significant exposure history to cigarette or biomass smoke (51). Overall, the diagnosis of ACO in adults remains uncertain and a challenge (52). This entity adds to the confusion, however, it brings back the importance of identifying a constellation of symptoms and looking for evidence of underlying pathophysiology, with the approach of targeting therapy in individuals according to "treatable traits" (2). Certainly, in children, the approach taken is that the presence of persistent airflow limitation in a child with presumed asthma should lead to referral to a specialist center and the search for alternative diagnoses. However, if no other diagnoses explain the child's symptoms and presentation, asthma with persistent airflow limitation is the diagnosis and the patient should be treated as such. It is important to remember, however, that therapy escalation to try to reach "normal" lung function may not be appropriate, especially if a child does not have evidence of eosinophilic airway inflammation. A trial of steroids to try to establish optimal lung function may be appropriate, but if there is no improvement and the child's symptoms are controlled, attempts to escalate steroid medication must be resisted in this exceptional scenario (53).

UTILITY OF LUNG FUNCTION TESTS OTHER THAN SPIROMETRY FOR ASTHMA DIAGNOSIS

The limitation of spirometry in children is prevalent because of the reliance on the ability of the child to adequately perform voluntary maneuvers. This is a particular challenge in the absence of computer aided incentive devices (54). Alternative effort independent lung function tests can therefore be used in children, but none of these are available in primary or secondary care and issues around technical competence and normal values are even more of an issue than for spirometry, even in specialist centers. As a result, the application of tidal breathing or effort independent tests is currently limited predominantly to the research setting and being tested mainly in preschool children being assessed at specialist centers. The assessment of airway obstruction in children with severe asthma has been reviewed elsewhere (55) and the utility of forced oscillation technique and impulse oscillometry for asthma diagnosis have also been reviewed (56).

Other lung function tests that can be used include plethysmography, multiple breath washout (to measure lung clearance index) and airway resistance using the interruptor technique (Rint). However, none of these are used routinely in clinical practice, certainly none are available for use in primary or secondary care. The test used most commonly in specialist centers is plethysmography, however this measures lung volumes, and the role of assessing lung volumes in asthma diagnosis remains controversial. Although there is evidence that lung volumes may be complementary to spirometry to assess asthma severity (57), plethysmography alone is not routinely used to make the diagnosis. Similarly, the other tests have been used in small studies, especially in populations where voluntary maneuvers cannot be reliably performed, but currently their use remains limited to research and specialist centers, without obvious evidence for their role in routine clinical practice, in either children or adults.

ASSESSMENT OF AIRWAY HYPERRESPONSIVENESS TO DIAGNOSE ASTHMA

As spirometry is often normal during stable disease in patients with a clinical picture consistent with asthma, an indirect bronchial provocation test to assess airway hyperresponsiveness can be used to help diagnostic confirmation. Various challenge agents can be used to induce hyperresponsiveness including histamine, methacholine, allergens, adenosine, and mannitol. However, the importance of optimal delivery of the inhaled agents to the airways to ensure reproducible data are generated has been highlighted (58). Inhaled methacholine, a direct cholinergic agonist, to evoke concentration-dependent airway smooth muscle contraction can be used and bronchoconstriction at low concentrations of methacholine (typically <4 mg/mL) suggest increased airway hyperresponsiveness. A novel method to report responsiveness using dose rather than concentration has recently been proposed (59). However, allergen challenge tests can only be undertaken in specialist centers and so are not routinely used for asthma diagnosis, but should be undertaken in patients with a symptom constellation suggestive of asthma, without evidence of reversible airflow obstruction or eosinophilic airway inflammation and without response to therapy.

In addition to inhaled challenge tests, another scenario that may uncover bronchoconstriction, and may also be supportive of an asthma diagnosis, is exercise. Exercise is a frequent precipitant of asthma symptoms, however an exercise test is of particular importance if this is the only trigger for symptoms in order to obtain objective confirmation of true bronchoconstriction and diagnose asthma, (60) and to exclude any contributory upper airway symptoms including exercise induced laryngeal obstruction which may be prevalent in both children and adults (61, 62). Importantly, the presence of exercise induced bronchoconstriction alone may not equate to a diagnosis of asthma as it may occur in people without asthma, the need to assess the complete clinical picture and airway inflammation remains essential.

ASSESSMENTS OF ATOPY IN ASTHMA DIAGNOSIS

Often a diagnosis of asthma is made clearer in the presence of associated allergic diseases including eczema, allergic rhinitis or food allergy. In children, allergic asthma is the most common phenotype (63) and therefore assessments of allergic sensitization, in the absence of disease manifestation, are undertaken to help support the diagnosis. However, what remains uncertain is how best to include tests of allergic sensitization into diagnostic algorithms for asthma (64). The presence of allergic sensitization, particularly to aeroallergens is supportive of the diagnosis, but the absence of sensitization does not rule out the disease. In school children, non-atopic asthma is rare and should be diagnosed after careful exclusion of other differential diagnoses (65).

The phenotype of "adult-onset asthma" is often non-atopic (66) and therefore atopy is not as central to the diagnosis in adults as in children. However, it must be remembered that atopy is not an all or nothing phenomenon and must itself be quantified in terms of severity (67). An absence of elevated specific IgE to a limited range of allergens may not exclude atopy, moreover, low peripheral IgE levels may not reflect low pulmonary mucosal IgE levels as has been shown by a reduction in bronchial IgE and associated improved lung function following omalizumab therapy in "non-atopic" adult asthmatics (68). As for blood eosinophils and other objective tests, the presence of allergic sensitization and indeed associated clinical manifestation of allergic diseases certainly supports a diagnosis of asthma in a patient with the correct symptom constellation, but the absence of atopy does not exclude asthma.

SHOULD WE HAVE DIAGNOSTIC ALGORITHMS/GUIDELINES FOR ASTHMA?

Unfortunately, we do not have a gold standard confirmatory test for asthma, so although objective markers may be used, they still all only provide evidence that is supportive of, or less indicative of asthma. Ultimately, a diagnosis at present can only be made based using a constellation of clinical features, supportive objective tests and frequently an assessment of response to therapy. The absence of a gold standard test, and the recognition that asthma constitutes a disease with an array of etiologies, phenotypes and clinical manifestations has led to the proposal that we should now diagnose "asthma" based on symptoms, and then identify pathological and physiological "treatable traits" to allow targeted and personalized therapy. Although in England the NICE guidelines have attempted to overcome the lack of utility of any objective tests to make a diagnosis of asthma, they remain restrictive, as the objective tests used assume the presence of predominantly eosinophilic airway inflammation and reversible airflow obstruction are required for the diagnosis. This approach has the risk of being too restrictive and potential for under diagnosis as numerous phenotypes and endotypes of the disease display either non-eosinophilic inflammation, or airflow limitation without obstruction. The inclusion of objective tests is important, and it should be remembered that a single test may not be enough to make a diagnosis, and a combination of tests demonstrating variable airflow obstruction and airway inflammation are needed. When applied to a cohort of 13–16 year old children spirometry, bronchodilator reversibility and exhaled nitric oxide were all normal in 24 of 56 children (43%) with current asthma defined epidemiologically (physician diagnosed asthma, current wheeze and prescribed asthma medication) (43). Moreover, the data question the cut-offs proposed for obstructive spirometry in children, the order in which the lung function tests are proposed and the position of bronchodilator reversibility within the algorithm. The authors plainly state the

NICE algorithm should not be used for an asthma diagnosis in children until better evidence of its utility is available (43).

DIFFERENTIAL DIAGNOSIS

Even though patients may present clinically with acute symptoms of breathlessness and wheeze, the long list of differential diagnoses that may cause these symptoms must be considered before asthma is diagnosed (69). Features in the history that are supportive of asthma include a positive family history in a parent or sibling, a history of atopy, including eczema, allergic rhinitis or food allergy and, for children, a symptom pattern that incorporates symptoms with several triggers such as exercise, cold air as well as upper respiratory infections. The important "red flags" in the clinical history and examination that should question the diagnosis in both children and adults have been clearly summarized in the British Thoracic Society/ Scottish Intercollegiate Network Guidelines (https://www.brit-thoracic.org.uk/document-library/clinical-information/asthma/btssign-asthma-guideline-quick-reference-guide-2016/). The initial structured clinical assessment should be used to help decide whether asthma is of high, intermediate or low probability. If any doubts about the diagnosis arise, it is essential that referral to a specialist is made prior to any diagnostic label being applied as the high risk of misdiagnosis and over diagnosis with the resulting undesirable consequences to the patient and inappropriate use of resources has become increasingly apparent (8).

SHOULD A TRIAL OF TREATMENT BE USED TO DIAGNOSE ASTHMA?

Given the difficulties associated with the absence of a gold standard diagnostic test for asthma, and especially in children, difficulties around appropriate lung function tests and assessments of airway inflammation, it has been argued that the only way to confirm the diagnosis is to assess response to a trial of asthma medication. However, this approach carries a significant risk of a misdiagnosis with the associated problems of inappropriate therapy. This is even more of a concern now since the BTS/SIGN guidance for the management of asthma suggests as required short acting bronchodilators should not be the starting point of treatment, but all patients should be commenced on anti-inflammatory treatment with low dose regular inhaled corticosteroids (70). Whenever possible, the diagnostic tests that have been outlined thus far to try to identify "treatable traits" such as evidence of eosinophilic airway inflammation and reversible airflow obstruction should be undertaken. This applies equally to children and adults. The concern is that a response of symptoms to a trial of therapy does not make a diagnosis. Indeed, a trial of therapy is not part of the diagnostic algorithm proposed by NICE in England (71). If a child or adult presents acutely with wheeze, then it is a priority to treat the symptoms and not wait for objective tests. However, once symptoms have been controlled, even if empirical maintenance therapy such as inhaled corticosteroids have been commenced, it remains important to undertake some objective testing once the patient is stable to help to confirm the diagnosis.

SPECIFIC CONSIDERATIONS

Diagnosing Asthma at the Extremes of Age

Preschool Wheeze

Making a diagnosis of asthma in preschool children is a huge challenge because objective tests of airway inflammation and lung function are either invasive (broncho-alveolar lavage for inflammation) or require voluntary maneuvers and cooperation (spirometry). In addition, children under 5 years old have phenotypes of wheezing that are distinct from allergic asthma. Some only wheeze with respiratory infections in acute episodes and others may have persistent symptoms during and in between episodes. The diagnostic term preschool wheeze is therefore used in preference to asthma for children under 5 years old. Guidelines and recommendations for diagnosis and management have been published (72, 73). Diagnosis currently relies predominantly on confirmation of wheeze (doctor diagnosed wheeze), history and symptom pattern (which relies on accurate parental recall) and tests of atopy. However, the pitfalls of relying predominantly on subjective markers to make a diagnosis and direct management have been highlighted (74). Increasing efforts are being made to identify biomarkers to help guide management in preschool wheezers. The most promising is recent evidence of children with aero-allergen sensitization and elevated blood eosinophils as differential responders to maintenance inhaled corticosteroids (75). The role of respiratory infection (both viral and bacterial) and neutrophilic airway inflammation in mediating symptoms is being increasingly recognized in this age group (76), but biomarkers that distinguish children with predominant eosinophilic and allergic airways disease compared to those with infection driven disease are currently lacking.

Asthma in the Elderly

It is important to recognize the impact of aging on lung physiology when diagnosing asthma in the elderly. Specifically, because aging impacts respiratory mechanics, the fixed threshold of <0.70 for the ratio FEV_1 to FVC frequently misclassifies normal-for-age spirometry as airflow obstruction. Such misclassification can occur in otherwise asymptomatic never-smokers, starting at about age 45–50 (77). It is not fully understood how FeNO varies with age in healthy individuals. One study has demonstrated three distinct phases in the evolution of FeNO throughout the age range 6–80 years (78). FeNO values increased linearly between 6 and 14 years of age in girls and between 6 and 16 years of age in boys. After that, FeNO levels plateaued in both genders until age 45 years in females and age 59 years in males, when they started to increase linearly again. This increase continued until age 80.

Smoking and Asthma Diagnosis

A smoking history should always be obtained as regardless of the underlying disease smoking cessation advice should be given. Current or past smoking, conventionally at least a 20 pack year history, opens up the potential diagnosis of a smoking asthmatic, COPD or ACO. To a certain extent these labels are arbitrary and of more importance is the identification of underlying treatable traits (79). Active smoking will lower FeNO measurements (80) and any trial of treatment with either ICS or OCS may be affected by the impact of smoking on the mechanism of action of corticosteroids (81). Current smoking should not have any impact on blood eosinophils, spirometry, or bronchodilator reversibility.

Occupational Asthma

Asthma either caused by occupation or aggravated by occupation should always be considered in people diagnosed with asthma during their working lives. Studies have suggested that up to 10% of people diagnosed with asthma in adult life have an occupational cause (82). Occupational asthma can be simply screened for in primary care by asking whether asthma symptoms improve at the weekend or when on holiday (83). If the answer to either of these questions is yes then a full occupational history including exposures should be obtained. The diagnosis of occupational asthma is extremely important given that moving away from the relevant exposure may allow for their asthma to be cured, providing that this occurs in a timely fashion. Everyone with occupational asthma should be referred to a specialist occupational lung disease unit who will perform detailed peak flow monitoring, potentially skin prick tests for the relevant allergens and on occasion challenge testing.

SUMMARY

There is definite consensus among adult physicians and pediatricians that asthma is a heterogeneous disease underpinned by numerous pathophysiological mechanisms. It is no longer acceptable to make a diagnosis in a patient of any age simply from a history and physical examination and by assessing a response to a trial of therapy. Young preschool aged children may not be able to undertake tests of lung function and inflammation that require voluntary maneuvers, but they can have assessments of atopy and blood eosinophils to help make a diagnosis and guide therapy. Children and adults above 5 years should all have at least some objective confirmation to support the diagnosis using lung function tests and non-invasive assessments of airway inflammation using exhaled nitric oxide. These tests can be undertaken in a primary or secondary care setting providing adequate education and training in the use and interpretation of the equipment is made available to health professionals. There is no gold standard test, but we now know that to avoid under diagnosis, over diagnosis and misdiagnosis, it is essential to undertake objective tests to support a diagnosis of asthma and to identify treatable traits of the airway disease.

AUTHOR CONTRIBUTIONS

All authors listed have made a substantial, direct and intellectual contribution to the work, and approved it for publication.

REFERENCES

1. Papi A, Brightling C, Pedersen SE, Reddel HK. Asthma. *Lancet.* (2018) 391:783–800. doi: 10.1016/S0140-6736(17)33311-1
2. Pavord ID, Beasley R, Agusti A, Anderson GP, Bel E, Brusselle G, et al. After asthma: redefining airways diseases. *Lancet.* (2018) 391:350–400. doi: 10.1016/S0140-6736(17)30879-6
3. Becker AB, Abrams EM. Asthma guidelines: the Global Initiative for Asthma in relation to national guidelines. *Curr Opin Allergy Clin Immunol.* (2017) 17:99–103. doi: 10.1097/ACI.0000000000000346
4. Patel SP, Jarvelin MR, Little MP. Systematic review of worldwide variations of the prevalence of wheezing symptoms in children. *Environ Health.* (2008) 7:57. doi: 10.1186/1476-069X-7-57
5. Spurgeon D. One third of diagnoses of asthma in Canada are wrong, study finds. *BMJ.* (2008) 337:a2665. doi: 10.1136/bmj.a2665
6. Stanbrook MB, Kaplan A. The error of not measuring asthma. *CMAJ.* (2008) 179:1099–102. doi: 10.1503/cmaj.081665
7. Pakhale S, Sumner A, Coyle D, Vandemheen K, Aaron S. (Correcting) misdiagnoses of asthma: a cost effectiveness analysis. *BMC Pulmonary Med.* (2011) 11:27. doi: 10.1186/1471-2466-11-27
8. Aaron SD, Vandemheen KL, FitzGerald JM, Ainslie M, Gupta S, Lemiere C, et al. Reevaluation of diagnosis in adults with physician-diagnosed asthma. *JAMA.* (2017) 317:269–79. doi: 10.1001/jama.2016.19627
9. MacNeil J, Loves RH, Aaron SD. Addressing the misdiagnosis of asthma in adults: where does it go wrong? *Expert Rev Respir Med.* (2016) 10:1187–98. doi: 10.1080/17476348.2016.1242415
10. Thorley J. NICE issues draft guideline for asthma diagnosis. *Lancet Respir Med.* (2015) 3:184. doi: 10.1016/S2213-2600(15)00038-7
11. Keeley D, Baxter N. Conflicting asthma guidelines cause confusion in primary care. *BMJ.* (2018) 360:k29. doi: 10.1136/bmj.k29
12. Barnes PJ, Dweik RA, Gelb AF, Gibson PG, George SC, Grasemann H, et al. Exhaled nitric oxide in pulmonary diseases: a comprehensive review. *Chest.* (2010) 138:682–92. doi: 10.1378/chest.09-2090
13. Dweik RA, Boggs PB, Erzurum SC, Irvin CG, Leigh MW, Lundberg JO, et al. An official ATS clinical practice guideline: interpretation of exhaled nitric oxide levels (FENO) for clinical applications. *Am J Respir Crit Care Med.* (2011) 184:602–15. doi: 10.1164/rccm.9120-11ST
14. Guo Z, Wang Y, Xing G, Wang X. Diagnostic accuracy of fractional exhaled nitric oxide in asthma: a systematic review and meta-analysis of prospective studies. *J Asthma.* (2016) 53:404–12. doi: 10.3109/02770903.2015.1101132
15. Garcia-Marcos L, Edwards J, Kennington E, Aurora P, Baraldi E, Carraro S, et al. Priorities for future research into asthma diagnostic tools: a PAN-EU consensus exercise from the European asthma research innovation partnership (EARIP). *Clin Exp Allergy.* (2018) 48:104–20. doi: 10.1111/cea.13080
16. Harnan S, Essat M, Gomersall T, Tappenden P, Wong R, Lawson R, et al. Exhaled nitric oxide for the diagnosis of asthma in adults and children: a systematic review. *Value Health.* (2015) 18:A345. doi: 10.1016/j.jval.2015.09.607
17. Peirsman EJ, Carvelli TJ, Hage PY, Hanssens LS, Pattyn L, Raes MM, et al. Exhaled nitric oxide in childhood allergic asthma management: a randomised controlled trial. *Pediatr Pulmonol.* (2014) 49:624–31. doi: 10.1002/ppul.22873
18. Sivan Y, Gadish T, Fireman E, Soferman R. The use of exhaled nitric oxide in the diagnosis of asthma in school children. *J Pediatr.* (2009) 155:211–6. doi: 10.1016/j.jpeds.2009.02.034
19. Paraskakis E, Brindicci C, Fleming L, Krol R, Kharitonov SA, Wilson NM, et al. Measurement of bronchial and alveolar nitric oxide production in normal children and children with asthma. *Am J Respir Crit Care Med.* (2006) 174:260–7. doi: 10.1164/rccm.200506-962OC
20. Sordillo JE, Webb T, Kwan D, Kamel J, Hoffman E, Milton DK, et al. Allergen exposure modifies the relation of sensitization to fraction of exhaled nitric

oxide levels in children at risk for allergy and asthma. *J Allergy Clin Immunol.* (2011) 127:1165–72.e1165. doi: 10.1016/j.jaci.2011.01.066

21. Rao DR, Phipatanakul W. An overview of fractional exhaled nitric oxide and children with asthma. *Expert Rev Clin Immunol.* (2016) 12:521–30. doi: 10.1586/1744666X.2016.1141049
22. Yancey SW, Keene ON, Albers FC, Ortega H, Bates S, Bleecker ER, et al. Biomarkers for severe eosinophilic asthma. *J Allergy Clin Immunol.* (2017) 140:1509–18. doi: 10.1016/j.jaci.2017.10.005
23. Korevaar DA, Westerhof GA, Wang J, Cohen JF, Spijker R, Sterk PJ, et al. Diagnostic accuracy of minimally invasive markers for detection of airway eosinophilia in asthma: a systematic review and meta-analysis. *Lancet Respir Med.* (2015) 3:290–300. doi: 10.1016/S2213-2600(15)00050-8
24. Westerhof GA, Korevaar DA, Amelink M, de Nijs SB, de Groot JC, Wang J, et al. Biomarkers to identify sputum eosinophilia in different adult asthma phenotypes. *Eur Respir J.* (2015) 46:688–96. doi: 10.1183/09031936.00012415
25. Petsky HL, Kew KM, Turner C, Chang AB. Exhaled nitric oxide levels to guide treatment for adults with asthma. *Cochrane Database Syst Rev.* (2016) 9:CD011440. doi: 10.1002/14651858.CD011440.pub2
26. Fleming L, Tsartsali L, Wilson N, Regamey N, Bush A. Longitudinal relationship between sputum eosinophils and exhaled nitric oxide in children with asthma. *Am J Respir Crit Care Med.* (2013) 188:400–2. doi: 10.1164/rccm.201212-2156LE
27. Aldrimer M, Ridefelt P, Rodoo P, Niklasson F, Gustafsson J, Hellberg D. Population-based pediatric reference intervals for hematology, iron and transferrin. *Scand J Clin Lab Invest.* (2013) 73:253–61. doi: 10.3109/00365513.2013.769625
28. Arbes SJ Jr., Calatroni A, Mitchell HE, Gergen PJ. Age-dependent interaction between atopy and eosinophils in asthma cases: results from NHANES 2005–2006. *Clin Exp Allergy.* (2013) 43:544–51. doi: 10.1111/cea.12069
29. Ullmann N, Bossley CJ, Fleming L, Silvestri M, Bush A, Saglani S. Blood eosinophil counts rarely reflect airway eosinophilia in children with severe asthma. *Allergy.* (2013) 68:402–6. doi: 10.1111/all.12101
30. van Bragt J, Vijverberg SJH, Weersink EJM, Richards LB, Neerincx AH, Sterk PJ, et al. Blood biomarkers in chronic airways diseases and their role in diagnosis and management. *Expert Rev Respir Med.* (2018) 12:361–74. doi: 10.1080/17476348.2018.1457440
31. FitzGerald JM, Bleecker ER, Menzies-Gow A, Zangrilli JG, Hirsch I, Metcalfe P, et al. Predictors of enhanced response with benralizumab for patients with severe asthma: pooled analysis of the SIROCCO and CALIMA studies. *Lancet Respir Med.* (2018) 6:51–64. doi: 10.1016/S2213-2600(17)30344-2
32. Hambleton K, Connolly CM, Borg C, Davies JH, Jeffers HP, Russell RE, et al. Comparison of the peripheral blood eosinophil count using near-patient testing and standard automated laboratory measurement in healthy, asthmatic and COPD subjects. *Int J Chronic Obstruct Pulmonary Dis.* (2017) 12:2771–5. doi: 10.2147/COPD.S147216
33. Gershon AS, Victor JC, Guan J, Aaron SD, To T. Pulmonary function testing in the diagnosis of asthma: a population study. *Chest.* (2012) 141:1190–6. doi: 10.1378/chest.11-0831
34. Holt NR, Thompson BR, Miller B, Borg BM. Substantial variation exists in spirometry interpretation practices for airflow obstruction in accredited lung function laboratories across Australian and New Zealand. *Intern Med J.* (2018) 49:41–7. doi: 10.1111/imj.14047
35. Lusuardi M, De Benedetto F, Paggiaro P, Sanguinetti CM, Brazzola G, Ferri P, et al. A randomized controlled trial on office spirometry in asthma and COPD in standard general practice: data from spirometry in Asthma and COPD: a comparative evaluation Italian study. *Chest.* (2006) 129:844–52. doi: 10.1378/chest.129.4.844
36. Sokol KC, Sharma G, Lin YL, Goldblum RM. Choosing wisely: adherence by physicians to recommended use of spirometry in the diagnosis and management of adult asthma. *Am J Med.* (2015) 128:502–8. doi: 10.1016/j.amjmed.2014.12.006
37. Cloutier MM, Salo PM, Akinbami LJ, Cohn RD, Wilkerson JC, Diette GB, et al. Clinician agreement, self-efficacy, and adherence with the guidelines for the diagnosis and management of asthma. *J Allergy Clin Immunol Pract.* (2018) 6:886–94.e4. doi: 10.1016/j.jaip.2018.01.018
38. Heffler E, Crimi C, Mancuso S, Campisi R, Puggioni F, Brussino L, et al. Misdiagnosis of asthma and COPD and underuse of spirometry in primary care unselected patients. *Respir Med.* (2018) 142:48–52. doi: 10.1016/j.rmed.2018.07.015
39. Dombkowski KJ, Hassan F, Wasilevich EA, Clark SJ. Spirometry use among pediatric primary care physicians. *Pediatrics.* (2010) 126:682–7. doi: 10.1542/peds.2010-0362
40. Zanconato S, Meneghelli G, Braga R, Zacchello F, Baraldi E. Office spirometry in primary care pediatrics: a pilot study. *Pediatrics.* (2005) 116:e792–7. doi: 10.1542/peds.2005-0487
41. Ayuk AC, Uwaezuoke SN, Ndukwu CI, Ndu IK, Iloh KK, Okoli CV. Spirometry in asthma care: a review of the trends and challenges in pediatric practice. *Clin Med Insights Pediatr.* (2017) 11:1179556517720675. doi: 10.1177/1179556517720675
42. Bush A, Fleming L, Saglani S. Severe asthma in children. *Respirology.* (2017) 22:886–97. doi: 10.1111/resp.13085
43. Murray C, Foden P, Lowe L, Durrington H, Custovic A, Simpson A. Diagnosis of asthma in symptomatic children based on measures of lung function: an analysis of data from a population-based birth cohort study. *Lancet Child Adolescent Health.* (2017) 1:114–23. doi: 10.1016/S2352-4642(17)30008-1
44. Latzin P, Fuchs O. Asthma diagnosis in children: more evidence needed. *Lancet Child Adolesc Health.* (2017) 1:83–5. doi: 10.1016/S2352-4642(17)30019-6
45. Brigham EP, West NE. Diagnosis of asthma: diagnostic testing. *Int Forum Allergy Rhinol.* (2015) 5 (Suppl 1):S27–30. doi: 10.1002/alr.21597
46. Vilozni D, Hakim F, Livnat G, Ofek M, Bar-Yoseph R, Bentur L. Assessment of airway bronchodilation by spirometry compared to airway obstruction in young children with asthma. *Can Respir J.* (2016) 2016:5394876. doi: 10.1155/2016/5394876
47. Tse SM, Gold DR, Sordillo JE, Hoffman EB, Gillman MW, Rifas-Shiman SL, et al. Diagnostic accuracy of the bronchodilator response in children. *J Allergy Clin Immunol.* (2013) 132:554–9.e555. doi: 10.1016/j.jaci.2013.03.031
48. Quanjer PH, Hall GL, Stanojevic S, Cole TJ, Stocks J. Age- and height-based prediction bias in spirometry reference equations. *Eur Respir J.* (2012) 40:190–7. doi: 10.1183/09031936.00161011
49. Krishnan S, Dozor AJ, Bacharier L, Lang JE, Irvin CG, Kaminsky D, et al. Clinical characterization of children with resistant airflow obstruction, a multicenter study. *J Asthma.* (2018) doi: 10.1080/02770903.2018.1477956. [Epub ahead of print].
50. Konstantellou E, Papaioannou AI, Loukides S, Patentalakis G, Papaporfyriou A, Hillas G, et al. Persistent airflow obstruction in patients with asthma: characteristics of a distinct clinical phenotype. *Respir Med.* (2015) 109:1404–9. doi: 10.1016/j.rmed.2015.09.009
51. Sin DD, Miravitlles M, Mannino DM, Soriano JB, Price D, Celli BR, et al. What is asthma-COPD overlap syndrome? Towards a consensus definition from a round table discussion. *Eur Respir J.* (2016) 48:664–73. doi: 10.1183/13993003.00436-2016
52. Leung JM, Sin DD. Asthma-COPD overlap syndrome: pathogenesis, clinical features, and therapeutic targets. *BMJ.* (2017) 358:j3772. doi: 10.1136/bmj.j3772
53. Bush A, Saglani S. Management of severe asthma in children. *Lancet.* (2010) 376:814–25. doi: 10.1016/S0140-6736(10)61054-9
54. Beydon N. Pulmonary function testing in young children. *Paediatr Respir Rev.* (2009) 10:208–13. doi: 10.1016/j.prrv.2009.03.001
55. Calogero C, Fenu G, Lombardi E. Measuring airway obstruction in severe asthma in children. *Front Pediatr.* (2018) 6:189. doi: 10.3389/fped.2018.00189
56. Galant SP, Komarow HD, Shin HW, Siddiqui S, Lipworth BJ. The case for impulse oscillometry in the management of asthma in children and adults. *Ann Allergy Asthma Immunol.* (2017) 118:664–71. doi: 10.1016/j.anai.2017.04.009
57. Luo J, Liu D, Chen G, Liang B, Liu C. Clinical roles of lung volumes detected by body plethysmography and helium dilution in asthmatic patients: a correlation and diagnosis analysis. *Sci Rep.* (2017) 7:40870. doi: 10.1038/srep40870
58. Lexmond AJ, Singh D, Frijlink HW, Clarke GW, Page CP, Forbes B, et al. Realising the potential of various inhaled airway challenge agents through improved delivery to the lungs. *Pulmonary Pharmacol Therapeut.* (2018) 49:27–35. doi: 10.1016/j.pupt.2018.01.004
59. Davis BE, Simonson SK, Blais CM, Cockcroft DW. Methacholine challenge testing: a novel method for measuring

PD20. *Chest.* (2017) 152:1251–7. doi: 10.1016/j.chest.2017.09.001
60. Aggarwal B, Mulgirigama A, Berend N. Exercise-induced bronchoconstriction: prevalence, pathophysiology, patient impact, diagnosis and management. *NPJ Primary Care Respir Med.* (2018) 28:31. doi: 10.1038/s41533-018-0098-2
61. Buchvald F, Phillipsen LD, Hjuler T, Nielsen KG. Exercise-induced inspiratory symptoms in school children. *Pediatr Pulmonol.* (2016) 51:1200–5. doi: 10.1002/ppul.23530
62. Walsted ES, Hull JH, Sverrild A, Porsbjerg C, Backer V. Bronchial provocation testing does not detect exercise-induced laryngeal obstruction. *J Asthma.* (2017) 54:77–83. doi: 10.1080/02770903.2016.1195843
63. Martinez FD, Vercelli D. Asthma. *Lancet.* (2013) 382:1360–72. doi: 10.1016/S0140-6736(13)61536-6
64. Oksel C, Custovic A. Development of allergic sensitization and its relevance to paediatric asthma. *Curr Opin Allergy Clin Immunol.* (2018) 18:109–16. doi: 10.1097/ACI.0000000000000430
65. Strina A, Barreto ML, Cooper PJ, Rodrigues LC. Risk factors for non-atopic asthma/wheeze in children and adolescents: a systematic review. *Emerg Themes Epidemiol.* (2014) 11:5. doi: 10.1186/1742-7622-11-5
66. de Nijs SB, Venekamp LN, Bel EH. Adult-onset asthma: is it really different? *Eur Respir Rev.* (2013) 22:44–52. doi: 10.1183/09059180.00007112
67. Marinho S, Simpson A, Marsden P, Smith JA, Custovic A. Quantification of atopy, lung function and airway hypersensitivity in adults. *Clin Transl Allergy.* (2011) 1:16. doi: 10.1186/2045-7022-1-16
68. Pillai P, Chan YC, Wu SY, Ohm-Laursen L, Thomas C, Durham SR, et al. Omalizumab reduces bronchial mucosal IgE and improves lung function in non-atopic asthma. *Eur Respir J.* (2016) 48:1593–601. doi: 10.1183/13993003.01501-2015
69. McCracken JL, Veeranki SP, Ameredes BT, Calhoun WJ. Diagnosis and management of asthma in adults: a review. *JAMA.* (2017) 318:279–90. doi: 10.1001/jama.2017.8372
70. *British Guideline on the Management of Asthma.* (2016). Available online at: https://wwwbrit-thoracicorguk/document-library/clinical-information/asthma/btssign-asthma-guideline-quick-reference-guide-2016/ (accessed January 15, 2019).
71. NIH. *Asthma: Diagnosis and Monitoring of Asthma in Adults, Children and Young People.* London: National Institute for Health and Care Excellence (2017).
72. Brand PL, Baraldi E, Bisgaard H, Boner AL, Castro-Rodriguez JA, Custovic A, et al. Definition, assessment and treatment of wheezing disorders in preschool children: an evidence-based approach. *EurRespir J.* (2008) 32:1096–110. doi: 10.1183/09031936.00002108
73. Brand PL, Caudri D, Eber E, Gaillard EA, Garcia-Marcos L, Hedlin G, et al. Classification and pharmacological treatment of preschool wheezing: changes since 2008. *Eur Respir J.* (2014) 43:1172–7. doi: 10.1183/09031936.00199913
74. Bush A, Grigg J, Saglani S. Managing wheeze in preschool children. *BMJ.* (2014) 348:g15. doi: 10.1136/bmj.g15
75. Fitzpatrick AM, Jackson DJ, Mauger DT, Boehmer SJ, Phipatanakul W, Sheehan WJ, et al. Individualized therapy for persistent asthma in young children. *J Allergy Clin Immunol.* (2016) 138:1608–18.e1612. doi: 10.1016/j.jaci.2016.09.028
76. Kwong CG, Bacharier LB. Microbes and the role of antibiotic treatment for wheezy lower respiratory tract illnesses in preschool children. *Curr Allergy Asthma Rep.* (2017) 17:34. doi: 10.1007/s11882-017-0701-6
77. Skloot GS, Busse PJ, Braman SS, Kovacs EJ, Dixon AE, Vaz Fragoso CA, et al. An Official American Thoracic Society Workshop Report: evaluation and management of asthma in the elderly. *Ann Am Thoracic Soc.* (2016) 13:2064–77. doi: 10.1513/AnnalsATS.201608-658ST
78. Jacinto T, Malinovschi A, Janson C, Fonseca J, Alving K. Evolution of exhaled nitric oxide levels throughout development and aging of healthy humans. *J Breath Res.* (2015) 9:036005. doi: 10.1088/1752-7155/9/3/036005
79. Agusti A, Bel E, Thomas M, Vogelmeier C, Brusselle G, Holgate S, et al. Treatable traits: toward precision medicine of chronic airway diseases. *Eur Respir J.* (2016) 47:410–9. doi: 10.1183/13993003.01359-2015
80. Habib SS, Ahmed SM, Al Drees AM, Husain A. Effect of cigarette smoking on fractional exhaled nitric oxide in Saudi medical college students. *JPMA.* (2011) 61:120–3.
81. Chalmers GW, Macleod KJ, Little SA, Thomson LJ, McSharry CP, Thomson NC. Influence of cigarette smoking on inhaled corticosteroid treatment in mild asthma. *Thorax.* (2002) 57:226–30. doi: 10.1136/thorax.57.3.226
82. Ghosh RE, Cullinan P, Fishwick D, Hoyle J, Warburton CJ, Strachan DP, et al. Asthma and occupation in the 1958 birth cohort. *Thorax.* (2013) 68:365–71. doi: 10.1136/thoraxjnl-2012-202151
83. Fishwick D, Barber C, Walker S, Scott A. Asthma in the workplace: a case-based discussion and review of current evidence. *Primary Care Respir J.* (2013) 22:244–8. doi: 10.4104/pcrj.2013.00038

15

Interventions on Adherence to Treatment in Children with Severe Asthma

Barbara Boutopoulou [1†], Despoina Koumpagioti [2†], Vasiliki Matziou [3], Kostas N. Priftis [1] and Konstantinos Douros [1]*

[1] Respiratory and Allergy Unit, 3rd Pediatric Department of National and Kapodistrian University of Athens, University General Hospital "Attikon," Athens, Greece, [2] 2nd Pediatric Department of National and Kapodistrian University of Athens, "P & A Kiriakou" Children Hospital, Athens, Greece, [3] Faculty of Nursing, National and Kapodistrian University of Athens, Athens, Greece

***Correspondence:**
Barbara Boutopoulou
bmpoutopoulou@gmail.com

† These authors have contributed equally to this work

Introduction: Poor adherence to inhaled medication is a commonly encountered problem among children with asthma. However, there is a relatively paucity of data regarding the adherence of children with severe asthma, as well as the merit of any interventions to improve this adherence.

Objectives: The aim of this systematic review was to identify the available literature on the rate of adherence and the influence of interventions in improving adherence to controller inhaled medication, in children with severe asthma.

Methods: A systematic literature search was performed in MEDLINE/PubMed, Cochrane Library, and Scopus databases. Studies were included in the present review if their target population were children and/or adolescents with severe asthma and presented data on medication adherence before and after a given intervention.

Results: A total of seven studies, conducted in USA, Canada, and UK, and published between 2012 and 2018, met the inclusion criteria. Adherence to controller medication was assessed via either objective or subjective measures (questionnaires), or a combination of them. Interventions included communication during pediatric visits and audio-taped medical visits, individualized care programs, electronic monitoring devices, interactive website and peak–flow prediction with feedback. Adherence rates for the baseline (before intervention) or for the control groups ranged from 28 to 67%. In general, there was a significant improvement of adherence after intervention with rates increasing to 49–81%.

Conclusion: Adherence rate in children with severe asthma is not satisfactory but it can be improved after proper interventions. Nevertheless, the heterogeneity among adherence assessment tools, and the variety of interventions, in combination with the lack of studies focusing on severe asthma, highlight the need for further research in this field.

Keywords: children, severe asthma, difficult asthma, inhaled treatment, adherence

INTRODUCTION

Asthma is a heterogeneous disease, usually characterized by chronic airway inflammation. It is defined by the history of respiratory symptoms such as wheeze, shortness of breath, chest tightness, and cough that vary over time and in intensity, together with variable expiratory airflow limitation (1). Asthma affects 1–18% of the population in different countries. It is one of the main causes of disability, health care services utilization, and quality of life impairment (2–5). It is estimated that about 14% of the children worldwide experience asthma symptoms. Asthma management aims to achieve good symptom control; maintain normal activities; minimize asthma attacks; reduce the side effects of treatment and as a result prevent the progression of obstructive lung damage during growth and then later in life (2).

Although the majority of asthma patients can be effectively controlled with the available medications, a substantial subset remains uncontrolled despite being offered the optimal therapy (6).

Severe asthma, according to European Respiratory Society (ERS)/American Thoracic Society (ATS) is asthma which requires Step 4 or 5 treatment [according to Global Initiative for Asthma (GINA) guidelines], e.g., high dose inhaled corticosteroids (ICS) and long-acting beta agonists (LABA) or leukotriene modifier/theophylline for the previous year or systemic ICS for $\geq$50% of the previous year to prevent it from becoming "uncontrolled" or which remains "uncontrolled" despite this therapy (6). Severe asthma includes patients with refractory or treatment-resistant asthma, or patients with incomplete response to treatment due to comorbidities (5). The primary approach of a child with problematic, severe respiratory symptoms, who is unresponsive to prescribed asthma therapy should be the confirmation of asthma diagnosis; secondly, one should explore if the child belongs to the category of "difficult-to-treat asthma" (2). The latter term is reserved for patients with ongoing factors that interfere with achieving good asthma control (allergen exposure, poor adherence), severe therapy-resistant asthma, asthma plus comorbidities (gastroesophageal reflux, obesity, obstructive apnea), or any combination of the above (7). Clinicians should also be aware of a prevalent cluster of chronic upper airway comorbidities, such as chronic rhinosinusitis and allergic rhinitis, which is recognized to patients with severe asthma but also seems that contribute to worsen asthma control and complicate asthma diagnosis and management (8). Distinguishing between severe asthma and uncontrolled asthma is crucial since the latter can be due to causes that can be more or less easily improved, such as the correction of a faulty inhaler technique and poor adherence (2, 9, 10).

Adherence is defined as the extent to which the patient's behavior matches the agreed recommendations from the prescriber. Patients can follow or not their doctors' recommendations, but failure to do so should not be a reason to blame the patient (11, 12). Adherence of asthmatics to long-term inhaled treatment has contributed substantial to asthma control and to morbidity reduction, yet, in general, it still remains suboptimal (13–16). The suboptimal adherence leads to poorer clinical outcomes and increased health care costs (17, 18).

Poor adherence (<60%) (19) to inhaled medication should be considered in all "difficult to control" patients. It has been reported that only 55% of children with moderate/severe persistent asthma use their controller medication daily (20).

Low adherence rates suggest an urgent need to increase adherence in order to reduce the burden of the disease. The improvement of adherence will result in better asthma control, and therefore, in a reduction of asthma severity (16, 21, 22). Shared decision making for medication/dose choice (23), inhaler reminders (24), home visits (25), prescribing ICS once daily versus twice (26), are all some of the interventions that are conducive to adherence improvement (2).

Although there are quite a few published reviews on the adherence of asthmatic children to controller medication and the effects of various interventions thereupon, there is still a lack of focus on severe asthma. Our aim in this systematic review was to identify the available literature on the rate of adherence and the influence of various interventions in improving adherence to controller inhaled medication, in children with severe asthma.

METHODS

This systematic review was based on the Preferred Reporting Items for Systematic Reviews and Meta—Analyses (PRISMA) statement, which aims to be the most accurate elaboration of a systematic review (27).

Two independent reviewers searched for publications in three of the most commonly used databases in medicine: Pubmed/Medline, Cochrane Library and Scopus. Key word combinations of "children," "severe asthma," "difficult asthma," "inhaled treatment," and "adherence," were used to retrieve articles with these key words in title and abstract.

The criteria included were as follows:

1) Articles which were published from January of 2012 to March of 2018;
2) Articles written in English;
3) Studies that targeted children and/or adolescents;
4) Studies which have focused on severe asthma (as their main aim or as a subcategory of the study population); and
5) Studies on the effect of an intervention on adherence rate (as their main aim or as a subcategory of the study population).

Data Extraction

The data extraction was conducted by two reviewers. The characteristics collected for each study were references, sample characteristics, study design, duration, adherence assessment, intervention tools, and outcomes. **Table 1** illustrates the main studies' characteristics.

RESULTS

Studies Selection

The search of the 3 databases retrieved 644 articles. Of these, 284 were duplicates and were excluded. The remaining 360 articles were screened for relevance. The full texts of 23 articles were

TABLE 1 | Study characteristics.

References	Sample characteristics	Study design	Duration	Adherence assessment	Intervention tool	Outcomes
Jochmann et al. (19)	93 children (STRA $n = 21$, Difficult asthma $n = 51$), 5–17 years, outpatient	Prospective observational cohort	6 months	Electronic monitoring device (smartinhaler) MARS-5 rating scale for self-reported adherence	Electronic monitoring	Median adherence for whole population was 74%. Good adherence (≥80%) in 42% of patients, Suboptimal adherence (<80%) in 58% ($p < 0.0065$).
Feldman et al. (14)	192 children (severe persistent $n = 52$), 7–15 years (feedback group), 7–12 years (no feedback group), outpatient	Prospective longitudinal	6 weeks	Doser CT (MediTrack)	PEF prediction with feedback	Adherence to PEF feedback group 48.8 ± 4.5(%) and to no PEF feedback group 27.5 ± 4.9 (%) ($p = 0.002$).
Duncan et al. (29)	48 youth (severe persistent $n = 8$), 9–15 years, outpatient	Randomized controlled trial	5 months	Electronic monitoring device (MDILog-II)	Teamwork intervention (TI) Asthma education (AE) Standard care (SC)	Mean daily adherence for TI group (20-weeks) was 81%, while for the AE group 33.6% and for the SC group 37%.
Sleath et al. (28)	259 children (moderate/severe persistent $n = 185$), 8–16 years, outpatient	Prospective interventional	1 month	Questionnaire	Audio-taped medical visit and home visit interview	Children reported average control medication adherence was 72.4% (SD = 32.9; range, 0–100), while caregivers reported average control medication adherence 84.7% (SD = 26.1; range, 0–100).
Christakis et al. (31)	603 children (severe persistent $n = 14$) , 2–10 years, outpatient	Randomized controlled trial	6 months	Questionnaire	Tailored interactive website	Controller medicine users with persistent asthma (intervention group) at both time points had significantly better adherence than the control group ($p = 0.01$).
Guénette et al. (32)	61 adolescents, 12–17 years ($N = 349$, aged 12–45 years)	Pragmatic controlled clinical trial	12 months	Morisky Medication Adherence Scale (MMAS –4) Medication Possession Rate (MPR)	Integrated care program	The integrated program had statistically significant effectiveness on ICS adherence, $p = 0.0197$ (mean MMAS-4 at baseline/12 month follow-up = 1.98/1.70, $p = 0.051$, mean MRP at baseline/12 month follow-up 19.41/22.86, $p = 0.0629$).
Ellis et al. (30)	167 adolescents, 12–16 years, outpatient	Randomized controlled trial	12 months	Medication Adherence subscale	Multisystemic Therapy-Health Care (MST-HC)	MST-HC was associated with better controller medication adherence at 6 months postintervention ($p < 0.01$).

STRA, Severe therapy-resistant asthma; ICS, Inhaled Corticosteroids; PEF, Peak expiratory flow.

assessed for eligibility; and finally 7 articles were chosen for the systematic review.

The reasons for the exclusions are listed on the flow chart (**Figure 1**) which also provides the publication retrieval process.

Studies Description

Seven articles were included in the systematic review. Five of them were conducted in USA (14, 28–31); 1 in Canada (32); and 1 in UK (19).

Three studies were randomized controlled clinical trials (29–31), 1 was a controlled pragmatic clinical trial (32), 1 was a prospective observational cohort (19), 1 was a prospective longitudinal study (14), and 1 was a prospective interventional study (28).

Patients' recruitment was held mainly during outpatient visits. Guénette et al. (32) recruited patients with mediation of community pharmacists. Patients were children and their age ranged from 2 to 16 years old.

The total sample for severe asthma from the 7 studies was $n = 508$ children/adolescents, with the lowest sample size being $n = 8$ (29) and the highest $n = 185$ (28).

Severe asthma was a subcategory of the selected sample in all seven studies (14, 19, 28–32).

Adherence Assessment

Adherence in ICS treatment was evaluated through objective (14, 29), or subjective measures (28, 30, 31) or as a combination of both (19, 32). Objective measures of adherence assessment included electronic monitoring devices (Smartinhaler, Doser CT, MDILog-II) used in 4 of the studies (14, 19, 29, 32) and Medication Possession Ratio (MPR) used by Guénette et al. (32).

All three pre-mentioned devices developed as a canister attachment that fits on top of the majority of inhalers. They can provide accurate information on medication usage, including timing and number of doses taken, and all these recorded data can be used to guide asthma management (19).

Medication Possession Ratio (MPR) is a validated objective measure based on pharmacy records expressing the percentage of days supply received divided by a period of time and has been found to be more accurate than self-report (33).

Questionnaires are subjective measures for assessing adherence that are convenient and relatively unobtrusive and rely on self-report (34). The questionnaires used in the studies reported in this review were:

(1) Brief Medication Questionnaire, a tool for screening patients' adherence as well as their barriers to adherence. The tool includes a 5-item Regimen Screen that asks patients how they took each medication in the past week, a 2-item Belief Screen that asks about drug effects and bothersome features, and a 2-item Recall Screen about potential difficulties remembering (35);

(2) Morisky medication adherence scale (MMAS-4) which is a generic self-reported, medication-taking behavior scale using four questions about past medication use patterns (36);

(3) Medication Adherence Rating Scale (MARS-5) is a self-reported measure which evaluates both attitudes about medications and actual medication-taking behavior and consists of 10 items (37); and

(4) Medication Adherence subscale which measures adherence to controller medication (38).

Intervention Tools

Among the 7 studies, 3 had as a main research objective the increase of adherence rate after an intervention (28, 29, 31) whereas in the other 4 studies (14, 19, 30, 32) the adherence improvement rate was a subcategory of the findings.

Interventions design addressed solely the children (14, 19, 32), or there was also an element of parental involvement (28–31).

Briefly, Sleath et al. (28) audio-taped and coded communication during pediatric visits whether the provider included child or caregiver input into the asthma management treatment plan. Individualized care programs where health teams assess patients' and their caregivers' individual needs, share information and improve knowledge on asthma, were implemented in 3 of the studies (29, 30, 32). Christakis et al. (31) created a web-based tailored intervention aiming to increase children's positive beliefs about asthma management and Feldman et al. (14) used a piece of equipment where peak—flow prediction with feedback encouraged children to receive daily their inhaled treatment. Electronic monitoring devices were used in 1 study as an intervention (19) with the perception that adherence could improve following a period of monitoring.

The mean duration of interventions was 22 weeks, whereas the maximum (30, 32) and minimum duration (28) was 48 and 4 weeks, respectively.

Outcomes

Across the 7 studies, adherence rates for the baseline (before intervention) or for the control groups ranged from 28 to 67% (14, 29, 31); there was a remarkable improvement after intervention with adherence rates increasing to 49–81% (14, 28, 29, 31).

Feldman et al. (14) found a significant positive difference between intervention and the control group ($p = 0.02$) using PEF prediction with feedback. Christakis et al. (31) using an interactive website, also showed a significant correlation between intervention and adherence improvement. Concerning the implementation of individualized care programs, Guénette et al. (32) showed statistically significant effectiveness measuring the adherence with MMAS-4 Scale ($p = 0.0151$). Statistically significant correlation was also demonstrated in Ellis et al. (30) measurements ($p < 0.01$). Team Intervention in Duncan et al. (29) study had a positive impact in adherence rate in comparison with Standard Care (81 vs. 37% respectively). Suboptimal adherence rates after intervention were presented in Jochman et al. (19) (median adherence was 74%) similarly with Sleath et al. (28) (average control medication adherence as reported by children was 72.4%).

DISCUSSION

This systematic review isolated seven articles from the recent literature, which focused on the improvement of adherence to inhaled medication after specific intervention, in children with severe asthma. Overall, the results of this systematic review

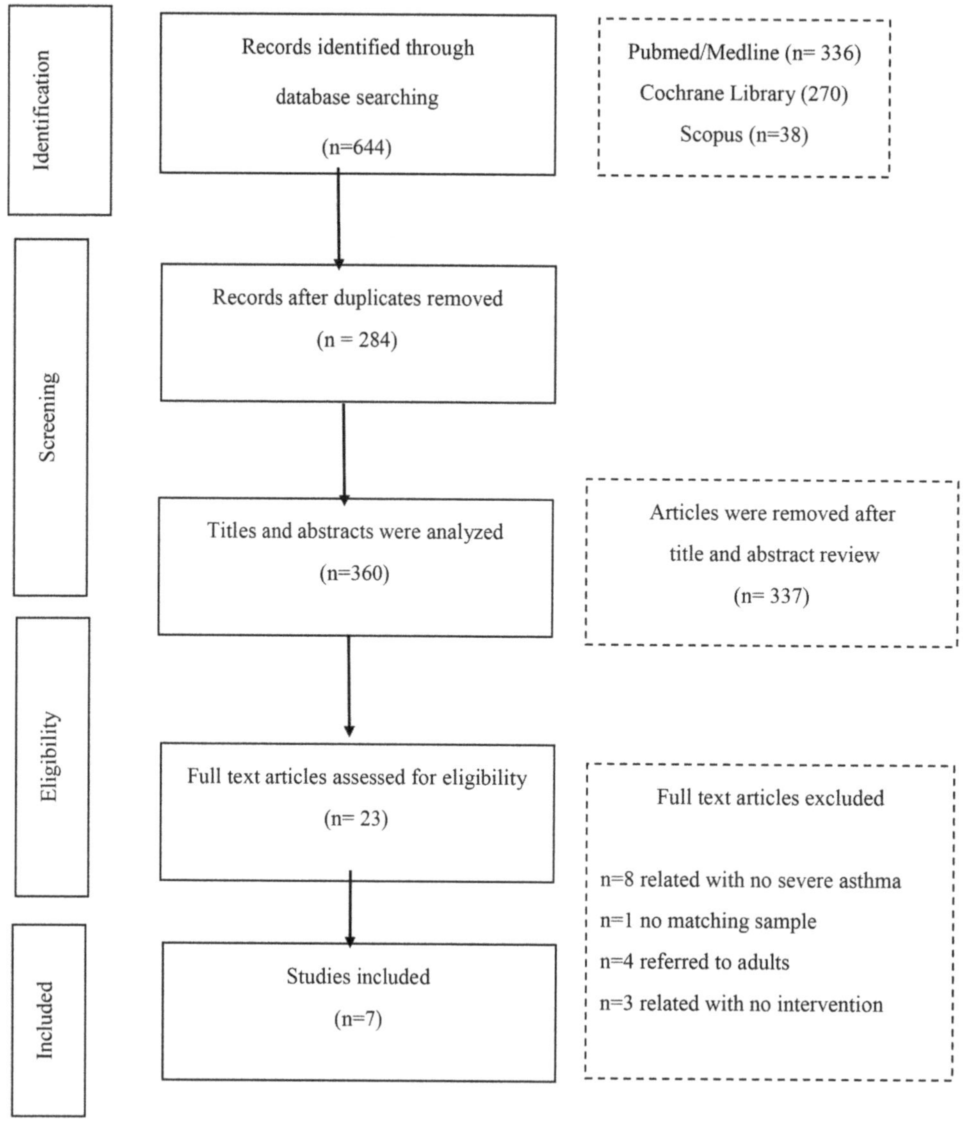

FIGURE 1 | Flow diagram of studies included in systematic review.

highlight the importance of interventions in respect of adherence improvement, in children suffering from severe asthma.

Adherence can be assessed with objective or subjective measures (34). Objective measures used in some of the studies included in the current review were different kinds of electronic monitoring devices and the Medication Possession Ratio. There have also been included studies that used questionnaires for the subjective assessment of adherence. Some of the main objective adherence measuring tools for asthma medication adherence are the electronic monitoring devices, the canister weight, and the pharmacy refill data (39). Electronic monitoring has been labeled as the "gold standard" for assessing adherence due to the objective and detailed data it provides, but the cost and technology requirements (e.g., equipment, staff training) prohibit its widespread routine clinical use (40, 41). At the same time, some of the subjective measuring tools are interviews, questionnaires and diary/self-reporting (34). Subjective measures are inexpensive, convenient, and relatively unobtrusive and have the potential to provide information on related issues. Although, they mostly rely on self-report, their accuracy depends on psychometric properties and may mask variability of adherence across regimen components if assessed globally (40–42). **Table 2** shows advantages and disavantages of methods for adherence assessment (34). As a great heterogeneity has appeared in asthma population regarding individualized capabilities, needs and preferences (43), researchers have concluded that more targeted and personalized methods of assessment are required (44).

Severe asthma in children is known to cause great morbidity, and raise asthma costs. The exact prevalence is unknown

TABLE 2 | Summary of objective and subjective methods for adherence assessment (34).

Objective methods
ELECTRONIC MONITORING
Advantages
• Potentially measuring a variety of adherence behaviors (e.g., timing of dose, technique)
Disadvantages
• Usually not measuring actual consumption of medication
• Difficult to use
• Costly
• Associated with technological issues (e.g., battery failure and malfunction)
• Doubtful acceptability to patients and families
PHARMACY REFILL DATA
Advantages
• Inexpensive
• Fairly accurate (correlating with electronic monitoring data)
Disadvantages
• Not measuring consumption
• May be patients use other pharmacies, stockpiling medications, or family members' medications
• Difficulty in logistics (e.g., staff time, privacy regulations) to obtain records
PILL COUNT/CANISTER WEIGHT
Advantages
• Inexpensive
• Fairly accurate (correlating with electronic monitoring data)
Disadvantages
• Patients may forget to bring their medication or miss their appointment
• May be manipulated by patient
• Not confirming that medication was taken
• Can be cumbersome for staff collecting and calculating
Subjective methods
INTERVIEWS
Advantages
• Can obtain extra information (e.g., regimen components, family issues), not only for medication use
• Can be administered over the telephone
Disadvantages
• Relies on self-report; subject to recall bias
• Psychometric properties and structure of the interview determine accuracy
DIARY/SELF-MONITORING
Advantages
• Reduces demands on memory
• Inexpensive
• Flexible-monitoring a range of variables in relation to a variety of adherence components
Disadvantages
• Relies on self-report; can be fabricated by patient
• Requires "adherence" to recording information, when adherence is a general concern
QUESTIONNAIRES
Advantages
• Inexpensive
• Convenient to be administered
Disadvantages
• Relies on self-report; subject to bias and social desirability
• May mask variability of adherence across regimen if assessed globally

although it is estimated that 2–5% of asthmatic children have severe disease (45, 46). There is an interrelated relationship between severe asthma and adherence and clinicians can overestimate the severity of asthma if they do not assess adherence. Furthermore, poor adherence can lead to severe asthma if it is not corrected (47). According to our findings, adherence rate at the baseline for children with severe asthma ranged between 28 and 67%, which is in agreement with Celano et al. (48) who studied children with persistent asthma. The adherence of children with any kind of asthma is approximately 30–70% (49).

In our systematic review, we retrieved studies with interventions aimed at improving adherence. Some of the intervention tools that had been used were: home interviews and audio-taped medical visits (28); individualized care programs (29, 30, 32); electronic monitoring device use (19); interactive website (31) and peak-flow prediction with feedback. In another systematic review and meta-analysis various behavioral interventions, e.g., providing families with specific strategies to manage the regimen; educational interventions providing basic information to families about the patient's illness and the importance of adherence; organizational interventions such as introducing calendars for self-monitoring and facilitating discussion with caregivers about their child's illness or supporting caregiver-health care provider interactions were meta-analyzed and discussed (50). Furthermore, two other studies investigated the efficacy and safety of text messages for dose reminding (51, 52).

Asthma control is associated with adherence level. Jochmann et al. (19) found that children with poor adherence maintained poor control, while Ellis et al. (30) showed that children with asthma knowledge and controller device use skills had better medication adherence. Similarly, in other studies, adolescents report that it is more likely to adhere to treatment when they feel hopeful (53), view management tasks as important and feel competent (54), or when they intend to follow treatment recommendations (55, 56). Increased levels of self-efficacy are associated with better adherence, as well (57, 58). Adherence to ICS was an independent strong predictor of long term asthma control, with highest levels of asthma control found when the adherence raised above 80% of prescribed doses (16).

Our review showed that adherence rate in children with severe asthma can be increased after a proper intervention. In the studies included in our review, there was a significant increase of adherence rate, from 28–67% to 49–81%. There is a relatively lack of studies focusing on severe asthma, but the above findings are in agreement with the results of studies dealing with all kinds of asthma in children (24, 59). Although, the majority of studies have shown a positive effect, there are some instances where intervention with electronic asthma medication reminders did not improve the adherence rate (32, 51). Also, a scheduled follow up visit in combination with a comprehensive asthma management care program implemented in preschool children with asthma in the Netherlands did not correct adherence rates (60). A systematic review and meta-analysis found the studies that applied adherence education as intervention achieved a benefit of 20% points over control, while electronic trackers or reminders led to better adherence rates of 10% points. Researchers concluded that interventions' results depend on the group target, method and duration of intervention (61).

The main limitations of this review is the lack of studies focusing on severe asthma in children as most of the studies investigate adherence in children in the community and adult severe asthmatics rather than severely asthmatic children. Additionally, there is heterogeneity in the definitions of severe asthma among studies, a problem that has already been noticed by other researchers (62). Studies used different adherence assessment tools, therefore results were presented in various ways.

A weak point of all 7 studies is that it is not clear whether the adherence improvement was clinically meaningful. Literature suggests that in order to maintain asthma control, adherence rates have to be in excess of 80% (63).

CONCLUSION

Adherence interventions have a positive impact on adherence rate in children with severe asthma. The remarkable heterogeneity between adherence assessment tools, and interventions, combined with the lack of studies focused on severe asthma, highlight the research gap in this field. There is a great need for further research focused exclusively on severe asthma and adherence treatment, in children.

AUTHOR CONTRIBUTIONS

BB and DK contributed equally to this review. They did the literature research and the main writing of the article. VM, KP, and KD did all the academic support and the corrections during the whole process. KD did the finally fixing in English also.

REFERENCES

1. Pavord ID, Beasley R, Agusti A, Anderson GP, Bel E, Brussell G, et al. After asthma: redefining airways diseases. *Lancet* (2017) 391:350–400. doi: 10.1016/S0140-6736(17)30879-6
2. ISAAC steering Committee. Worldwide variations in the prevalence of asthma symptoms: the Intrenational Study of Asthma and Allergies in Childhood (ISAAC). *Eur Respir J.* (1998) 12:315–35. doi: 10.1183/09031936.98.12020315
3. Bender BG, Rand C. Medication non-adherence and asthma treatment cost. *Curr Opin Allergy Clin Immunol.* (2004) 4:191–5. doi: 10.1097/01.all.0000129449.73727.cf
4. Engelkes M, Janssens HM, de Jongste JC, Sturkenboom MC, Verhamme KM. Medication adherence and the risk of severe asthma exacerbations: a systematic review. *Eur Respir J.* (2015) 45:396–407. doi: 10.1183/09031936.00075614
5. GINA Report, Global Strategy for Asthma Management and Prevention. *From the Global Strategy for Asthma Management and Prevention, Global Initiative for Asthma (GINA)* (2018). Available online at: http://www.ginaasthma.org (Accessed April 4, 2018).
6. Chung KF, Wenzel SE, Brozek JL, Bush A, Castro M, Sterk PJ, et al. International ERS/ATS guidelines on definition, evaluation and treatment of severe asthma. *Eur Respir J.* (2014) 43:343–73. doi: 10.1183/09031936.00202013
7. Bush A, Fleming L, Saglani S. Severe asthma in children. *Respirology* (2017) 22:886–97. doi: 10.1111/resp.13085
8. Licari A, Brambilla I, De Filippo M, Poddighe D, Castagnoli R, Marseglia GL. The role of upper airway pathology as a co-morbidity in severe asthma. *Expert Rev Respir Med.* (2017) 11:855–65. doi: 10.1080/17476348.2017.1381564
9. Melani AS, Bonavia M, Cilenti V, Cinti C, Lodi M, Martucci P, et al. Inhaler mishandling remains common in real life and is associated with reduced disease control. *Respir Med.* (2011) 105:930–8. doi: 10.1016/j.rmed.2011.01.005
10. Boulet LP, Vervloet D, Magar Y, Foster JM. Adherence: the goal to control asthma. *Clin Chest Med.* (2012) 33:405–17. doi: 10.1016/j.ccm.2012.06.002
11. Haynes RB. Determinants of compliance: the disease and the mechanics of treatment. In: Haynes RB, Taylor DW, Sackett DL, editors. *Compliance in Health Care.* Baltimore, MD: Johns Hopkins University Press (1979). p. 49–62.
12. Horne R. Compliance, adherence and concordance: Implications for asthma treatment. *Chest* (2006) 130:65–72. doi: 10.1378/chest.130.1_suppl.65S
13. Klok T, Kaptein AA, Duiverman EJ, Brand PL. High inhaled corticosteroids adherence in childhood asthma: the role of medication beliefs. *Eur Respir J.* (2012) 40:1149–55. doi: 10.1183/09031936.00191511
14. Feldman JM, Kutner H, Matte L, Lupkin M, Steinberg D, Sidora-Arcoleo K, et al. Prediction of peak flow values followed by feedback improves perception of lung function and adherence to inhaled corticosteroids in children with asthma. *Thorax* (2012) 67:1040–5. doi: 10.1136/thoraxjnl-2012-201789
15. Vasbinder E, Dahhan N, Wolf B, Zoer J, Blankman E, Bosman D, et al. The association of ethnicity with electronically measured adherence to inhaled corticosteroids in children. *Eur J Clin Pharmacol.* (2013) 69:683–90. doi: 10.1007/s00228-012-1380-9
16. Klok T, Kaptein AA, Duiverman EJ, Brand PL. Long-term adherence to inhaled corticosteroids in children with ashma: observational study. *Respir Med.* (2015) 109:1114–9. doi: 10.1016/j.rmed.2015.07.016
17. Kew KM, Normansell R, Stovold E. Intervention to improve adherence to inhaled steroids for asthma. *Cochrane Database Syst Rev.* (2016) 6:CD012226. doi: 10.1002/14651858.CD012226.
18. World Health Organization. *Adherence to Long-Term Therapies: Evidence for Action.* Geneva: World Health Organization (2003). Available online at: http://www.who.int/chp/knowledge/publications/adherence_report/en/ (Assessed April 8, 2018).
19. Jochmann A, Artusio L, Jamalzadeh A, Nagakumar P, Delgado-Eckert E, Saglani S, et al. Electronic monitoring of adherence to inhaled corticosteroids: an essential tool in identifying severe asthma in children. *Eur Respir J.* (2017) 50:1700910. doi: 10.1183/13993003.00910-2017
20. Diette GB, Skinner EA, Markson LE, Algatt-Bergstrom P, Nguyen TT, Clark RD, et al. Consistency of care with national guidelines for children with asthma in managed care. *J Pediatr.* (2001) 138:59–64. doi: 10.1067/mpd.2001.109600
21. Jentzsch NS, Camargos P, Sarinho E, Bousquet J. Adherence rate to beclomethasone dipropionate and the level of asthma control. *Respir Med.* (2012) 106:338–43. doi: 10.1016/j.rmed.2011.12.001
22. Klok T, Kaptein AA, Duiverman EJ, Brand PL. It's adherence, stupid (that determines asthma control in preschool children) *Eur Respir J.* (2014) 43:783–91. doi: 10.1183/09031936.00054613
23. Wilson SR, Strub P, Buist AS, Knowles SB, Lavori PW, Lapidus J, et al. Shared treatment decision making improves adherence: systematic review and meta-analysis. *BMJ* (2003) 326:1308–9. doi: 10.1164/rccm.200906-0907OC
24. Chan AH, Stewart AW, Harrison J, Camargo CA Jr, Black PN, Mitchell EA. The effect of an electronic monitoring device with audiovisual reminder function on adherence to inhaled corticosteroids and school attendance in children with asthma: a randomised controlled trial. *Lancet Respir Med.* (2015) 3:210–9. doi: 10.1016/S2213-2600(15)00008-9
25. Otsuki M, Eakin MN, Rand CS, Butz AM, Hsu VD, Zuckerman IH, et al. Adherence feedback to improve asthma outcomes among inner-city children: a randomized trial. *Pediatrics* (2009) 124:1513–21. doi: 10.1542/peds.2008-2961
26. Price D, Robertson A, Bullen K, Rand C, Horne R, Staudinger H. Improved adherence with once-daily versus twice-daily dosing of mometasone furoate administered via a dry powder inhaler: a randomized open-label study. *BMC Pulm Med.* (2010) 10:1. doi: 10.1186/1471-2466-10-1
27. Moher D, Shamseer L, Clarke M, Ghersi D, Liberati A, Petticrew M, et al.

Preferred reporting items for systematic review and meta-analysis protocols (PRISMA-P) 2015 statement. *Syst Rev.* (2015) 4:1. doi: 10.1186/2046-4053-4-1

28. Sleath B, Carpenter DM, Slota C, Williams D, Tudor G, Yeatts K, et al. Communication during pediatric asthma visits and self-reported asthma medication adherence. *Pediatrics* (2012) 130:627–33. doi: 10.1542/peds.2012-0913
29. Duncan CL, Hogan MB, Tien KJ, Graves MM, Chorney JM, Zettler MD, et al. Efficacy of a parent-youth teamwork intervention to promote adherence in pediatric asthma. *J Pediatr Psychol.* (2012) 38:617–28. doi: 10.1093/jpepsy/jss123
30. Ellis DA, King P, Naar-King S. Mediators of treatment effects in a randomized clinical trial of multisystemic therapy-health care in adolescents with poorly controlled asthma: disease knowledge and device use skills. *J Pediatr Psychol.* (2016) 41:522–30. doi: 10.1093/jpepsy/jsv114
31. Christakis DA, Garrison MM, Lozano P, Meischke H, Zhou C, Zimmerman FJ. Improving parental adherence with asthma treatment guidelines: a randomized controlled trial of an interactive website. *Acad Pediatr.* (2012) 12:302–11. doi: 10.1016/j.acap.2012.03.006
32. Guénette L, Breton MC, Grégoire JP, Jobin MS, Bolduc Y, Boulet LP, et al. Effectiveness of an asthma integrated care program on asthma control and adherence to inhaled corticosteroids. *J Asthma* (2015) 52:638–45. doi: 10.3109/02770903.2014.999084
33. Modi AC, Lim CS, Yu N, Geller D, Wagner MH, Quittner AL. A multi-method assessment of treatment adherence for children with cystic fibrosis. *J Cyst Fibros* (2006) 5:117–85. doi: 10.1016/j.jcf.2006.03.002
34. Duncan CL, Mentrikoski JM, Wu YP, Fredericks EM. Practice-based approach to assessing and treating nonadherence in pediatric regimens. *Clin Pract Pediatr Psychol.* (2014) 2:322–36. doi: 10.1037/cpp0000066
35. Svarstad BL, Chewning BA, Sleath BL, Claesson C. The Brief Medication Questionnaire: a tool for screening patient adherence and barriers to adherence. *Patient Educ Couns.* (1999) 37:113–24.
36. Morisky DE. Nonadherence to medical recommendations for hypertensive patients: problems and potential solutions. *J Compliance Health Care* (1986) 1:5–32.
37. Horne R, Weinman J. Self-regulation and self-management in asthma: exploring the role of 'illness perceptions and treatment beliefs in explaining non-adherence to preventer medication. *Psychol Health* (2002) 17:17–32. doi: 10.1080/08870440290001502
38. Morisky DE, Ang A, Krousel-Wood M, Ward HJ. Predictive validity of a medication adherence measure in an outpatient setting. *J Clin Hypertens (Greenwich)* (2008) 10(5):348-54.
39. Jentzsch NS, Camargos PA. Methods of assessing adherence to inhaled corticosteroid therapy in children and adolescents: adherence rates and their implications for clinical practice. *J Bras Pneumol.* (2008) 34:614-21. doi: 10.1590/S1806-37132008000800012
40. Hommel KA, Greenley RN, Maddux MH, Gray WN, Mackner LM. Self-management in pediatric inflammatory bowel disease: a clinical report of the North American Society for Pediatric Gastroenterology, Hepatology, and Nutrition. *J Pediatr Gastroenterol Nutr.* (2013) 57:250–7. doi: 10.1097/MPG.0b013e3182999b21
41. Quittner AL, Modi AC, Lemanek KL, Ievers-Landis CE, Rapoff MA. Evidence-based assessment of adherence to medical treatments in pediatric psychology. *J Pediatr Psychol.* (2008) 33:916–36. doi: 10.1093/jpepsy/jsm064
42. Garfield S, Clifford S, Eliasson L, Barber N, Willson A. Suitability of measures of self-reported medication adherence for routine clinical use: a systematic review. *BMC Med Res Methodol.* (2011) 11:149. doi: 10.1186/1471-2288-11-149
43. Thomas M. Why aren't we doing better in asthma: time for personalized medicine? *NPJ Prim Care Respir Med.* (2015) 25:15004. doi: 10.1038/npjpcrm.2015.4
44. van Boven JF, Trappenburg JC, van der Molen T, Chavannes NH. Towards tailored and targeted adherence assessment to optimise asthma management. *NPJ Prim Care Respir Med.* (2015) 25:15046. doi: 10.1038/npjpcrm.2015.46
45. Lang A, Carlsen KH, Haaland G, Devulapalli CS, Munthe-Kaas M, Mowinckel P, et al. Severe asthma in childhood: assessed in 10 year olds in a birth cohort study. *Allergy* (2008) 63:1054–60. doi: 10.1111/j.1398-9995.2008.01672.x
46. Nordlund B, Melen E, Schultz ES, Gronlund H, Hedlin G, Kull I. Prevalence of severe childhood asthma according to the WHO. *Respir Med.* (2014) 108:1234–37. doi: 10.1016/j.rmed.2014.05.015
47. Pike KC, Levy ML, Moreiras J, Fleming L. Managing problematic severe asthma: beyond the guidelines. *Arch Dis Child.* (2018) 103:392–397. doi: 10.1136/archdischild-2016-311368
48. Celano MP, Linzer JF, Demi A, Bakeman R, Smith CO, Croft S, et al. Treatment adherence among low-income, African American children with persistent asthma. *J Asthma* (2010) 47:317–322. doi: 10.3109/02770900903580850
49. Jentzsch NS, Camargos PA, Colosimo EA, Bousquet J. Monitoring adherence to beclomethasone in asthmatic children and adolescents through four different methods. *Allergy* (2009) 64:1458–62. doi: 10.1111/j.1398-9995.2009.02037.x
50. Wu YP, Pai AL. Health care provider-delivered adherence promotion interventions: a meta-analysis. *Pediatrics* (2014) 133:1698–707. doi: 10.1542/peds.2013-3639
51. Mosnaim G, Li H, Martin M, Richardson D, Belice PJ, Avery E, et al. The impact of peer support and mp3 messaging on adherence to inhaled corticosteroids in minority adolescents with asthma: a randomized, controlled trial. *J Allergy Clin Immunol Pract.* (2013) 1:485–493. doi: 10.1016/j.jaip.2013.06.010
52. Kenyon CC, Gruschow SM, Quarshie WO, Griffis H, Leach MC, Zorc JJ, et al. Controller adherence following hospital discharge in high risk children: A pilot randomized trial of text message reminders. *J Asthma* (2018) 13:1–9. doi: 10.1080/02770903.2018.1424195
53. Burgess SW, Sly PD, Morawska A, Devadason SG. Assessing adherence and factors associated with adherence in young children with asthma. *Respirology* (2008) 13:559–63. doi: 10.1111/j.1440-1843.2008.01292.x
54. Armstrong ML, Duncan CL, Stokes JO, Pereira D. Association of caregiver health beliefs and parenting stress with medication adherence in preschoolers with asthma. *J Asthma* (2014) 51:366–72. doi: 10.3109/02770903.2013.876431
55. Capo-Ramos DE, Duran C, Simon AE, Akinbami LJ, Schoendorf KC. Preventive asthma medication discontinuation among children enrolled in fee-for-service Medicaid. *J Asthma* (2014) 51:618–26. doi: 10.3109/02770903.2014.895010
56. Mulvaney SA, Ho YX, Cala CM, Chen Q, Nian H, Patterson BL, et al. Assessing adolescent asthma symptoms and adherence using mobile phones. *J Med Internet Res.* (2013) 15:141. doi: 10.2196/jmir.2413
57. Edgecombe K, Latter S, Peters S, Roberts G. Health experiences of adolescents with uncontrolled severe asthma. *Arch Dis Child.* (2010) 95:985–91. doi: 10.1136/adc.2009.171579
58. Blaakman SW, Cohen A, Fagnano M, Halterman JS. Asthma medication adherence among urban teens: a qualitative analysis of barriers, facilitators and experiences with school-based care. *J Asthma* (2014) 51:522–9. doi: 10.3109/02770903.2014.885041
59. Vasbinder EC, Goossens LM, Rutten-van Mölken MP, de Winter BC, van Dijk L, Vulto AG, et al. e-Monitoring of asthma therapy to improve compliance in children (e-MATIC): a randomised controlled trial. *Eur Respir J.* (2016) 48:758–67. doi: 10.1183/13993003.01698-2015
60. Keemink YS, Klok T, Brand PL. Long-term adherence to daily controller medication in children with asthma: the role of outpatient clinic visits. *Pediatr Pulmonol.* (2015) 50:1060–4. doi: 10.1002/ppul.23138
61. Normansell R, Kew KM, Stovold E. Interventions to improve adherence to inhaled steroids for asthma. *Cochrane Database Syst Rev.* (2017) 4:CD012226. doi: 10.1002/14651858.CD012226.pub2
62. Hedlin G, Bush A, Lødrup Carlsen K, Wennergren G, De Benedictis FM, Melén E, el al. Problematic severe asthma in children, not one problem but many: a GA2LEN initiative. *Eur Respir J.* (2010) 36:196–201. doi: 10.1183/09031936.00104809
63. Lasmar L, Camargos P, Champs NS, Fonseca MT, Fontes MJ, Ibiapina C, et al. Adherence rate to inhaled corticosteroids and their impact on asthma control. *Allergy* (2009) 64:784–9. doi: 10.1111/j.1398-9995.2008.01877.x

16

Two Sides of the Same Coin?—Treatment of Chronic Asthma in Children and Adults

Li Ping Chung[1*] *and James Y. Paton*[2]

[1] *Department of Respiratory Medicine, Fiona Stanley Hospital, Perth, WA, Australia,* [2] *School of Medicine, College of Medical, Veterinary, and Life Sciences, University of Glasgow, Glasgow, United Kingdom*

Globally, asthma is one of the most common chronic conditions that affect individuals of all ages. When poorly controlled, it negatively impacts patient's ability to enjoy life and work. At the population level, effective use of recommended strategies in children and adults can reduce symptom burden, improve quality of life and significantly reduce the risk of exacerbation, decline of lung function and asthma-related death. Inhaled corticosteroid as the initial maintenance therapy, ideally started within 2 years of symptom onset, is highly effective in both children and adults and across various degrees of asthma severity. If asthma is not controlled, the choice of subsequent add-on therapies differs between children and adults. Evidence supporting pharmacological approach to asthma management, especially for those with more severe disease, is more robust in adults compared to children. This is, in part, due to various challenges in the diagnosis of asthma, in the recruitment into clinical trials and in the lack of objective outcomes in children, especially those in the preschool age group. Nevertheless, where evidence is emerging for younger children, it seems to mirror the observations in adults. Clinicians need to develop strategies to implement guideline-based recommendations while taking into consideration individual variations in asthma clinical phenotypes, pathophysiology and treatment responses at different ages.

Keywords: chronic asthma, pharmacotherapy, treatment, adult, children, guidelines

INTRODUCTION

Asthma Burden

Asthma is a chronic inflammatory disease of the airways with typical symptoms of wheezing, breathlessness and cough and variable airflow obstruction. The WHO estimates that some 235 million people currently suffer from asthma (1) and it is the commonest chronic disease of children worldwide. Asthma causes long term effects: it affects patient's quality of life, daily activities, their work and school attendance; it causes anxiety—to the patients themselves, and to their families and caregivers; it imposes a substantial economic burden on families and societies; and it causes death. Yet, with appropriate management most people with asthma can enjoy excellent symptom control and a good quality of life (1).

Control of asthma symptoms, reduction of future risk in terms of asthma attacks, and prevention of decline in lung function are recognized as the key goals of asthma management (**Figure 1**). These goals are relevant to all patients with asthma irrespective of age. Pharmacological therapies are the main tools for controlling asthma but non-pharmacological interventions such as allergen or

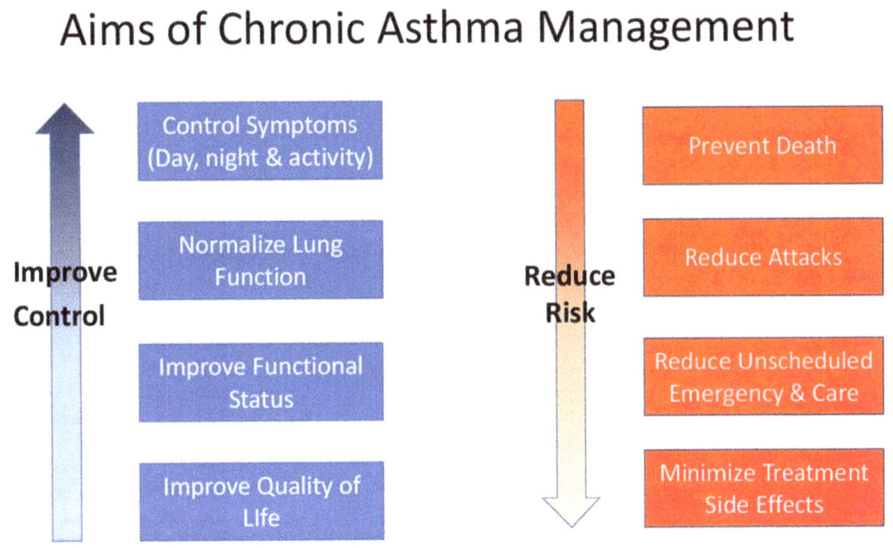

FIGURE 1 | Aims of asthma management.

irritant (especially tobacco smoke) avoidance, and education about the disease, inhaler device use and self-management strategies are also important.

Asthma Phenotypes

There is increasing recognition of different clinical and patho-physiological patterns of asthma ('phenotypes') in both children and adults.

The most striking asthma phenotype is found in young children who present with wheezing attacks associated with viral infection, particularly rhinovirus infection, often with no symptoms between attacks. For many of these children, the wheezing attacks stop in later childhood (2). In older children, a more classic asthma pattern of attacks with chronic interval symptoms usually with an atopic background emerges (3). However, these patterns overlap and are unstable, at least in early childhood, and may change from one to another over times scales as short as a year (4, 5). Lung function testing in young children is generally not possible and making a diagnosis of asthma without objective testing has been criticized (6). The implications for the choice of treatments of the different phenotypes is complex and has resulted in a wide variety of approaches often compounded by a lack of evidence (7).

In adults, the pattern of airway inflammation is more diverse and the clinical presentation is often clouded by co-existing comorbidities especially in those with severe asthma (8, 9). Currently an emerging concept, but an important focus of asthma management in adults is the identification and management of pulmonary, extrapulmonary and behavioral "treatable traits". The hope is that treatment of these modifiable elements (e.g., bronchodilator reversibility, eosinophilic airway inflammation, depression) even in the absence of a deeper understanding of the mechanisms of airway inflammation will improve patient outcomes (10). Although the concept of treatable traits has been developed in relation to adults it is also likely to be useful in children with asthma.

There are some patients, both adult and children, with "discordant" disease who suffer substantial symptom burden with little evidence of eosinophilic inflammation or those with high level of inflammation but few symptoms (11). However, the majority of patients will have asthma symptoms that parallel the degree of inflammation in which step-wise guideline recommended approach is likely to be effective.

This review summarizes evidence about differences in the approaches to asthma treatments in adults and children as currently recommended in commonly used asthma guidelines (12, 13) (**Table 1**).

GUIDELINE RECOMMENDED APPROACH FOR CHRONIC ASTHMA

Step 1: As Needed SABA

For patients of all ages, as needed short acting beta2 agonist (SABA) reliever therapy is highly effective for rapid relief of asthma symptoms. SABA as the sole treatment is now only recommended for those with the mild and intermittent symptoms (<2 per week and no nocturnal awakenings), no history of asthma attacks in the previous year and normal lung function.

Historically, there has been a perception that patients with intermittent symptoms are not at risk of asthma attacks, a view increasingly challenged. Evidence from adult studies showed that airways inflammation occurs at a very early stage of the disease even in patients with intermittent asthma, albeit at a lower level than in those with persistent asthma (14, 15). Furthermore, early introduction of once daily inhaled corticosteroid (ICS) in adults and children > 5years with mild asthma symptoms

TABLE 1 | Comparison of recommended treatments for chronic asthma in adults and children from widely used international guidelines (12, 13).

Asthma guideline treatment steps	Similarities in recommendations	Differences in recommendations, effectiveness or safety profile
Step 1	• As needed SABA effective for all ages • Consider early use of ICS for adults and children ≥ 6 years old	
Step 2	• Regular low dose ICS for all ages	• Potential concern for effect of ICS on linear growth in children • Intermittent ICS may improve symptom control in adults and adolescents • Intermittent ICS in children < 5 years with viral induced wheezing reduces the risk of severe asthma attacks.
Step 3	• Regular ICS recommended for all age groups • LTRA inferior to LABA or higher dose ICS in adults and children respectively • Allergen immunotherapy limited to carefully selected adults and children.	• Addition of LABA to low dose ICS as first preferred option in adolescents and adults • Moderate dose ICS preferred in children • Concern for LTRA-related neuropsychiatric effects in children and adolescents • ICS/formoterol as single maintenance and reliever therapy is another option for adolescents and adults; insufficient evidence for use in children <12 years old
Step 4	• ICS/LABA + SABA prn or ICS/fomoterol as single maintenance and reliever therapy recommended for adults and adolescents. • Higher dose ICS monotherapy provides little additional benefit in children and adults • Tiotropium is a safe, alternative add-on therapy for adults and adolescents; emerging supportive data for younger children • Theophylline no longer recommended for adults and children.	• Insufficient data for ICS/formoterol as single inhaler therapy use in children <12 years old • Specialist review recommended for children
Step 5	• Referral to specialist recommended for all ages • Review of medication adherence, comorbidities and risk factors important for all ages groups • Anti-IgE monoclonal therapy can be used for patients ≥ 6 years old • Anti-IL5 monoclonal therapy (mepolizumab) can be used in patients ≥18 years old and has been approved for use in children ≥ 6 years	• Use of anti-IL5 (mepolizumab) more extensively researched in adolescents and adults; use of younger children (≥ 6years old) approved based on extrapolated data. • Other advanced therapies such as macrolides and bronchial thermoplasty are recommended for adults; lacks data in children or adolescents.

ICS, inhaled corticosteroid; LABA, long acting beta2 agonist; LTRA, leukotriene receptor antagonist; SABA, short acting beta2 agonist.

reduced the risk of severe asthma exacerbation by almost half, with better asthma control although it did not affect lung function (16, 17).

This has led widely used international guidelines (12, 13) to update their recommendation for the consideration of ICS use as Step 1 treatment in all adults, adolescents and children over 6 years with mild asthma, even those with infrequent symptoms, to reduce the risk of severe, potentially life-threatening exacerbations (18–20).

Step 2: Regular Low Dose ICS Plus as Needed SABA

Adults and Children (Age >5years)

Regular low dose ICS significantly improves lung function, quality of life and reduces asthma exacerbations in both adults and children with mild persistent asthma (13, 18). O'Byrne et al showed that introduction of low dose budesonide reduced the risk of asthma exacerbation by 60% and improved asthma control days by half (19). Selected studies in adults also showed less rescue SABA use (18). It was suggested that duration of therapy of at least 4 weeks may be an important determinant of overall treatment response (18).

The greatest benefits of ICS in adults and children older than 5 years old have been achieved when ICS therapy was started within 2 years of symptom onset (21, 22); this effectively halved the overall risk of severe or life-threatening exacerbations (16, 17). After this time, higher ICS doses are required for adults and there is a negative correlation between duration of symptoms and maximal increases in lung function (22–24). Low dose ICS appears protective against potential long-term decline in lung function following severe exacerbations. Interestingly, this effect is only seen in adults and children but not adolescents (25). It is unclear if this is due to the relatively small number of adolescents studied or relates to the improvements in asthma that have been noted during adolescence (26). Early initiation of ICS also improves asthma control and diminished subsequent needs for additional maintenance therapy (24).

One important difference in children compared with adults is a persistent concern about the impact of regular ICS in children on linear growth. As an example, in the START study Pauwels et al. reported that children aged 5–15years treated with budesonide showed reduced growth especially in the first year of treatment (16). However, other studies found that children attain normal projected adult height while on prolonged inhaled budesonide (21, 22).

The evidence on linear growth in children treated with ICS has recently been updated to take account of newer inhaled steroid molecules. The regular use of ICS at low or medium daily doses was found to be associated with statistically significant growth suppression during a 1-year treatment period in children with mild to moderate persistent asthma. The mean growth reduction was 0.48 cm/year in linear growth velocity and 0.61 cm change from baseline height during a one year treatment period. ICS-induced growth suppression appears to be maximal during the first year of treatment and less pronounced in subsequent years and appears to be more strongly associated with ICS molecule than with the device or dose in the low to medium dose range (27). A second review looking at dose response effects found a small but statistically significant group difference in growth velocity between low doses and low to medium doses, favoring the use of low-dose ICS (28). Thus the evidence confirms the relative safety of ICS in relation to growth effects but supports the use of the lowest effective dose of ICS, with regular monitoring of linear growth. It is surprising how many gaps still exist in the current evidence base about ICS and growth (29).

Preschool Children (Age <5years)

There is also strong and consistent evidence to support the use of daily ICS for preventing exacerbations in preschool children with recurrent wheeze, especially in those with persistent asthma symptoms (30). The effect of ICS appears to be stronger in those with a diagnosis of asthma compared with recurrent wheezing and is independent of age (pre-schoolers vs. infants), atopic condition, type of ICS, and mode of delivery (spacer vs. nebulizer) (31).

The evidence about growth suppression in pre-school children is limited. Nevertheless, because of concerns about side effects, an important question is whether ICS therapy can be targeted to those children most likely to respond? One recent study in children requiring step 2 treatment showed that while individual treatment responses were phenotypically diverse, children with aeroallergen sensitization and increased blood eosinophil counts responded best to a daily ICS as opposed to a leukotriene receptor antagonist (LTRA) or as needed-ICS. Daily ICS was associated with more asthma control days and fewer exacerbation (32). However, a very recent real-world study of large matched cohort analysis of anonymized UK medical record data found no evidence that stepping up therapy by adding ICS or monteleukast, compared with as-needed use of SABA, reduced wheezing/asthma attacks in a diverse population of preschool children with at least two documented prior wheezing episodes (33). In the absence of better tools to help target treatments, and in light of improved outcomes over time in preschool children a "wait-and-see approach" may be a clinically prudent approach for many with infrequent, intermittent attacks.

Alternative Options

Low Dose Combination ICS/Long Acting Beta2 Agonist (LABA)

For steroid-naïve adults and adolescents with mild persistent asthma, ICS/LABA works faster in achieving GINA-defined good asthma control compared to ICS alone. However, there is little difference in exacerbation rate between the two therapies. In practice, the additional cost for ICS/LABA compared to low dose ICS may be an important consideration for the individual patient (34). Data as to whether there would be similar benefits in children is not available.

Intermittent ICS Regimes

Regular use of ICS raises concerns from patients and clinicians about adherence and steroid side effects. Poor adherence to ICS potentially results in patients relying on SABAs to control symptoms, possibly resulting in overuse.

Recently, it was shown that adults and adolescents with mild asthma using as-needed combination ICS and fast acting LABA had better asthma symptom control measured by an electronic diary compared to as-needed SABA (35). However, the magnitude of effect was inferior to regular low dose ICS therapy. A second trial in a similar cohort reported no difference in exacerbation rate when comparing ICS/formoterol as needed vs. regular ICS (36).

There is less evidence about the use of as needed ICS treatment in children. One study in children from 5 years upwards with mild well-controlled asthma stepping down from daily ICS found ICS and SABAs as needed more effective at reducing attacks than SABA use alone (37). Liner growth was 1.1 cm a year less when ICS was used regularly but not when used on an as needed basis.

In children under 5 years, the most common asthma phenotype is intermittent viral triggered wheezing attacks with no interval symptoms. In this group, intermittent ICS, usually as high-dose ICS at the first sign of an URTI for 7 to 10 days led to a 35% reduction in severe attacks (30). Intermittent ICS were associated with greater linear growth of 0.41 cm per year (i.e., less growth suppression) compared with daily treatment (38).

Oral Leukotriene Receptor Antagonist (LTRA) in Preschool Children

Because of concerns about ICS side effects and difficulties using inhaled therapies in young children, oral montelukast has been widely prescribed as an alternative to regular ICS. While early studies showed it to be effective, the most recent review found no evidence of benefit from the use of montelukast, continuously or intermittently on the number of wheezing episodes, unscheduled medical attendance, or oral corticosteroid use in preschool children with recurrent wheeze (39). There is also little evidence of benefit for other secondary outcomes (7).

Step 3: One or two Maintenance Treatments Plus as Needed Reliever Therapy

For adults and adolescents with suboptimal symptom control or more than 1 exacerbation in the previous year despite treatment with low dose ICS, guidelines recommend low dose ICS/LABA as maintenance therapy plus SABA or ICS/formoterol as single inhaler therapy (12, 13). In children, at present, moderate dose ICS plus as needed SABA is the preferred treatment for children.

ICS/LABA Maintenance Plus SABA as Required

Historically, there were concerns that LABA may mask airway inflammation leading to potential adverse events including asthma exacerbations. To the contrary, the addition of LABA to ICS significantly increases the odds of achieving good overall asthma control as defined by guidelines (34). Combination low dose ICS/LABA therapy was highly effective at reducing the risk of exacerbations needing oral corticosteroid (19, 40, 41) and hospitalizations (40, 42, 43) in symptomatic adults and adolescents with mild to moderate asthma compared to ICS alone. The addition of LABA also leads to improvement in lung function (especially in those with lower baseline FEV_1), proportion of symptom-free days (19, 44) and a slight reduction in rescue SABA use compared to same or higher dose of ICS (41, 43).

The advantages of adding a LABA have been less clear in children. In children with persistent asthma, the addition of LABA to ICS was not associated with a significant reduction in the rate of exacerbations requiring systemic steroids, but it was superior for improving lung function compared with the same or higher doses of ICS. There were no differences in adverse effects, with the exception of significantly lower linear growth over a year in the children treated with a higher ICS dose, with a mean difference of 1.21cm/yr. A trend toward an increased risk of hospital admission with LABA, irrespective of the dose of ICS, was noted as a matter for concern (45).

ICS/Formoterol as Single Maintenance and Reliever Therapy

Combination of ICS with formoterol as fast acting bronchodilator allows patients to use their regular maintenance inhaler also for rapid relief of symptoms. Single inhaler therapy is more effective at reducing mild to moderate exacerbations while providing similar levels of asthma control compared with medium dose ICS monotherapy or fixed dose of ICS/LABA and as required SABA (46–50). It has been suggested that using single inhaler for both maintenance and reliever therapy may improve adherence but definitive data is lacking.

The role of single maintenance and reliever therapy in children age 12 years and below is unclear at present and requires further study. It is not currently licensed for use in this way in this age group.

Alternative Treatment Options

Higher dose ICS

At the population level, further escalation to higher dose ICS use in adults and adolescents provides little added benefit but rather greater adrenal suppression (51, 52). Higher dose of ICS is inferior to combination ICS/LABA in reducing the risk of exacerbations requiring oral corticosteroids. Combination therapy is also superior in improving lung function, symptom control, and use of rescue SABA than a higher dose of ICS alone (44, 47).

In the past, written action plans commonly included advice about a temporary increase in inhaled steroid dose—usually doubling—in the early stages of an asthma exacerbation to reduce the severity of the attack and to prevent the need for oral steroids or hospital admission. The accumulated evidence suggested that this doubling approach was not effective (53).

However, the concept of intermittent ICS dose escalation to prevent asthma exacerbations has recently been revisited in two large studies. In a pragmatic and unblinded trial, McKeever et al. randomized adults and adolescents ($N = 1922$) on ICS maintenance therapy to receive a personalized management plan that included a temporary quadrupling of ICS when asthma control started to deteriorate compared to remaining on their usual ICS dose (54). They showed that a temporary quadrupling at the time of worsening asthma control resulted in a lower rate of severe exacerbations of asthma than no increase in the dose (45% vs. 52%).

In contrast, Jackson et al. studied children 5 to 11 years of age ($n = 254$) with mild to moderate asthma already on low dose ICS therapy and reported no difference in rates of exacerbation in those treated with quintupled dose of ICS compared with their usual ICS dose at the earliest sign of asthma deterioration (55).

The reasons for the differences in outcomes between these two studies are not completely clear. Differences in the size of study cohort and fewer than expected exacerbations in the pediatric study may be one reason and there may be differences in pathophysiology during exacerbations between adults and children. A more plausible explanation may lie in the fact the study by McKeever et al. was a pragmatic open label study with no monitoring of compliance. Increasing the ICS dose at the start of an exacerbation may have merely resulted in the patients starting a treatment they had been poorly compliant with before. In contrast, Jackson's study was a randomized control trial with electronic diary recording of treatment. Diary completion was > 70% during usual treatment and rose to around 98% of the days during the treatment (55, 56). Thus there may have been no headroom for a further impact of the increased ICS dose.

Given the bioequivalence dose of inhaled to oral corticosteroid and subsequent potential effects on adrenal suppression, it is also debatable whether the very high steroid dose used in the quadrupling or quintupling approach is necessarily better than a standard course of oral prednisolone (57).

Leukotriene receptor antagonists (LTRA)

Leukotriene receptor antagonists inhibit the pro-inflammatory effect of leukotrienes not completely suppressed by corticosteroid therapy. The addition of LTRA to symptomatic adult asthmatics already treated with regular ICS monotherapy leads to reduced exacerbations, better asthma control and better lung function (58, 59).

It is unclear if LTRA is superior to higher doses of ICS monotherapy (58) except in adults with aspirin-intolerant asthma. However, asthma symptoms, lung function, and rescue medication use are improved when LTRA is added to high doses of ICS (60). In this specific patient cohort, aspirin desensitization is also a safe, and effective option (61).

The addition of LTRA is less effective than adding LABA to ICS when one looks at comparative benefits in lung function, asthma symptoms, rescue medication use, and asthma related quality of life (62). The effect on oral corticosteroid-treated exacerbation was statistically superior with the addition of LABA than LTRA to ICS but with only an absolute difference of 2% between groups. However, this meta-analysis was dominated by 16 trials that included 6872 adults and adolescents; only 2 studies included 336 children (age 6–17 years). As such, it is unclear which adjunct therapy is best for children.

An earlier Cochrane 2013 analysis concluded there was no difference in asthma exacerbations needing oral corticosteroid or hospitalization comparing LTRA to same or higher dose ICS in children and adolescents with mild to moderate asthma (63). The paucity of randomized trials and heterogeneity in study design and reporting of published studies make it difficult to support its use as add-on therapy in children with moderate asthma (step 3 treatment).

In preschool children, there are as yet no trials comparing LTRA, or LABA, as an add on therapy to ICS.

Neuropsychiatric side effects have been reported as not uncommon in young children started on montelukast. One study ($n = 106$) found montelukast had been stopped in 16% of children because of neuropsychiatric effects (irritability, aggressiveness, and sleep disturbance), mostly within 2 weeks of starting therapy (64). Long term use in adults is not recommended unless there is clear symptomatic improvement after a trial of therapy (65).

Allergen immunotherapy

Allergen immunotherapy (AIT) is still the only-disease modifying treatment strategy for IgE-mediated allergic disease (66). Studies using both subcutaneous (SCIT) and sublingual treatments (SLIT) have shown some benefit in reducing asthma symptoms and bronchial hyper-reactivity in adults and children.

GINA guideline recommend SLIT for adults with rhinitis and allergy to house dust mite with exacerbations despite ICS, provided FEV_1 is > 70% predicted (12). It reduces exacerbation rates in adults with moderate asthma but has minimal effect on asthma symptom control or quality of life (67). Its role in adults with compromised lung function requires further clarification. In a randomized control trial of subjects 14 years or older with mild to moderate asthma, those treated with sublingual house dust mite immunotherapy were able to reduce their ICS dose while maintaining asthma control (68).

In children, the most up to date evidence noted that there were no studies that evaluated asthma symptom using a validated tool and both study characteristics and outcomes were reported heterogeneously. There is moderate-strength evidence that SCIT may reduce long term asthma controller medication use in children with allergic asthma (68). Studies of SLIT have only studied children with mild/moderate asthma mono-sensitized to house dust mite. Local and systemic allergic reactions were common but anaphylaxis was reported rarely (69).

Current recommendations advise that allergen immunotherapy should not be given to patients with severe or uncontrolled asthma who are at increased risk for systemic reactions (70).

Step 4: Two or More Maintenance Therapies Plus as Needed Reliever Medication

For adults and adolescents whose asthma is inadequately controlled on low dose ICS/LABA maintenance therapy, the two recommended step-up approaches are low dose ICS/formoterol single maintenance and reliever therapy or medium dose ICS/LABA as maintenance plus as needed SABA (44). In contrast, for children < 12 years old because of concerns regarding medication side effects and the lack of sound evidence base, current guidelines recommend referral for specialist review (12).

Post hoc analysis of five large clinical trials suggests that ICS/formoterol as single maintenance and reliever inhaler may be the preferred option compared to guideline recommended treatment for various stages of asthma severity using low dose ICS monotherapy or same or higher fixed dose ICS/LABA regime (50). The magnitude of difference is more marked for those with more severe disease requiring GINA Step 4 treatment. Single maintenance and inhaler therapy prolongs the time to first exacerbation and reduces the overall risk of exacerbations at relatively low doses of ICS compared with higher fixed dose of ICS/LABA and as-needed SABA (46, 47, 50). The effect on hospitalization is less clear. Secondary outcomes such as lung function, rescue SABA use, symptom free days, and quality of life were also superior for single maintenance and reliever therapy than higher fixed dose ICS/LABA regime.

Again, the best option in children younger than 12 years old is unclear due to insufficient data.

Alternative and/or Additional Treatment Options

Several alternative options are available for adults and adolescents. However, robust data for their use in younger children is again currently lacking.

High dose ICS/LABA

While high dose ICS/LABA may be considered in adults and adolescents, the increase in ICS dose generally provides little additional benefit (34, 41, 71), and there is an increased risk of side effects, including adrenal suppression (72). A high dose is recommended only on a trial basis for up to 6 months when good asthma control cannot be achieved with medium dose ICS/LABA and /or a third controller (12).

Long acting muscarinic antagonist (LAMA)

The long-acting anticholinergic tiotropium, delivered once daily via a mist inhaler, is approved for the treatment of asthma in the EU and the USA with the license recently extended to include children with severe asthma over 6 years of age. The GINA guidelines currently position tiotropium as an add on therapy option at step 4 in patients aged ≥12years with a history of exacerbations (12).

For adults treated with ICS, LAMA prescribed as add on therapy has been shown to reduce the risk of exacerbations and improve lung function but made no difference in quality of life (73). In a study of 210 moderate asthmatics, tiotropium bromide added to ICS offered marginal improvements in peak flow and symptoms compared to doubling dose of ICS. The effect was considered non-inferior to salmeterol. However, there was the possibility of carry-over effects due to the cross-over design (74, 75). Cochrane analysis of 3 trials (76–78) comparing addition of tiotropium mist inhaler in adults with severe asthma already treated with ICS/LABA combination therapy showed definitive improvement in trough FEV_1 and fewer exacerbations (79).

In children over 6 years with symptomatic moderate or severe asthma, tiotropium treatment led to improvement in lung function and asthma control (80), similar to that found in adult studies. However, the data in children is less extensive and generally short term with the longest study lasting 48 weeks (81). In younger children, one small 12 week RCT of children aged 1–5years study showed tiotropium was safe, led to a reduction in asthma attacks but did not improve daily asthma symptom scores. These findings need to be confirmed in larger studies (82).

Both in adults and children tiotropium has a safety profile comparable to placebo.

Theophylline

The addition of slow release theophylline to low dose budesonide for moderate asthma is just as effective as high dose budesonide in improving lung function and reducing symptoms and rescue SABA use in adults but has little effect on exacerbation rate over 3 months duration (83). Theophylline is a less effective bronchodilator than beta2 agonists and associated with high risk of adverse effects.

In the past, oral xanthines were used as a first line preventer treatment (at Step 2) for children with asthma. Although there is weak evidence that theophyllines were better than placebo, they are no longer used because ICS were shown to be more effective at improving symptoms and reducing asthma attacks (84). When low dose ICS fail to control asthma, oral theophyllines have been used as one of the available add-on options and there is weak evidence that adding theophylline to ICS treatment improves symptom control and reduces exacerbations (85). However, current recommendations are that theophyllines should only be tried when the addition of LABA and LTRA have both failed.

Theophyllines have adverse effects including headaches and nausea if therapeutic concentrations are exceeded. There are also significant interactions with some commonly used drugs which inhibit theophylline clearance e.g., erythromycin which can result in increased theophylline levels and resulting toxicity.

Step 5: Refer for Expert Review and Add-On Therapy

The great majority of adults with severe asthma not responding to high dose treatments are "difficult-to-treat" because of comorbidities and risk factors that mimic or worsen asthma control (86, 87) and the management of these other factors is as important as the asthma treatments in improving the outcomes of patients with severe asthma. The situation is similar in children where only the minority will have genuinely therapy resistant asthma (88).

Poor adherence with treatment is a particularly important cause of difficult to treat asthma in both adults and children. Improving adherence is difficult. A variety of interventions have been shown to lead to improvements including adherence education, the use of electronic trackers or reminders, simplified drug regimens and school-based directly observed therapy. However, because of uncertain and inconsistent impact on clinical outcomes such as quality of life and asthma control the clinical relevance of the improvements has been less clear with many studies affected by concerns about risk of bias and inconsistency (89). The most recent studies in adults and children have shown that a combination of electronic monitoring and biofeedback can improve adherence and asthma outcomes (90–92). In one adult study, a programme of adherence and inhaler technique assessment resulted in only 27% remaining refractory to their asthma treatment (92). Hence, such approaches may offer a more effective approach in the future.

A number of add-on options are available for those with severe therapy resistant asthma. But prior to the use of these therapies, it is important to follow a systematic approach in the assessment and management of "difficult-to-treat" severe asthma—to confirm diagnosis, address poor adherence and to identify and manage comorbidities and risk factors (93, 94).

The following add-on options are best reserved for well-phenotyped patients with "severe treatment-refractory" asthma. The bulk of the evidence for their use at present is in adults and adolescents.

Anti-IgE Monoclonal Therapy

Omalizumab can be used for adults and children over 6 years of age with inadequately controlled severe allergic asthma despite optimized therapies (12, 13). The published data mostly related to adolescents and adults with only 3 randomized studies exclusive to children or adolescents (95–97). Most of the published data included subjects with moderate to severe asthma where omalizumab appears equally effective across different ages at reducing the risk of exacerbations and hospitalizations (98–100). Benefits are also seen in asthma symptom control for adults and children whilst other outcomes such as quality of life and rescue medication use have mainly been assessed in adults with modest improvements.

In addition, omalizumab allows for reduction or withdrawal of inhaled corticosteroid use but the latter option must be considered with caution (98). In children with severe disease omalizumab can reduce the burden of corticosteroids (101) and might be an effective alternative to oral corticosteroids (OCS) although a large direct OCS-sparing trial in children is required to confirm this.

In clinical use in both adults and children omalizumab has proved safe with few serious adverse effects (98).

Anti-interleukin 5 (IL-5) Monoclonal Therapy

Newer therapies targeted at IL-5 (mepolizumab, reslizumab) or the IL-5 receptor (benralizumab) are effective for adolescents and adults with severe eosinophilic asthma at high risk of exacerbations or with high symptom burden despite high dose ICS and another maintenance therapy (102). The effectiveness of subcutaneous mepolizumab (103, 104) and benralizumab (105, 106) in reducing exacerbations and hospitalizations is well-documented. They also improve asthma control, quality of life with modest gain in lung function and reduce the need for oral corticosteroid (106–108). Similar benefits were demonstrated with reslizumab only when administered intravenously which may impact its use in clinical practice (109, 110).

Randomized trials for all three anti-IL-5 therapies recruited patients over 12 years and included a few adolescents; studies using mepolizumab in children age between 6 and 11yr are underway. The EMA has recently approved mepolizumab for use in children 6–17years but this is based on an extrapolation of data from the efficacy and safety data from the Phase III studies in the mepolizumab severe asthma development programme for patients 12 and over.

Possible Alternatives for Adults Not Included in Guidelines: Macrolides, Bronchial Thermoplasty

Macrolides

Macrolides have antibacterial, antiviral and immunomodulatory effects and are shown to be effective in different asthma phenotypes (111). Adults with persistent asthma despite two or more maintenance therapies including ICS have fewer exacerbations and better quality of life when treated with azithromycin for 6-12months (111, 112). Macrolides are well-tolerated but microbial resistance is a potential concern with long term use. To date, there is no reported increase in infections related to macrolide use.

At present, there is no evidence that regular treatment with macrolides improves asthma control in children. Intermittent use of azithromycin in preschool children at the time of asthma attacks has been investigated. One study found that Azithromycin shortened the duration of episodes of asthma-like symptoms in young children aged 1–3years (113); in a second study in preschool children presenting to an emergency department, 5 days azithromycin (vs. placebo) neither reduced the duration of respiratory symptoms nor time to respiratory exacerbation in the following 6 months after treatment (114).

Bronchial thermoplasty

Bronchial thermoplasty is a non-pharmacological, endoscopic treatment for subjects aged ≥18 years with severe persistent asthma that is not well-controlled with ICS and LABA. Bronchial thermoplasty provides lower rates of exacerbations and modest improvements in quality of life but no difference in asthma control scores in patients with moderate to severe asthma (115–117). The procedure may be associated with temporary deterioration in asthma control needing hospitalization but is not associated with significant adverse respiratory effects on follow up out with the treatment phase. Its role in adult patients with severe asthma remains unclear especially in those with poor lung function. Based on current data, bronchial thermoplasty is not recommended by guidelines and it should only be used in carefully considered patients in the setting of a registry to allow independent data collection and in centers experienced in the technique. At present, there is no data on the use of bronchial thermoplasty in young people with severe asthma <18years of age.

Chromones (nedocromial sodium and sodium cromoglycate)

Chromones have favorable safety profile but low clinical efficacy compared to ICS in adults and children (118). The most recent Cochrane systematic review of studies in children judged there was insufficient evidence to be sure about the efficacy of sodium chromoglycate over placebo and was concerned that publication bias is likely to have overestimated the beneficial effects of sodium chromoglycate as maintenance therapy in childhood asthma in the past. They may have some role in those with exercise induced bronchospasm who are unresponsive to SABA pre-exercise and regular ICS for underlying asthma, as well as those intolerant of bronchodilators (119).

Approach to Adjusting Maintenance Treatment

Pharmacological management of asthma is based on continuous cycle of assessment, treatment and review to allow up or down titration of maintenance therapies to maximize patient outcomes using minimal treatment at various stage of the disease (12, 13).

Control Based Treatment Adjustment

Most guidelines recommend a change in management based on measures of symptom control with or without other risk factors such as compromised lung function or a history of exacerbations. Symptom based approaches are essentially all that is available in young children because of the fact they cannot co-operate with standard lung function tests.

For many patients in primary care, symptom control is a good guide to reduced risk of exacerbations. However, it is important to be mindful that in some patients, there may be discordance between responses in symptom control and asthma attacks. In preschool children, particularly, many children will have severe attacks of wheezing but no symptoms in between attacks.

Alternative Strategies for Adjusting Asthma Treatment Based on Eosinophilic Markers (Sputum Eosinophil Count or Exhaled Nitric Oxide)

Airways inflammation in asthma can be predominantly eosinophilic or non-eosinophilic. While ICS are the major preventer treatment to control symptoms, ICS are more effective in reducing symptoms in patients with eosinophilic inflammation than in those with neutrophilic inflammation (120). There has therefore been interest in whether tailoring asthma treatment based on objective eosinophilic inflammation improved asthma outcomes. Two approaches have been used to date: examination of eosinophil counts in induced sputum samples; or the measurement of exhaled nitric oxide.

The most up-to-date synthesis of the evidence concluded that children and adults randomized to either eosinophilic marker strategy were significantly less likely to experience an exacerbation during the follow-up period (4.5–24months). The exacerbation rate was also lower in adults with either strategy compared to controls, but not in children. For both strategies in adults and children, there was no difference for all secondary outcomes (FEV_1, asthma control test score, asthma quality of life, beta agonist use). There was also no difference in the final ICS use in either adults or children for either strategy (121).

Exacerbations are one, albeit important, asthma outcome; other outcomes such as symptom control and lung function also need consideration. Why there is discrepancy between exacerbations and other asthma outcomes is not understood but it has been noted in other studies involving the newer monoclonal drugs targeted at eosinophilic allergic pathways such as mepolizumab (103).

Currently, sputum induction is restricted to laboratories and clinics with specific expertise. It is technically demanding and time consuming and not always successful, particularly in younger children. Universal use of FeNO would be a substantial extra cost if used for all asthma patients and there is a yet no evidence-based algorithm on how to adjust treatment based on FeNO levels. Such an approach is most likely to benefit those with frequent asthma exacerbations.

In studies limited to non-smoking adults, FeNO >50ppb was predictive of good short-term response to ICS (122). However, there are no studies examining the long-term safety with regard to exacerbations or withholding ICS in patients with low initial FeNO.

Asthma Treatment at Different Ages – Challenges to Asthma Guidelines

The evidence base for the management of children with asthma, particularly young children, is often quite limited and has been compounded by a number of problems. Children under the age of 5–6years are usually not able to co-operate with lung function test and as result objective outcomes are commonly not available. Trials of treatment are more problematic without objective outcomes. New drugs are usually not tested in children until they have been extensively tested in adult patients. Recruiting and retaining children and their parents into randomized studies is difficult and as a result trials are often more limited in scale and duration. The consequence is that the evidence base for asthma treatments is often much smaller than available for adults. However, when an evidence base does emerge it is surprising how often it mirrors the that from adult studies. The value of ICS in preventing asthma exacerbations in young children would be an obvious example.

Asthma Guidelines summarize "population level" evidence and provide broad and generalized recommendations about asthma management (12, 13). However, it is now accepted that asthma is a heterogeneous disease and adjusting asthma treatment that takes account of differing phenotypes is one of the most important current challenges.

Despite publication of many evidence-based guidelines and the availability of effective therapies, there is widespread concern that asthma control in adults and children often remains poor and that asthma attacks and even deaths from asthma are not improving (123, 124). This is largely because there is a need to take account of "patient level" factors and tailor treatments to individuals. Such factors include any individual characteristics, preferences, risk factors, comorbidities or phenotype that predict or influence a patient's likely response to treatment, together with practical issues such as ability to use a particular inhaler, adherence, and affordability. Finally, patients with asthma, including children and their parents, often have different treatment goals from their physicians and want to balance the aims of optimizing asthma management against the side effects or inconvenience of taking regular medication necessary to achieve asthma control (13).

CONCLUSION

Asthma can significantly impact on all facets of life for patients across all age groups. Effective management strategies are broadly summarized by local and international guidelines. Overall, the evidence for pharmacological approach are more extensive and more robust for adults than that for younger children. For milder disease, the use of ICS as the initial maintenance therapy and SABA as needed appears universally effective for children, adolescents and adults. However, the preferred choice of subsequent add-on therapies differs and the evidence base for advanced therapeutic options is mostly based on studies in adolescents and adults. Clinicians are currently challenged with the need to develop management strategies that best caters for individual differences in asthma presentation and management. Accounting for differences in pathophysiological mechanisms, asthma phenotypes and treatment responses at different ages remains one of the most significant of these challenges.

AUTHOR CONTRIBUTIONS

Both authors contributed to the conception and preparation of this manuscript. LC contributed to the first draft and the content relating to asthma management in adults. JP provided his summary and expertise on treatment of asthma in children. Both authors contributed to manuscript revisions, read and approved the submitted version.

ACKNOWLEDGMENTS

We would like to acknowledge the contributions from Dr. Quentin Summers for his comments and suggestions for the overall content of this paper.

REFERENCES

1. World Health Organisation. Asthma–Key Facts. (2017). Available online at: http://www.who.int/news-room/fact-sheets/details/asthma (Accessed September 8, 2018).
2. Martinez FD, Wright AL, Taussig LM, Holberg CJ, Halonen M, Morgan WJ. Asthma and wheezing in the first six years of life. the group health medical associates. *N Engl J Med.* (1995) 332:133–8. doi: 10.1056/NEJM199501193320301
3. Silverman M. Out of the mouths of babes and sucklings: lessons from early childhood asthma. *Thorax.* (1993) 48:1200–4. doi: 10.1136/thx.48.12.1200
4. Schultz A, Devadason SG, Savenije OE, Sly PD, Le Souef PN, Brand PL. The transient value of classifying preschool wheeze into episodic viral wheeze and multiple trigger wheeze. *Acta Paediatr.* (2010) 99:56–60. doi: 10.1111/j.1651-2227.2009.01508.x
5. Garden FL, Simpson JM, Mellis CM, Marks GB, Investigators C. Change in the manifestations of asthma and asthma-related traits in childhood: a latent transition analysis. *Eur Respir J.* (2016) 47:499–509. doi: 10.1183/13993003.00284-2015
6. National Institute for Health and Care Excellence. *Asthma: Diagnosis, Monitoring and Chronic Asthma Management.* NICE guideline (2017). Available online at: www.nice.org.uk/guideance/ng80 (Accessed January 1, 2019).
7. Castro-Rodriguez JA, Custovic A, Ducharme FM. Treatment of asthma in young children: evidence-based recommendations. *Asthma Res Pract.* (2016) 2:5–16. doi: 10.1186/s40733-016-0020-z
8. Schleich F, Manise M, Sele J, Henket M, Seidel L, Louis R. Distribution of sputum cellular phenotype in a large asthma cohort: predicting factors for eosinophilic vs neutrophilic inflammation. *BMC Pulm Med.* (2013) 2013:11–8. doi: 10.1186/1471-2466-13-11
9. Clark VL, Gibson PG, Genn G, Hiles SA, Pavord ID, McDonald VM. Multidimensional assessment of severe asthma: a systematic review and meta-analysis. *Respirology.* (2017) 22: 1262–75. doi: 10.1111/resp.13134
10. Agusti A, Bafadhel M, Beasley R, Bel EH, Faner R, Gibson PG, et al. Precision medicine in airway diseases: moving to clinical practice. *Eur Respir J.* (2017) 50:1701655. doi: 10.1183/13993003.01655-2017
11. Haldar P, Pavord ID, Shaw DE, Berry MA, Thomas M, Brightling CE, et al. Cluster analysis and clinical asthma phenotypes. *Am J Respir Crit Care Med.* (2008) 178:218–24. doi: 10.1164/rccm.200711-1754OC
12. Global Initiative for Asthma. *Global Strategy for Asthma Management and Prevention.* 2018. (Available online at: http://www.ginaasthma.org (Accessed September 10, 2018).
13. British Thoracic Society. *British Guideline on the Management of Asthma.* (2016). Available online at: http://www.brit-thoracic.org.uk (Accessed September 12, 2018).
14. Vignola AM, Chanez P, Campbell AM, Souques F, Lebel B, Enander I, et al. Airway inflammation in mild intermittent and in persistent asthma. *Am J Respir Crit Care Med.* (1998) 157:403–9. doi: 10.1164/ajrccm.157.2.96-08040
15. Haahtela T, Selroos O, O'Byrne P. Revisiting early intervention in adult asthma. *ERJ Open Res.* (2015) 1:00022-2015. doi: 10.1183/23120541.00022-2015
16. Pauwels RA, Pedersen S, Busse WW, Tan WC, Chen YZ, Ohlsson SV, et al. Early intervention with budesonide in mild persistent asthma: a randomised, double-blind trial. *Lancet.* (2003) 361:1071–6. doi: 10.1016/S0140-6736(03)12891-7
17. Busse WW, Pedersen S, Pauwels RA, Tan WC, Chen YZ, Lamm CJ, et al. The Inhaled steroid treatment as regular therapy in early asthma (START) study 5-year follow-up: effectiveness of early intervention with budesonide in mild persistent asthma. *J Allergy Clin Immunol.* (2008) 121:1167–74. doi: 10.1016/j.jaci.2008.02.029
18. Adams NP, Bestall JB, Malouf R, Lasserson TJ, Jones PW. Inhaled beclomethasone versus placebo for chronic asthma. *Cochrane Database Syst Rev.* (2005) 1:CD002738. doi: 10.1002/14651858.CD002738.pub2
19. O'Bryne P, Barnes P, Rodrizuez-Roisin R, Runnerstrom E, Sandstrom T, Svensson K, et al. Low dose inhaled budesonide and formoterol in mild persistent asthma: the OPTIMA Randomized Trial. *Am J Respir Crit Care Med.* (2001) 164:1392–7. doi: 10.1164/rccm2104102
20. Reddel HK, Busse WW, Pedersen S, Tan WC, Chen Y-Z, Jorup C, et al. Should recommendations about starting inhaled corticosteroid treatment for mild asthma be based on symptom frequency: a *post-hoc.* efficacy analysis of the START study. *Lancet.* (2017) 389:157–66. doi: 10.1016/S0140-6736(16)31399-X
21. Agertoft L, Pedersen S. Effects of long-term treatment with an inhaled corticosteroid on growth and pulmonary function in asthmatic children. *Respir Med.* (1994) 88:373–81. doi: 10.1016/0954-6111(94)90044-2
22. Selroos O, Pietinalho A, Lofroos A, Riske H. Effect of early vs late intervention with inhaled corticosteroid in asthma. *Chest.* (1995) 108:1228–34. doi: 10.1378/chest.108.5.1228
23. Selroos O. Effect of disease duration on dose-response of inhaled budesonide in asthma. *Respir Med.* (2008) 102:1065–72. doi: 10.1016/j.rmed.2007.12.029
24. Selroos O, Lofroos A, Pietinalho A, Riska H. Asthma control and steroid doses 5 years after early or delayed introduction of inhaled corticosteroids in asthma: a real-life study. *Respir Med.* (2004) 98:254–62. doi: 10.1016/j.rmed.2003.10.007
25. O'Byrne PM, Pedersen S, Lamm CJ, Tan WC, Busse WW. Severe exacerbations and decline in lung function in asthma. *Am J Respir Crit Care Med.* (2009) 179:19–24. doi: 10.1164/rccm.200807-1126OC
26. Phelan PD, Robertson CF, Olinsky A. The melbourne asthma study: (1964)-(1999). *J Allergy Clin Immunol.* (2002) 109:189–94. doi: 10.1067/mai.2002.120951
27. Zhang L, Prietsch SO, Ducharme FM. Inhaled corticosteroids in children with persistent asthma: effects on growth. *Evid Based Child Health.* (2014) 9:829–930. doi: 10.1002/ebch.1988
28. Pruteanu AI, Chauhan BF, Zhang L, Prietsch SO, Ducharme FM. Inhaled corticosteroids in children with persistent asthma: dose-response effects on growth. *Evid Based Child Health.* (2014) 9:931–1046. doi: 10.1002/ebch.1989
29. Zhang L, Pruteanu AI, Prietsch SO, Chauhan BF, Ducharme FM. Cochrane in context: Inhaled corticosteroids in children with persistent asthma: effects on growth and dose-response effects on growth. *Evid Based Child Health.* (2014) 9:1047–51. doi: 10.1002/ebch.1984
30. Kaiser SV, Huynh T, Bacharier LB, Rosenthal JL, Bakel LA, Parkin PC, et al. Preventing exacerbations in preschoolers with recurrent wheeze: a meta-analysis. *Pediatrics.* (2016) 137:e–20154496. doi: 10.1542/peds.2015-4496
31. Castro-Rodriguez JA, Rodrigo GJ. Efficacy of inhaled corticosteroids in infants and preschoolers with recurrent wheezing and asthma: a systematic review with meta-analysis. *Pediatrics.* (2009) 123:e519–25. doi: 10.1542/peds.2008-2867
32. Fitzpatrick AM, Jackson DJ, Mauger DT, Boehmer SJ, Phipatanakul W, Sheehan WJ, et al. Individualized therapy for persistent asthma in young children. *J Allergy Clin Immunol.* (2016) 138:1608–18. doi: 10.1016/j.jaci.2016.09.028
33. Grigg J, Nibber A, Paton J, Chisholm A, Guilbert T, Kaplan A, et al. Matched cohort study of therapeutic strategies to prevent preschool wheezing/asthma attacks. *J Asthma Allergy.* (2018) 11:309–21. doi: 10.2147/JAA.S178531
34. Bateman ED, Boushey H, Bousquet J, Busse WW, Clark T, Pauwels R, et al. Can guideline-defined asthma control be achieved? the gaining optimal asthma control study. *Am J Respir Crit Care Med.* (2004) 170:836–44. doi: 10.1164/rccm.200401-033OC
35. O'Byrne PM, FitzGerald JM, Bateman ED, Barnes PJ, Zhong N, Keen C, et al. Inhaled combined budesonide–formoterol as needed in mild asthma. *N Engl J Med.* (2018) 378:1865–76. doi: 10.1056/NEJMoa1715274
36. Bateman ED, Reddel HK, O'Byrne PM, Barnes PJ, Zhong N, Keen C, et al. As-needed budesonide-formoterol versus maintenance budesonide in mild asthma. *N Engl J Med.* (2018) 378:1877–87. doi: 10.1056/NEJMoa1715275
37. Martinez FD, Chinchilli VM, Morgan WJ, Boehmer SJ, Lemanske RF, Jr., Mauger DT, et al. Use of beclomethasone dipropionate as rescue treatment for children with mild persistent asthma (TREXA): a randomised, double-blind, placebo-controlled trial. *Lancet.* (2011) 377:650–7. doi: 10.1016/S0140-6736(10)62145-9
38. Chauhan B, Chartrand C, Ducharme FM. Intermittent versus daily inhaled corticosteroids for persistent asthma in children and adults. *Cochrane Database Syst Rev.* (2013) 2:CD009611. doi: 10.1002/14651858.CD009611.pub3
39. Hussein HR, Gupta A, Broughton S, Ruiz G, Brathwaite N, Bossley CJ. A meta-analysis of montelukast for recurrent wheeze in preschool

children. *Eur J Pediatr.* (2017) 176:963–9. doi: 10.1007/s00431-017-2936-6

40. Ducharme FM, Ni Chroinin M, Greenstone I, Lasserson TJ. Addition of long-acting beta2-agonists to inhaled corticosteroids versus same dose inhaled corticosteroids for chronic asthma in adults and children. *Cochrane Database of Syst Rev.* (2010) 5:CD005535. doi: 10.1002/14651858.CD005535.pub2
41. Pauwels R, Lofdahl C, Postma D, Tattersfield A, O'Bryne P, Barnes P, et al. Effect of inhaled formoteol and budesonide on exacerbations of asthma. Formoterol and Corticosteroids establishing therapy (FACET) International Study Group. *N Engl J Med.* (1997) 337:1405–11.
42. Peters SP, Bleecker ER, Canonica GW, Park YB, Ramirez R, Hollis S, et al. Serious asthma events with budesonide plus formoterol vs. budesonide alone. *N Engl J Med.* (2016) 375:850–60. doi: 10.1056/NEJMoa1511190
43. Stempel DA, Raphiou IH, Kral KM, Yeakey AM, Emmett AH, Prazma CM, et al. Serious Asthma Events with fluticasone plus salmeterol versus fluticasone alone. *N Engl J Med.* (2016) 374:1822–30. doi: 10.1056/NEJMoa1511049
44. O'Byrne PM, Naya IP, Kallen A, Postma DS, Barnes PJ. Increasing doses of inhaled corticosteroids compared to adding long-acting inhaled beta2-agonists in achieving asthma control. *Chest.* (2008) 134:1192–9. doi: 10.1378/chest.08-1018
45. Chauhan BF, Chartrand C, Ni Chroinin M, Milan SJ, Ducharme FM. Addition of long-acting beta2-agonists to inhaled corticosteroids for chronic asthma in children. *Cochrane Database Syst Rev.* (2015) 11:CD007949. doi: 10.1002/14651858.CD007949.pub2
46. Cates CJ, Karner C. Combination formoterol and budesonide as maintenance and reliever therapy versus current best practice (including inhaled steroid maintenance), for chronic asthma in adults and children. *Cochrane Database Syst Rev.* (2013) 4:CD007313. doi: 10.1002/14651858.CD007313.pub3
47. Kew KM, Karner C, Mindus SM, Ferrara G. Combination formoterol and budesonide as maintenance and reliever therapy versus combination inhaler maintenance for chronic asthma in adults and children. *Cochrane Datab Syst Rev.* (2013) 12:CD009019. doi: 10.1002/14651858.CD009019.pub2
48. Patel M, Pilcher J, Pritchard A, Perrin K, Travers J, Shaw D, et al. Efficacy and safety of maintenance and reliever combination budesonide–formoterol inhaler in patients with asthma at risk of severe exacerbations: a randomised controlled trial. *Lancet Resp Med.* (2013) 1:32–42. doi: 10.1016/S2213-2600(13)70007-9
49. Papi A, Corradi M, Pigeon-Francisco C, Baronio R, Siergiejko Z, Petruzzelli S, et al. Beclometasone–formoterol as maintenance and reliever treatment in patients with asthma: a double-blind, randomised controlled trial. *Lancet Resp Med.* (2013) 1:23–31. doi: 10.1016/S2213-2600(13)70012-2
50. Bateman ED, Harrison TW, Quirce S, Reddel HK, Buhl R, Humbert M, et al. Overall asthma control achieved with budesonide/formoterol maintenance and reliever therapy for patients on different treatment steps. *Respir Res.* (2011) 12:38 doi: 10.1186/1465-9921-12-38
51. Szefler SJ, Martin RJ, King TS, Boushey HA, Cherniack RM, Chinchilli VM, et al. Significant variability in response to inhaled corticosteroids for persistent asthma. *J Allergy Clin Immunol.* (2002) 109:410–8. doi: 10.1067/mai.2002.122635
52. Ducharme FM, Ni Chroinin M, Greenstone I, Lasserson TJ. Addition of long-acting beta2-agonists to inhaled steroids versus higher dose inhaled steroids in adults and children with persistent asthma. *Cochrane Database Syst Rev.* (2010) 4:CD005533. doi: 10.1002/14651858.CD005533.pub2
53. Kew KM, Quinn M, Quon BS, Ducharme FM. Increased versus stable doses of inhaled corticosteroids for exacerbations of chronic asthma in adults and children. *Cochrane Database Syst Rev.* (2016) 6:CD007524. doi: 10.1002/14651858.CD007524.pub4
54. McKeever T, Mortimer K, Wilson A, Walker S, Brightling C, Skeggs A, et al. Quadrupling inhaled glucocorticoid dose to abort asthma exacerbations. *N Engl J Med.* (2018) 378:902–10. doi: 10.1056/NEJMoa1714257
55. Jackson DJ, Bacharier LB, Mauger DT, Boehmer S, Beigelman A, Chmiel JF, et al. Quintupling Inhaled Glucocorticoids to Prevent Childhood Asthma Exacerbations. N Engl J Med. (2018) 378:891–901. doi: 10.1056/NEJMoa1710988
56. Zeiger RS, Mauger DT, Bacharier LB, Guilbert T, Martinez FD, Lemanske RF, Jr., et al. Daily or intermittent budesonide in preschool children with recurrent wheezing. *N Engl J Med.* (2011) 365:1990–2001. doi: 10.1056/NEJMoa1104647
57. Toogood J, Baskerville J, Jennings B, Lefcoe N, Johansson S. Bioequivalent doses of budesonide and prednisolone in moderate and severe asthma. *J Allergy Clin Immunol.* (1989) 84:688–700. doi: 10.1016/0091-6749(89)90297-2
58. Chauhan BF, Jeyaraman MM, Singh Mann A, Lys J, Abou-Setta AM, Zarychanski R, et al. Addition of anti-leukotriene agents to inhaled corticosteroids for adults and adolescents with persistent asthma. *Cochrane Database Syst Rev.* (2017) 3:CD010347. doi: 10.1002/14651858.CD010347.pub2
59. Vaquerizo M, Casan P, Castillo J, Perpina M, Sanchis J, Sobradillo V, et al. Effect of montelukast added to inhaled budesonide on control of mild to moderate asthma *Thorax.* (2003) 58:204–10. doi: 10.1136/thorax.58.3.204
60. Dahlen S-E, Malmstrom K, Nizankowska E, Dahlen B, Kuna P, Kowaski M, et al. Improvement of aspirin-intolerant asthma by montelukast, a leukotriene antagonist, a randomized, double-blind, placebo-controlled trial. *Am J Respir Crit Care Med.* (2002) 165:9–14. doi: 10.1164/ajrccm.165.1.2010080
61. Walter K, Waldram J, Woessner K, White A. Long-term clinical outcomes of aspirin desensitisation with continuous daily aspirin therapy in aspirin-exacerbated respiratory disease. *Am J Rhinol Allergy.* (2018) 32:280–86. doi: 10.1177/1945892418770260
62. Chauhan BF, Ducharme FM. Addition to inhaled corticosteroids of long-acting beta2-agonists versus anti-leukotrienes for chronic asthma. *Cochrane Datab Syst Rev.* (2014) 1:CD003137. doi: 10.1002/14651858.CD003137.pub5
63. Chauhan BF, Ben Salah R, Ducharme FM. Addition of anti-leukotriene agents to inhaled corticosteroids in children with persistent asthma. *Cochrane Datab Syst Rev.* (2013) 10:CD009585. doi: 10.1002/14651858.CD009585.pub2
64. Benard B, Bastien V, Vinet B, Yang R, Krajinovic M, Ducharme FM. Neuropsychiatric adverse drug reactions in children initiated on montelukast in real-life practice. *Eur Respir J.* (2017) 50:1702135. doi: 10.1183/13993003.00148-2017
65. National Asthma Council Australia. *Australian Asthma Handbook, Version 1.3. Melbourne: National Asthma Council Australia.* (2017) Available online at: http://www.asthmahandbook.org.au. (Accessed October 01, 2018).
66. Tosca MA, Licari A, Olcese R, Marseglia G, Sacco O, Ciprandi G. Immunotherapy and Asthma in Children. *Front Pediatr.* (2018) 6:231. doi: 10.3389/fped.2018.00231
67. Virchow J, Backer V, Kuna P, Prieto L, Nolte H, Villesen H, et al. Efficacy of house dust mite sublingual allergen immunotherapy tablet in adults with allergic asthma: a randomised clinical trial. *JAMA.* (2016) 315:1715–25. doi: 10.1001/jama.2016.3964
68. Mosbech H, Deckelmann R, de Blay F, Pastorello EA, Trebas-Pietras E, Andres LP, et al. Standardized quality (SQ) house dust mite sublingual immunotherapy tablet (ALK) reduces inhaled corticosteroid use while maintaining asthma control: A randomized, double-blind, placebo-controlled trial. *J Allergy Clin Immunol.* (2014) 134:568–75. doi: 10.1016/j.jaci.2014.03.019
69. Rice JL, Diette GB, Suarez-Cuervo C, Brigham EP, Lin SY, Ramanathan M Jr, et al. Allergen-specific immunotherapy in the treatment of pediatric asthma: a systematic review. *Pediatrics.* (2018) 141:e20173833. doi: 10.1542/peds.2017-3833
70. Cox L, Nelson H, Lockey R, Calabria C, Chacko T, Finegold I, et al. Allergen immunotherapy: a practice parameter third update. *J Allergy Clin Immunol.* (2011) 127:S1–55. doi: 10.1016;j.jaci.2010.09.034
71. Powell H, Gibson P. Inhaled corticosteroid doses in asthma: an evidence-based approach. *Med J Aust.* (2003) 178:223–5.
72. Broersen L, Pereira A, Jorgensen J, Dekkers O. Adrenal insufficiency in corticosteroid. use: Systemic review and meta-analysis. *J Clin Endocrinol Metab.* (2015) 100:2171–80. doi: 10.1210/jc.2015-1218
73. Anderson DE, Kew KM, Boyter AC. Long-acting muscarinic antagonists (LAMA) added to inhaled corticosteroids (ICS) versus the same dose of ICS alone for adults with asthma. *Cochrane Database Syst Rev.* (2015) 8:CD011397. doi: 10.1002/14651858.CD011397.pub2

74. Peters S, Kunselman S, Icitovic N, Moore WC, Pascual R, Ameredes BT, et al. Tiotropium bromide step-up therapy for adults with uncontrolled asthma. *N Engl J Med.* (2010) 363:1715–26. doi: 10.1056/NEJMoa1008770
75. Evans DJ, Kew KM, Anderson DE, Boyter AC. Long-acting muscarinic antagonists (LAMA) added to inhaled corticosteroids (ICS) versus higher dose ICS for adults with asthma. *Cochrane Database Syst Rev.* (2015) 7:CD011437. doi: 10.1002/14651858.CD011437.pub2
76. Kerstjens HA, Engel M, Dahl R, Paggiaro P, Beck E, Vandewalker M, et al. Tiotropium in asthma poorly controlled with standard combination therapy. *N Engl J Med.* (2012) 367:1198–207. doi: 10.1056/NEJMoa1208606
77. Kerstjens HAM, Casale TB, Bleecker ER, Meltzer EO, Pizzichini E, Schmidt O, et al. Tiotropium or salmeterol as add-on therapy to inhaled corticosteroids for patients with moderate symptomatic asthma: two replicate, double-blind, placebo-controlled, parallel-group, active-comparator, randomised trials. *Lancet Resp Med.* (2015) 3:367–76. doi: 10.1016/S2213-2600(15)00031-4
78. Ohta K, Ichinose M, Tohda Y, Engel M, Moroni-Zentgraf P, Kunimitsu S, et al. Long-term once-daily tiotropium respimat® is well tolerated and maintains efficacy over 52 weeks in patients with symptomatic asthma in Japan: a randomised, placebo-controlled study. *PLoS ONE.* (2015) 10:e0124109 doi: 10.1371/journal.pone.0124109
79. Kew KM, Dahri K. Long-acting muscarinic antagonists (LAMA) added to combination long-acting beta2-agonists and inhaled corticosteroids (LABA/ICS) versus LABA/ICS for adults with asthma. *Cochrane Database Syst Rev.* (2016) 1:CD011721. doi: 10.1002/14651858.CD011721.pub2
80. Hamelmann E, Szefler SJ. Efficacy and safety of tiotropium in children and adolescents. *Drugs.* (2018) 78:327–38. doi: 10.1007/s40265-018-0862-1
81. Hamelmann E, Bateman ED, Vogelberg C, Szefler SJ, Vandewalker M, Moroni-Zentgraf P, et al. Tiotropium add-on therapy in adolescents with moderate asthma: A 1-year randomized controlled trial. *J Allergy Clin Immunol.* (2016) 138:441–50. doi: 10.1016/j.jaci.2016.01.011
82. Vrijlandt E, El Azzi G, Vandewalker M, Rupp N, Harper T, Graham L, et al. Safety and efficacy of tiotropium in children aged 1–5 years with persistent asthmatic symptoms: a randomised, double-blind, placebo-controlled trial. *Lancet Respir Med.* (2018) 6:127–37. doi: 10.1016/S2213-2600(18)30012-2
83. Evans D, Taylor D, Zetterstrom O, Chung K, O'Connor B, Barnes P. A comparison of low dose inhaled budesonide plus theophylline and high dose inhaled budesonide for moderate asthma. *N Engl J Med.* (1997) 337:1412–8.
84. Castro-Rodriguez JA, Rodrigo GJ, Rodriguez-Martinez CE. Principal findings of systematic reviews for chronic treatment in childhood asthma. *J Asthma.* (2015) 52:407–16. doi: 10.3109/02770903.2014.971968
85. Turner SW, Friend AJ, Okpapi A. Asthma and other recurrent wheezing disorders in children (chronic). *BMJ Clin Evid.* (2012) 2012:0302.
86. Hekking P-PW, Wener RR, Amelink M, Zwinderman AH, Bouvy ML, Bel EH. The prevalence of severe refractory asthma. *J Allergy ClinImmunol.* (2015) 135:896–902. doi: 10.1016/j.jaci.2014.08.042
87. Tay T, Lee J, Hew M. Diagnosis of severe asthma. *Med J Aust.* (2018) 209:S3–10. doi: 10.5694/mja18.00125
88. Bush A, Saglani S, Fleming L. Severe asthma: looking beyond the amount of medication. *Lancet Respir Med.* (2017) 5:844–6. doi: 10.1016/S2213-2600(17)30379-X
89. Normansell R, Kew KM, Stovold E. Interventions to improve adherence to inhaled steroids for asthma. *Cochrane Database Syst Rev.* (2017) 4:CD012226. doi: 10.1002/14651858.CD012226.pub2
90. Jochmann A, Artusio L, Jamalzadeh A, Nagakumar P, Delgado-Eckert E, Saglani S, et al. Electronic monitoring of adherence to inhaled corticosteroids: an essential tool in identifying severe asthma in children. *Eur Respir J.* (2017) 50:1700910. doi: 10.1183/13993003.00910-2017
91. Chan AH, Stewart AW, Harrison J, Camargo CA Jr., Black PN, Mitchell EA. The effect of an electronic monitoring device with audiovisual reminder function on adherence to inhaled corticosteroids and school attendance in children with asthma: a randomised controlled trial. *Lancet Respir Med.* (2015) 3:210–9. doi: 10.1016/S2213-2600(15)00008-9
92. Sulaiman I, Greene G, MacHale E, Seheult J, Mokoka M, D'Arcy S, et al. A randomised clinical trial of feedback on inhaler adherence and technique in patients with severe uncontrolled asthma. *Eur Respir J.* (2018) 51:1701126. doi: 10.1183/13993003.01126-2017
93. Gibson PG, McDonald VM. Management of severe asthma: targeting the airways, comorbidities and risk factors. *Intern Med J.* (2017) 47:623–31. doi: 10.1111/imj.13441
94. Bush A, Fleming L, Saglani S. Severe asthma in children. *Respirology.* (2017) 22:886–97. doi: 10.1111/resp.13085
95. Lanier B, Brideges T, Kulus M, Taylor A, Berhane I, Vidaurre C. Omalizuamb for the treatment of exacerations in children with inadequately controlled allergic (IgE-mediated) asthma. *J Allergy Clin Immunol.* (2009) 124:1210–6. doi: 10.1016/j.jaci.2009.09.021
96. Busse W, Morgan W, Gergen P, Mitchell H, Gern J, Liu A, et al. Randomized trial of omalizumab (anti-IgE) for asthma in inner-city children. *N Engl J Med.* (2011) 364:1005–15. doi: 10.1056/NEJMoa1009705
97. Milgron H, Berger W, Nayak A, Gupta N, Pollard S, McAlary M, et al. Treatment of childhood asthma with anti-immunoglobulin E antibody (omalizumab). *Pediatrics.* (2001) 108:E36. doi: 10.1542/peds.108.2.e36
98. Normansell R, Walker S, Milan SJ, Walters EH, Nair P. Omalizumab for asthma in adults and children. *Cochrane Database of Syst Rev.* (2014):CD003559. doi: 10.1002/14651858.CD003559.pub4
99. Rodrigo G, Neffen H. Systematic review on the use of omalizumab for the treatment of asthmatic children and adolescents. *Pediatr Allergy Immunol.* (2015) 26:551–6. doi: 10.1111/pai.12405
100. Chipps BE, Lanier B, Milgrom H, Deschildre A, Hedlin G, Szefler SJ, et al. Omalizumab in children with uncontrolled allergic asthma: review of clinical trial and real-world experience. *J Allergy Clin Immunol.* (2017) 139:1431–44. doi: 10.1016/j.jaci.2017.03.002
101. Brodlie M, McKean MC, Moss S, Spencer DA. The oral corticosteroid-sparing effect of omalizumab in children with severe asthma. *Arch Dis Child.* (2012) 97:604–9. doi: 10.1136/archdischild-2011-301570
102. Farne HA, Wilson A, Powell C, Bax L, Milan SJ. Anti-IL5 therapies for asthma. *Cochrane Database Syst Rev.* (2017) 9:CD010834. doi: 10.1002/14651858.CD010834.pub3
103. Pavord ID, Korn S, Howarth P, Bleecker ER, Buhl R, Keene ON, et al. Mepolizumab for severe eosinophilic asthma (DREAM): a multicentre, double-blind, placebo-controlled trial. *Lancet.* (2012) 380:651–9. doi: 10.1016/S0140-6736(12)60988-X
104. Ortega HG, Liu MC, Pavord ID, Brusselle GG, FitzGerald JM, Chetta A, et al. Mepolizumab treatment in patients with severe eosinophilic asthma. *N Engl J Med.* (2014) 371:1198–207. doi: 10.1056/NEJMoa1403290
105. FitzGerald JM, Bleecker ER, Nair P, Korn S, Ohta K, Lommatzsch M, et al. Benralizumab, an anti-interleukin-5 receptor α monoclonal antibody, as add-on treatment for patients with severe, uncontrolled, eosinophilic asthma (CALIMA): a randomised, double-blind, placebo-controlled phase 3 trial. *Lancet.* (2016) 388:2128–41. doi: 10.1016/S0140-6736(16)31322-8
106. Bleecker ER, FitzGerald JM, Chanez P, Papi A, Weinstein SF, Barker P, et al. Efficacy and safety of benralizumab for patients with severe asthma uncontrolled with high-dosage inhaled corticosteroids and long-acting β2-agonists (SIROCCO): a randomised, multicentre, placebo-controlled phase 3 trial. *Lancet.* (2016) 388:2115–27. doi: 10.1016/S0140-6736(16)31324-1
107. Bel EH, Wenzel SE, Thompson PJ, Prazma CM, Keene ON, Yancey SW, et al. Oral glucocorticoid-sparing effect of mepolizumab in eosinophilic asthma. *N Engl J Med.* (2014) 371:1189–97. doi: 10.1056/NEJMoa1403291
108. Nair P, Wenzel S, Rabe KF, Bourdin A, Lugogo NL, Kuna P, et al. Oral glucocorticoid-sparing effect of benralizumab in severe asthma. *N Engl J Med.* (2017) 376:2448–58. doi: 10.1056/NEJMoa1703501
109. Castro M, Zangrilli J, Wechsler ME, Bateman ED, Brusselle GG, Bardin P, et al. Reslizumab for inadequately controlled asthma with elevated blood eosinophil counts: results from two multicentre, parallel, double-blind, randomised, placebo-controlled, phase 3 trials. *Lancet Resp Med.* (2015) 3:355–66. doi: 10.1016/S2213-2600(15)00042-9
110. Bjermer L, Lemiere C, Maspero J, Weiss S, Zangrilli J, Germinaro M. Reslizumab for inadequately controlled asthma with elevated blood eosinophil levels: a randomized phase 3 study. *Chest.* (2016) 150:789–98. doi: 10.1016/j.chest.2016.03.032
111. Gibson PG, Yang IA, Upham JW, Reynolds PN, Hodge S, James AL, et al. Effect of azithromycin on asthma exacerbations and quality of life in adults with persistent uncontrolled asthma (AMAZES): a randomised, double-blind, placebo-controlled trial. *Lancet.* (2017) 390:659–68. doi: 10.1016/S0140-6736(17)31281-3

112. Brusselle GG, VanderStichele C, Jordens P, Deman R, Slabbynck H, Ringoet V, et al. Azithromycin for prevention of exacerbations in severe asthma (AZISAST): a multicentre randomised double-blind placebo-controlled trial. *Thorax.* (2013) 68:322–9. doi: 10.1136/thoraxjnl-2012-202698
113. Stokholm J, Chawes BL, Vissing NH, Bjarnadottir E, Pedersen TM, Vinding RK, et al. Azithromycin for episodes with asthma-like symptoms in young children aged 1–3 years: a randomised, double-blind, placebo-controlled trial. *Lancet Respir Med.* (2016) 4:19–26. doi: 10.1016/S2213-2600(15)00500-7
114. Mandhane PJ, Paredes Zambrano de Silbernagel P, Aung YN, Williamson J, Lee BE, Spier S, et al. Treatment of preschool children presenting to the emergency department with wheeze with azithromycin: a placebo-controlled randomized trial. *PLoS ONE.* (2017) 12:e0182411. doi: 10.1371/journal.pone.0182411
115. Torrego A, Solà I, Munoz AM, Roqué i Figuls M, Yepes-Nuñez JJ, Alonso-Coello P, et al. Bronchial thermoplasty for moderate or severe persistent asthma in adults. *Cochrane Datab Syst Rev.* (2014).CD(0099)10. doi: 10.(1002)/(1465)(1858).CD(0099)10.pub2
116. Castro M, Rubin AS, Laviolette M, Fiterman J, De Andrade Lima M, Shah PL, et al. Effectiveness and safety of bronchial thermoplasty in the treatment of severe asthma: a multicenter, randomized, double-blind, sham-controlled clinical trial. *Am J Respir Crit Care Med.* (2010) 181:116–24. doi: 10.1164/rccm.200903-0354OC
117. Chupp G, Laviolette M, Cohn L, McEvoy C, Bansal S, Shifren A, et al. Long-term outcomes of bronchial thermoplasty in subjects with severe asthma: a comparison of 3-year follow-up results from two prospective multicentre studies. *Eur Respir J.* (2017) 50:1750017. doi: 10.1183/13993003.000 17-2017
118. Guevara JP, Ducharme FM, Keren R, Nihtianova S, Zorc J. Inhaled corticosteroids versus sodium cromoglycate in children and adults with asthma. *Cochrane Database Syst Rev.* (2006) CD003558. doi: 10.1002/14651858.CD003558.pub2
119. Aggarwal B, Mulgirigama A, Berend N. Exercise-induced bronchoconstriction: prevalence, pathophysiology, patient impact, diagnosis and management. *NJP Prim Care Respir Med.* (2018) 28:31–9. doi: 10.1038/s41533-018-0098-2
120. Berry M, Morgan A, Shaw DE, Parker D, Green R, Brightling C, et al. Pathological features and inhaled corticosteroid response of eosinophilic and non-eosinophilic asthma. *Thorax.* (2007) 62:1043–9. doi: 10.1136/thx.2006.073429
121. Petsky HL, Cates CJ, Lasserson TJ, Li AM, Turner C, Kynaston JA, et al. A systematic review and meta-analysis: tailoring asthma treatment on eosinophilic markers (exhaled nitric oxide or sputum eosinophils). *Thorax.* (2012) 67:199–208. doi: 10.1136/thx.2010.135574
122. Dweik RA, Boggs PB, Erzurum SC, Irvin CG, Leigh MW, Lunberg JO, et al. An official ATS clinical practice guideline: Interpretation of exhaled nitric oxide levels (FENO) for clinical applications. *A J Respir Crit Care Med.* (2011) 184:602–15. doi: 10.1164/rccm.9120-11ST
123. Lenney W, Bush A, Fitzgerald DA, Fletcher M, Ostrem A, Pedersen S, et al. improving the global diagnosis and management of asthma in children. *Thorax.* (2018) 73:662–9. doi: 10.1136/thoraxjnl-2018-211626
124. Royal College of Physicians. *Why Asthma Still Kills: the National Review of Asthma Deaths (NRAD) Confidential Enquiry Report.* London (2014). Available online at: http://www.rcplondon.ac.uk/projects/outputs/why-asthma-still-kills (Accessed October 2, 2018).

17

Macrophage Phagocytosis and Allergen Avoidance in Children with Asthma

Neeta Kulkarni[1], Ahmad Kantar[2], Silvia Costella[3], Vincenzo Ragazzo[4], Giorgio Piacentini[5], Attilio Boner[5] and Christopher O'Callaghan[6]*

[1] *Department of Infection, Immunity and Inflammation, Institute for Lung Health, University of Leicester, Leicester, United Kingdom,* [2] *Pediatric Cough and Asthma Center, Istituti Ospedalieri Bergamaschi, University and Research Hospitals, Bergamo, Italy,* [3] *High Altitude Paediatric Asthma Centre in Misurina, Pio XII Institute, Belluno, Italy,* [4] *Department of Pediatrics, Versilia Hospital, Lido di Camaiore, Italy,* [5] *Pediatrics Section, Department of Surgery, Dentistry, Paediatrics, and Gynaecology, University of Verona, Verona, Italy,* [6] *Respiratory, Critical Care and Anaesthesia, UCL Great Ormond Street Institute of Child Health, NIHR Great Ormond Street Hospital Biomedical Research Centre, Great Ormond Street Children's Hospital, London, United Kingdom*

Correspondence:
Ahmad Kantar
kantar@centropediatricotosse.com

Background and Objective: Airway macrophages perform the crucial functions of presenting antigens, clearing pathogens, and apoptotic cells. Macrophage phagocytosis is increased in adults with mild asthma and allergen exposure is known to activate macrophages. However, it is not clear whether the mechanism behind this is due to a primary defect or environmental factors such as allergen or lipopolysaccaride (LPS) exposure. Our aim was to assess the phagocytic function of airway macrophages in children with mild to moderate asthma after residence in a low allergen\LPS environment at high altitude.

Methods: Sputum induction was performed in children with asthma at baseline and after residence for a 3 weeks' period at a high-altitude asthma center that has very low ambient allergen levels. The markers of eosinophilic inflammation (including percentage of macrophage cytoplasm with red hue) and phagocytosis of fluorescein isothiocyanate-labeled, heat-killed *Staphylococcus aureus* by airway macrophages was analyzed. Internalized bacteria were quantified using confocal microscopy.

Results: The median bacterial count [mean (standard deviation)] per macrophage was significantly lower [39.55 (4.51) vs. 73.26 (39.42) ($p = 0.006$)] after residence at high altitude. No association was observed between markers of eosinophilic inflammation and bacterial phagocytosis.

Conclusions: The results suggest that the mechanism behind the enhanced phagocytosis of bacteria in childhood asthma may be secondary to allergen or possibly LPS exposure.

Keywords: macrophages, phagocytosis, asthma, children, allergen avoidance

INTRODUCTION

In recent years, knowledge of macrophage biology has vastly improved. The normally protective alveolar macrophages can turn into pathogenic cells in adverse lung environment demonstrating their plasticity (1). The transcriptome and epigenetic landscape of tissue macrophages have been demonstrated as being determined by the tissue-specific microenvironment. Macrophages are constantly sensing the milieu of the adjacent stroma to regulate the tissue homeostasis both during steady and inflammatory states. (2). Lavin at all have shown that local tissue environment can alter the macrophages to acquire the identity and function of tissue resident macrophages e.g., transfer of bone marrow derived alveolar macrophages or mature peritoneal macrophages into alveolar space converted to alveolar macrophage-like cells (3).

Irrespective of the origin of macrophages (fetal, adult or differentiated tissue) once in lung environment they can fully function as alveolar macrophages and are similar at genomic and epigenomic levels (4, 5). Various studies have revealed that the development and resolution of lung injury is accompanied by remarkable changes in the numbers and types of macrophages (6, 7).

The lung is exposed to the environmental toxins like, microorganisms, chemical agents (including environmental LPS), allergens, and antigens. The alveolar and airway macrophages perform a dual role of activation and suppression of inflammation (8).

Asthma research has long been focused on cells that appear to be the major contributors of airway inflammation, including eosinophils, neutrophils, and lymphocytes. However, few studies have endorsed the mechanisms of function and regulation of macrophages that may orchestrate the inflammatory process. Macrophages are front line defenders of innate immunity and also play a crucial role in organ development, tissue turnover, and regeneration (9). The macrophages are capable of sensing viral, microbial, parasitic antigens, immune complexes, and apoptotic or necrotic cells which helps in immune surveillance (9–11).

Airway macrophage phagocytosis in adults with mild asthma is increased compared to healthy individuals and is possibly related to higher levels of activation of macrophages (12). The enhanced phagocytic function could be related to increased levels of cysteinyl leukotrienes in allergic lung (13) or other inflammatory mechanisms. However, Alexis et al. (12) observed adults with mild asthma, and those with higher eosinophil counts had lower phagocytosis (12). This suggests that macrophage phagocytic function may be related to an interaction with allergen and eosinophilic inflammation. Thus far, there have been no studies on allergen exposure reduction to test this as a possible cause of enhanced phagocytosis. In addition, LPS is well known to activate macrophages resulting in increased chemotactic and phagocytic activity (14) and therefore reduction of LPS would reduce phagocytic activity.

Because of the low relative humidity at high altitudes, the environment is free of house dust mites and molds (15). A number of studies in children (16–20) and adults with asthma have revealed a beneficial effect of high altitude residence on symptoms, lung function, and eosinophilic inflammation (21). However, no study has explored the effect of high altitude on macrophage phagocytosis, which results in a marked reduction in allergen and also possibly LPS exposure.

In adults with high levels of airway eosinophilic inflammation (defined as a sputum eosinophil count greater than 5%), macrophage phagocytosis has been shown to be lower, indicating that eosinophilic inflammation may affect phagocytosis (12). The toxic effect of eosinophil proteins on the epithelium and other cells (22, 23) is well known. These proteins may impair macrophage function.

We have previously shown, however, that sputum eosinophil count alone may be insufficient to identify ongoing eosinophilia (24). In children with asthma glucocorticoid treatment results in reduction of sputum eosinophil count, this could also be due to drop in recruitment of eosinophils because of natural resolution of disease process. Corticosteroid therapy increases eosinophil apoptosis and uptake by macrophages, thereby increasing the eosinophil protein content within the macrophages. To differentiate between these processes and to identify ongoing eosinophilia, we recently developed a novel marker of eosinophilic inflammation (eosinophil protein content in airway macrophages) (24).

In this study we hypothesized that airway macrophage phagocytosis would be lower after reduction of allergen exposure in children with mild to moderate asthma. To test our hypothesis, we compared airway macrophage phagocytosis before and after allergen avoidance during residence at the High Altitude Paediatric Asthma Centre in Misurina (1,756 m), which offers residential treatment for children with asthma. In addition, we assessed the relationship between airway macrophage phagocytosis and markers of eosinophilic inflammation (including eosinophilic proteins in airway macrophages) before their high-altitude residence. According to our understanding, this is the first study that explores the effect of a high altitude, with allergen and possibly LPS avoidance, on the phagocytic function of sputum macrophages in pediatric or adult asthma.

MATERIALS AND METHODS

Study Patients

The study enrolled children aged 7–17 years ($n = 62$) admitted to Istituto Pio XII, Misurina, Belluno (High Altitude Paediatric Asthma Centre) from various cities in Italy between June and September 2010. Children with a diagnosis of asthma and residing in the center for 3 weeks or more were included. The diagnosis of asthma was supported by clinical symptoms and reversibility testing (> 12% increase in FEV_1 after short acting bronchodilator treatment) (25). The exclusion criteria were respiratory infection in the preceding 6 weeks, congenital heart disease and chronic suppurative lung disease, or associated respiratory conditions such as cystic fibrosis and primary ciliary dyskinesia.

Study Design

On the day of arrival (T0) the demographic data, exposure to tobacco smoke, and medications including the doses of inhaled steroids were recorded. All children underwent clinical examination; spirometry, FeNO, and skin prick tests were performed. Spirometry was carried out as per the American Thoracic Society Guidelines (26). Sputum induction and blood eosinophil blood counts were performed within 2 days of arrival. At the end of the stay (T1) the symptoms during the stay and the treatment received were recorded and sputum induction was performed. The inhaled corticosteroid dose was converted to an estimated equipotent daily dose, in accordance with the guidelines of the Global Initiative for Asthma (GINA) (25) to compare the groups. Ethical approval was obtained by the Ethics Committee for Clinical Research of the Local Heath Authority in Belluno, and the parents provided written informed consent for the study. Our investigation was restricted to children with asthma because no healthy children resided at a high altitude for the time required by the study.

METHODS

Reagents and Chemicals

All reagents, culture media, and latex beads were purchased from Sigma–Aldrich (Milan, Italy) unless otherwise specified.

EXHALED NITRIC OXIDE MEASUREMENT

FeNO was measured using a standard technique complying with the recommendations of the European Respiratory Society/American Thoracic Society (27), using a chemiluminescence analyzer (Logan LR 2149; Logan Research Ltd., Rochester, Kent, UK), and expressed as parts per billion (ppb).

SPUTUM INDUCTION AND PROCESSING

Sputum was induced and processed as described previously (28, 29). Air-dried cytospins were stained with Diff-Quik. The total cell count, cell viability, and level of squamous cell contamination were assessed. The eosinophil differential count was obtained by counting 400 non-squamous cells and expressed as a percentage. The children were divided into 2 groups depending on the differential count on arrival (T0): eosinophilic ($\geq 3\%$) and non-eosinophilic ($< 3\%$).

Macrophage Eosinophil Protein Content

The image analysis method used was as previously described (24). Please refer to the online supporting information for details.

Macrophage Culture and Phagocytosis Assays

The macrophage culture and phagocytosis are described in the online supporting information.

CONFOCAL MICROSCOPY AND IMAGE ANALYSIS OF *STAPHYLOCOCCUS AUREUS* PHAGOCYTOSIS

After adherence, macrophages were incubated for 2 h with fluorescein isothiocyanate conjugated, heat-killed *Staphylococcus aureus* (Invitrogen Milan Italy) resuspended in RPMI 1640 supplemented with 5% FBS (10:1 ratio of staph aureus/Airway Macrophage). Please refer to online supporting information for details of further processing of sample, confocal microscopy, and image analysis to quantify internalized bacteria. The median bacterial count/airway macrophage and median maximum intensity\airway macrophage was calculated for each subject.

Latex Bead Phagocytosis: Phagocytic Index

After adherence, macrophages were incubated with 2-μm latex beads (airway macrophage: bead = 1:10) resuspended in RPMI 1640 (supplemented with 5% FBS) for 2 h. Please refer to the online supporting information for details on the counting of internalized bacteria. The phagocytic index (beads/100 airway macrophages) and number of phagocytic macrophages were calculated.

Statistics

Statistical analysis was performed using GraphPad Prism 6 (GraphPad, San Diego, CA, USA). Patient characteristics are presented as mean (standard error), median (range or interquartile range) or percentages. The between-group comparisons for non-parametric data were made using the Mann–Whitney test for unpaired data and the Wilcoxon matched-pair test for paired data as appropriate and proportions were assessed using Fisher's exact/chi-square test. Differences were considered significant when $p < 0.05$. Linear regression and Spearman's co-relations were used to explore the association between the macrophage eosinophil protein content and phagocytosis.

RESULTS

Patient Characteristics

The clinical characteristics of 54 children who produced adequate sputum for cell counts on arrival (T0) are as shown in **Table 1**. All children were in GINA Groups 1–3 (with 77.7% of children in GINA Groups 1 and 2) depending on the treatment in the previous 3 months prior to the start of residency. Thirty children had sputum eosinophil counts over 3% and were therefore assigned to the eosinophilic group, with 24 in the non-eosinophilic group. The median (range) sputum eosinophil content in the eosinophilic group was 12% (3–52%). Boys were predominant in the eosinophilic group. No difference was observed in FEV_1 between the groups. However, the predicted $FEF_{25-75}\%$ was lower and blood eosinophil and FeNo content were higher in the eosinophilic phenotype (**Table 1**).

Fifty children produced adequate sputum samples on both occasions (T0 and T1) for differential counts. No statistical difference was observed in lung function measurements before or after their high-altitude stay in a very low ambient allergen environment. However, after exposure to a high altitude (T1), they had a significantly lower FeNO ($p < 0.001$) and eosinophil counts ($p = 0.001$) (**Table 2**, **Figure 1d**). No difference was observed in percentage cell viability (**Table 1**) (all cell types) in the eosinophilic and non-eosinophilic groups or in the T0 or T1 samples. The patients who produced an adequate sample for phagocytosis assay did not differ from those who did in age, lung function parameters, blood eosinophil counts, or sputum cell counts. The equipotent inhaled corticosteroid dose was reduced ($p = 0.01$) (**Table 2**) during their stay at the center because the children were exhibiting fewer symptoms.

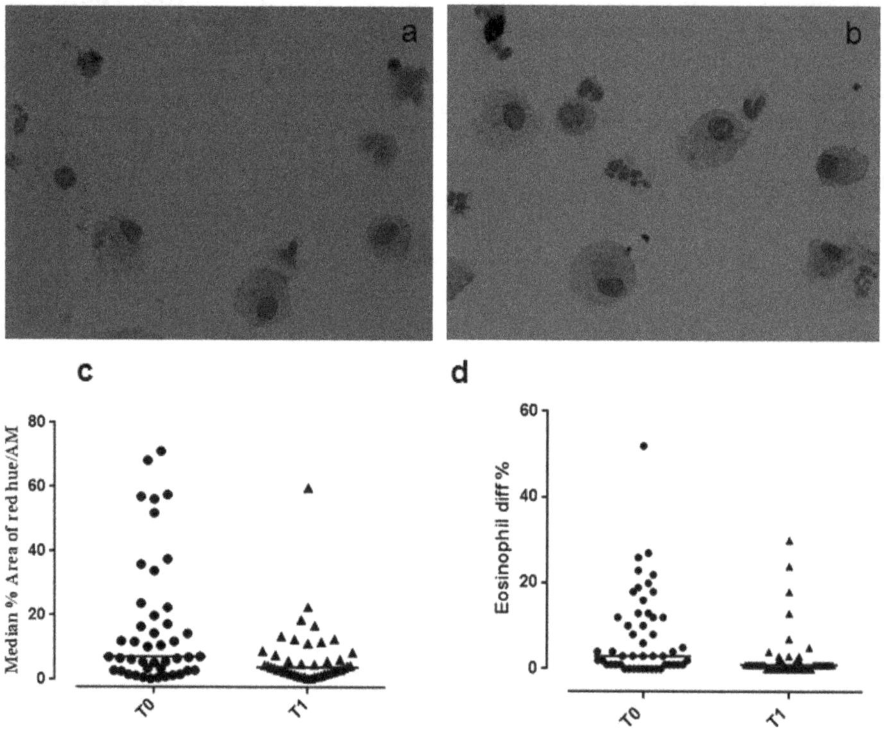

FIGURE 1 | Eosinophilic staining of macrophages at **(a)** T0 and **(b)** T1. Graphs showing **(c)** the median % red hue/airway macrophage ratio, and **(d)** sputum eosinophil differential counts at T0 and T1.

Macrophage Eosinophilic Proteins

Example images of red hue in macrophages before and after residence in Misurina, as an index of eosinophil uptake, are shown in **Figures 1a,b**. No significant difference was observed ($p = 0.39$) between median airway macrophage red hue percentage in eosinophilic ($n = 30$) [median (range)] [5.9 (0.6–57.6)] and non-eosinophilic asthma ($n = 24$) [8.7 (0.34–71.2)]. After time spent at a high altitude (T1), the children ($n = 43$ pairs) had a significantly lower airway macrophage red hue percentage [$p = 0.005$] than before T0 (**Table 2**, **Figure 1c**).

Macrophage Phagocytosis

Examples of confocal images showing internalized bacteria and light microscopy images showing latex beads are presented in **Figures 2**, **3**, respectively. No significant difference ($p = 0.3$) was observed between the median bacterial counts in eosinophilic ($n = 16$) and non-eosinophilic asthma ($n = 8$) at T0. After exposure to a high altitude (T1), the children ($n = 19$ pairs) exhibited significantly lower median bacterial counts [Mean (standard deviation)] [$p = 0.006$, 39.55 (4.51) vs. 73.26 (39.42)] than at T0 (**Table 3**).

Eosinophilic Inflammation and Phagocytosis

No significant correlation or association was observed between age, FeNo, pre- and post-bronchodilator lung function (FEV_1% predicted, FVC% predicted, FEF_{25-75}% predicted), blood counts (total white count, eosinophil count), or sputum parameters (viability, eosinophil and neutrophil counts) and bacterial uptake by macrophages (median bacterial count) and median maximum intensity (bacterial fluorescence). Latex bead phagocytosis (number of phagocytic macrophages (%) and phagocytic index) were significantly positively associated with FeNo ($p = 0.028$) and blood eosinophils ($p = 0.028$), but were not associated with any other parameter. There was a positive correlation between number of phagocytic macrophages (%) and blood eosinophils ($r = 0.508$, $p = 0.046$). The median airway macrophage red hue area percentage was not associated with bacterial or latex phagocytosis parameters. Please refer to online Supplement Figures 1–4.

DISCUSSION

Alveolar macrophages line the luminal surface and are primary defense mechanism to protect the lungs from invading pathogens and pollutants. They initiate and evolve the immune response in the lung. Overall, the number of macrophages in patients with asthma is similar to that in healthy individuals (30).

In asthma, two major functionally distinct subsets of macrophages have been intensively investigated: the M1 and M2 macrophages. Macrophages have been grouped into M1 and M2 types depending on their function in subjects with asthma. M1 macrophages are differentiated by bacteria-derived mediators such as interferon-c and lipopolysaccaride (LPS)

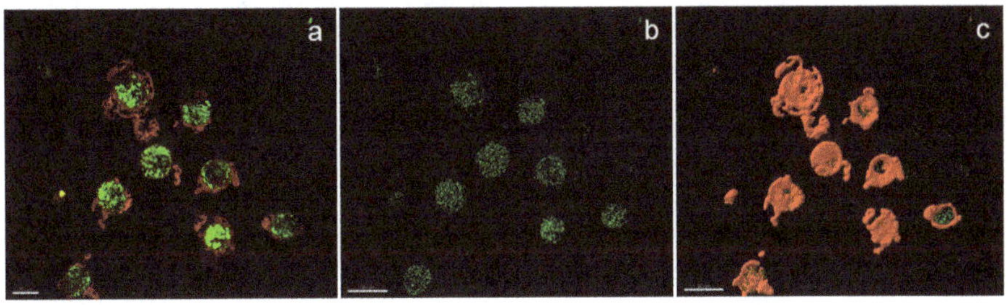

FIGURE 2 | Confocal image of sputum macrophages cultured with heat-killed fluorescein isothiocyanate-labeled *Staphylococci aureus* (airway macrophage:bacteria = 1:10) showing internalized bacteria. **(a)** Confocal image of bacteria (green) and cytoplasm (red), **(b)** bacteria alone, and **(c)** the surface view of macrophages showing that a majority of the bacteria are internalized.

TABLE 1 | Baseline characteristics of patients.

	Eosinophilic group ($n = 30$)	Non-eosinophilic group ($n = 24$)	*p*-value
Mean age (yr) (SD)	13.51 (± 3.1)	13.02 (± 2.9)	0.55
Sex (male), No. (%)	25 (83.3)	13 (54.1)	**0.034**
BMI	18.99 (14.4–31.9)	19.99 (12.8–41.1)	0.7
Smoking in house (yes) No. (%)	12 (40)	7 (29.2)	0.56
Food allergy (yes) No. (%)	14 (46.6)	9 (37.5)	0.58
GINA Classification No. (%)			0.30
1	6 (20)	9 (37.5)	
2	17 (56.7)	10 (41.7)	
3	7 (23.3)	4 (16.7)	
5	0	1 (4.1)	
FEV_1 % predicted mean (SE)	106.8 (2.97)	113.7 (3.7)	0.13
FVC% predicted mean (SE)	104.5 (2.22)	107.2 (2.8)	0.45
FEF_{25-75}% predicted Mean (SE)	98.27 (5.03)	115.9 (6.5)	**0.034**
Blood eosinophils (%)	7.8 (3.9–12.1)	5.05 (1.9–13.1)	**0.014**
Median FeNo (ppb) (range)	23.75 (6.3–79.3)	12.8 (12.7–41.1)	**0.001**
MEDIAN INDUCED SPUTUM (RANGE)			
Total cell count × 10^6 \g sputum	2.3 (0.39–9.5)	1.7 (0.05–7.2)	0.48
Cell viability (%)	86.5 (59.7–96.4)	88.9 (57.9–100)	0.27
Macrophages (%)	62.5 (1–88)	72.5 (14–97)	0.17
Neutrophils (%)	22 (8–72)	26.5 (3–86)	0.46

(Eosinophilic group ≥ 3% sputum eosinophil differential count). Bold P-values indicates $p < 0.05$.

TABLE 2 | Lung function, FeNo, sputum differential counts, inhaled corticosteroids, and macrophage red hue percentage results on arrival (T0), and after the allergen reduction intervention (3-week residence at a high-altitude asthma center) (T1).

	T0 ($n = 50$)	T1 ($n = 50$)	*p*-value
FEV_1 % predicted mean (SE)	109.5 (2.4)	116.0 (2.04)	0.67
FVC% predicted mean (SE)	105.8 (1.81)	105.6 (1.89)	0.91
FEV/FVC ratio % predicted mean (SE)	103.1 (1.29)	101.8 (1.3)	0.56
FEF_{25-75}% predicted mean (SE)	105.3 (4.38)	102.9 (4.01)	0.72
Median FeNo (ppb) (range)	18.85 (2.6–79.3)	11.5 (2.1–52.2)	**0.0004**
ICS treatment*			**0.01**
No ICS treatment No. (%)	13 (26)	20 (40)	
Low daily dose No. (%)	21 (42)	26 (52)	
Medium daily dose No. (%)	16 (32)	4 (8)	
MEDIAN INDUCED SPUTUM (RANGE)			
Total cell count × 10^6\g sputum	2.2 (05–9.5)	2.25 (0.26–11.2)	0.24
Macrophages (%)	65 (1–97)	63 (6–87)	0.15
Neutrophils (%)	24.5 (3–86)	32.5 (11–90)	**0.006**
Eosinophils (%)	3 (0–52)	1 (0–30)	**0.001**
Lymphocytes (%)	0 (0–2)	0 (0–8)	0.7
Median % area red hue/airway macrophage (range) ($n = 43$ pairs)	7.04 (0.72–71.23)	3.82 (0.41–59.82)	**0.005**

**GINA classification of equipotent daily dose of inhaled glucocorticosteroids for children older than 5 years (25). Bold P-values indicates $p < 0.05$.*

and release various inflammatory cytokines and chemokines, whereas M2 macrophages have increased phagocytic activity but are poor at clearing intracellular pathogens. Moreover, experimental data suggests both M1 and M2 subsets are involved in asthma (31). In addition there are regulatory macrophages performing different physiological functions and develop in response to different stimuli (32). These are vital in regulating immune responses and reduce inflammation (33). Macrophages are critical for both innate and acquired immunity and play a pivotal role in lung defense. Lung macrophages recognize a wide variety of pathogenic antigens, immune complexes, and apoptotic or necrotic cells (11). Increased infection in asthma has led to increased investigation of the clearance of bacterial, cellular, and inhaled particles by macrophages in patients with asthma.

Alexis et al. have demonstrated that phagocytosis of opsonised particles in subjects with mild asthma with airway eosinophilia was lower as compared to those without eosinophilia. Overall phagocytosis was comparable between controls and those with mild intermittent asthma (12). In a similar subjects, phagocytic

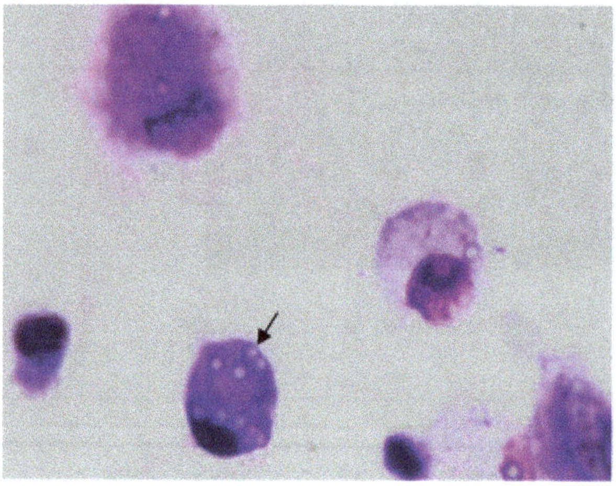

FIGURE 3 | Image of airway macrophages cultured with latex beads (airway macrophage: bead = 1:10) for 2 h. External beads were digested with xylene. Internalized beads are preserved (arrow).

TABLE 3 | Phagocytosis assay on arrival (T0) and after the allergen reduction intervention (T1) (3-week residence at a high-altitude asthma center).

Bacterial phagocytosis (n = 19 pairs)	**T0**	**T1**	p
Mean bacterial count mea (SD)	73.26 (39.42)	39.55 (4.51)	**0.006**
Mean max intensity (SD)	0.044 (0.010)	0.038 (0.01)	0.08
LATEX BEAD PHAGOCYTOSIS (n = 10 pairs)			
Median beads/100 cells (range)	201.0 (71.56–1268)	44.52 (9.8–246.8)	**0.003**
Mean % phagocytic AM (SD)	57.70 (16.24)	27.86 (16.36)	**0.001**

Bold P-values indicates $p < 0.05$.

activity in airway macrophages decreased by about 50% 6 h after endotoxin (LPS) inhalation (34).

Fitzpatrick et al. sampled bronchoalveolar lavage macrophages from children with severe asthma and demonstrated impaired phagocytosis of *S. Aureus.* Interestingly this remained unchanged after LPS stimulation. Moreover, they have shown that children with severe asthma also had increased alveolar macrophage apoptosis (35). These later findings were attributed to imbalance in glutathione homeostasis (36). Similar findings of reduced phagocytosis of *H influenzae* and *S aureus* were seen in bronchoalveolar lavage and monocyte-derived macrophages from adults with severe asthma (37). Not only bacterial uptake but apoptotic cell clearance by lavage macrophages is reduced in severe asthma as compared to healthy controls or mild-moderate asthma patients (38).

Studies have demonstrated that severe asthma is associated with inflammatory mediators such as prostaglandin E2 and D2, which can suppress the phagocytic activity of alveolar macrophages (39–41). Recently, Brugha et al. investigated the phagocytosis of inhalable carbonaceous particle matter by airway macrophages obtained from the induced sputum of asthmatic children. Their results demonstrated a 51% lower carbon content in the macrophages of children with moderate to severe asthma compared with mild asthma and healthy children (42). Moreover, the study demonstrated an inverse association between alveolar macrophage carbon and urinary metabolites of prostaglandin E2 and prostaglandin D2.

The effect of a high altitude on improvement of asthma symptoms has been attributed to the very low levels of ambient allergens. In this study, we described for the first time the effect of residence at a high altitude with markedly reduced allergens and possibly pollutants (e.g., LPS) on the phagocytic function of sputum macrophages and markers of eosinophilic inflammation in children with mild to moderate asthma. According to our understanding, this is the original study exploring the effect of reduced allergen\LPS exposure on the phagocytic function of sputum macrophages in pediatric or adult asthma. The phagocytosis of heat-killed bacteria in this group of children decreased after residence at a high altitude and was similar in eosinophilic and non-eosinophilic phenotypes. We also found that bacterial phagocytosis was not associated with parameters of eosinophilic inflammation, including the median airway macrophage red hue percentage.

Our study strongly suggests that allergen and possibly LPS exposure is a major contributor to enhanced macrophage phagocytosis in asthma. The induced sputum macrophage capacity to phagocytose particles has been demonstrated to be higher in subjects with mild asthma (12, 43) than in healthy controls. One possible explanation is that activation of macrophages is enhanced in asthma. Silva et al showed that cysteinyl leukotrienes enhanced Fcγ-mediated phagocytosis in sensitized rats (13). **(author?)** (28) showed that children with asthma, after residence in a very low ambient allergen environment at a high altitude had lower exhaled breath cysteinyl leukotrienes and leukotriene B4 (28). This might partially explain our finding of reduced phagocytosis in children with mild asthma staying in similar conditions. Along with reduction in allergens there is also possibility of lower level of ambient pollution including LPS. LPS is known to stimulate macrophages and therefore reduction would lower phagocytic capacity.

Fitzpatrick et al. sampled bronchoalveolar lavage macrophages from children with severe asthma and demonstrated impaired phagocytosis (35) but did not include children with mild asthma. We were unable to compare our results of phagocytosis assays with other studies assessing sputum macrophage phagocytosis because this is the first such study on children with asthma. In addition, no studies have included reduction of allergens as an intervention to assess phagocytosis of sputum macrophages. No difference was observed in the viability of sputum cells on arrival or after residence at a high altitude that could have affected the macrophage phagocytic function.

We recently described a novel marker (macrophage eosinophil protein content measured as red hue percentage) that identifies ongoing sputum eosinophilia in patients with asthma and a normal sputum eosinophil count (24). On admission, children without sputum eosinophilia had similar airway macrophage red hue percentages as those with sputum eosinophilia. This suggests the presence of ongoing eosinophilia in the non-eosinophilic group. Because airway macrophages acquire eosinophilic proteins by phagocytizing apoptotic eosinophils, a lower airway macrophage red hue suggests that macrophages have ingested fewer eosinophils. Therefore, the combination of low airway macrophage red hue and low sputum eosinophil counts suggests a reduction of eosinophil recruitment to the airways. The reduction of sputum eosinophilia after residence at a high altitude has previously been demonstrated (20, 28). In children with asthma glucocorticoid treatment results in reduction of sputum eosinophil count, this could also be due to drop in recruitment of eosinophils because of natural resolution of disease process. Corticosteroid therapy increases eosinophil apoptosis and uptake by macrophages, thus increasing the eosinophil protein content within macrophages. It could be argued that when admitted to the center that supervises administration of treatment, the improved adherence to therapy could have contributed to the reduction in eosinophilic inflammation. However, this is unlikely because the airway macrophage red hue percentage dropped after residence at a high altitude, suggesting reduction of eosinophil ingestion by sputum macrophages and reduced recruitment. Therefore, using the macrophage red hue measurement has the added value of helping to differentiate between a reduced sputum eosinophil count related to treatment and that related to reduced recruitment of eosinophils.

Although evidence (12) indicates that increased eosinophilic inflammation is inversely associated with phagocytosis, we did not find an association between bacterial phagocytosis and markers of eosinophilic inflammation (including the eosinophilic proteins in airway macrophages). However, this relationship must be explored further in children with severe asthma who have persistent inflammation.

Our study had some limitations. We were unable to recruit healthy children because they did not reside for 4 weeks at the high-altitude asthma center. Because of the small amount of sputum samples obtained from the children, insufficient numbers of macrophages were obtained to analyze the macrophages for cell surface markers of activation. It is possible that *in vivo* phagocytosis may be affected by other factors that we did not measure. However, our study results indicating higher phagocytosis in patients with mild asthma are like those of inhaled particles in adults in *in vivo* experiments (43).

In conclusion, induced sputum was successfully used to study macrophage phagocytosis in children with asthma. The sputum macrophages in children with mild to moderate asthma after allergen and possibly lipopolysaccaride avoidance at a high altitude are less phagocytic. Because activation of macrophages by allergens in mild asthma enhances phagocytosis, removal of this stimulus appears to reduce phagocytosis. No association was observed between phagocytosis and eosinophilic inflammation markers. Further research is essential to dissect the mechanism of various types of alveolar macrophage phagocytosis in asthma.

AUTHOR CONTRIBUTIONS

All authors listed have made a substantial, direct and intellectual contribution to the work, and approved it for publication.

ACKNOWLEDGMENTS

The authors thank all staff at High Altitude Children's Asthma Center in Misurina, Claire Smith, Louise Donnelly (Imperial College London for advice on methodology), Will Monteiro (Institute for Lung Health in Glenfield Hospital). This research is supported by the NIHR GOSH BRC. The views expressed are those of the author(s) and not necessarily those of the NHS, the NIHR or the Department of Health. NK is the recipient of a European Respiratory Society Fellowship (Number 774).

REFERENCES

1. Joshi N, Walter JM, Misharin AV. Alveolar macrophages. *Cell Immunol.* (2018). doi: 10.1016/j.cellimm.2018.01.005. [Epub ahead of print].
2. Lavin Y, Mortha A, Rahman A, Merad M. Regulation of macrophage development and function in peripheral tissues *Nat Rev Immunol.* (2015) 15:731–44. doi: 10.1038/nri3920
3. Lavin Y, Winter D, Blecher-Gonen R, David E, Keren-Shaul H, Merad M, et al. Tissue-resident macrophage enhancer landscapes are shaped by the local microenvironment. *Cell* (2014) 159:1312–26. doi: 10.1016/j.cell.2014.11.018
4. Janssen WJ, Barthel L, Muldrow A, Oberley-Deegan RE, Kearns MT, Jakubzick C, et al. Fas determines differential fates of resident and recruited macrophages during resolution of acute lung injury. *Am J Respir Crit Care Med.* (2011) 184:547–60. doi: 10.1164/rccm.201011-1891OC
5. van de Laar L, Saelens W, De Prijck S, Martens L, Scott CL, Van Isterdael G, et al. Yolk sac macrophages, fetal liver, and adult monocytes can colonize an empty niche and develop into functional tissue-resident macrophages. *Immunity* (2016) 44:755–68. doi: 10.1016/j.immuni.2016.02.017
6. Alber A, Howie SE, Wallace WA, Hirani N. The role of macrophages in healing the wounded lung. *Int J Exp Pathol.* (2012) 93:243–51. doi: 10.1111/j.1365-2613.2012.00833.x
7. Misharin AV, Scott Budinger GR, Perlman H. The lung macrophage: a Jack of all trades. *Am J Respir Crit Care Med.* (2011) 184:497–8. doi: 10.1164/rccm.201107-1343ED
8. Pappas K, Papaioannou AI, Kostikas K, Tzanakis N. The role of macrophages in obstructive airways disease: chronic obstructive pulmonary disease and asthma. *Cytokine* (2013) 64:613–25. doi: 10.1016/j.cyto.2013.09.010
9. Akira S, Misawa T, Satoh T, Saitoh T. Macrophages control innate inflammation. *Diabetes Obesity Metab.* (2013) 15(Suppl. 3):10–8. doi: 10.1111/dom.12151
10. Forbes SJ, Rosenthal N. Preparing the ground for tissue regeneration: from mechanism to therapy. *Nat Med.* (2014) 20:857–69. doi: 10.1038/nm.3653
11. Roszer T. Understanding the mysterious M2 macrophage through activation markers and effector mechanisms. mediators of inflammation. (2015) 2015:816460. doi: 10.1155/2015/816460
12. Alexis NE, Soukup J, Nierkens S, Becker S. Association between airway hyperreactivity and bronchial macrophage dysfunction in individuals with

mild asthma. *Am J Physiol Lung Cell Mol Physiol.* (2001) 280:L369–75. doi: 10.1152/ajplung.2001.280.2.L369

13. Silva RC, Landgraf MA, Hiyane MI, Pacheco-Silva A, Camara NO, Landgraf RG. Leukotrienes produced in allergic lung inflammation activate alveolar macrophages. *Cell Physiol Biochem.* (2010) 26:319–26. doi: 10.1159/000320555
14. Wu T-T, Chen T-L, Chen R-M. Lipopolysaccharide triggers macrophage activation of inflammatory cytokine expression, chemotaxis, phagocytosis, and oxidative ability via a toll-like receptor 4-dependent pathway: validated by RNA interference. *Toxicol. Lett.* (2009) 191:195–202. doi: 10.1016/j.toxlet.2009.08.025
15. Spieksma FT, Zuidema P, Leupen MJ. High altitude and house-dust mites. *Br Med J.* (1971) 1:82–4.
16. Boner AL, Niero E, Antolini I, Valletta EA, Gaburro D. Pulmonary function and bronchial hyperreactivity in asthmatic children with house dust mite allergy during prolonged stay in the Italian Alps (Misurina, 1756 m). *Ann. Allergy* (1985) 54:42–5.
17. Grootendorst DC, Dahlen SE, Van Den Bos JW, Duiverman EJ, Veselic-Charvat M, Vrijlandt EJ, et al. Benefits of high altitude allergen avoidance in atopic adolescents with moderate to severe asthma, over and above treatment with high dose inhaled steroids. *Clin Exp Allergy* (2001) 31:400–8. doi: 10.1046/j.1365-2222.2001.01022.x
18. Peroni DG, Piacentini GL, Costella S, Pietrobelli A, Bodini A, Loiacono A, et al. Mite avoidance can reduce air trapping and airway inflammation in allergic asthmatic children. *Clin Exp Allergy* (2002) 32:850–5. doi: 10.1046/j.1365-2222.2002.01372.x
19. Peroni DG, Piacentini GL, Vicentini L, Costella S, Pietrobelli A, Boner AL. Effective allergen avoidance reduces residual volume and sputum eosinophils in children with asthma. *J Allergy Clin Immunol.* (2001) 108:308. doi: 10.1067/mai.2001.117174
20. Piacentini GL, Del Giudice MJ, Bodini A, Costella S, Vicentini L, Peroni D, et al. Exhaled NO reduced on allergen avoidance. *Allergy* (2001) 56:251–2. doi: 10.1034/j.1398-9995.2001.056003251.x
21. Rijssenbeek-Nouwens LH, Bel EH. High-altitude treatment: a therapeutic option for patients with severe, refractory asthma? *Clin Exp Allergy* (2011) 41:775–82. doi: 10.1111/j.1365-2222.2011.03733.x
22. Frigas E, Motojima S, Gleich GJ. The eosinophilic injury to the mucosa of the airways in the pathogenesis of bronchial asthma. *Eur Respir J.* (1991) 13:123s–35s.
23. Maeda T, Kitazoe M, Tada H, de Llorens R, Salomon DS, Ueda M, et al. Growth inhibition of mammalian cells by eosinophil cationic protein. *Eur J Biochem.* (2002) 269:307–16. doi: 10.1046/j.0014-2956.2001.02653.x
24. Kulkarni NS, Hollins F, Sutcliffe A, Saunders R, Shah S, Siddiqui S, et al. Eosinophil protein in airway macrophages: a novel biomarker of eosinophilic inflammation in patients with asthma. *J Allergy Clin Immunol.* (2010) 126:61–9 e3. doi: 10.1016/j.jaci.2010.03.026
25. GINA. *Gobal Strategy for Asthma Management and Prevention. Global Initiative for Asthma* (GINA); Available online at www.ginasthma.org (Accessed March 3, 2014). (2009).
26. ATS. Standardization of Spirometry, 1994 Update. American Thoracic Society. *Am J Respir Crit Care Med.* (1995) 152:1107–36.
27. American Thoracic Society, European Respiratory Society. ATS/ERS recommendations for standardized procedures for the online and offline measurement of exhaled lower respiratory nitric oxide and nasal nitric oxide, 2005. *Am J Respir Crit Care Med.* (2005) 171:912–30. doi: 10.1164/rccm.200406-710ST
28. Bodini A, Peroni D, Vicentini L, Loiacono A, Baraldi E, Ghiro L, et al. Exhaled breath condensate eicosanoids and sputum eosinophils in asthmatic children: a pilot study. *Pediatr Allergy Immunol.* (2004) 15:26–31. doi: 10.1046/j.0905-6157.2003.00097.x
29. Brightling CE, Ward R, Woltmann G, Bradding P, Sheller JR, Dworski R, et al. Induced sputum inflammatory mediator concentrations in eosinophilic bronchitis and asthma. *Am J Respir Crit Care Med.* (2000) 162(3 Pt 1):878–82. doi: 10.1164/ajrccm.162.3.9909064
30. Donnelly LE, Barnes PJ. Defective phagocytosis in airways disease. *Chest* (2012) 141:1055–62. doi: 10.1378/chest.11-2348
31. Moreira AP, Hogaboam CM. Macrophages in aller7gic asthma: fine-tuning their pro- and anti-inflammatory actions for disease resolution. *J Interf Cytokine Res.* (2011) 31:485–91. doi: 10.1089/jir.2011.0027
32. Fleming BD, Mosser DM. Regulatory macrophages: setting the threshold for therapy. *Eur J Immunol.* (2011) 41:2498–502. doi: 10.1002/eji.201141717
33. Yang M, Kumar RK, Hansbro PM, Foster PS. Emerging roles of pulmonary macrophages in driving the development of severe asthma. *J Leukocyte Biol.* (2012) 91:557–69. doi: 10.1189/jlb.0711357
34. Alexis NE, Eldridge MW, Peden DB. Effect of inhaled endotoxin on airway and circulating inflammatory cell phagocytosis and CD11b expression in atopic asthmatic subjects. *J Allergy Clin Immunol.* (2003) 112:353–61. doi: 10.1067/mai.2003.1651
35. Fitzpatrick AM, Holguin F, Teague WG, Brown LA. Alveolar macrophage phagocytosis is impaired in children with poorly controlled asthma. *J Allergy Clin Immunol.* (2008) 121:1372–8.e1–3. doi: 10.1016/j.jaci.2008.03.008
36. Fitzpatrick AM, Teague WG, Burwell L, Brown MS, Brown LA. Program NNSAR. Glutathione oxidation is associated with airway macrophage functional impairment in children with severe asthma. *Pediatr Res.* (2011) 69:154–9. doi: 10.1203/PDR.0b013e3182026370
37. Liang Z, Zhang Q, Thomas CM, Chana KK, Gibeon D, Barnes PJ, et al. Impaired macrophage phagocytosis of bacteria in severe asthma. *Respiratory Res.* (2014) 15:72. doi: 10.1186/1465-9921-15-72
38. Huynh ML, Malcolm KC, Kotaru C, Tilstra JA, Westcott JY, Fadok VA, et al. Defective apoptotic cell phagocytosis attenuates prostaglandin E2 and 15-hydroxyeicosatetraenoic acid in severe asthma alveolar macrophages. *Am J Respir Crit Care Med.* (2005) 172:972–9. doi: 10.1164/rccm.200501-035OC
39. Aggarwal S, Moodley YP, Thompson PJ, Misso NL. Prostaglandin E2 and cysteinyl leukotriene concentrations in sputum: association with asthma severity and eosinophilic inflammation. *Clin Exp Allergy* (2010) 40:85–93. doi: 10.1111/j.1365-2222.2009.03386
40. Aronoff DM, Canetti C, Peters-Golden M. Prostaglandin E2 inhibits alveolar macrophage phagocytosis through an E-prostanoid 2 receptor-mediated increase in intracellular cyclic AMP. *J Immunol.* (2004) 173:559–65. doi: 10.4049/jimmunol.173.1.559
41. Profita M, Sala A, Bonanno A, Riccobono L, Siena L, Melis MR, et al. Increased prostaglandin E2 concentrations and cyclooxygenase-2 expression in asthmatic subjects with sputum eosinophilia. *J Allergy Clin Immunol.* (2003)112:709–16. doi: 10.1016/S0091
42. Brugha RE, Mushtaq N, Round T, Gadhvi DH, Dundas I, Gaillard E, et al. Carbon in airway macrophages from children with asthma. *Thorax* (2014) 69:654–9. doi: 10.1136/thoraxjnl-2013-204734
43. Lay JC, Alexis NE, Zeman KL, Peden DB, Bennett WD. *In vivo* uptake of inhaled particles by airway phagocytes is enhanced in patients with mild asthma compared with normal volunteers. *Thorax* (2009) 64:313–20. doi: 10.1136/thx.2008.096222

18

New Drugs for Pediatric Asthma

Marco Maglione [1,2], Marco Poeta [1,2] and Francesca Santamaria [1,2]*

[1] *Department of Translational Medical Sciences, Federico II University, Naples, Italy,* [2] *Department of Pediatrics, Federico II University, Naples, Italy*

***Correspondence:**
Francesca Santamaria
santamar@unina.it

Asthma is the most common chronic disease in children. As suggested by international guidelines, the main goals of asthma treatment are symptoms control and lung function preservation, through a stepwise and control-based approach. The first line therapy based on inhaled corticosteroids may fail to reach control in more than one third of patients, especially adolescents, and in these lung function and quality of life may progressively worsen. Treatment with omalizumab, the first anti-immunoglobulin E recombinant humanized monoclonal antibody, has been definitely approved in pediatric uncontrolled asthma. In this review, we discuss the mechanisms and potential roles of emerging therapies for pediatric severe asthma. Novel biologic drugs (i.e., dupilumab, mepolizumab, reslizumab, and benralizumab) seem to be promising in reducing annual exacerbation rates and steroid-use in glucocorticoid-dependent cases, but available data are few and limited to adolescents and adults. Evidences on the use of the muscarinic antagonist tiotropium as controller medication in pediatric settings are progressively growing, sustaining an application as asthma maintenance treatment in children aged >6 years and in preschool children with persistent asthmatic symptoms, but well powered trials are needed to confirm its safety and efficacy. New inhaled corticosteroids (i.e., ciclesonide and mometasone) are effective as once-daily controller therapy, but long-term studies in the different pediatric ages are needed to compare effectiveness and safety to usual treatments. At present, the role of macrolides in pediatric severe asthma is controversial and their administration is not recommended routinely, but may be considered in children with neutrophilic asthma for reducing daily oral steroids administration and improving lung function. Despite the availability of several novel therapeutic strategies for uncontrolled asthma, future trials targeted at specific pediatric age subgroups are needed to support evidences of safety and efficacy also in children.

Keywords: severe asthma, therapy, biologics, inhaled corticosteroids, muscarinic antagonists, macrolides, children, adolescents

INTRODUCTION

Asthma is the most common chronic condition of childhood, and its management represents part of the daily activity of most professionals who deal with pediatric care. At any age, the main purposes of asthma treatment are to reduce exacerbations and to limit the progressive loss of lung function, thus decreasing the use of health resources and improving quality of life. In few words, asthma therapy aims to achieve good symptom control (1).

National and international guidelines on asthma management of adults and children agree in indicating inhaled corticosteroids (ICS) as the most effective and safe medications, which may be used alone or associated with other controller therapies, in a stepwise, control-based approach (2–4).

Nevertheless, despite this approach, in more than one third of all patients with asthma the persistence of clinical symptoms, often associated with overt lung function abnormalities, indicate poor control, with the proportion increasing to >50% in adolescents (5, 6). This variability in treatment response is partly genetically determined. Pharmacogenomic studies, through the characterization of genes relevant in asthma treatment response, are paving the way toward the personalization of therapy. This would entail a dramatic change in asthma treatment from the actual "one size fits all" approach to the so called "precision medicine," that is the tailoring of healthcare to the individual through the identification of clinical, biological, or genetic markers (7). Therefore, the interest in the development of new drugs and in the application of therapies currently used in other conditions for pursuing asthma control is high. This is particularly true in the pediatric setting, due to the lack of adequately designed trials including children. Indeed, even though results from adult studies may be sometimes translated to adolescents, this is not the case for younger asthmatic patients for whom evidence on the safety and efficacy of new treatments is still sparse.

The present review will go through the new therapeutic approaches to pediatric asthma, highlighting available evidence on their efficacy, the related risks, and the areas of uncertainty that in many cases still limit their regular application in the clinical practice.

BIOLOGICS

Over the last decades, the development of monoclonal antibodies specifically designed to bind determined targets has deeply changed the approach to a number of conditions, also affecting children (8). In pediatric respiratory medicine, this novelty has been embodied by omalizumab, a recombinant DNA-derived humanized anti-IgE monoclonal antibody, which is the only biologic drug recommended in children with moderate-to-severe asthma (3, 9). Omalizumab, which was approved by the United States (US) and the European Union in 2003 and 2005, respectively, is able to decrease the quantity of cell-bound IgE, to downregulate the IgE receptors on mast cells, basophils, and dendritic cells, thus preventing mediator release from effector cells (10, 11). At present, its use is licensed as an add-on treatment for patients aged > 6 years with severe persistent allergic asthma and positive skin test or specific IgE to perennial aeroallergens, FEV_1 < 80% predicted, frequent daytime symptoms, or nighttime awakenings, and multiple severe asthma exacerbations despite traditional maintenance therapy (12, 13). In comparison to the robust body of literature supporting the efficacy and safety of omalizumab in severe, inadequately controlled adult asthma (14, 15), evidence in children is far more limited. Nevertheless, even though no studies have been published to date in preschoolers, only few well-designed clinical trials have addressed the role of omalizumab in uncontrolled asthma affecting children older than 6 years. A large, multicenter randomized controlled trial (RCT) assessed the efficacy of omalizumab in 419 subjects (mean age 10.9 years) with persistent allergic asthma, and showed that anti-IgE treatment increases the number of symptoms-free days and reduces the number of exacerbations and the need for controller therapies (16). Similar results were achieved by other pediatric studies which have strengthened the role of omalizumab in limiting asthma exacerbations, and to a lesser extent, in improving patients' lung function (17–21). Despite reported cases of anaphylaxis in children (22), which warrant hospital administration, omalizumab is basically safe, whereas high cost represents a more relevant issue.

The scenario of biologics applied to asthma treatment has recently added to the more "consolidated" omalizumab, a number of novel drugs for which evidence of safety and efficacy is still very sparse and generally limited to adult studies. Dupilumab, an anti–interleukin-4 receptor α monoclonal antibody blocking both interleukin-4 and interleukin-13 signaling, is probably the most promising for a future application in pediatric asthma, as shown by two recent trials (23, 24). These large, multicenter RCT have enrolled patients aged >12 years with moderate-to-severe uncontrolled asthma (23) or glucocorticoid-dependent severe asthma (24). In such subjects dupilumab has proven effective in decreasing exacerbations and improving asthma control, also resulting in better lung function. Similar results have been provided for mepolizumab, which has been recently approved for severe eosinophilic asthma in adults and adolescents. This anti-interleukin-5 antibody has been shown to reduce severe asthma exacerbations (25) and need for oral steroids (26), even though evidence for its use in children < 12 years is virtually absent. Mepolizumab is not the only anti-interleukin-5 antibody under investigation for improving asthma control. Reslizumab and benralizumab are anti-interleukin-5 antibodies whose efficacy has been evaluated by few recent studies including patients with asthma aged >12 years (27–31). Both treatments have proven safe and effective in improving asthma control and lung function in selected patients with severe uncontrolled asthma and high blood eosinophil count, but, again, available data are few and limited to adolescents and adults.

MUSCARINIC ANTAGONISTS

The increased cholinergic tone typical of asthma makes muscarinic receptors an obvious target for therapeutic strategies aimed at reducing airway hyperresponsiveness. In children with severe asthma exacerbations, inhaled short-acting antimuscarinic agents, namely ipratropium, are a widely accepted therapeutic option whose efficacy on lung function is well documented (32). Used in addition to nebulized albuterol, ipratropium has proven effective in reducing the risk for hospital admission as well as in improving spirometry in children with asthma exacerbations (33). Less frequent is the use of muscarinic antagonists as controller therapy, even though tiotropium, the most widely used long-acting muscarinic antagonist is mentioned as a possible add-on therapeutic option in step 4 of GINA guidelines for children older than 12 years taking the combined treatment of ICS and long-acting beta^2-agonists (LABA), but still reporting inadequate asthma control (3). Inhaled tiotropium (Spiriva Respimat®), first indicated in adult COPD treatment, was shown to improve pulmonary function and respiratory symptoms in adult moderate-to-severe asthma (34, 35). Nevertheless, when added to ICS, tiotropium appears to be slightly less effective in improving quality of life in comparison to the traditional combination ICS/LABA (36). Tiotropium was recently approved by the US Federal Drug Administration (FDA) as an asthma maintenance treatment in children aged >6 years (37), whereas in Europe its use is still limited to adults. However, available evidence in children and adolescents is progressively growing, thus making a future wider application in pediatric asthma likely. In particular, school-aged children with severe symptomatic asthma have shown improvement of lung function and good tolerability and safety when tiotropium was added to medium or high-doses of ICS (38, 39). Furthermore, positive trends in asthma control and FEV_1 were also observed in adolescents with moderately severe asthma treated with tiotropium as an add-on drug to ICS and other controllers for 3 months (40, 41). Finally, a recent small RCT showed the potential to reduce asthma exacerbation risk in children aged 1–5 years with persistent asthmatic symptoms, with tolerability similar to that of placebo, although mean daytime asthma symptom scores were not significantly different between groups (42). Despite its debated role within the group of controller drugs in childhood asthma, tiotropium remains an attractive option, both for the possibility of once-daily administration and for its peculiar way of delivery. Indeed, the drug is administered by a device named Respimat® in form of a mist of extremely fine particles (diameter $< 6\,\mu m$), whose main advantages are the lower speed of delivery, the limited pharyngeal deposition and the enhanced pulmonary deposition in comparison to the common metered dose inhalers. Additional well powered trials are needed to further assess the safety and efficacy of tiotropium especially in young children with uncontrolled asthma symptoms.

NEW INHALED CORTICOSTEROIDS

Inhaled corticosteroids represent the cornerstone of asthma therapy at all ages (3). Despite the long and large experience with traditional molecules such as beclometasone, flunisolide, fluticasone, and budesonide, all with high safety and efficacy profiles, some new ICS have been recently approved, but only few of these are allowed for the pediatric use.

Ciclesonide, licensed from age 4 years in the US and from age 12 years in Europe, is a pro-drug activated by esterases within the lung to form the active compound (des-ciclesonide). The possibility of a single daily administration, and evidence supporting its efficacy in improving asthma control and in reducing airway inflammation make this steroid a valid option as asthma controller therapy (43). Nonetheless, given the lack of relevant differences in the efficacy of ciclesonide vs. fluticasone or budesonide, long-term superiority trials are needed to identify the usefulness and safety of ciclesonide compared to other ICS (44). Similarly, mometasone, which has the same FDA approval as ciclesonide and may be used down to the age of 4 years also in Europe, has proven effective as once-daily controller therapy in several pediatric studies (45), with evidence supporting a significant functional improvement in school-aged children with persistent asthma (46).

MACROLIDE ANTIBIOTICS

Macrolides are widely used antibiotics with both antimicrobial and anti-inflammatory activities (47). Indeed, in addition to their well-known antibiotic effect, there is evidence that macrolides modulate the expression of cellular adhesion molecules, may attenuate inflammatory cell migration and inhibit the respiratory burst in polymorphonuclear cells. Furthermore, macrolides clearly affect neutrophil function, even though the exact mechanisms have not been elucidated (48). For these reasons, macrolides have been initially recommended in diffuse panbronchiolitis (49), cystic fibrosis (50), and non-cystic fibrosis bronchiectasis (51). As airways infection is a possible cause for asthma, macrolides have been supposed to be used as long-term treatment for improving the disease control and reducing the need for steroids (52). Actually, the early troleandomycin—no longer recommended because of adverse effects on liver function tests—was reported to work as "steroid-sparing" drug by reducing the catabolism of steroids, but indeed no steroid reduction was demonstrated (53). Most recently, clarithromycin was found to widely suppress severe, steroid-insensitive allergic airways disease in a mouse model through its anti-inflammatory effects on tumor necrosis factor-α/interleukin-17 immune responses that are largely independent of its antimicrobial effects (54). Indeed, macrolides may reduce airway inflammation either by acting on pro-inflammatory cytokines or by controlling intracellular infection which may trigger and maintain inflammation (55).

At present, the role of macrolides in severe asthma is controversial. In a large multicentre RCT azithromycin did not reduce the rate of severe exacerbations and lower respiratory tract infections in a population of severe asthma adults not including children or adolescents (56). Finally, a systematic review and meta-analysis did not show a benefit of macrolides over placebo on rates of exacerbations, quality of life or participants' need for rescue medications (57).

Looking specifically at the pediatric literature, *Chlamydia pneumoniae* and *Mycoplasma pneumoniae* have been suggested to play a role in the pathogenesis of severe asthma (58). Preschool-aged children with frequent, severe exacerbations may benefit from sporadic use of azithromycin (59). Regrettably, very few RCTs investigated the role of macrolides in school-age children or adolescents with asthma, and failed to demonstrate a beneficial effect probably because of the low power of the study

TABLE 1 | Summary of novel drugs for treatment of severe pediatric asthma.

Drug	Mechanism of action	Novel evidence in children
BIOLOGICS		
Dupilumab	Anti–IL-4 receptor α monoclonal antibody, blocks both IL-4 and IL-13 signaling.	Two trials also involving children >12 years. Decreases exacerbations and improves lung function in moderate-to-severe uncontrolled asthma (22). In glucocorticoid-dependent asthma reduces steroid use (23).
Mepolizumab	Anti-IL-5 monoclonal antibody, selectively inhibits eosinophilic inflammation.	Two trials also involving children >12 years. Effective and well tolerated. Reduces the risk of asthma exacerbations in patients with severe eosinophilic asthma (24, 25).
Reslizumab	Anti-IL-5 monoclonal antibody, inhibits activity within the IL-5 signaling pathway and reduces blood and tissue eosinophils.	Three trials also involving children >12 years (26, 27, 29). Improves lung function, asthma control and symptoms, quality of life in uncontrolled asthma.
Benralizumab	Anti-IL-5 receptor α monoclonal antibody, induces direct, rapid, and nearly complete depletion of eosinophils.	Two trials also involving children >12 years (28, 30). Significantly reduces annual exacerbation rates in patients with severe, uncontrolled asthma with blood eosinophils >300 cells per μL.
MUSCARINIC ANTAGONISTS		
Tiotropium	Long-acting muscarinic antagonist, decreases airway tone binding the muscarinic receptors.	Evidence of improved lung function in children >12 years receiving tiotropium in addition to standard therapy (39, 40), as well as in children aged 6–11 years (37, 38). Weaker evidence of reduction in exacerbations rate in children aged 1–5 years (41).
NEW INHALED CORTICOSTEROIDS		
Ciclesonide	Reduces airway inflammation through a single day administration	Improves airway inflammation and asthma control in atopic children (42). Longer-term trials needed to identify the usefulness and safety compared to other ICS (43).
Mometasone	Reduces airway inflammation through a single day administration	Functional improvement in school-aged children with persistent asthma (45).
MACROLIDES		
	Reduce airway inflammation by acting on pro-inflammatory cytokines or by controlling intracellular infection.	May reduce daily oral steroid administration and improve FEV_1 (63). Routine use not recommended in children or adolescents with severe asthma (8, 62).

(60–62). Actually, the possibility that macrolides work well in pediatric severe asthma is not definitely excluded, yet at present the evidence is quite poor. It should be also kept in mind that an inappropriate use of macrolides unavoidably results in antibiotic resistance that is a major worldwide concern, especially in the pediatric population where the respiratory infection rate is as high as in the elderly (63).

Although an official document and a recent pragmatic review do not recommend the routine use of macrolides for children with severe asthma (9, 64), they may be useful for reducing daily oral steroid administration and improving FEV_1 (65), and, for this reason, can be proposed as *ex-juvantibus* trial in children with neutrophilic asthma (66). In conclusion, further well-designed and large RCTs are warranted before routine use of macrolides is recommended or definitely condemned in pediatric severe asthma.

A list of new medications for treating children with severe, uncontrolled asthma, also including the novel evidence for their use, is provided in **Table 1**.

OTHER INTERVENTIONS

Immunosuppressive drugs including cyclosporine, azathioprine and methotrexate, commonly used in several immune-mediated disorders, have been proposed for severe asthma management, but no recommendation may be formulated at present due to the insufficiency of data, particularly in children (3).

Allergen immunotherapy has proven effective in improving symptom control in mild to moderate asthmatic children, especially in the presence of a clear association between symptoms and exposure to a specific allergen, but its applicability in the clinical practice is strongly limited by the requirement for patients to have stable (and not uncontrolled) asthma symptoms due to the risk of severe reaction (67).

A surgical procedure named bronchial thermoplasty, consisting in the ablation of the airway smooth muscle layer, has shown to provide some benefits in adults unresponsive to conventional therapies (68). Nevertheless, evidence in children or adolescents is completely lacking at present, and such intervention is therefore not recommended in these age groups.

Finally, the association between worse symptom control and fungal sensitization in severe asthma has led to studies assessing the efficacy of antifungal drugs on asthma outcomes. However, data are still conflicting and not conclusive and insufficient to support formal recommendations (69).

CONCLUSIONS

Severe asthma identifies children or adolescents who need high-dose ICS therapy and a second controller therapy in the previous year, or systemic corticosteroids for 50% of the year, to prevent asthma from being uncontrolled or that remains uncontrolled notwithstanding these medications (9). Unfortunately, once excluded any comorbidity or optimized patients' adherence to treatment and inhalation technique, about 5–10% of the asthmatic pediatric population continue to have severe symptoms or signs and the loss of lung function may be progressive and irreversible (70). The latter point is of paramount importance in view of the fact that a stringent relationship between the childhood insults to the lung and the accelerated aging that can occur in adult chronic obstructive lung disease has been postulated (71). Finally, asthma not responding to treatment may result in significant morbidity and frequent healthcare utilization (1, 72). For all the above, there is considerable need for robust studies of children with uncontrolled asthma confirming the clinical efficacy and safety of medications increasingly used in the adult population, but not allowed in patients <12 years of age because of the paucity of literature data.

AUTHOR CONTRIBUTIONS

MM has made substantial contributions to conception and design, has been involved in drafting the manuscript, and has given final approval of the version to be published. MP conceived the idea, has been involved in drafting the manuscript and has given final approval of the version to be published. FS has made substantial contributions to conception and design, has been involved in drafting the manuscript and revising it critically for important intellectual content, and has given final approval of the version to be published.

REFERENCES

1. O'Byrne PM, Pedersen S, Schatz M, Thoren A, Ekholm E, Carlsson LG, et al. The poorly explored impact of uncontrolled asthma. *Chest* (2016) 143:511–23. doi: 10.1378/chest.12-0412
2. British Thoracic Society, Scottish Intercollegiate Guidelines Network. British guideline on the management of asthma. *Thorax* (2014) 69 (Suppl. 1):1–192.
3. Global Initiative for Asthma. *GINA Report: Global Strategy for Asthma Management and Prevention* (2017). Available online at: https://ginasthma.org/gina-reports/ (Accessed October 14, 2018).
4. National Heart, Lung, and Blood Institute, National Asthma Education and Prevention Program. *Expert Panel Report 3: Guidelines for the Diagnosis and Management of Asthma* (2007). Available online at: http://www.nhlbi.nih.gov/files/docs/guidelines/asthgdln.pdf (Accessed October 0 3, 2018).
5. Schmier JK, Manjunath R, Halpern MT, Jones ML, Thompson K, Diette GB. The impact of inadequately controlled asthma in urban children on quality of life and productivity. *Ann Allergy Asthma Immunol.* (2007) 98:245–51. doi: 10.1016/S1081-1206(10)60713-2
6. Licari A, Brambilla I, Marseglia A, De Filippo M, Paganelli V, Marseglia GL. Difficult vs. severe asthma: definition and limits of asthma control in the pediatric population. *Front Pediatr.* (2018) 6:170. doi: 10.3389/fped.2018.00170
7. Kersten ET, Koppelman GH. Pharmacogenetics of asthma: toward precision medicine. *Curr Opin Pulm Med.* (2017) 23:12–20. doi: 10.1097/MCP.0000000000000335
8. Katial RK, Bensch GW, Busse WW, Chipps BE, Denson JL, Gerber AN, et al. Changing paradigms in the treatment of severe asthma: the role of biologic therapies. *J Allergy Clin Immunol Pract.* (2017) 5:S1–14. doi: 10.1016/j.jaip.2016.11.029
9. Chung KF, Wenzel SE, Brozek JL, Bush A, Castro M, Sterk PJ, et al. International ERS/ATS guidelines on definition, evaluation and treatment of severe asthma. *Eur Respir J.* (2014) 43:343–73. doi: 10.1183/09031936.00202013
10. Djukanović R, Wilson SJ, Kraft M, Jarjour NN, Steel M, Chung KF, et al. Effects of treatment with anti-immunoglobulin E antibody omalizumab on airway inflammation in allergic asthma. *Am J Respir Crit Care Med.* (2004) 170:583–93. doi: 10.1164/rccm.200312-1651OC
11. Holgate S, Casale T, Wenzel S, Bousquet J, Deniz Y, Reisner C. The anti-inflammatory effects of omalizumab confirm the central role of IgE in allergic inflammation. *J Allergy Clin Immunol.* (2005) 115:459–65. doi: 10.1016/j.jaci.2004.11.053
12. Federal Drug Administration Advisory for Omalizumab. Available online at:http://www.fda.gov/Drugs/DevelopmentApprovalProcess/HowDrugsareDevelopedandApproved/ApprovalApplications/TherapeuticBiologicApplications/default.htm (Accessed October 14, 2018).
13. European Medicines Agency: assessment report for Xolair. Available online at: https://www.ema.europa.eu/medicines/human/EPAR/xolair (Accessed October 14, 2018).
14. Humbert M, Beasley R, Ayres J, Slavin R, Hébert J, Bousquet J, et al. Benefits of omalizumab as add-on therapy in patients with severe persistent asthma who are inadequately controlled despite best available therapy (GINA 2002 step 4 treatment): INNOVATE. *Allergy* (2005) 60:309–16. doi: 10.1111/j.1398-9995.2004.00772.x
15. Normansell R, Walker S, Milan SJ, Walters EH, Nair P. Omalizumab for asthma in adults and children. *Cochrane Database Syst Rev.* (2014) 1:CD003559. doi: 10.1002/14651858.CD003559.pub4
16. Busse WW, Morgan WJ, Gergen PJ, Mitchell HE, Gern JE, Liu AH, et al. Randomized trial of omalizumab (anti-IgE) for asthma in inner-city children. *N Engl J Med.* (2011) 364:1005–15. doi: 10.1056/NEJMoa1009705
17. Lanier B, Bridges T, Kulus M, Taylor AF, Berhane I, Vidaurre CF. Omalizumab for the treatment of exacerbations in children with inadequately controlled allergic (IgE-mediated) asthma. *J Allergy Clin Immunol.* (2009) 124:1210–6. doi: 10.1016/j.jaci.2009.09.021
18. Odajima H, Ebisawa M, Nagakura T, Fujisawa T, Akasawa A, Ito K, et al. Omalizumab in Japanese children with severe allergic asthma uncontrolled with standard therapy. *Allergol Int.* (2015) 64:364–70. doi: 10.1016/j.alit.2015.05.006
19. Milgrom H, Berger W, Nayak A, Gupta N, Pollard S, McAlary M, et al. Treatment of childhood asthma with anti-immunoglobulin E antibody (omalizumab). *Pediatrics* (2001) 108:E36. doi: 10.1542/peds.108.2.e36
20. Deschildre A, Marguet C, Salleron J, Pin I, Rittié JL, Derelle J, et al. Add-on omalizumab in children with severe allergic asthma: a 1-year real life survey. *Eur Respir J.* (2013) 42:1224–33. doi: 10.1183/09031936.00149812
21. Teach SJ, Gill MA, Togias A, Sorkness CA, Arbes SJ Jr., Calatroni A, et al. Preseasonal treatment with either omalizumab or an inhaled corticosteroid

boost to prevent fall asthma exacerbations. *J Allergy Clin Immunol.* (2015) 136:1476–85. doi: 10.1016/j.jaci.2015.09.008

22. Limb SL, Starke PR, Lee CE, Chowdhury BA. Delayed onset and protracted progression of anaphylaxis after omalizumab administration in patients with asthma. *J Allergy Clin Immunol.* (2007) 120:1378–81. doi: 10.1016/j.jaci.2007.09.022
23. Castro M, Corren J, Pavord ID, Maspero J, Wenzel S, Rabe KF, et al. Dupilumab efficacy and safety in moderate-to-severe uncontrolled asthma. *N Engl J Med.* (2018) 378:2486–96. doi: 10.1056/NEJMoa1804092
24. Rabe KF, Nair P, Brusselle G, Maspero JF, Castro M, Sher L, et al. Efficacy and safety of dupilumab in glucocorticoid-dependent severe asthma. *N Engl J Med.* (2018) 378:2475–85. doi: 10.1056/NEJMoa1804093
25. Ortega HG, Liu MC, Pavord ID, Brusselle GG, FitzGerald JM, Chetta A, et al. Mepolizumab treatment in patients with severe eosinophilic asthma. *N Engl J Med.* (2014) 371:1198–207. doi: 10.1056/NEJMoa1403290
26. Bel EH, Ortega HG, Pavord ID. Glucocorticoids and mepolizumab in eosinophilic asthma. *N Engl J Med.* (2014) 371:2434. doi: 10.1056/NEJMoa1403291
27. Brusselle G, Germinaro M, Weiss S, Zangrilli J. Reslizumab in patients with inadequately controlled late-onset asthma and elevated blood eosinophils. *Pulm Pharmacol Ther.* (2017) 43:39–45. doi: 10.1016/j.pupt.2017.01.011
28. Murphy K, Jacobs J, Bjermer L, Fahrenholz JM, Shalit Y, Garin M, et al. Long-term safety and efficacy of reslizumab in patients with eosinophilic asthma. *J Allergy Clin Immunol Pract.* (2017) 5:1572–81. doi: 10.1016/j.jaip.2017.08.024
29. Bleecker ER, FitzGerald JM, Chanez P, Papi A, Weinstein SF, Barker P, et al. Efficacy and safety of benralizumab for patients with severe asthma uncontrolled with high-dosage inhaled corticosteroids and long-acting β2-agonists (SIROCCO): a randomised, multicentre, placebo-controlled phase 3 trial. *Lancet* (2016) 388:2115–27. doi: 10.1016/S0140-6736(16)31324-1
30. Bjermer L, Lemiere C, Maspero J, Weiss S, Zangrilli J, Germinaro M. Reslizumab for inadequately controlled asthma with elevated blood eosinophil levels: a randomized phase 3 study. *Chest* (2016) 150:789–98. doi: 10.1016/j.chest.2016.03.032
31. FitzGerald JM, Bleecker ER, Nair P, Korn S, Ohta K, Lommatzsch M, et al. Benralizumab, an anti-interleukin-5 receptor α monoclonal antibody, as add-on treatment for patients with severe, uncontrolled, eosinophilic asthma (CALIMA): a randomised, double-blind, placebo-controlled phase 3 trial. *Lancet* (2016) 388:2128–41. doi: 10.1016/S0140-6736(16)31322-8
32. Qureshi F, Zaritsky A, Lakkis H. Efficacy of nebulized ipratropium in severely asthmatic children. *Ann Emerg Med.* (1997) 29:205–11. doi: 10.1016/S0196-0644(97)70269-5
33. Rodrigo GJ, Castro-Rodriguez JA. Anticholinergics in the treatment of children and adults with acute asthma: a systematic review with meta-analysis. *Thorax* (2005) 60:740–6. doi: 10.1136/thx.2005.047803
34. Kerstjens HA, Disse B, Schröder-Babo W, Bantje TA, Gahlemann M, Sigmund R, et al. Tiotropium improves lung function in patients with severe uncontrolled asthma: a randomized controlled trial. *J Allergy Clin Immunol.* (2011) 128:308–14. doi: 10.1016/j.jaci.2011.04.039
35. Kerstjens HA, Engel M, Dahl R, Paggiaro P, Beck E, Vandewalker M, et al. Tiotropium in asthma poorly controlled with standard combination therapy. *N Engl J Med.* (2012) 367:1198–207. doi: 10.1056/NEJMoa1208606
36. Kew KM, Evans DJ, Allison DE, Boyter AC. Long-acting muscarinic antagonists (LAMA) added to inhaled corticosteroids (ICS) versus addition of long-acting beta2-agonists (LABA) for adults with asthma. *Cochrane Database Syst Rev.* (2015) 6:CD011438. doi: 10.1002/14651858.CD011438
37. Boehringer Ingelheim International GmbH. *Spiriva Respimat, Highlights of Prescribing Information.* (2017). Available online at: http://docs.boehringer-ingelheim.com/Prescribing Information/PIs/SpirivaRespimat/spirivarespimat.pdf (Accessed October 13, 2018).
38. Vogelberg C, Moroni-Zentgraf P, Leonaviciute-Klimantaviciene M, Sigmund R, Hamelmann E, Engel M, et al. A randomised dose-ranging study of tiotropium Respimat® in children with symptomatic asthma despite inhaled corticosteroids. *Respir Res.* (2015) 16:20. doi: 10.1186/s12931-015-0175-9
39. Szefler SJ, Murphy K, Harper T III, Boner A, Laki I, Engel M, et al. A phase III randomized controlled trial of tiotropium add-on therapy in children with severe symptomatic asthma. *J Allergy Clin Immunol.* (2017) 140:1277–87. doi: 10.1016/j.jaci.2017.01.014
40. Hamelmann E, Bernstein JA, Vandewalker M, Moroni-Zentgraf P, Verri D, Unseld A, et al. A randomised controlled trial of tiotropium in adolescents with severe symptomatic asthma. *Eur Respir J.* (2017) 49:1601100. doi: 10.1183/13993003.01100-2016
41. Hamelmann E, Bateman ED, Vogelberg C, Szefler SJ, Vandewalker M, Moroni-Zentgraf P, et al. Tiotropium add-on therapy in adolescents with moderate asthma: a 1-year randomized controlled trial. *J Allergy Clin Immunol.* (2016) 138:441–50. doi: 10.1016/j.jaci.2016.01.011
42. Vrijlandt EJLE, El Azzi G, Vandewalker M, Rupp N, Harper T, Graham L, et al. Safety and efficacy of tiotropium in children aged 1–5 years with persistent asthmatic symptoms: a randomised, double-blind, placebo-controlled trial. *Lancet Respir Med.* (2018) 6:127–37. doi: 10.1016/S2213-2600(18)30012-2
43. Mallol J, Aguirre V, Gallardo A, Cortez E, Sánchez C, Riquelme C, et al. Effect of once-daily generic ciclesonide on exhaled nitric oxide in atopic children with persistent asthma. *Allergol Immunopathol.* (2016) 44:106–12. doi: 10.1016/j.aller.2015.01.011
44. Kramer S, Rottier BL, Scholten RJ, Boluyt N. Ciclesonide vs. other inhaled corticosteroids for chronic asthma in children. *Cochrane Database Syst Rev.* (2013) 2:CD010352. doi: 10.1002/14651858.CD010352
45. Milgrom H. Mometasone furoate in children with mild to moderate persistent asthma: a review of the evidence. *Paediatr Drugs* (2010) 12:213–21. doi: 10.2165/11316220-000000000-00000
46. Amar NJ, Shekar T, Varnell TA, Mehta A, Philip G. Mometasone furoate (MF) improves lung function in pediatric asthma: a double-blind, randomized controlled dose-ranging trial of MF metered-dose inhaler. *Pediatr Pulmonol.* (2017) 52:310–8. doi: 10.1002/ppul.23563
47. Steel HC, Theron AJ, Cockeran R, Anderson R, Feldman C. Pathogen- and host-directed anti-inflammatory activities of macrolide antibiotics. *Mediators Inflamm.* (2012) 2012:584262. doi: 10.1155/2012/584262
48. Sharma S, Jaffe A, Dixon G. Immunomodulatory effects of macrolide antibiotics in respiratory disease: therapeutic implications for asthma and cystic fibrosis. *Pediatr Drugs* (2007) 9:107–18. doi: 10.2165/00148581-200709020-00004
49. Koyama H, Geddes DM. Erythromycin and diffuse panbronchiolitis. *Thorax* (1997) 52:915–18. doi: 10.1136/thx.52.10.915
50. Equi A, Balfour-Lynn IM, Bush A, Rosenthal M. Long term azithromycin in children with cystic fibrosis: a randomised, placebo-controlled crossover trial. *Lancet* (2002) 360:978–84. doi: 10.1016/S0140-6736(02)11081-6
51. Choo JM, Abell GCJ, Thomson R, Morgan L, Waterer G, Gordon DL, et al. Impact of long-term erythromycin therapy on the oropharyngeal microbiome and resistance gene reservoir in non-cystic fibrosis bronchiectasis. *mSphere* (2018) 3:e00103-18. doi: 10.1128/mSphere.00103-18
52. Wong EH, Porter JD, Edwards MR, Johnston SL. The role of macrolides in asthma: current evidence and future directions. *Lancet Respir Med.* (2014) 2:657–70. doi: 10.1016/S2213-2600(14)70107-9
53. Siracusa A, Brugnami G, Fiordi T, Areni S, Severini C, Marabini A. Troleandomycin in the treatment of difficult asthma. *J Allergy Clin Immunol.* (1993) 92:677–82. doi: 10.1016/0091-6749(93)90010-D
54. Essilfie AT, Horvat JC, Kim RY, Mayall JR, Pinkerton JW, Beckett EL, et al. Macrolide therapy suppresses key features of experimental steroid-sensitive and steroid-insensitive asthma. *Thorax* (2015) 70:458–67. doi: 10.1136/thoraxjnl-2014-206067
55. Zimmermann P, Ziesenitz VC, Curtis N, Ritz N. The immunomodulatory effects of macrolides-a systematic review of the underlying mechanisms. *Front Immunol.* (2018) 9:302. doi: 10.3389/fimmu.2018.00302
56. Brusselle GG, Vanderstichele C, Jordens P, Deman R, Slabbynck H, Ringoet V, et al. Azithromycin for prevention of exacerbations in severe asthma (AZISAST): a multicentre randomised double-blind placebo-controlled trial. *Thorax* (2013) 68:322–9. doi: 10.1136/thoraxjnl-2012-202698
57. Kew KM, Undela K, Kotortsi I, Ferrara G. Macrolides for chronic asthma. *Cochrane Database Syst Rev.* (2015) 9:CD002997. doi: 10.1002/14651858.CD002997.pub4
58. Iramain R, De Jesús R, Spitters C, Jara A, Jimenez J, Bogado N, et al. Chlamydia pneumoniae, and mycoplasma pneumoniae: are they related to severe asthma in childhood? *J Asthma* (2016) 53:618–21. doi: 10.3109/02770903.2015.1116085
59. Bacharier LB, Guilbert TW, Mauger DT, Boehmer S, Beigelman A, Fitzpatrick AM, et al. Early administration of azithromycin and prevention of severe

lower respiratory tract illnesses in preschool children with a history of such illnesses: a randomized clinical trial. *JAMA* (2015) 314:2034–44. doi: 10.1001/jama.2015.13896

60. Kamada AK, Hill MR, Iklé DN, Brenner AM, Szefler SJ. Efficacy and safety of low-dose troleandomycin therapy in children with severe, steroid-requiring asthma. *J Allergy Clin Immunol.* (1993) 91:873–82.
61. Piacentini GL, Peroni DG, Bodini A, Pigozzi R, Costella S, Loiacono A, et al. Azithromycin reduces bronchial hyperresponsiveness and neutrophilic airway inflammation in asthmatic children: a preliminary report. *Allergy Asthma Proc.* (2007) 28:194–8. doi: 10.2500/aap.2007.28.2958
62. Strunk RC, Bacharier LB, Phillips BR, Szefler SJ, Zeiger RS, Chinchilli VM, et al. Azithromycin or montelukast as inhaled corticosteroid-sparing agents in moderate-to-severe childhood asthma study. *J Allergy Clin Immunol.* (2008) 122:1138–44.e4. doi: 10.1016/j.jaci.2008.09.028
63. Malhotra-Kumar S, Lammens C, Coenen S, Van Herck K, Goossens H. Effect of azithromycin and clarithromycin therapy on pharyngeal carriage of macrolide-resistant streptococci in healthy volunteers: a randomised, double-blind, placebo-controlled study. *Lancet* (2007) 369:482–90. doi: 10.1016/S0140-6736(07)60235-9
64. Barsky EE, Giancola LM, Baxi SN, Gaffin JM. A practical approach to severe asthma in children. *Ann Am Thorac Soc.* (2018) 15:399–408. doi: 10.1513/AnnalsATS.201708-637FR
65. Mikailov A, Kane I, Aronoff SC, Luck R, Delvecchio MT. Utility of adjunctive macrolide therapy in treatment of children with asthma: a systematic review and meta-analysis. *J Asthma Allergy* (2013) 6:23–9. doi: 10.2147/JAA.S38652
66. Bush A, Pedersen S, Hedlin G, Baraldi E, Barbato A, de Benedictis F, et al. Pharmacological treatment of severe, therapy-resistant asthma in children: what can we learn from where? *Eur Respir J.* (2011) 38:947–58. doi: 10.1183/09031936.00030711
67. Cox L, Nelson H, Lockey R, Calabria C, Chacko T, Finegold I, et al. Allergen immunotherapy: a practice parameter third update. *J Allergy Clin Immunol.* (2011) 127:S1–55. doi: 10.1016/j.jaci.2010.09.034
68. Castro M, Rubin AS, Laviolette M, Fiterman J, De Andrade Lima M, Shah PL, et al. AIR2 Trial Study Group. Effectiveness and safety of bronchial thermoplasty in the treatment of severe asthma: a multicenter, randomized, double-blind, sham-controlled clinical trial. *Am J Respir Crit Care Med.* (2010) 181:116–24. doi: 10.1164/rccm.200903-0354OC
69. Parulekar AD, Diamant Z, Hanania NA. Antifungals in severe asthma. *Curr Opin Pulm Med.* (2015) 21:48–54. doi: 10.1097/MCP.0000000000000117
70. Mirra V, Montella S, Santamaria F. Pediatric severe asthma: a case series report and perspectives on anti-IgE treatment. *BMC Pediatr.* (2018) 18:73. doi: 10.1186/s12887-018-1019-9
71. McGeachie MJ, Yates KP, Zhou X, Guo F, Sternberg AL, Van Natta ML, et al. Patterns of growth and decline in lung function in persistent childhood asthma. *N Engl J Med.* (2016) 374:1842–52. doi: 10.1056/NEJMoa1513737
72. Montella S, Baraldi E, Cazzato S, Aralla R, Berardi M, Brunetti LM, et al. Severe asthma features in children: a case-control online survey. *Ital J Pediatr.* (2016) 42:9. doi: 10.1186/s13052-016-0217-z

19

Pathophysiological Mechanisms of Asthma

*Andrew Bush**

Departments of Paediatrics and Paediatric Respiratory Medicine, Royal Brompton Harefield NHS Foundation Trust and Imperial College, London, United Kingdom

Correspondence:
Andrew Bush
a.bush@imperial.ac.uk
orcid.org/0000-0001-6756-9822

The recent *Lancet* commission has highlighted that "asthma" should be used to describe a clinical syndrome of wheeze, breathlessness, chest tightness, and sometimes cough. The next step is to deconstruct the airway into components of fixed and variable airflow obstruction, inflammation, infection and altered cough reflex, setting the airway disease in the context of extra-pulmonary co-morbidities and social and environmental factors. The emphasis is always on delineating treatable traits, including variable airflow obstruction caused by airway smooth muscle constriction (treated with short- and long-acting β-2 agonists), eosinophilic airway inflammation (treated with inhaled corticosteroids) and chronic bacterial infection (treated with antibiotics with benefit if it is driving the disease). It is also important not to over-treat the untreatable, such as fixed airflow obstruction. These can all be determined using simple, non-invasive tests such as spirometry before and after acute administration of a bronchodilator (reversible airflow obstruction); peripheral blood eosinophil count, induced sputum, exhaled nitric oxide (airway eosinophilia); and sputum or cough swab culture (bacterial infection). Additionally, the pathophysiology of risk domains must be considered: these are risk of an asthma attack, risk of poor airway growth, and in pre-school children, risk of progression to eosinophilic school age asthma. Phenotyping the airway will allow more precise diagnosis and targeted treatment, but it is important to move to endotypes, especially in the era of increasing numbers of biologicals. Advances in -omics technology allow delineation of pathways, which will be particularly important in TH2 low eosinophilic asthma, and also pauci-inflammatory disease. It is very important to appreciate the difficulties of cluster analysis; a patient may have eosinophilic airway disease because of a steroid resistant endotype, because of non-adherence to basic treatment, and a surge in environmental allergen burden. Sophisticated –omics approaches will be reviewed in this manuscript, but currently they are not being used in clinical practice. However, even while they are being evaluated, management of the asthmas can and should be improved by considering the pathophysiologies of the different airway diseases lumped under that umbrella term, using simple, non-invasive tests which are readily available, and treating accordingly.

Keywords: biomarker, transcriptomics, bronchial biopsy, bronchial brushings, induced sputum, airway inflammation, asthma phenotype, endotype

INTRODUCTION: APPROACHING AIRWAYS DISEASE

The recent Lancet *Asthma* Commission (1) was predicated on the assumption that the term "asthma" was no more a diagnosis than is "arthritis" or "anemia." It is an umbrella term that should be used to describe a constellation of clinical symptoms, namely wheeze, breathlessness, chest tightness and cough, and should be followed by the question "what sort of asthma is this?" Dissecting out the individual asthmas is increasingly important as novel biologicals with different modes of action are increasingly being deployed. The ultimate aim is to discover endotypes of asthma, but currently we have not yet got to this point. The importance of endotyping is illustrated by the extraordinary achievements when the endotypes and the gene-class specific sub-endotypes of cystic fibrosis (CF) were first separated from the generality of conditions with chronic airflow infection and inflammation. The result has been the specific, molecular therapies (2–4), none of which would have come to the bedside if they had been tested on every child with a chronic wet cough. It is also important, but largely outside the scope of this chapter, to set airway disease in the context of extra-pulmonary co-morbidities such as obesity, and environmental and lifestyle factors, such as adverse environmental exposures and adherence (5).

The conventional view of at least school age and adult asthma is that the root cause is airway inflammation, which leads to airway hyper-responsiveness, and, secondary to repeated episodes of inflammation, airway remodeling. However, a critical review of the evidence shows that this view is untenable. There is only a weak correlation at baseline between eosinophilic inflammation and bronchial hyper-responsiveness (6, 7). The anti-IgE monoclonal omalizumab reduces airway eosinophilia, but has no effect on bronchial hyper-responsiveness (8), whereas the anti-TNF monoclonal etanercept reduces hyper-responsiveness but has no effect on airway inflammation (9). Furthermore, there is no relationship between the extent of airway remodeling, specifically reticular basement membrane thickness, and the degree or duration of any inflammatory parameter (10). Indeed, there is evidence that remodeling may be protective under some circumstances, discussed in more detail below. Thus, the relationships between the three classic components of asthma are more complex than previously thought, and this is highly relevant to considerations of pathophysiology.

FIRST PRINCIPLE: DECONSTRUCTING AIRWAY DISEASE

Adverse stimuli can affect any biological tube in relatively limited and stereotypical ways. These are:

- Narrowing to cause fixed obstruction
- Narrowing to cause variable obstruction which changes spontaneously over time, and with treatment
- Inflammation with various cell types predominant; inflammation may be harmful or beneficial
- The tube may become infected with combinations of bacterial, viral and fungal pathogens
- There may be increased "twitchiness" of the tube—this is different from variable obstruction. An increased reflex expulsive effort (cough) may not be accompanied by transient airflow obstruction
- The tube contents may be abnormal: including being too wet, too many solids, or too dry.

Furthermore, there are domains of risk, which also need to be considered in any discussion of pathophysiology:

- Risk of acute asthma attacks, which may be fatal
- Risk of impaired trajectories of lung growth, which may sometimes but not inevitably be associated with asthma attacks
- (in pre-school children) risk of progressing from episodic wheeze to eosinophilic atopic school age asthma
- A fourth risk, about which little is known and will not be discussed here, is the risk of failing to remit

Clearly not all are relevant to all pediatric airways diseases: the hallmark of CF is the effects of the airway being too dry ["low volume hypothesis" (11)] and infection and neutrophilic inflammation, whereas some at least of the asthmas are dominated by eosinophilic airway inflammation. What is also clear is that we need modern-omics or genetic tools to try to dissect out these components—and these are sadly lacking. Indeed, currently we are not even trying routinely to identify treatable traits in airway disease, instead haphazardly making diagnoses and embarking on therapeutic trials without making simple measurements in order objectively to phenotype the airway disease. The three important treatable traits, which will be considered in turn, are:

- Does the child have the treatable trait of eosinophilic airway inflammation which is likely to respond to inhaled corticosteroids (ICS)?
- Does the child have the treatable trait of (usually short-acting, β-2 agonist sensitive) reversible airflow obstruction? And conversely, does the child have the untreatable trait, meaning treatment should be discontinued, of fixed airflow obstruction?
- Does the child have the treatable trait of bacterial infection which is driving the disease and can be treated with antibiotics?

The contention of this chapter is that the isolated questions "does my child have asthma?" and (for example) "do survivors of preterm birth have a higher risk of asthma?" are meaningless in isolation. The correct questions are "does this child have an airway disease at all, or are the symptoms in fact due to deconditioning or some other cause (12)?" and, if the child has an airway disease, "what is the nature of this particular airway disease?"

CURRENT BEST PRACTICE: PHENOTYPING THE AIRWAY

A phenotype is defined as the set of observable characteristics of an individual resulting from the interaction of its genotype with the environment. It is important to make the distinction between phenotyping which is of clinical value (changes treatment, prognostic value) from those determining mechanistic pathways. However, if phenotyping does not help in either domain, it cannot be said to be useful. An endotype is defined as a subtype of a condition, which is defined by a distinct functional or pathobiological mechanism. In general, phenotyping leads to rather non-specific treatment, whereas endotyping opens up an exciting vista of pathway specific therapies, as I will show.

Airway Inflammation, and the Potentially Treatable Trait of Airway Eosinophilia

Airway Eosinophilia

ICS are amongst the most effective agents in the whole of therapeutics for the vast majority of children with eosinophilic asthma. Low dose treatment, if taken efficiently and regularly, will result in complete control of asthma in most children (13), while accepting there are steroid resistant phenotypes. The most direct evidence of airway eosinophilia is of course obtained at fibreoptic bronchoscopy (FOB) with broncho-alveolar lavage (BAL) and endobronchial biopsy. This is of course not ethical or practical in most children, and non-invasive methods must be used. Induced sputum was initially the most popular technique, and although this is time-consuming, it is perfectly feasible as a diagnostic test for infection even in resource poor areas (14). Although in older children sputum and BAL eosinophilia are tightly correlated (15), this is not the case in pre-schoolers (16). Furthermore, there is a failure rate of up to 20% (17), and induced sputum does not reflect mucosal inflammation.

Of the other non-invasive methods, peripheral blood eosinophil count has become most popular. It reflects BAL eosinophilia (15, 18), and, even more importantly, is an excellent biomarker predicting response to anti-TH2 monoclonal antibody strategies (19–21). Peripheral blood eosinophil count can be measured on a finger prick sample with point of care equipment (22). Significantly, in the first attempt at personalized medicine in pre-school children, the combination of a peripheral blood eosinophil count $>300/\mu\lambda$ and aeroallergen sensitization was the strongest predictor of response to ICS (23). Exhaled nitric oxide (FeNO) has also been used as a surrogate for airway eosinophilia. The utility of this method in reducing asthma attacks has been demonstrated (24), but although there is a relationship with induced sputum eosinophil count, it varies between individuals and is inconsistent in the same individual over time (25). Clearly FeNO and induced sputum are complimentary and useful, but exactly how they should be used in combination is unclear.

However, the presence of airway eosinophils should prompt critical thought. Firstly, airway eosinophilia, although often related to Type 2 inflammation, is not synonymous with that endotype, and this needs to be borne in mind when contemplating anti-TH2 monoclonal therapies. In our cohort of severe, therapy resistant asthmatics, those with steroid resistant airway eosinophilia had very little evidence of ongoing secretion of the signature TH2 cytokines interleukin (IL)-4, IL-5 and IL-13, in either induced sputum supernatant, BAL or immunohistochemistry of endobronchial biopsy (26). Also, the U-BIOPRED group, using sputum transcriptomics in adult asthmatics documented a group which included patients with moderate sputum eosinophilia, who instead of having the expected TH2 handprint, were characterized by genes of metabolic pathways, ubiquitination and mitochondrial function, as well as, in another study, an IL-6 modulated pathway (below).

Furthermore, if eosinophils are present in the airway, their role or otherwise in disease causation should be carefully considered. In adults at least, eosinophilic bronchitis is a cause of chronic cough, but with no evidence of reversible airflow obstruction; treatment is with ICS, but not β-2 agonists (27). In a challenging study, airway biopsies were compared in patients with active asthma, normal controls, and patients who by any criteria had outgrown their previously diagnosed asthma (28). The airway wall histology, in terms of eosinophilia and reticular basement membrane thickness was the same irrespective of whether the patient had active asthma or had "outgrown" the disease. This leads to the challenging question as to what is the "X-factor" that is needed to convert airway eosinophilia into airway disease? At the moment this remains completely unknown.

Having said all this, clearly if there is no airway eosinophilia, it seems to make little sense to prescribe an anti-eosinophil strategy such as ICS. Although it is true that corticosteroids have numerous genomic and non-genomic effects (29) which hypothetically could be beneficial in airway disease, this has never been shown, and there may be potentially adverse effects in at least some airway diseases, for example reducing neutrophil apoptosis and prolonging the survival of this cell in the airway (30). Surely in the twenty-first century we should not prescribe anti-eosinophilic medications if there is no airway eosinophilia to treat, any more than anti-hypertensives should be prescribed to people who have a normal blood pressure?

Neutrophilic Asthma?

This is another area which illustrates the danger of extrapolating adult studies to children. Asthma characterized by mucosal and sputum neutrophilia is well described in adults (31), who tend also to have severe asthma with less evidence of atopy. Unsurprisingly, neutrophilic asthma is steroid non-responsive. By contrast, in our cohort of children with severe asthma, multiple atopic sensitization was common, but there was no evidence of mucosal, sputum or BAL neutrophilia (26). However, in a subgroup of patients neutrophils were found within the epithelium (32), and, quite unlike what might be expected from adult data, these patient had better symptom control (Asthma control test, ACT) and better first second forced expired volume (FEV_1) while being prescribed a lower dose of ICS. Although it is always dangerous to move from cross-sectional associations to hypotheses, nonetheless it would seem that, whatever the role of neutrophils in adult asthma, in pediatric asthma neutrophils are having a beneficial effect. This raises the intriguing possibility that bacterial infection may have a role in some pediatric asthmas. Again highly speculatively, is it possible that excessively high doses of ICS might actually worsen "bacterial asthma" (if it exists!) by causing topical mucosal immunosuppression (33), leading to a positive feedback loop of worsening symptoms leading to higher ICS doses leading to worsening symptoms? Further data are needed to explore this. However, a practical clinical message is that the finding of BAL or mucosal neutrophilia should prompt a search for another diagnosis.

Fixed and Variable Airflow Obstruction

Variable Airflow Obstruction

Wheeze is a frequently sought, and often misinterpreted sound. Even when a polyphonic, musical predominantly expiratory noise is heard by the physician, all it betokens is narrowing of the airway lumen. It is not synonymous with airway smooth muscle constriction. Causes include intraluminal airway secretions; airway malacia which may be localized or generalized; and extraluminal compression, for example by a mass of lymph nodes. Most of the asthmas as defined above have the hallmark of either or both of obstructive physiology which improves with acute administration of a short acting β-2 agonist, or normal physiology but with an exaggerated response to stimuli such as cold air or allergen challenge.

In terms of variable airflow obstruction, as a profession we have been remiss in failing to document this objectively. Even pre-school children can perform spirometry, and criteria for adequate curves (34) and definitions of bronchodilator responsiveness (35) for this age group have been published. Simple field tests, like acute response to a short acting β-2 agonist, a short period of home peak flow or increasingly electronic spirometry monitoring, and an exercise challenge may be informative. Although there is no one definitive diagnostic test for asthma, and all the above have a high specificity but low sensitivity for asthma (36), the more tests that fail to demonstrated variable airflow obstruction, the less likely is the treatable trait of bronchodilator responsive airflow obstruction to be present.

AHR correlates poorly with inflammation (above), but of course there is a relationship which is best described by a two-component model, "inflammatory" and "anatomical." Three major longitudinal studies (37–39) have measured AHR very early in life, before any significant exposure to infection or allergen, and certainly before there is any evidence of airway inflammation or remodeling (40). Each has shown a strong association between early AHR and adverse long term respiratory outcomes. The likely pathological basis is increased airway length and reduced radius, leading to a baseline increase in airway resistance (41), which with further narrowing by a constrictor stimulus leads to an exaggerated reduction in airflow. There is also evidence in later life that airway inflammation causes a component of AHR, and that anti-inflammatory therapies can improve AHR (42).

In terms of the practical value of measuring AHR in the clinic, population studies have shown that, although in group data, AHR relates to asthma severity, many normal people can be shown to have AHR but have no symptoms (43). Thus, "abnormal" AHR of itself does not lead to disease; by analogy with the airway eosinophil story, what is the "X-factor" that converts asymptomatic AHR to an airway disease? Again, this is completely unknown. However, what is certain is that failure to demonstrate AHR in a patient said to be symptomatic with asthma should lead to reconsideration of the diagnosis; certainly, if a child is thought to have eosinophilic airway inflammation but AHR cannot be demonstrated, then the child's symptoms are not due to eosinophilic asthma.

Fixed Airflow Obstruction

The importance of this *untreatable* trait is that ICS and other therapies should not be escalated when there is no hope of benefit. There is no generally accepted pediatric definition of fixed airflow obstruction. In general, it should be defined as an abnormal FEV_1 (more than 1.96 Z-scores below normal) after a systemic corticosteroid trial and the acute administration of short-acting β-2 agonist, but neither the dose, duration or route of administration of systemic steroids, nor the dose of short-acting β-2 agonist is agreed. We use a single injection of intramuscular triamcinolone (40 mg in a child weighing <40 kgm, 80 mgm in the rest) to ensure adherence, and 1 mgm of salbutamol via a spacer (44). We found very little evidence of benefit from adding extra doses of triamcinolone (45). It should be noted that the measurement of steroid responsiveness in children with asthma encompasses more than just measuring spirometry; we use a multi-domain approach (46, 47).

One component of airway obstruction is determined antenatally. Maternal nicotine exposure (active and passive smoking, vaping) has been shown in animal models and humans to lead to structural changes with a readout of airflow obstruction shortly after birth, before the first viral infection (41, 48–52). Other adverse factors include maternal exposure to environmental pollution (53), maternal hypertension (54), and any factor leading to a low birth weight or prematurity or both (55, 56). The second component is the structural airway wall changes in established asthma, including increased airway smooth muscle, reticular basement membrane thickening, increased numbers of goblet cells and increased airway vascularity. Conventionally, these are considered to result from cycles of airway inflammation and contribute to airflow obstruction (above). However, at least in pediatrics, most studies linking inflammation and remodeling are cross-sectional and observational, and demonstrating association is a long step from proving causation. It is currently not possible to synthesis a coherent account of the pathophysiology of remodeling, and one can only present a few statements which require integration and explanation.

1. At least some aspects of remodeling, for example increased reticular basement membrane thickening, plateau in childhood, and are non-progressive into adult life (10).
2. No pediatric studies have shown eosinophilic airway inflammation with no evidence of remodeling. Remodeling has been described in the absence of current airway eosinophilia, but these children have been prescribed usually high dose ICS, and these data are equally consistent with the hypothesis of ICS having successfully treated airway eosinophilia as the alternative, that remodeling precedes airway eosinophilia (57).
3. Although airway remodeling can be partially attenuated by prolonged use of high-dose ICS (58, 59), the changes are much more steroid resistant than is airway eosinophilia.

4. Reticular basement thickening is inversely correlated with AHR, (60) and thus may be a protective response of the airway, protecting against life-threatening bronchoconstriction.
5. It is at least conceivable that reticular basement membrane thickening is a protective measure designed to limit penetration of cytokines and chemokines into the systemic circulation, and possibly also protect the airway mucosa from tissue damaging enzymes within the lumen (61).
6. On the other hand, the increase in airway smooth muscle in asthma (62), and the beneficial responses seen in adults with bronchial thermoplasty together with reduction in smooth muscle in animals submitted to thermoplasty (63, 64), suggests this aspect of remodeling is adverse.

Airway Infection and the Asthmas

This is another area that is currently difficult to understand. Some issues are clear; acute attacks of wheeze are usually precipitated by respiratory viral infections at all ages (65). Recent studies have shown that bacteria are isolated equally frequently during a wheeze attack (66), but it is unclear whether bacteria cause the attack, or are the result of a transient mucosal immunoparesis secondary to viral infection or iatrogenic as a result of ICS treatment (33). The general failure of antibiotics to impact acute wheeze attacks to any great degree is a strong pointer against a causal role for bacteria. We also know that the airway microbiome differs between normal and asthmatic children (67), and that airway neutrophilia in children appears to be beneficial rather than the reverse (32), implying a more important role of infection than previously thought. It is also clear that very early nasopharyngeal bacterial colonization with bacteria is associated with a mixed TH1/TH2/TH17 mucosal response, and subsequent adverse respiratory outcomes (68–72), although whether bacterial colonization is causal, or a marker of a subtle immune deficiency, is unclear. In a study using bronchoscopy and BAL to measure airway inflammation and infection, and the airway microbiota, in severe pre-school wheezers, we demonstrated two separate microbiota-based clusters; a Moraxella positive, airway neutrophilic group, and a mixed microbiota, macrophage and lymphocyte predominant group (73). Interestingly, these did not relate to clinical phenotype or markers of atopic status. Long term follow up will be needed to determine the significance of these clusters. There are some *in vitro* data lending plausibility to a link between bacterial infection and airway eosinophilia; in a nasal polyp model, *Staph aureus* binds via TLR2 leading to epithelial release of the alarmins TSLP and IL33, and the TH2 signature cytokines IL5 and IL13 (74). However, we need more data about the role of bacteria and the interactions with airway eosinophilia to try to understand asthma pathophysiology.

Of more immediate practical clinical significance is the need to determine whether the child with respiratory symptoms has an underlying chronic bacterial infection which will respond to oral antibiotics ["persistent bacterial bronchitis (PBB)"] (75, 76). Typically the symptoms are of wet cough not wheeze, but secretions narrowing the lumen may cause wheeze, and non-wheeze noises may be misinterpreted by the family. For most of these children, invasive sampling is not appropriate. We have shown that the yield of organisms is much greater with induced sputum, even in young children, compared to cough swabs, and indeed induced sputum results are comparable to FOB (16). It should be noted that PBB, like bronchiectasis, is a description not a diagnosis, and should prompt a focused diagnostic work-up (77).

The Time Domain: Often Unappreciated

The two important pathophysiological areas are firstly, the stability of measurements over time, and secondly, the extent to which sophisticated analysis of simple measurements over a long time period can help us understand asthma pathophysiology and understand risk.

Temporal Stability of Measurements

Adult studies in which sputum cell counts are used to guide treatment have given promising results, in particular in the reduction of asthma attack frequency (78). When we attempted to replicate this study in pediatric asthma (79), we actually found that sputum cellular phenotypes were very variable in the same individual over time, in both severe and mild-moderate asthma (80). These discrepancies are unexplained, but underscore the importance of not critically extrapolating from adults to children. Likely sputum cell counts reflect not merely the underlying disease, but environmental factors and treatment adherence. The U-BIOPRED group used breath-omics (the eNose) to define three clusters, but also noted that many patients changed cluster as peripheral blood eosinophil count changed over time (81). Cluster stability is discussed in more detail below.

Fluctuation Analyses

The first major paper used time series analyses of fluctuations in peak flow to develop a quantitative basis for objective risk prediction of acute asthma attacks and for evaluating treatment effectiveness (82). Subsequent manuscripts from this group confirmed that by considering measurements of peak flow and spirometry in isolation, rather than as part of a series, resulted in important information being lost. These and other mathematical techniques could be used to predict the response to β-2 agonists (83) and whether ICS withdrawal was likely to be successful (84). Furthermore, the method distinguished between asthma and healthy controls, partly independent of atopy, and inflammation but related to the *17q21* locus (85). These mathematical techniques have not found their way into the routine asthma clinic, but clearly this sort of mathematical analysis is giving potentially important information about asthma pathophysiology which may aid management.

Summary: What Is Current Best Practice?

The days of diagnosing and treating asthma without making objective measurements are past. Is there any other chronic condition in which simple tests are available, but are routinely not performed before committing a child to long term treatment? We should use our knowledge of the pathophysiology of asthma to phenotype the airway, even in young children, focusing on the treatable traits. It is out with the scope of this article, but we should also consider any extra-pulmonary co-morbidities and social and environmental factors when planning management.

SPECIAL "ASTHMAS": HOW DOES THE LANCET COMMISSION HELP US?

Most of the phenotyping issues arise in children who solely have an airway disease. However, there are some situations in which airway phenotyping is helpful in understanding pathophysiology and planning treatment.

Pre-school Wheeze: Is It Asthma, Dr?

As discussed, this question is without meaning, as is the statement that asthma cannot be diagnosed until a given and entirely arbitrary age. The proper approach is to determine which (if any) treatable traits the infant exhibits. The INFANT study (23) was discussed above; so at the very least, rather than asking pointless questions or making fatuous statements, a blood eosinophil count should be performed and aeroallergen sensitization determined. Ideally spirometry should be measured, but at the very least, if the child becomes acutely wheezy, this should be documented by a physician, and the response of wheeze intensity and oxygen saturation to inhaled β-2 agonist determined. If airway infection and PBB is suspected, documentation with cough swab or induced sputum that there is actually infection present should be mandatory, especially if multiple or prolonged antibiotic courses are being used.

Wheeze in the First Year of Life: What Is It, Dr?

Very little is known about this asthma. We know it is not related to airway eosinophilia (40), so ICS should not be prescribed. We know it is common, and the prevalence across the world is highly variable (86). This is an area where a lot more work is needed on pathophysiology.

Does the Child With Another Pulmonary or a Systemic Disease Also Have Asthma?

Very frequently, ICS are prescribed to children with reasons other than asthma for being symptomatic, often either preceding the realization that a non-asthma disease is present, or on the "just in case" principle. This is to be deplored; ICS have potential serious adverse events, not least the increased risk of pneumonia (87), tuberculous (88) and non-tuberculous *Mycobacterial* infection (89), at least from adult studies.

"Asthma" in Other Pulmonary Diseases

The classical quandary is whether survivors of premature birth have "asthma" (90). Again, phenotyping resolves this. It is clear from a number of studies that these children have fixed and variable airflow obstruction (91, 92). However, FeNO is normal not raised, even in the absence of ICS (93), nor is there an elevation of exhaled breath temperature (94), a non-specific sign of inflammation ("calor" in the parlance of yesteryear). Thus, unless there is evidence in a given individual of a second diagnosis of atopic, allergic asthma (raised FeNO and peripheral blood eosinophil count, aeroallergen sensitization), ICS should not be prescribed. The same principles of investigation apply to other airway diseases, such as obliterative bronchiolitis and the airway disease after neuroendocrine cell hyperplasia of infancy; these are discussed in detail elsewhere (95).

"Asthma" in Children With a Systemic Disease

Exemplar diseases are CF, primary ciliary dyskinesia (PCD) and sickle cell anemia (SCD). We have shown that the prescription of ICS in PCD is haphazard and bears no relationship to any marker of atopic sensitization or airway eosinophilia (96). In both CF and PCD, where there is evidence that airway neutrophilia leads to tissue damage from the release of proteases and other enzymes, inhibiting neutrophil apoptosis with ICS (above) may have particularly adverse consequences. In these situations also, determining the presence or otherwise of the treatable traits airway eosinophilia and β-2 responsive bronchoconstriction should be used to determine treatment. SCD is a particularly interesting airway disease. Compared with controls, SCD children had fixed but not variable airflow obstruction, and no evidence of AHR or airway eosinophilia (97) we speculate that the airway disease may be on the basis of airway ischaemia due to microinfarcts secondary to sickling, analogous to what is seen more dramatically when the bronchial arteries are stripped off the airway during the unifocalisation procedure (98). So in all systemic conditions, if a treatable trait is present it should be treated, but treatment for a non-existent problem should be withheld.

Obesity Asthma—Not Lean Asthma in a Fat Body

The impact of the obesity epidemic across the world is well known, and the question as to whether obesity "causes" asthma is hotly debated (99). Again, phenotyping and looking at pathophysiology sheds light on the subject. The first question in a child who is breathless and obese is, does the child have an airway disease at all? Even in lean children, exertional breathlessness is more often due to deconditioning than asthma or exercise-induced laryngeal obstruction (EILO), and many non-asthmatics were treated with inhaled medication (12). A cardiopulmonary exercise test with measurements of any post-exercise bronchoconstriction may be informative.

If the obese child truly has an airway disease, then its nature should be characterized. Of course, obesity does not prevent the development of atopy, and the child may have standard atopic, eosinophilic pediatric asthma. However, obese asthma may be relatively ICS resistant, suggestive of another phenotype in some cases. Dysanaptic airway growth is defined as a normal FEV_1 with a greater than normal FVC, and thus a reduced FEV_1/FVC ratio (100). Essentially airways are of normal caliber but increased length, the latter thought to be determined by lung size. In a study of six adult cohorts, four with longitudinal data, dysanapsis was found to be commoner in the obese, and associated with worse outcomes including severe asthma attacks and use of oral prednisolone. Studies on whether obese asthma is associated with Type 2 inflammation are conflicting (101, 102). It is well known that obesity is a pro-inflammatory condition. There are intriguing data suggesting that the airway may be the target of systemic inflammation, instead of the source of inflammatory cytokines spilling into the systemic circulation. In a study of two adult cohorts, plasma IL-6 was measured as a marker of systemic inflammation and related to BMI and asthma outcomes (103) Patients who were IL-6 high were more likely (but not inevitably) obese, and had worse FEV_1 and more likely a history of asthma attacks. There was no relationship between IL-6 and serum IgE or sputum eosinophils, demonstrating that the effects of systemic inflammation were not mediated via Type 2 inflammation. Again these studies indicate the need to go back to pathophysiology, and the utility of airway phenotyping when considering airway disease, especially if it is non-responsive to conventional therapy.

THE PATHOPHYSIOLOGY OF ASTHMA RISK

Increasingly the importance of future risk as a domain to be considered in asthma management[1]. If risk is to be managed, it must be measured, and the underlying pathophysiology of the risk be understood.

Asthma Attacks

Asthma attacks are all too common, may cause death, impair quality of life, incur a huge burden of health care cost and are associated with worsening respiratory and lung growth trajectories. Asthma attacks are not "exacerbations," a futile word implying a reversible inconvenience (104, 105); they are lung attacks. A recent meta-analysis of the risk factors for an asthma lung attack (106), as did the UK National Review of Asthma Deaths[2], highlighted that having had one bad attack, the patient was at high risk of having another. Many asthma fatalities related to social factors, such as poor adherence and failure to engage with regular follow up reviews. However, the underlying pathophysiology of asthma attacks is also important. Specifically, the concept that asthma control may be good, but risk of a future attack high, is pivotal.

Asthma attacks may be driven purely by respiratory viral infection, with no background Type 2 inflammation, usually in pre-school children with episodic viral wheeze (107). A huge surge in environmental allergen burden in the absence of viral infection may also rarely cause acute asthma attacks, as in the Barcelona soya bean epidemics (108), and thunderstorm asthma (109). The vast majority of attacks are respiratory viral driven in patients who have background ongoing type 2 inflammation; thus the combination of respiratory viral infection, allergic sensitization and allergen exposure was very strongly predictive of an asthma attack (110). It has been shown that using FeNO and (in adults) induced sputum eosinophil count to titrate ICS treatment leads to a reduction in asthma attacks (24). Inadequate ICS treatment (usually related to non-adherence) was another strong predictor of an asthma attack (106). Omalizumab therapy in the summer given to children on step 5 therapy who had had an asthma attack in the previous year ameliorated the autumnal rise in asthma attacks driven by returning to school and winter viral infections (111). Finally, in a proof of concept, double blind, randomized controlled study, mite impermeable bedding led to a reduction in oral corticosteroid use in the year after an asthma attack in children sensitized to house dust mite (112). This allows a risk prediction index for asthma attacks (112). The Seasonal Asthma Exacerbation Prediction Index (SAEPI) has been validated as a means of predicting children at risk for an asthma attack (113, 114). For those aeroallergen sensitized, an attack in the prior season and reduced spirometry predict a further asthma attack irrespective of season. Measures such as increased numbers of positive allergen skin prick tests, high prescribed ICS doses, increased FeNO, blood eosinophil counts and total and specific IgE levels may predict a seasonal asthma exacerbation. In summary, uncontrolled Type 2 inflammation, even in the face of good asthma symptom control, is a major risk factor for future asthma attacks.

There are other factors of importance which have been reviewed elsewhere (115). There are some asthma patients who never have an attack, implying either genetic protection or susceptibility factors, which are poorly understood. One example is the gene for the epithelial protein CDHR3, which is the receptor for RV-C (116), and gene mutations may convey increased susceptibility to attacks (117, 118). Indoor and outdoor air pollution, including tobacco, and vitamin D deficiency potentially through multiple immunological and other pathways (119), are all associated with increased risk of asthma attacks.

Interestingly, many severe asthma patients never have an attack, for reasons which are unclear. Analysis of the SARP-3 cohort showed that nearly half never had an asthma attack, but a quarter had at least three attacks per year (120). Peripheral blood eosinophil count, body mass index, and bronchodilator responsiveness were positively associated with frequency of attacks, but not asthma duration, age, sex, race, and socioeconomic status. The findings were replicated in previous SARP patient cohorts.

Adverse Trajectories of Lung Function

There is an extensive literature on tracking of lung function, from a series of overlapping birth cohorts (121). Although there are discrepancies, some due to methodological issues such as lung function measurements in infancy, the balance of the evidence is that spirometry tracks from the pre-school years to late middle age at least, with possible deviations from tracking if puberty is late with a subsequent fast growth trajectory (122). In summary, spirometry rises to a plateau at about 20–25 years of age and thereafter declines (123). Adult studies have shown that failure to reach a normal spirometric plateau carries a 26% risk of COPD, compared with a 6% risk in those who attain their full growth potential (and who develop COPD because of an abnormally rapid rate of decline of spirometry) (124). A number of cohort studies have shown that some children have persistently low spirometry during childhood, putting them in the high risk category. The pathophysiology of this phenotype is poorly understood (125–127). The Tucson group used latent class analysis to determine that there were two trajectories, normal, and low lung function. Risk factors for the low lung function group included a history of maternal asthma (20.0 vs. 9.9%; $P = 0.02$); early life RSV lower respiratory tract infection

[1] https://ginasthma.org/

[2] https://www.rcplondon.ac.uk/projects/national-review-asthma-deaths/

(41.2 vs. 21.4%; $P = 0.001$); and physician-diagnosed active asthma (whatever the value of that label) at age 32 years (43.9 vs. 16.2%; $P < 0.001$) (125). In the Tasmanian cohort (126), there were three low trajectories (early below average, accelerated decline; persistently low; and below average); predictors included childhood asthma, bronchitis, pneumonia, allergic rhinitis, eczema, parental asthma, and maternal smoking. This group were followed up into the sixth decade, and COPD risk could be calculated. Odds ratios were 35·0, 95% CI 19·5-64·0 (early below average, accelerated decline): 9·5, 4·5–20·6 (persistently low); and 3·7, 1·9–6·9 (below average). In a combined analysis of the MAAS and ALSPAC cohorts (127), the persistently low trajectory was associated with severe wheeze attacks, early allergic sensitization, and tobacco smoke exposure. However, although it is clear that there is a group of asthmatics with low trajectory lung function who are at risk of COPD, it is not clear that anything can be done to reverse this. The Tasmanian group showed that risks were exacerbated in those children who went on to smoke, and certainly general advice should be given about risk avoidance; but this is clearly an area of asthma pathophysiology which merits further work. Also of note, and meriting further work is the association of high early all-cause mortality in populations with impaired spirometry (128, 129); it may well be that low spirometry should be used as an important signal of systemic disease (130).

Risk of Progressive Disease

Many if not all children who develop atopic eosinophilic asthma by school age start with acute discrete episodes of pre-school wheeze before progressing to a multiple trigger pattern of symptoms. A proportion of children with viral wheeze progress to school age eosinophilic airway disease. The pathways to progression are very poorly understood (40, 107, 131, 132). Important factors associated with progression include multiple early atopic sensitization and severe attacks of wheeze (133). We know that those with no personal or family atopic history are unlikely to progress, but although predictive indices (134–136) have a good negative predictive value, unfortunately the positive predictive value not much better than 50%. Currently we know that in the pre-school years those who develop school age asthma lose lung function, which is never regained throughout life (137, 138); and they develop airway remodeling and eosinophilic inflammation. Although there is active research in the field (139) we do not have good predictive biomarkers nor do we understand the endotypes of progression or regression of the disease, nor do we have any therapeutic interventions. We know that ICS used early are not disease-modifying (140–142), but we do not know what might be useful. There are tantalizing hints that risk reduction is possible, from a randomized controlled trial of fish-oil supplementation (143) and the differences in atopic risk between the Amish and Hutterite communities, related to environmental exposures (144). This is another aspect of pathophysiology that requires more work.

Risk of Side-Effects

Clearly ICS doses should be the minimum required to control Type 2 inflammation. There is some evidence that the risk of side-effects relates more to an excessive dose of ICS relative to the degree of airway inflammation rather than the absolute dose prescribed. In a group of adult asthmatics, there was no difference in the pharmacokinetics of an intravenous dose of fluticasone, with similar area under the curves (145). However, when the same dose was given by inhalation, there was far greater absorption into the systemic circulations in the non-asthmatics. There was unfortunately no objective measurement of inflammation, but it is not unreasonable to suppose that overdosing relative to inflammation leads to side-effects.

CONCLUSION: AIRWAY PHENOTYPING

Clearly we can learn a lot about the pathophysiology of the asthmas, and use this knowledge to improve diagnosis and treatment. We are still not achieving this in routine clinical practice, and this is shameful. However, even if we were phenotyping all patients and understanding pathophysiology with currently available tools, we need to progress to the next step, namely endotyping. The current position is described in the next section of this article.

OUR TARGET: ENDOTYPING THE AIRWAY

The general approach to airway endotyping has been to collect and characterize as far as possible large groups of patients, for example the U-BIOPRED (146, 147) and SARP (148) cohorts, and use sophisticated—omics technologies to perform cluster analyses to try to determine the endotypes driving disease. However, caution is needed; whether a child is in a particular cluster will be driven by the underlying endotype, but also the effects of adverse environmental, infective or other factors which may vary over time, the contrasting effects of prescribed treatment, and whether the treatment is actually used by the patient. Environmental factors are unstable over time, and changes may be dramatic (108, 109, 149, 150). Treatment adherence is highly variable, difficult to measure and will affect the airway. Hence an eosinophilic airway may be the final common pathway of combinations of a steroid resistant endotype; poor adherence to ICS treatment; and increased environmental allergen exposure. Clearly the management of these three factors is very different. Very few groups have studied longitudinal stability of phenotypes or endotypes, and a second, validation cohort is rarely used; when done, the evidence for stability is weak (151). Thus, our challenge is to differentiate what truly reflects a real endotype and what represents non-disease attributes (above). This is rarely addressed or even often identified as a problem.

Furthermore, most of these analyses are in patients with severe asthma, because mild asthma hardly merits study. However, most patients referred with "severe" asthma would have mild asthma if they took their treatment (152–154). In this regard, in a recent GWAS there was substantial overlap between mild and moderate to severe asthma (155). Although the authors speculated that this related to epigenetic silencing of genes, and was therefore not reflective of gene expression, an alternative explanation is that many diagnosed as moderate to severe asthma in fact were non-adherent to treatment.

Endoyping Asthma With Omics Technology

The U-BIOPRED (146, 147) and SARP (148) investigators, who have largely focused on severe asthma, albeit with additional controls, are the major groups exploiting -omics technology. Systems biology is increasingly used to allow clusters and phenotypes to emerge from the data (103, 156) using an unbiased analysis, not confounded by pre-set ideas. This is impossible; there is inevitable investigator bias in selecting the data to collect and analyse. For example, until relatively recently, bacterial infection was not thought relevant to asthma, but this has been challenged (above); prior to this work, bacterial samples would not have been collected and analyzed.

Cluster Analyses: What Do They Tell Us?

The SARP investigators (157) identified four clusters: mild to moderate early onset asthma, normal body mass index and no or eosinophilic airway inflammation; the second had the same inflammatory characteristics, but the patients older, more likely to be obese, with impaired airway obstruction on spirometry and African Americans were over-represented. The last two exhibited had predominantly neutrophilic sputum; sputum eosinophilia was also sometimes seen. One of these clusters also contained older patients who were more likely to be obese and have severe asthma, obstructive spirometry and to be treated with oral corticosteroids. The final cluster was the oldest, with males over-represented, and more likely to be obese and prescribed complex medication regimes. As well as a lack of replication and assessment of cluster stability over time, the investigators could not dissociate the effects of disease from those of treatment. Furthermore, association does not prove causation, which could not be determined. Critically, this sort of cluster analysis did not appear to help us make progress in understanding or treating disease. This last point is underscored by another SARP analysis revealing this time five clusters (120) with no differences in outcomes, again questioning the usefulness of this approach.

The U-BIOPRED investigators identified four clusters in adults using sputum cell transcriptomics (158, 159). They used clinical clustering and training and validation cohorts to define phenotypes (159) which were then used to assess differences in sputum proteomics and transcriptomics data. The first were well-controlled patients with moderate-to-severe asthma. The second was in smokers with late onset severe asthma, further characterized by chronic airflow obstruction. The only difference between this and the third cluster was that the latter contained non-smokers. The fourth cluster contained obese women who had uncontrolled severe asthma, normal lung function but multiple asthma attacks. There were differences in gene expression in these clusters, which adds validity to their findings.

Assessment of the temporal stability of clusters was performed by the ADEPT group (160). They performed a baseline cluster analysis in adults which were then re-assessed over time and also validated in a U-BIOPRED subset (161). They used sophisticated mathematical techniques which included fuzzy-partition-around-medoid clustering. They included including clinical and biomarker profiles. They also classified the patients into $TH2_{hi}$ and $TH2_{lo}$ using gene expression profiles on bronchial biopsies. They identified four phenotypic clusters. The first was characterized by mild, early onset disease, good spirometry, and little in the way of inflammation; that present was predominantly Type 2. The second contained moderately well controlled asthmatics who had mild airflow limitation and moderate airway responsiveness; they also had Type 2 inflammation. The third group were only moderately well controlled, had minor Type 2 inflammation or a non-eosinophilic, neutrophilic phenotype airway phenotype with predominantly fixed airflow obstruction. The fourth cohort had severe asthma with uncontrolled reversible airflow obstruction, a mixed and type 2 inflammatory picture. However, there was huge overlap between the clusters for almost every marker; this does not invalidate the study, but suggests that cluster analysis may be excellent for determining groups linked by common mechanisms, but has yet to been shown in any cluster analysis. Hence the role of cluster analyses is yet to be defined. There are commonalities and differences between studies, and they have not delivered endotypes.

Asthma Diagnosis Using Omics Technology

It is well known that asthma is poorly diagnosed (162–164), often objective diagnostic tests are not used, and those that are available are so crude when compared with the gene signature approaches used, for example, in tuberculosis diagnostics (165, 166). Blood transcriptomics would be the ideal. Red cedarwood triggered asthma in adults has a gold standard diagnostic test, unlike most of the asthmas outside the workplace, namely bronchial challenge. In a small study split into two cohorts, discovery and validation, adults with red cedarwood asthma could be reliably diagnosed using a gene signature in peripheral blood (167). Confirmation in other settings is needed, but a gene signature approach would be a major step change on current diagnostic approaches.

The U-BIOPRED group (168) also used a training and validation set. They identified 1693 genes differentially expressed in adult asthmatics as against controls, with a bigger effect size in severe asthmatics. Unfortunately, and reducing the value of this approach, around 90% of the differences could be related solely to differences in peripheral blood white cell count. Pathway analysis showed that genes related to chemotaxis, migration and myeloid cell trafficking, and decreased development of B-cells, haematopoietic progenitor cells and lymphoid organs were involved in the differences, in both training and validation cohorts. The results were similar but less pronounced in mild-moderate asthmatics. Gene signatures of corticosteroid responsiveness also differed. However, the transcriptomics did not map to any clinical cluster (169). Again this calls into question the utility of this approach, certainly as a clinical tool, and highlights our lack of understanding of the complexity of asthma. It is possible that the results might have been different if airway cells had been used, as being closer to the pathological process.

Asthma Pathophysiology: Hypothesis Generating Studies

Gene expression is regulated in part by non-coding RNA, and this has been a subject of asthma research. In adults with severe asthma, activation status of CD4 and CD8 lymphocytes was related to non-coding RNA expression. There were significant changes in CD8 but not CD4 cells, Multiple pathways involved in T-cell activation were enhanced and there were many changes in miRNA expression (170). This is observational study, and very preliminary, but an important starting point. The rapidly expanding field of the role of micro-RNAs has been reviewed in detail elsewhere (171).

Asthma Pathophysiology: Exploring Endotypes of Inflammation

Although the ideal is one endotype susceptible to a single biological, the reality is likely to be much more complex. Cytokines and chemokines were measured in sputum from subjects in the SARP group with varying severities of asthma, and unbiased factor analysis was used to try to define specific inflammatory pathways (172). There were complex inflammatory protein interactions identified by factor analysis. Severe asthma patients had nine increased and four decreased proteins compared to mild asthma subjects. Twenty-six mediators were significantly associated with an increasing single induced sputum leucocyte type: sixteen with neutrophils; 5 with lymphocytes; IL-15 and CCL15/MIP1δ with macrophages; interestingly, only IL-5 with eosinophils; and IL-4 and TNFSF10/TRAIL with airway epithelial cells. Forty three cytokines, chemokines, and growth factors which had no missing data were mapped onto the first 10 factors, containing mixes of Th1, Th2, Th9, and Th17 inflammatory and anti-inflammatory proteins, rather than pure pathways. Hence focus on a single specific mediator or pathway is likely an oversimplification of the complex reality of the asthmatic airway.

In a further study, the U-BIOPRED investigators started by defining phenotypes from sputum cytology, either eosinophil- and neutrophil-predominant. Next, they used sputum plugs to generate Affymetrix arrays and analyzed the data were analyzed using hierarchical, unsupervised clustering. They identified three transcript associated clusters (TACs). The first was contained oral corticosteroid dependent patients who had frequent asthma attacks, severe airflow obstruction, and the highest sputum eosinophil counts and FeNO levels. Immunologically, the receptors Il33R, CCR3 and TSLPR were upregulated and there was the strongest IL-13/TH2 and ILC2 gene signatures. The second cluster was clinically characterized by sputum neutrophilia, a raised serum CRP and eczema, and immunologically by IFN-, TNF-α- and inflammasome related genes being upregulated. The final cluster had moderate sputum eosinophilia and better spirometry, but despite sputum eosinophilia was immunologically characterized by upregulation of genes of metabolic pathways, ubiquitination and mitochondrial, with surprisingly, no TH2 signature. This important paper again highlights that eosinophilia is not synonymous with TH2 activation, confirming our own findings in severe asthma (26).

A pioneering study used transcriptomics of bronchial brushings and biopsies to determine $TH2_{hi}$ and $TH2_{lo}$ subgroups of mild to moderate asthmatics based on TH2 gene signatures (173). The $TH2_{hi}$ subgroup had elevated peripheral blood levels of periostin (which is also derived from growing bone, so cannot be used in pediatrics), CLCA1 and Serpin B2, and eosinophilic airway inflammation which was ICS responsive. A subsequent study (174) using airway epithelial cell gene expression in adults confirmed this finding, but found that non-invasive biomarkers such as periostin were not sufficiently sensitive. The U-BIOPRED subsequently identified two steroid-resistant, eosinophilic subgroups in severe asthmatics (175); one with high mucosal eosinophilia, raised FeNO, asthma attacks and oral corticosteroid use; by contrast, the second eosinophilic group was more obese. We previously noted that sputum and BAL eosinophils correlate with each other, but not with mucosal biopsy eosinophils (15), but which is most important under what circumstances has not been determined. The U-BIOPRED investigators also described two non-eosinophilic groups, and developed model to predict the likelihood of the patient being steroid responsive. It is very clear that there are non-inflammatory phenotypes of severe asthma, and also that mucosal and BAL eosinophilia is not synonymous with Type 2 inflammation (176).

A further U-BIOPRED study highlighted the IL6 pathway as a potential cause of eosinophilic inflammation independent of TH2 cytokines (177). Activation of IL-6 trans signaling in air-liquid interface cultures of bronchial epithelial cells reduced the integrity of the epithelium. Associated with this was a specific signature enriched in airway remodeling genes. This signature identified a subgroup of adult asthmatics with increased epithelial expression of these inducible genes in the absence of systemic inflammation. There was an overrepresentation of patients with frequent attacks, peripheral blood eosinophilia, and submucosal of T cells and macrophage infiltration. TLR receptor pathway genes were upregulated, but cell junction genes expression was reduced. Sputum sIL6R and IL6 levels correlated with sputum markers of innate immune activation and airway remodeling. This study further evidence that there is a subset of asthmatic patients with no evidence of Type 2 inflammation; it may be that IL6 is driving airway inflammation and epithelial dysfunction in this group of patients.

The IL1 pathway may also be important (178). Sputum transcriptomics were compared in severe and mild-moderate adult asthmatics with eosinophilic and neutrophilic asthma. The investigators reported that IL1RL1 gene expression was associated with severe eosinophilic asthma, whereas NLRP3 inflammasome expression was highest in those with severe, neutrophilic asthma. These changes were only seen in induced sputum, not in bronchial brushings or biopsy specimens, underscoring the need to study multiple tissues if pathophysiology is to be understood.

Finally, FeNO is a well-known as an asthma biomarker, but whether more than one pathway results in increases has been little studied. The SARP team used a microarray platform to relate FeNO to bronchial airway epithelial cell gene expression (179). They identified 549 genes whose expression correlated with FeNO. They used k-means to cluster the patient samples and found that a total of 1,384 genes were identified in nine gene groups. Although type 2 inflammation genes were present, novel pathways, including those related to neuronal function, WNT pathways, and actin cytoskeleton, were also discovered, suggesting novel and as yet poorly characterized inflammatory pathways were at play in asthma.

Taken together, these studies suggest that in particular in severe asthma, there are multiple endotypes, possibly co-existing in some patients. There is far more to asthma pathophysiology than Type 2 inflammation. We have much more to learn from harnessing omics technology to the study of the asthmas.

Asthma Pathophysiology: Persistent Airflow Limitation

As discussed above, there are multiple contributory factors to persistent airflow limitation, including congenital and acquired remodeling, so it is likely that multiple genes are involved. The UBIOPRED group (180) used Gene Set Variation Analysis (GSVA), as a means of detecting underlying endotypes in such heterogeneous samples. Severe adult asthma patients from the U-BIOPRED cohort with persistent airflow limitation defined as post-bronchodilator FEV_1/FVC below the lower limit of normal) were compared with asthmatics with normal spirometry. Gene expression was assessed on the total RNA of sputum cells, nasal brushings, and endobronchial brushings and biopsies. Fourteen differentially enriched gene signatures were identified that were associated with ICS, eosinophils, IL13, IFN-α, specific $CD4^+$ T-cells and airway remodeling. There was a differentially expressed gene network associated with remodeling solely in the airway wall.

Asthma Attacks: Can We Do Better?

Chitinase-like protein YKL-40 modulates airway inflammation and serum levels are associated with asthma severity (181). In another SARP study (182), adult asthmatics were analyzed to determine if there were clusters based on YKL-40 levels, and the findings were validated in SARP. Sputum transcriptome analysis were used to demonstrate molecular pathways associated with YKL-40 clusters, of which four could be identified. Those with high serum YKL-40 were associated with earlier onset and longer duration of disease, severe airflow obstruction, and near-fatal asthma attacks. The cluster with the highest serum YKL-40 levels had adult onset disease and less airflow obstruction, but frequent attacks. Interestingly, and despite the fact that attack frequency was an important correlate of these clusters, an airway transcriptome analysis showed activation of non-type 2 inflammatory pathways. This study provides further evidence for the importance of non-TH2 pathways, and, although this needs validation, possibly suggests that serum YKL-40 levels may help risk-stratify patients.

Future Risks: Progression From Pre-school Episodic Wheeze to School Age Eosinophilic Airway Disease

This is an extremely complicated subject which is largely beyond the scope of this review. We know that antenatal and postnatal tobacco and pollution exposure are important factors impacting future lung health, but we know little or nothing of the molecular pathways to disease [see review Bush (121)]. Furthermore, although we can predict who are low risk children, we are poor at predicting high risk, what the pathways to eosinophilic asthma actually are, and how we can reduce risk, either on a population or individual level. We have some largely descriptive -omics data which hint at pathways, but our knowledge gaps are huge.

Gene expression profiles were studied in transient and persistent wheezers using peripheral CD4+ve cells, and compared to normal, non-wheezing controls (183). The study was observational and descriptive, but did describe differences in gene expression between the two wheezing groups, with some commonalities in the paths involving proliferation and apoptosis of T-cells. Another group prospectively followed 202 preschool wheezers to school age, and testing the hypothesis that the use of volatile organic compounds (VOCs) and exhaled breath condensate would enhance the prognostic value of conventional predictive indices (184). They showed that VOCs and possibly inflammation related genes (TLR-4, catalase, TNF-α) improved predictive of persistent wheeze, but this study is also realm, and hypothesis generating, requiring validation in another cohort.

HOW WILL WE MAKE OMICS WORK IN PRACTICE?

When clinically indicated, invasive techniques can be used to discover novel mechanisms and pathways, but these will be only applicable in really severe cases, not in more mildly affected infants and children. For most cases, non-invasive approaches must be found, especially in children. Blood, urine and induced sputum can and should be routine clinical tests, there are other accessible biosamples which should be evaluated. Exhaled breath analysis is non-invasive, requires only passive co-operation, and with modern analytical techniques can give point of care answers. Investigators can distinguish different airway diseases in adults (COPD, asthma) from a breathprint of VOCs (185, 186). In children, 8 of 945 compounds studied could differentiate asthmatics from controls with a sensitivity of 89% and a specificity of 95% (187). There has been considerable interest in sophisticated mass spectrometry techniques, which can be applied for example to skin secretions, in order to detect airway infection in CF (188). The true test of the utility of these techniques will be whether they can differentiate children with non-specific respiratory symptoms from true asthmatics, and predict steroid responsiveness in the asthmatics. Perhaps in the future we will have a pediatric "Breathalyzer" which will give a readout of the important biomarkers to tell us the diagnosis, what endotypes are at play, and how best to treat the child.

SUMMARY AND CONCLUSIONS

There is no doubt we have incredible opportunities within reach to transform the diagnosis and treatment of the asthmas. We have powerful tools and -omics technologies available to us, as well as pathway specific monoclonals. These need to be targeted rationally. We need to reflect that the specific designer molecules which are transforming CF (2–4) would have been discarded as ineffective if they had been applied indiscriminately to all CF patients, and not to gene class specific sub-endotypes. The CF community are progressing to *ex vivo* testing of novel compounds (189, 190) and we must do the same for the asthmas, to produce truly personalized airway medicine.

There are questions specifically pertaining to the asthmas that we need to address. We need to understand steroid resistant, particularly non-TH2 driven eosinophilia, and apparently non-inflammatory asthma pathways. We have argued elsewhere that children with refractory difficult asthma (for example, those persistently not taking basic medications) should not be denied biologicals to prevent them from dying (191); even in this group, identification of the endotype will be needed to ensure the right child gets the right biological. But we also need to appreciate the diversity of the asthmas—Type 2 inflammation, although obviously important, is only one part of the picture, and we need to better are specific appreciate the whole.

But finally we must appreciate that the more sophisticated and expensive approaches to monitoring and treatment are available, the more clinical skills become relevant (192). We will need better get the basics right, rather than immediately deploy the latest gene probe test and expensive therapeutic molecule. At bottom, most pediatric asthma is a simple disease to diagnose and treat if basic measurements are made and the child is given low dose therapy appropriately and regularly. We should never lose sight of this reality, and never stop using our clinical skills, and honing those skills, to get the basics right, working in a multidisciplinary team alongside the child and family.

AUTHOR CONTRIBUTIONS

The author confirms being the sole contributor of this work and has approved it for publication.

REFERENCES

1. Pavord ID, Beasley R, Agusti A, Anderson GP, Bel E, Brusselle G, et al. After asthma - redefining airways diseases. A *Lancet* commission. *Lancet*. (2018) 391:350–400. doi: 10.1016/S0140-6736(17)30879-6
2. Ramsey BW, Davies J, McElvaney NG, Tullis E, Bell SC, Drevínek P, et al. A CFTR potentiator in patients with cystic fibrosis and the G551D mutation. *N Engl J Med*. (2011) 365:1663–72. doi: 10.1056/NEJMoa1105185
3. Wainwright CE, Elborn JS, Ramsey BW, Marigowda G, Huang X, Cipolli M, et al. Lumacaftor-Ivacaftor in Patients with Cystic Fibrosis Homozygous for Phe508del CFTR. *N Engl J Med*. (2015) 373:220–31. doi: 10.1056/NEJMoa1409547
4. Davies JC, Moskowitz SM, Brown C, Horsley A, Mall MA, McKone EF, et al. VX-659-tezacaftor-ivacaftor in patients with cystic fibrosis and one or two Phe508del alleles. *N Engl J Med*. (2018)379:1599–611. doi: 10.1056/NEJMoa1807119
5. Agusti A, Bel E, Thomas M, Vogelmeier C, Brusselle G, Holgate S, et al. Treatable traits: toward precision medicine of chronic airway diseases. *Eur Respir J*. (2016) 47:410–9. doi: 10.1183/13993003.01359-2015
6. Crimi E, Spanevello A, Neri M, Ind PW, Rossi GA, Brusasco V. Dissociation between airway inflammation and airway hyperresponsiveness in allergic asthma. *Am J Respir Crit Care Med*. (1998) 157:4–9. doi: 10.1164/ajrccm.157.1.9703002
7. Wilson NM, James A, Uasuf C, Payne DN, Hablas H, Agrofioti C, et al. Asthma severity and inflammation markers in children. *Pediatr Allergy Immunol*. (2001) 12:125–32. doi: 10.1034/j.1399-3038.2001.012003125.x
8. Djukanović R, Wilson SJ, Kraft M, Jarjour NN, Steel M, Chung KF, et al. Effects of treatment with anti-immunoglobulin E antibody omalizumab on airway inflammation in allergic asthma. *Am J Respir Crit Care Med*. (2004) 170:583–93. doi: 10.1164/rccm.200312-1651OC
9. Berry MA, Hargadon B, Shelley M, Parker D, Shaw DE, Green RH, et al. Evidence of a role of tumor necrosis factor alpha in refractory asthma. *N Engl J Med*. (2006) 354:697–708. doi: 10.1056/NEJMoa050580
10. Payne DN, Rogers AV, Adelroth E, Bandi V, Guntupalli KK, Bush A, et al. Early thickening of the reticular basement membrane in children with difficult asthma. *Am J Respir Crit Care Med*. (2003) 167:78–82. doi: 10.1164/rccm.200205-414OC
11. Matsui H, Grubb BR, Tarran R, Randell SH, Gatzy JT, Davis CW, et al. Evidence for periciliary liquid layer depletion, not abnormal ion composition, in the pathogenesis of cystic fibrosis airways disease. *Cell*. (1998) 95:1005–15. doi: 10.1016/S0092-8674(00)81724-9
12. Johansson H, Norlander K, Berglund L, Janson C, Malinovschi A, Nordvall L, et al. Prevalence of exercise-induced bronchoconstriction and exercise-induced laryngeal obstruction in a general adolescent population. *Thorax*. (2015) 70:57–63. doi: 10.1136/thoraxjnl-2014-205738
13. Lemanske RF Jr, Mauger DT, Sorkness CA, Jackson DJ, Boehmer SJ, Martinez FD, et al. Step-up therapy for children with uncontrolled asthma receiving inhaled corticosteroids. *N Engl J Med*. (2010) 362:975–85. doi: 10.1056/NEJMoa1001278
14. Zar HJ, Hanslo D, Apolles P, Swingler G, Hussey G. Induced sputum versus gastric lavage for microbiological confirmation of pulmonary tuberculosis in infants and young children: a prospective study. *Lancet*. (2005) 365:130–4. doi: 10.1016/S0140-6736(05)17702-2
15. Lex C, Ferreira F, Zacharasiewicz A, Nicholson AG, Haslam PL, Wilson NM, et al. Airway eosinophilia in children with severe asthma: predictive values of non-invasive tests. *Am J Respir Crit Care Med*. (2006) 174:1286–91. doi: 10.1164/rccm.200603-352OC
16. Jochmann A, Artusio L, Robson K, Nagakumar P, Collins N, Fleming L, et al. Infection and inflammation in induced sputum from preschool children with chronic airways diseases. *Pediatr Pulmonol*. (2016) 51:778–86. doi: 10.1002/ppul.23366
17. Lex C, Payne DN, Zacharasiewicz A, Li A, Wilson NM, Hansel TT, et al. Sputum induction in children with difficult asthma: safety, feasibility, and inflammatory cell profiles. *Pediatr Pulmonol*. (2005) 39:318–24. doi: 10.1002/ppul.20159
18. Grootendorst DC, Sont JK, Willems LN, Kluin-Nelemans JC, Van Krieken JH, Veselic-Charvat M, et al. Comparison of inflammatory cell counts in asthma: induced sputum vs bronchoalveolar lavage and bronchial biopsies. *Clin Exp Allergy*. (1997) 27: 769–79. doi: 10.1046/j.1365-2222.1997.890900.x
19. Pavord ID, Chanez P, Criner GJ, Kerstjens HAM, Korn S, Lugogo N, et al. Mepolizumab for eosinophilic chronic obstructive pulmonary disease. *N Engl J Med*. (2017) 377:1613–29. doi: 10.1056/NEJMoa1708208
20. Busse W, Chupp G, Nagase H, Albers FC, Doyle S, Shen Q, et al. Anti-IL-5 treatments in patients with severe asthma by blood eosinophil thresholds: indirect treatment comparison. *J Allergy Clin Immunol*. (2018) 143:190–200.e20. doi: 10.1016/j.jaci.2018.08.031
21. Castro M, Corren J, Pavord ID, Maspero J, Wenzel S, Rabe KF, et al. Dupilumab efficacy and safety in moderate-to-severe uncontrolled asthma. *N Engl J Med*. (2018) 378:2486–96. doi: 10.1056/NEJMoa1804092

22. Heffler E, Terranova G, Chessari C, Frazzetto V, Crimi C, Fichera S, et al. Point-of-care blood eosinophil count in a severe asthma clinic setting. *Ann Allergy Asthma Immunol.* (2017) 119:16–20. doi: 10.1016/j.anai.2017.05.016
23. Fitzpatrick AM, Jackson DJ, Mauger DT, Boehmer SJ, Phipatanakul W, Sheehan WJ, et al. Individualized therapy for persistent asthma in young children. *J Allergy Clin Immunol.* (2016) 138:1608–18. doi: 10.1016/j.jaci.2016.09.028
24. Petsky HL, Cates CJ, Kew KM, Chang AB. Tailoring asthma treatment on eosinophilic markers (exhaled nitric oxide or sputum eosinophils): a systematic review and meta-analysis. *Thorax.* (2018) 73:1110–19. doi: 10.1136/thoraxjnl-2018-211540
25. Fleming L, Tsartsali L, Wilson N, Regamey N, Bush A. Longitudinal relationship between sputum eosinophils and exhaled nitric oxide in children with asthma. *Am J Respir Crit Care Med.* (2013) 188:400–2. doi: 10.1164/rccm.201212-2156LE
26. Bossley C, Fleming L, Gupta A, Regamey N, Frith J, Oates T, et al. Pediatric severe asthma is characterized by eosinophilia and remodeling without TH2 cytokines. *J Allergy Clin Immunol.* (2012) 129:974–82. doi: 10.1016/j.jaci.2012.01.059
27. Brightling CE. Chronic cough due to nonasthmatic eosinophilic bronchitis: ACCP evidence-based clinical practice guidelines. *Chest.* (2006) 129(Suppl. 1):116S–121S. doi: 10.1378/chest.129.1_suppl.116S
28. van den Toorn LM, Overbeek SE, de Jongste JC, Leman K, Hoogsteden HC, Prins JB. Airway inflammation is present during clinical remission of atopic asthma. *Am J Respir Crit Care Med.* (2001) 164:2107–13. doi: 10.1164/ajrccm.164.11.2006165
29. de Benedictis FM, Bush A. Corticosteroids in respiratory diseases in children. *Am. J. Respir. Crit. Care Med.* (2012) 185:12–23. doi: 10.1164/rccm.201107-1174CI
30. Meagher LC, Cousin JM, Seckl JR, Haslett C. Opposing effects of glucocorticoids on the rate of apoptosis in neutrophilic and eosinophilic granulocytes. *J Immunol.* (1996) 156:4422–8.
31. Wenzel SE, Schwartz LB, Langmack EL, Halliday JL, Trudeau JB, Gibbs RL, et al. Evidence that severe asthma can be divided pathologically into two inflammatory subtypes with distinct physiologic and clinical characteristics. *Am J Respir Crit Care Med·* (1999) 160:1001–8. doi: 10.1164/ajrccm.160.3.9812110
32. Andersson CK, Adams A, Nagakumar P, Bossley C, Gupta A, De Vries D, et al. Intra-epithelial neutrophils in paediatric severe asthma are associated with better lung function. *J Allergy Clin Immunol.* (2017) 139:1819–29. doi: 10.1016/j.jaci.2016.09.022
33. Sabroe I, Postma D, Heijink I, Dockrell DH. The yin and the yang of immunosuppression with inhaled corticosteroids. *Thorax.* (2013) 68:1085–7. doi: 10.1136/thoraxjnl-2013-203773
34. Aurora P, Stocks J, Oliver C, Saunders C, Castle R, Chaziparasidis G, et al. on behalf of LCCF. Quality control for spirometry in preschool children with and without lung disease. *Am J Respir Crit Care Med.* (2004) 169:1152–9. doi: 10.1164/rccm.200310-1453OC
35. Busi LE, Restuccia S, Tourres R, Sly PD. Assessing bronchodilator response in preschool children using spirometry. *Thorax.* (2017) 72:367–72. doi: 10.1136/thoraxjnl-2015-207961
36. Siersted HC, Mostgaard G, Hyldebrandt N, Hansen HS, Boldsen J, Oxhøj H. Interrelationships between diagnosed asthma, asthma-like symptoms, and abnormal airway behaviour in adolescence: the Odense Schoolchild Study. *Thorax.* (1996) 51:503–9. doi: 10.1136/thx.51.5.503
37. Young S, Le Souëf PN, Geelhoed GC, Stick SM, Turner KJ, Landau LI. The influence of a family history of asthma and parental smoking on airway responsiveness in early infancy. *N Engl J Med.* (1991) 324:1168–73. doi: 10.1056/NEJM199104253241704
38. Clarke JR, Salmon B, Silverman M. Bronchial responsiveness in the neonatal period as a risk factor for wheezing in infancy. *Am J Respir Crit Care Med.* (1995) 151:1434–40. doi: 10.1164/ajrccm.151.5.7735597
39. Bisgaard H, Jensen SM, Bønnelykke K. Interaction between asthma and lung function growth in early life. *Am J Respir Crit Care Med.* (2012) 185:1183–9. doi: 10.1164/rccm.201110-1922OC
40. Saglani S, Malmstrom K, Pelkonen AS, Malmberg LP, Lindahl H, Kajosaari M, et al. Airway remodeling and inflammation in symptomatic infants with reversible airflow obstruction. *Am J Respir Crit Care Med.* (2005) 171:722–7. doi: 10.1164/rccm.200410-1404OC
41. Wongtrakool C, Wang N, Hyde DM, Roman J, Spindel ER. Prenatal nicotine exposure alters lung function and airway geometry through α7 nicotinic receptors. *Am J Respir Cell Mol Biol.* (2012) 46:695–72. doi: 10.1165/rcmb.2011-0028OC
42. Deykin A, Wechsler ME, Boushey HA, Chinchilli VM, Kunselman SJ, Craig TJ, et al. Combination therapy with a long-acting beta-agonist and a leukotriene antagonist in moderate asthma. *Am J Respir Crit Care Med.* (2007) 175:228–34. doi: 10.1164/rccm.200601-112OC
43. Godfrey S. Bronchial hyper-responsiveness in children. *Paediatr Respir Rev.* (2000) 1:148–55. doi: 10.1053/prrv.2000.0042
44. Bush A, Saglani S. Management of severe asthma in children. *Lancet.* (2010) 376:814–25. doi: 10.1016/S0140-6736(10)61054-9
45. Cartledge N, Brown S, Bossley C, Gupta A, Fleming L, Saglani S, et al. Is a single intramuscular dose of triamcinolone and acute bronchodilator sufficient to determine optimal lung function in children with severe, therapy resistant asthma? *Thorax.* (2011) 66(Suppl. 4):A101–2. doi: 10.1136/thoraxjnl-2011-201054c.83
46. Bossley CJ, Fleming L, Ullmann N, Gupta A, Adams A, Nagakumar P, et al. Assessment of corticosteroid response in paediatric severe asthma using a multi-domain approach. *J Allergy Clin Immunol.* (2016) 137:624–6. doi: 10.1016/j.jaci.2015.12.1347
47. Fleming L, Koo M, Bossley CJ, Nagakumar P, Bush A, Saglani S. The utility of a multidomain assessment of steroid response for predicting clinical response to omalizumab. *J Allergy Clin Immunol.* (2016) 138:292–4. doi: 10.1016/j.jaci.2015.12.1317
48. Sekhon HS, Keller JA, Proskocil BJ, Martin EL, Spindel ER. Maternal nicotine exposure upregulates collagen gene expression in fetal monkey lung. Association with alpha7 nicotinic acetylcholine receptors. *Am J Respir Cell Mol Biol.* (2002) 26:31–4. doi: 10.1165/ajrcmb.26.1.4170
49. Fu XW, Wood K, Spindel ER. Prenatal nicotine exposure increases GABA signaling and mucin expression in airway epithelium. *Am J Respir Cell Mol Biol.* (2011) 44:222–9. doi: 10.1165/rcmb.2010-0109OC
50. Wongtrakool C, Roser-Page S, Rivera HN, Roman J. Nicotine alters lung branching morphogenesis through the alpha7 nicotinic acetylcholine receptor. *Am J Physiol Lung Cell Mol Physiol.* (2007) 293:L611–8. doi: 10.1152/ajplung.00038.2007
51. Sekhon HS, Jia Y, Raab R, Kuryatov A, Pankow JF, Whitsett JA, et al. Prenatal nicotine increases pulmonary alpha7 nicotinic receptor expression and alters fetal lung development in monkeys. *J Clin Invest.* (1999) 103:637–47. doi: 10.1172/JCI5232
52. Elliot J, Carroll N, Bosco M, McCrohan M, Robinson P. Increased airway responsiveness and decreased alveolar attachment points following in utero smoke exposure in the guinea pig. *Am J Respir Crit Care Med.* (2001) 163:140–4. doi: 10.1164/ajrccm.163.1.9805099
53. Morales E, Garcia-Esteban R, de la Cruz OA, Basterrechea M, Lertxundi A, de Dicastillo MD, et al. Intrauterine and early postnatal exposure to outdoor air pollution and lung function at preschool age. *Thorax.* (2015) 70:64–73. doi: 10.1136/thoraxjnl-2014-205413
54. Mirzakhani H, Carey VJ, McElrath TF, Qiu W, Hollis BW, O'Connor GT, et al. Impact of preeclampsia on the relationship between maternal asthma and offspring asthma. An observation from the VDAART clinical trial. *Am J Respir Crit Care Med.* (2019) 199:32–42. doi: 10.1164/rccm.201804-0770OC
55. Sonnenschein-van der Voort AM, Arends LR, de Jongste JC, Annesi-Maesano I, Arshad SH, Barros H, et al. Preterm birth, infant weight gain, and childhood asthma risk: a meta-analysis of 147,000 European children. *J Allergy Clin Immunol.* (2014) 133:1317–29. doi: 10.1016/j.jaci.2013.12.1082
56. Mu M, Ye S, Bai MJ, Liu GL, Tong Y, Wang SF, et al. Birth weight and subsequent risk of asthma: a systematic review and meta-analysis. *Heart Lung Circ.* (2014) 23:511–9. doi: 10.1016/j.hlc.2013.11.018
57. Castro-Rodriguez JA, Saglani S, Rodriguez-Martinez CE, Oyarzun MA, Fleming L, Bush A. The relationship between inflammation and remodeling in childhood asthma: a systematic review. *Pediatr Pulmonol.* (2018) 53:824–35. doi: 10.1002/ppul.23968
58. Sont JK, Willems LN, Bel EH, van Krieken JH, Vandenbroucke JP, Sterk PJ. Clinical control and histopathologic outcome of asthma when using airway hyperresponsiveness as an additional guide to long-term treatment.

The AMPUL study group. *Am J Respir Crit Care Med.* (1999) 159:1043–51. doi: 10.1164/ajrccm.159.4.9806052

59. Ward C, Walters H. Airway wall remodelling: the influence of corticosteroids. *Curr Opin Allergy Clin Immunol.* (2005) 5:43–8. doi: 10.1097/00130832-200502000-00009
60. Milanese M, Crimi E, Scordamaglia A, Riccio A, Pellegrino R, Canonica GW, et al. On the functional consequences of bronchial basement membrane thickening. *J Appl Physiol.* (2001) 91:1035–40. doi: 10.1152/jappl.2001.91.3.1035
61. Regamey N, Jeffery PK, Alton EW, Bush A, Davies JC. Airway remodelling and its relationship to inflammation in cystic fibrosis. *Thorax.* (2011) 66:624–9. doi: 10.1136/thx.2009.134106
62. Regamey N, Ochs M, Hilliard TN, Muhlfeld C, Cornish N, Fleming L, et al. Increased airway smooth muscle mass in children with asthma, cystic fibrosis and bronchiectasis. *Am J Respir Crit Care Med.* (2008) 177:837–43. doi: 10.1164/rccm.200707-977OC
63. Castro M, Rubin AS, Laviolette M, Fiterman J, De Andrade Lima M, Shah PL, et al. Effectiveness and safety of bronchial thermoplasty in the treatment of severe asthma: a multicenter, randomized, double-blind, sham-controlled clinical trial. *Am J Respir Crit Care Med.* (2010) 181:116–24. doi: 10.1164/rccm.200903-0354OC
64. Wechsler ME, Laviolette M, Rubin AS, Fiterman J, Lapa e Silva JR, Shah PL,et al. Bronchial thermoplasty: Long-term safety and effectiveness in patients with severe persistent asthma. *J Allergy Clin Immunol.* (2013) 132:1295–302. doi: 10.1016/j.jaci.2013.08.009
65. Johnston SL, Pattemore PK, Sanderson G, Smith S, Lampe F, Josephs L, et al. Community study of role of viral infections in exacerbations of asthma in 9-11 year old children. *BMJ.* (1995) 310:1225–9. doi: 10.1136/bmj.310.6989.1225
66. Bisgaard H, Hermansen MN, Bønnelykke K, Stokholm J, Baty F, Skytt NL, et al. Association of bacteria and viruses with wheezy episodes in young children: prospective birth cohort study. *BMJ.* (2010) 341: c4978. doi: 10.1136/bmj.c4978
67. Hilty M, Burke C, Pedro H, Cardenas P, Bush A, Bossley C, et al. Disordered microbial communities in asthmatic airways. *PLoS ONE.* (2010) 5: e857. doi: 10.1371/journal.pone.0008578
68. Bisgaard H, Hermansen MN, Buchvald F, Loland L, Halkjaer LB, Bønnelykke K, et al. Childhood asthma after bacterial colonization of the airway in neonates. *N Engl J Med.* (2007) 357:1487–95. doi: 10.1056/NEJMoa052632
69. Følsgaard NV, Schjørring S, Chawes BL, Rasmussen MA, Krogfelt KA, Brix S, Bisgaard H. Pathogenic bacteria colonizing the airways in asymptomatic neonates stimulates topical inflammatory mediator release. *Am J Respir Crit Care Med.* (2013) 187:589–95. doi: 10.1164/rccm.201207-1297OC
70. Larsen JM, Brix S, Thysen AH, Birch S, Rasmussen MA, Bisgaard H. Children with asthma by school age display aberrant immune responses to pathogenic airway bacteria as infants. *J Allergy Clin Immunol.* (2014) 133:1008–13. doi: 10.1016/j.jaci.2014.01.010
71. Vissing NH, Chawes BL, Bisgaard H. Increased risk of pneumonia and bronchiolitis after bacterial colonization of the airways as neonates. *Am J Respir Crit Care Med.* (2013) 188:1246–52. doi: 10.1164/rccm.201302-0215OC
72. Linstow ML, Schønning K, Hoegh AM, Sevelsted A, Vissing NH, Bisgaard H. Neonatal airway colonization is associated with troublesome lung symptoms in infants. *Am J Respir Crit Care Med.* (2013) 188:1041–2. doi: 10.1164/rccm.201302-0395LE
73. Robinson PFM, Pattaroni C, Cook J, Gregory L, Alonso AM, Fleming LJ, et al. Lower airway microbiota associates with inflammatory phenotype in severe preschool wheeze. *mJ Allergy Clin Immunol.* (2018). doi: 10.1016/j.jaci.2018.12.985
74. Lan F, Zhang N, Holtappels G, De Ruyck N, Krysko O, Van Crombruggen K, et al. Staphylococcus aureus induces a mucosal type 2 immune response via epithelial cell-derived cytokines. *Am J Respir Crit Care Med.* (2018) 198:452–63. doi: 10.1164/rccm.201710-2112OC
75. Chang AB, Upham JW, Masters IB, Redding GR, Gibson PG, Marchant JM, et al. Protracted bacterial bronchitis: the last decade and the road ahead. *Pediatr Pulmonol.* (2016) 51:225–42. doi: 10.1002/ppul.23351
76. Bush A. Persistent bacterial bronchitis: time to venture beyond the umbrella. *Front. Pediatr.* (2017) 5:264. doi: 10.3389/fped.2017.00264
77. Chang AB, Bush A, Grimwood K. Bronchiectasis in children: diagnosis and treatment. *Lancet.* (2018) 392:866–79. doi: 10.1016/S0140-6736(18)31554-X
78. Green RH, Brightling CE, McKenna S, Hargadon B, Parker D, Bradding P, et al. Asthma exacerbations and sputum eosinophil counts: a randomised controlled trial. *Lancet.* (2002) 360:1715–21. doi: 10.1016/S0140-6736(02)11679-5
79. Fleming L, Wilson N, Regamey N, Bush A. Use of sputum eosinophil counts to guide management in children with severe asthma. *Thorax.* (2012) 67:193–8. doi: 10.1136/thx.2010.156836
80. Fleming L, Tsartsali L, Wilson N, Regamey N, Bush A. Sputum inflammatory phenotypes are not stable in children with asthma.*Thorax.* (2012) 67:675–81. doi: 10.1136/thoraxjnl-2011-201064
81. Brinkman P, Wagener AH, Hekking PP, Bansal AT, Maitland-van der Zee AH, Wang Y, et al. U-BIOPRED Study Group. Identification and prospective stability of eNose derived inflammatory phenotypes in severe asthma. *J Allergy Clin Immunol.* (2018). doi: 10.1016/j.jaci.2018.10.058. [Epub ahead of print].
82. Frey U, Brodbeck T, Majumdar A, Taylor DR, Town GI, Silverman M, et al. Risk of severe asthma episodes predicted from fluctuation analysis of airway function. *Nature.* (2005) 438:667–70. doi: 10.1038/nature04176
83. Thamrin C, Stern G, Strippoli MP, Kuehni CE, Suki B, Taylor DR, et al. Fluctuation analysis of lung function as a predictor of long-term response to beta2-agonists. *Eur Respir J.* (2009) 33:486–93. doi: 10.1183/09031936.00106208
84. Thamrin C, Taylor DR, Jones SL, Suki B, Frey U. Variability of lung function predicts loss of asthma control following withdrawal of inhaled corticosteroid treatment. *Thorax.* (2010) 65:403–8. doi: 10.1136/thx.2009.129668
85. Delgado-Eckert E, Fuchs O, Kumar N, Pekkanen J, Dalphin JC, Riedler J, et al. Functional phenotypes determined by fluctuation-based clustering of lung function measurements in healthy and asthmatic cohort participants. *Thorax.* (2018) 73:107–15. doi: 10.1136/thoraxjnl-2016-209919
86. Mallol J, García-Marcos L, Solé D, Brand P, EISL Study Group. International prevalence of recurrent wheezing during the first year of life: variability, treatment patterns and use of health resources. *Thorax.* (2010) 65:1004–9. doi: 10.1136/thx.2009.115188
87. Crim C, Calverley PMA, Anderson JA, Celli B, Ferguson GT, Jenkins C, et al. Pneumonia risk in COPD patients receiving inhaled corticosteroids alone or in combination: TORCH study results. *Eur Respir J.* (2009) 34: 641–7. doi: 10.1183/09031936.00193908
88. Brassard P, Suissa S, Kezouh A, Ernst P. Inhaled corticosteroids and risk of tuberculosis in patients with respiratory diseases. *Am J Respir Crit Care Med.* (2011) 183: 675–8. doi: 10.1164/rccm.201007-1099OC
89. Andréjak C, Nielsen R, Thomsen VØ, Duhaut P, Sørensen HT, Thomsen RW. Chronic respiratory disease, inhaled corticosteroids and risk of non tuberculous mycobacteriosis. *Thorax.* (2013) 68: 256–62. doi: 10.1136/thoraxjnl-2012-201772
90. Bush A, Bolton C. Longer term sequelae of prematurity: the adolescent and young adult. In: Hibbs AM, Muhlebach MS, editors. *Respiratory Outcomes in Preterm Infants From Infancy to Childhood.* New York, NY: Publ Humana Press (2017). p. 99–118. doi: 10.1007/978-3-319-48835-6_7
91. Vollsaeter M, Roksund OD, Eide GE, Markestad T, Halvorsen T. Lung function after preterm birth: development from mid-childhood to adulthood. *Thorax.* (2013) 68:767–76. doi: 10.1136/thoraxjnl-2012-202980
92. Fawke J, Lum S, Kirkby J, Hennessy E, Marlow N, Rowell V, et al. Lung function and respiratory symptoms at 11 years in children born extremely preterm: the EPICure study. *Am J Respir Crit Care Med.* (2010) 182:237–45. doi: 10.1164/rccm.200912-1806OC
93. E, Bonetto G, Zachello F, Filippone M. Low exhaled nitric oxide in school-age children with bronchopulmonary dysplasia and airflow limitation. *Am J Respir Crit Care Med.* (2005) 171:68–72. doi: 10.1164/rccm.200403-298OC
94. Carraro S, Piacentini G, Lusiani M, Uyan ZS, Filippone M, Schiavon M, et al. Exhaled air temperature in bronchopulmonary dysplasia. *Pediatr Pulmonol.* (2010) 45:1240–5. doi: 10.1002/ppul.21317
95. Bush A, Nagakumar P. Preschool wheezing phenotypes. *Eur Med J.* (2016) 1:93–101. Available online at: https://www.emjreviews.com/respiratory/article/preschool-wheezing-phenotypes/

96. Dehlink E, Richardson C, Marsh G, Lee K, Jamalzadeh A, Bush A, et al. Are inhaled corticosteroids prescribed rationally in primary ciliary dyskinesia? *Eur Respir J.* (2018) 51:1702221. doi: 10.1183/13993003.02221-2017
97. Chaudry R, Rosenthal R, Bush A, Crowley S. Reduced forced expiratory flow but not increased exhaled nitric oxide or airway responsiveness to methacholine characterises paediatric sickle cell airway disease. *Thorax.* (2014) 69:580–5. doi: 10.1136/thoraxjnl-2013-204464
98. Schulze-Neick I, Ho Y, Bush A, Rosenthal M, Franklin RC, Redington A, et al. Severe airflow limitation after the unifocalization procedure: clinical and morphological correlates. *Circulation.* (2000) 102 (Suppl. 111):111–142–111–147.
99. Lang JE. Obesity and childhood asthma. *Curr Opin Pulm Med.* (2019) 25:34–43. doi: 10.1097/MCP.0000000000000537
100. Forno E, Weiner DJ, Mullen J, Sawicki G, Kurland G, Han YY, et al. Obesity and airway dysanapsis in children with and without asthma. *Am J Respir Crit Care Med.* (2017) 195:314–23. doi: 10.1164/rccm.201605-1039OC
101. van Huisstede A, Rudolphus A, van Schadewijk A, Cabezas MC, Mannaerts GH, Taube C, et al. Bronchial and systemic inflammation in morbidly obese subjects with asthma: a biopsy study. *Am J Respir Crit Care Med.* (2014) 190:951–4. doi: 10.1164/rccm.201407-1225LE
102. Desai D, Newby C, Symon FA, Haldar P, Shah S, Gupta S, et al. Elevated sputum interleukin-5 and submucosal eosinophilia in obese individuals with severe asthma. *Am J Respir Crit Care Med.* (2013) 188:657–63. doi: 10.1164/rccm.201208-1470OC
103. Peters MC, McGrath KW, Hawkins GA Hastie AT, Levy BD, Israel E, et al. Plasma interleukin-6 concentrations, metabolic dysfunction, and asthma severity: a cross-sectional analysis of two cohorts. *Lancet Respir Med.* (2016) 4:574–84. doi: 10.1016/S2213-2600(16)30048-0
104. FitzGerald JM. Targeting lung attacks. *Thorax.* (2011) 66:365–66. doi: 10.1136/thx.2010.156760
105. Bush A, Pavord I. Following Nero: fiddle while Rome burns, or is there a better way? *Thorax.* (2011) 66:367. doi: 10.1136/thx.2011.160861
106. Buelo A, McLean S, Julious S, Flores-Kim J, Bush A, Henderson J, et al. At-risk children with asthma (ARC): a systematic review. *Thorax.* (2018) 73:813–24.
107. Brand PL, Baraldi E, Bisgaard H, Boner AL, Castro-Rodriguez JA, Custovic A, et al. Definition, assessment and treatment of wheezing disorders in preschool children: an evidence-based approach. *Eur Respir J.* (2008) 32:1096–110. doi: 10.1183/09031936.00002108
108. Antó JM, Sunyer J, Rodriguez-Roisin R, Suarez-Cervera M, Vazquez L. Community outbreaks of asthma associated with inhalation of soybean dust. Toxicoepidemiological Committee. *N Engl J Med.* (1989) 320:1097–102. doi: 10.1056/NEJM198904273201701
109. Celenza A, Fothergill J, Kupek E, Shaw RJ. Thunderstorm associated asthma: a detailed analysis of environmental factors. *BMJ.* (1996) 312:604–7. doi: 10.1136/bmj.312.7031.604
110. Murray CS, Poletti G, Kebadze T, Morris J, Woodcock A, Johnston SL, et al. Study of modifiable risk factors for asthma exacerbations: virus infection and allergen exposure increase the risk of asthma hospital admissions in children. *Thorax.* (2006) 61:376–82. doi: 10.1136/thx.2005.042523
111. Teach SJ, Gill MA, Sorkness CA, Togias A, Arbes SJ, Calatroni A, et al.Preseasonal treatment with either omalizumab or an inhaled corticosteroid boost to prevent fall asthma exacerbations. *J Allergy Clin Immunol.* (2015) 136:1476–85. doi: 10.1016/j.jaci.2015.09.008
112. Murray CS, Foden P, Sumner H, Shepley E, Custovic A, Simpson A. Preventing severe asthma exacerbations in children. a randomized trial of mite-impermeable bedcovers. *Am J Respir Crit Care Med.* (2017) 196:150–8. doi: 10.1164/rccm.201609-1966OC
113. Teach SJ, Gergen PJ, Szefler SJ, Mitchell HE, Calatroni A, Wildfire J, et al. Seasonal risk factors for asthma exacerbations among inner city children. *J Allergy Clin Immunol.* (2015) 135:1465–73. doi: 10.1016/j.jaci.2014.12.1942
114. Hoch HE, Calatroni A, West JB, Liu AH, Gergen PJ, Gruchalla RS, et al. Can we predict fall asthma exacerbations? Validation of the seasonal asthma exacerbation index. *J Allergy Clin Immunol.* (2017) 140:1130–7. doi: 10.1016/j.jaci.2017.01.026
115. Puranik S, Forno E, Bush A, Celedón JC. Predicting severe asthma exacerbations in children. *Am J Respir Crit Care Med.* (2017) 195:854–59. doi: 10.1164/rccm.201606-1213PP
116. Bochkov YA, Watters K, Ashraf S, Griggs TF, Devries MK, Jackson DJ, et al. Cadherin-related family member 3, a childhood asthma susceptibility gene product, mediates rhinovirus C binding and replication. *Proc Natl Acad Sci USA.* (2015) 112:5485–90. doi: 10.1073/pnas.1421178112
117. Bønnelykke K, Sleiman P, Nielsen K, Kreiner-Møller E, Mercader JM, Belgrave D, et al. A genome-wide association study identifies CDHR3 as a susceptibility locus for early childhood asthma with severe exacerbations. *Nat Genet.* (2014) 46:51–5. doi: 10.1038/ng.2830
118. Bønnelykke K, Coleman AT, Evans MD, Thorsen J, Waage J, Vissing NH, et al. Cadherin-related Family Member 3 Genetics and Rhinovirus C Respiratory Illnesses. *Am J Respir Crit Care Med.* (2018) 197:589–94. doi: 10.1164/rccm.201705-1021OC
119. Gupta A, Bush A, Hawrylowicz C, Saglani S. Vitamin d and asthma in children. *Paediatr Respir Rev.* (2012) 13:236–43. doi: 10.1016/j.prrv.2011.07.003
120. Denlinger LC, Phillips BR, Ramratnam S, Ross K, Bhakta NR, Cardet JC, et al. Inflammatory and comorbid features of patients with severe asthma and frequent exacerbations. *Am J Respir Crit Care Med.* (2017) 195:302–13. doi: 10.1164/rccm.201602-0419OC
121. Bush A. Lung development and aging. *Ann Am Thorac Soc.* (2016) 13(Suppl. 5): S438–46. doi: 10.1513/AnnalsATS.201602-112AW
122. Mahmoud O, Granell R, Tilling K, Minelli C, Garcia-Aymerich J, Holloway JW, et al. Association of height growth in puberty with lung function: a longitudinal study. *Am J Respir Crit Care Med.* (2018). doi: 10.1164/rccm.201802-0274OC. [Epub ahead of print].
123. Quanjer PH, Stanojevic S, Cole TJ, Baur X, Hall GL, Culver BH, et al. Multi-ethnic reference values for spirometry for the 3-95-yr age range: the global lung function 2012 equations. *Eur Respir J.* (2012) 40:1324–43. doi: 10.1183/09031936.00080312
124. Lange P, Celli B, Agustí A, Boje Jensen G, Divo M, Faner R, et al. Lung-function trajectories leading to chronic obstructive pulmonary disease. *N Engl J Med.* (2015) 373:111–22. doi: 10.1056/NEJMoa1411532
125. Berry CE, Billheimer D, Jenkins IC, Lu ZJ, Stern DA, Gerald LB, et al. A distinct low lung function trajectory from childhood to the fourth decade of life. *Am J Respir Crit Care Med.* (2016) 194:607–12. doi: 10.1164/rccm.201604-0753OC
126. Bui DS, Lodge CJ, Burgess JA, Lowe AJ, Perret J, Bui MQ, et al. Childhood predictors of lung function trajectories and future COPD risk: a prospective cohort study from the first to the sixth decade of life. *Lancet Respir Med.* (2018) 6:535–44. doi: 10.1016/S2213-2600(18)30100-0
127. Belgrave DCM, Granell R, Turner SW, Curtin JA, Buchan IE, Le Souëf PN, et al. Lung function trajectories from pre-school age to adulthood and their associations with early life factors: a retrospective analysis of three population-based birth cohort studies. *Lancet Respir Med.* (2018) 6:526–34. doi: 10.1016/S2213-2600(18)30099-7
128. Vasquez MM, Zhou M, Hu C, Martinez FD, Guerra S. Low lung function in young adult life is associated with early mortality. *Am J Respir Crit Care Med.* (2017) 195:1399–401. doi: 10.1164/rccm.201608-1561LE
129. Agustí A, Noell G, Brugada J, Faner R. Lung function in early adulthood and health in later life: a transgenerational cohort analysis. *Lancet Respir Med.* (2017) 5:935–45. doi: 10.1016/S2213-2600(17)30434-4
130. Bush A. Low lung function in young adult life is associated with early mortality. *Am J Respir Crit Care Med.* (2017) 197:538–9. doi: 10.1164/rccm.201707-1416LE
131. Saglani S, Payne DN, Zhu J, Wang Z, Nicholson AG, Bush A, et al. Early detection of airway wall remodelling and eosinophilic inflammation in preschool wheezers. *Am J Respir Crit Care Med.* (2007) 176:858–64. doi: 10.1164/rccm.200702-212OC
132. Brand PL, Caudri D, Eber E, Gaillard EA, Garcia-Marcos L, Hedlin G, et al. Classification and pharmacological treatment of preschool wheezing: changes since 2008. *Eur Respir J.* (2014) 43:1172–7. doi: 10.1183/09031936.00199913
133. Belgrave DC, Buchan I, Bishop C, Lowe L, Simpson A, Custovic A. Trajectories of lung function during childhood. *Am J Respir Crit Care Med.* (2014) 189:1101–9. doi: 10.1164/rccm.201309-1700OC
134. Castro-Rodríguez JA, Holberg CJ, Wright AL, Martinez FD. A clinical index to define risk of asthma in young children with recurrent wheezing. *Am J Respir Crit Care Med.* (2000) 162:1403–6. doi: 10.1164/ajrccm.162.4.9912111

135. Guilbert TW, Morgan WJ, Krawiec M, Lemanske RF Jr, Sorkness C, Szefler SJ, et al. The Prevention of Early Asthma in Kids study: design, rationale and methods for the Childhood Asthma research and education network. *Control Clin Trials*. (2004) 25:286–310. doi: 10.1016/j.cct.2004.03.002
136. Devulapalli CS, Carlsen KC, Håland G, Munthe-Kaas MC, Pettersen M, Mowinckel P, et al. Severity of obstructive airways disease by age 2 years predicts asthma at 10 years of age. *Thorax*. (2008) 63:8–13. doi: 10.1136/thx.2006.060616
137. Morgan WJ, Stern DA, Sherrill DL, Guerra S, Holberg CJ, Guilbert TW, et al. Outcome of asthma and wheezing in the first 6 years of life: follow-up through adolescence. *Am J Respir Crit Care Med*. (2005) 172:1253–8. doi: 10.1164/rccm.200504-525OC
138. Tai A, Tran H, Roberts M, Clarke N, Wilson J, Robertson CF. The association between childhood asthma and adult chronic obstructive pulmonary disease. *Thorax*. (2014) 69:805–10. doi: 10.1136/thoraxjnl-2013-204815
139. Turner S, Custovic A, Ghazal P, Grigg J, Gore M, Henderson J, et al. Pulmonary epithelial barrier and immunological functions at birth and in early life - key determinants of the development of asthma? A description of the protocol for the Breathing Together study. *Wellcome Open Res*. (2018) 3:60. doi: 10.12688/wellcomeopenres.14489.1
140. Guilbert TW, Morgan WJ, Zeiger RS, Mauger DT, Boehmer SJ, Szefler SJ, et al. Long-term inhaled corticosteroids in preschool children at high risk for asthma. *N Engl J Med*. (2006) 354:1985–97. doi: 10.1056/NEJMoa051378
141. Murray CS, Woodcock A, Langley SJ, Morris J, Custovic A, IFWIN study team. Secondary prevention of asthma by the use of Inhaled Fluticasone propionate in Wheezy INfants (IFWIN): double-blind, randomised, controlled study. *Lancet*. (2006) 368:754–62. doi: 10.1016/S0140-6736(06)69285-4
142. Bisgaard H, Hermansen MN, Loland L, Halkjaer LB, Buchvald F. Intermittent inhaled corticosteroids in infants with episodic wheezing. *N Engl J Med*. (2006) 354:1998–2005. doi: 10.1056/NEJMoa054692
143. Bisgaard H, Stokholm J, Chawes BL, Vissing NH, Bjarnadóttir E, Schoos AM, et al. Fish oil-derived fatty acids in pregnancy and wheeze and asthma in offspring. *N Engl J Med*. (2016) 375:2530–9. doi: 10.1056/NEJMoa1503734
144. Stein MM, Hrusch CL, Gozdz J, Igartua C, Pivniouk V, Murray SE, et al. Innate immunity and asthma risk in amish and hutterite farm children. *N Engl J Med*. (2016) 375:411–421. doi: 10.1056/NEJMoa1508749
145. Brutsche MH, Brutsche IC, Munawar M, Langley SJ, Masterson CM, Daley-Yates PT, et al. Comparison of pharmacokinetics and systemic effects of inhaled fluticasone propionate in patients with asthma and healthy volunteers: a randomised crossover study. *Lancet*. (2000) 356:556–61. doi: 10.1016/S0140-6736(00)02581-2
146. Shaw DE, Sousa AR, Fowler SJ, Fleming LJ, Roberts G, Corfield J, et al. U-BIOPRED Study Group. Clinical and inflammatory characteristics of the European U-BIOPRED adult severe asthma cohort. *Eur Respir J*. (2015) 46:1308–21. doi: 10.1183/13993003.00779-2015
147. Fleming L, Murray C, Bansal AT, Hashimoto S, Bisgaard H, Bush A, et al. The burden of severe asthma in childhood and adolescence: results from the paediatric U-BIOPRED cohorts. *Eur Respir J*. (2015) 46:1322–33. doi: 10.1183/13993003.00780-2015
148. Jarjour NN, Erzurum SC, Bleecker ER, Calhoun WJ, Castro M, Comhair SA, et al. Severe asthme. lessons learned from the national heart, lung, and blood institute severe asthma research program. *Am J Respir Crit Care Med*. (2012) 185:356–62. doi: 10.1164/rccm.201107-1317PP
149. Wark PA, Simpson J, Hensley MJ, Gibson PG. Airway inflammation in thunderstorm asthma. *Clin Exp Allergy*. (2002) 32:1750–6. doi: 10.1046/j.1365-2222.2002.01556.x
150. Almqvist C, Wickman M, Perfetti L, Berglind N, Renström A, Hedrén M et al. Worsening of asthma in children allergic to cats, after indirect exposure to cat at school. *Am J Respir Crit Care Med*. (2001) 163:694–8. doi: 10.1164/ajrccm.163.3.2006114
151. Yan X, Liu Q, Gomez JV, Holm C, Cohn L, Chupp G, et al. Longitudinal RNA sequencing data of induced sputum in asthma patients reveals stable transcriptional endotypes of asthma associated with asthma severity (abstract). *Am J Respir Crit Care Med*. (2017) 195(Suppl.):A4908.
152. Bracken MB, Fleming L, Hall P, Van Stiphout N, Bossley CJ, Biggart E, et al. The importance of nurse led home visits in the assessment of children with problematic asthma. *Arch Dis Child*. (2009) 94:780–4. doi: 10.1136/adc.2008.152140
153. Cook J, Beresford F, Fainardi V, Hall P, Housley G, Jamalzadeh A, et al. Managing the paediatric patient with refractory asthma: a multidisciplinary approach. *J Asthma Allergy*. (2017) 10:123–30. doi: 10.2147/JAA.S129159
154. Bush A, Fleming L, Saglani S. Severe asthma in children. *Respirology*. (2017) 22:886–97. doi: 10.1111/resp.13085
155. Shrine N, Portelli MA, John C, Soler Artigas M, Bennett N, Hall R, Lewis J, et al. Moderate-to-severe asthma in individuals of European ancestry: a genome-wide association study. *Lancet Respir Med*. (2019) 7:20–34. doi: 10.1016/S2213-2600(18)30389-8
156. Auffray C, Adcock IM, Chung KF, Djukanovic R, Pison C, Sterk PJ. An integrative systems biology approach to understanding pulmonary diseases. *Chest*. (2010) 137:1410–6. doi: 10.1378/chest.09-1850
157. Bourdin A, Molinari N, Vachier I, Varrin M, Marin G, Gamez AS, et al. Prognostic value of cluster analysis of severe asthma phenotypes. *J Allergy Clin Immunol*. (2014) 1234:1043–50. doi: 10.1016/j.jaci.2014.04.038
158. Kuo C-HS, Pavlidis S, Loza M, Baribaud F, Rowe A, Pandis I, et al. T-helper cell type 2 (Th2) and non-Th2 molecular phenotypes of asthma using sputum transcriptomics in U-BIOPRED. *Eur Respir J*. (2017) 49:1602135. doi: 10.1183/13993003.02135-2016
159. Lefaudeux D, de Meulder B, Loza MJ, Peffer N, Rowe A, Baribaud F, et al. U-BIOPRED clinical asthma clusters linked to a subset of sputum omics. *J Allergy Clin Immunol*. (2016) 139:1797–807. doi: 10.1016/j.jaci.2016.08.048
160. Silkoff PE, Strambu I, Laviolette M, Singh D, FitzGerald JM, Lam S, et al. Asthma characteristics and biomarkers from the Airways Disease Endotyping for Personalized Therapeutics (ADEPT) longitudinal profiling study. *Respir Res*. (2017) 16:142. doi: 10.1186/s12931-015-0299-y
161. Loza MJ, Djukanovic R, Chung KF, Horowitz D, Ma K, et al. Validates and longitudinally stable asthma phenotypes based on cluster analysis of the ADEPT study. *Respir Res*. (2016) 17:165. doi: 10.1186/s12931-016-0482-9
162. Aaron SD, Vandemheen KL, FitzGerald JM, Ainslie M, Gupta S, Lemière C, et al. Reevaluation of diagnosis in adults with physician-diagnosed Asthma. *JAMA*. (2017) 317:269–79. doi: 10.1001/jama.2016.19627
163. Looijmans-van den Akker I, van Luijn K, Verheij T. Overdiagnosis of asthma in children in primary care: a retrospective analysis. *Br J Gen Pract*. (2016) 66:e152–7. doi: 10.3399/bjgp16X683965
164. Lenney, W, Bush A, Fitzgerald DA, Fletcher M, Ostrem A, Pedersen S, et al. Improving the global diagnosis and management of asthma in children. *Thorax*. (2018) 73:662–9. doi:10.1136/thoraxjnl-2018-211626
165. Xie YL, Chakravorty S, Armstrong DT, Hall SL, Via LE, Song T, et al. Evaluation of a rapid molecular drug-susceptibility test for tuberculosis. *N Engl J Med*. (2017) 377:1043–54. doi: 10.1056/NEJMoa1614915
166. Anderson ST, Kaforou M, Brent AJ, Wright VJ, Banwell CM, Chagaluka G, et al. Diagnosis of childhood tuberculosis and host RNA expression in Africa. *N Engl J Med*. (2014) 370:1712–23. doi: 10.1056/NEJMoa1303657
167. Yang CXY, Singht A, Kim YW, et al. Diagnosis of western red cedar asthma using a blood-based gene expression biomarker panel. *Am J Respir Crit Care Med*. (2017) 196:1615–17. doi: 10.1164/rccm.201608-1740LE.
168. Bigler J, Boedigheimer M, Schofield JPR, et al. A severe asthma disease signature from gene expression profiling of peripheral blood from UBIOPRED cohorts. *Am J Respir Crit Care Med*. (2017) 195:1311–20. doi: 10.1164/rccm.201604-0866OC
169. Altman MC, Busse WW. A deep dive into asthma transcriptomics. Lessons from U-BIOPRED. *Am J Respir Crit Care Med*. (2017) 195:1279–80. doi: 10.1164/rccm.201611-2387ED
170. Tsitsiou E, Williams AE, Moschos SA, Patel K, Rossios C, Jiang X, et al. Transcriptome analysis shows activation of circulating $CD8^{+}$ T-cells in patients with severe asthma. *J Allergy Clin Immunol*. (2012) 129:95–103. doi: 10.1016/j.jaci.2011.08.011
171. Heffler E, Allegra A, Pioggia G, Picardi G, Musolino C, Gangemi S, et al. MicroRnas profiling in asthma: potential biomarkers and therapeutic targets. *Am J Resp Cell Mol Biol*. (2017) 57:642–50. doi: 10.1165/rcmb.2016-0231TR.
172. Hastie AT, Steele C, Dunaway CW, Moore WC, Rector BM, Ampleford E, et al. Complex association patterns for inflammatory mediators in induced sputum from subjects with asthma. *Clin Exp Allergy*. (2018) 48:787–97. doi: 10.1111/cea.13129

173. Kuo C-HS, Pavlidis S, Loza M, Baribaud F, Rowe A, Pandis I, et al. A transcriptome-driven analysis of epithelial brushings and bronchial biopsies to define asthma phenotypes in U-BIOPRED. *Am J Respir Crit Care Med.* (2017) 195:444–55. doi: 10.1164/rccm.201512-2452OC
174. Pavlidis S, Takahashi K, Kwong FNK, Xie J, Hoda U, Sun K, et al. "T2-high" in severe asthma related to blood eosinophil, exhaled nitric oxide and serum periostin. *Eur Respir J.* (2018) 53:1800938. doi: 10.1183/13993003.00938-2018
175. Woodruff PG, Modrek B, Choy DF, , Jia G, Abbas AR, Ellwanger A, et al. T-helper type 2-driven inflammation defines major subphenotypes of asthma. *Am J Respir Crit Care Med.* (2009) 180:388–95. doi: 10.1164/rccm.200903-0392OC
176. Wilson SJ, Ward JA, Sousa AR, Corfield J, Bansal AT, De Meulder B, et al. Severe asthma exists despite suppressed tissue inflammation: findings of the U-BIOPRED study. *Eur Respir J.* (2016) 48:1307–19. doi: 10.1183/13993003.01129-2016
177. Jevnikar Z, Östling J, Ax E, Calvén J, Thörn K, Israelsson E, et al. Epithelial IL-6 trans-signaling defines a new asthma phenotype with increased airway inflammation. *J Allergy Clin Immunol.* (2018) 143:577–90. doi: 10.1016/j.jaci.2018.05.026
178. Rossios C, Pavlidis S, Hoda U, Kuo CH, Wiegman C, Russell K, et al. Sputum transcriptomics reveal upregulation of IL-1 receptor family members in patients with severe asthma. *J Allergy Clin Immunol.* (2017) 141:560–70. doi: 10.1016/j.jaci.2017.02.045
179. Modena BD, Tedrow JR, Milosevic J, Bleecker ER, Meyers DA, Wu W, et al. Gene expression in relation to exhaled nitric oxide identifies novel asthma phenotypes with unique biomolecular pathways. *Am J Respir Crit Care Med.* (2014) 190:1363–72. doi: 10.1164/rccm.201406-1099OC
180. Hekking PP, Loza MJ, Pavlidis S, De Meulder B, Lefaudeux D, Baribaud F, et al. Transcriptomic gene signatures associated with persistent airflow limitation in patients with severe asthma. *Eur Respir J.* (2017) 50:1602298. doi: 10.1183/13993003.02298-2016
181. Chupp GL, Lee CG, Jarjour N, Shim YM, Holm CT, He S, et al. A chitinase-like protein in the lung and circulation of patients with severe asthma. *N Engl J Med.* (2007) 357:2016–27. doi: 10.1056/NEJMoa073600
182. Gomez JL, Yan X, Holm CT, Grant N, Liu Q, Cohn L, et al; SARP Investigators. Characterisation of asthma subgroups associated with circulating YKL-40 levels. *Eur Respir J.* (2017) 50:1700800. doi: 10.1183/13993003.00800-2017
183. Kapitein B, Hoekstra MO, Nijhuis EHJ, Hijnen DJ, Arets HG, Kimpen JL, et al. Gene expression in CD4+ T-cells reflects heterogeneity in infant wheezing phenotypes. *Eur Respi J.* (2008) 32:1203–12. doi: 10.1183/09031936.00020108
184. Klassen EMM, van de Kant KDG, Jobsis Q, van Schayck OC, Smolinska A, Dallinga JW, et al. Exhaled biomarkers and gene expression at preschool age improve asthma predcition at 6 years of age. *Am J Respir Crit Care Med.* (2015) 191:201–7. doi: 10.1164/rccm.201408-1537OC
185. Ibrahim, Basanta M, Cadden P, Singh D, Douce D, Woodcock A, et al. Non-invasive phenotyping using exhaled volatile organic compounds in asthma. *Thorax.* (2011) 66:804–9. doi: 10.1136/thx.2010.156695
186. Fens N, Roldaan AC, van der Schee MP, Boksem RJ, Zwinderman AH, Bel EH, et al. External validation of exhaled breath profiling using an electronic nose in the discrimination of asthma with fixed airways obstruction and chronic obstructive pulmonary disease. *Clin Exp Allergy.* (2011) 41:1371–8. doi: 10.1111/j.1365-2222.2011.03800.x
187. Dallings JW, Robroeks CMHHT, van Berkel JJ, Moonen EJ, Godschalk RW, Jöbsis Q, et al. Volatile organic compounds in exhaled breath as a diagnostic tool for asthma in children. *Clin Exp Allergy.* (2009) 40:68–76. doi: 10.1111/j.1365-2222.2009.03343.x
188. Bardin EE, Cameron SJS, Perdones-Montero A, Hardiman K, Bolt F, Alton EWFW, et al. Metabolic phenotyping and strain characterisation of pseudomonas aeruginosa isolates from cystic fibrosis patients using rapid evaporative ionisation mass spectrometry. *Sci Rep.* (2018) 8:10952. doi: 10.1038/s41598-018-28665-7
189. Dekkers JF, Berkers G, Kruisselbrink E, Vonk A, de Jonge HR, Janssens HM, et al. Characterizing responses to CFTR-modulating drugs using rectal organoids derived from subjects with cystic fibrosis. *Sci Transl Med.* (2016) 8:344ra84. doi: 10.1126/scitranslmed.aad8278
190. Pranke I, Hatton A, Masson A, Flament T, Le Bourgeois M, Urbach V, et al. Might brushed nasal cells be a surrogate for CFTR modulator clinical response? *Am J Respir Crit Care Med.* (2019) 199:123–6. doi: 10.1164/rccm.201808-1436LE
191. Bush A, Saglani S, Fleming L. Severe asthma: looking beyond the amount of medication. *Lancet Respir Med.* (2017) 5:844–6. doi: 10.1016/S2213-2600(17)30379-X
192. Szefler SJ. Asthma across the lifespan: time for a paradigm shift. *J Allergy Clin Immunol.* (2018) 142:773–80. doi: 10.1016/j.jaci.2018.03.010

20

Astragalus Oral Solution Ameliorates Allergic Asthma in Children by Regulating Relative Contents of $CD4^{+}CD25^{high}CD127^{low}$ Treg Cells

Wei Wang*, Wei Jing and Qingbin Liu

Department of Pediatric, Affiliated Hospital of Changchun University of Chinese Medicine, Changchun, China

***Correspondence:**
Wei Wang
wangweicutcm@126.com

Objective: To explore the effects of *Astragalus* oral solution (AOS) on allergic asthma in children by investigating relative contents of $CD4^{+}CD25^{high}CD127^{low}$ Treg cells.

Methods: The contents of Astragaloside A in AOS were detected by using HPLC. Eighty children with allergic asthma were recruited from February 2016 to June 2017, and randomly assigned into the control group (received placebo, 0.1% quinine chloride in deionized water, daily) and the AOS group (received 10 mL AOS daily). After 6-month treatment, therapeutic results were compared between the two groups. Serum levels of IL-10 and TGF-beta, Th1 cytokines (IL-2 and IFN-γ), and Th2 cytokines (IL-4 and IL-6) were measured by using ELISA kits. Relative contents of $CD4^{+}CD25^{high}CD127^{low}$ Treg cells were determined by using flow cytometry.

Results: Astragaloside A was the main ingredient of AOS with 0.216 ± 0.027 mg/mL from six-batch samples. After 6-month therapy, the AOS group showed improved forced expiratory volume in 1 s (FEV1) and the Pediatric Asthma Quality of Life Questionnaire (PAQLQ) scores compared with the control group ($P < 0.05$). Serum level of IL-10 was higher and the levels of TGF-beta, Th1 cytokines (IL-2 and IFN-γ), and Th2 cytokines (IL-4 and IL-6) were lower in the AOS group than in the control group ($P < 0.05$). AOS treatment increased the percentage of gated $CD4^{+}$ T cells, $CD4^{+}CD25^{+}$ T cells, $CD4^{+}CD25^{high}$ Treg cells, $CD4^{+}CD25^{+}FoxP3^{+}$ Treg cells and $CD4^{+}CD25^{high}CD127^{low}$ Treg cells when compared with the control group ($P < 0.05$).

Conclusions: Astragaloside A was the main component of AOS, and AOS ameliorated allergic asthma in children by regulating relative contents of $CD4^{+}CD25^{high}CD127^{low}$ Treg cells.

Keywords: ***Astragalus*** **oral solution, Astragaloside A, allergic asthma, $CD4^{+}CD25^{high}CD127^{low}$ Treg cells, children**

BACKGROUND

Asthma is a common inflammatory disorder of the lungs and is often characterized by reversible airflow obstruction and bronchospasm. Allergic asthma is a main threat to public health as it perturbs children's respiratory system. More than 300 million people worldwide have allergic asthma (1, 2). According to the data from the World Health Organization (WHO), asthma affects most children, and the number is expected to increase to 400 million in 2025 (3). With the development of society and industrialization, the incidence and mortality of allergic asthma in children have been increasing. Approximately 30–90% of children with allergic asthma have allergic rhinitis (AR) (4). AR is one of the related factors in the pathogenesis of allergic asthma, which leads to a direct result of asthma onset (5). With their similarities in etiology, location, pathogenesis, and pathophysiology, both AR and allergy asthma should be treated together (6). Seasonal perennial allergens, such as grass, trees, pollen, house dust (HD), mold, and animal fur, can often cause allergic asthma in children (7, 8). In allergic patients, respiratory allergies often lead to systemic allergies. In nasal allergic inflammation, Th1, Th2, and Th17 cells migrate into the bone marrow, stimulating the production of inflammatory cells, mast cells, IL-5, IL-13, IL-17, IL-22, and IL-33 (9). Inflammatory cells and cytokines enter the nasal mucosa and lungs, triggering respiratory airway inflammation and causing allergic symptoms (10). At the same time, they can also increase the expression of adhesion molecules in the nasal and bronchial mucosa, thereby aggravating respiratory allergies (11).

Studies have shown that eosinophils and mast cells play important roles in the pathogenesis of allergic asthma (12). Th2-like cytokines are mainly secreted by T cells and regulate asthma airway inflammation. T cells and interleukins have been found to play an important role in the progression of allergic asthma (13).

The regulatory T cell (Treg) is a subpopulation of T cells that regulate the immune system, maintain tolerance to self-antigens, and prevent autoimmune disorders. An earlier report found decreased Treg cells in patients with asthma, and there was a significant correlation between change in airway Tregs cells and asthma. Improving Treg cells may be a novel strategy in the prevention of asthma and other allergic disorders (14). $CD4^{+}CD25^{+}$ Treg cells are a unique population of Treg cells that can independently modulate adaptive and innate autoimmune responses (15). Foxp3 is a cell marker of $CD4^{+}CD25^{+}$ Treg cells and is closely related to the differentiation and function of regulatory Treg cells (16, 17), which can regulate the immune responses. In the pathogenesis of asthma, Treg cells secrete a variety of cytokines that can suppress the proliferation of T cells and the synthesis of IgE through the transmission of inflammatory cells, such as IL-10 and TGF-β. In different stages of allergic asthma, the analysis of the effects of cytokines and chemokines becomes very important for asthma prevention and treatment.

Astragalus, a large genus of herbs, belongs to the legume family Fabaceae and has potent immune boosting and health-promoting properties (18, 19). *Astragalus membranaceus* (AM) has been widely used for thousands of years in China to treat asthma. Animal model tests showed that the extracts of AM can increase the levels of $CD4^{+}$ $CD25^{high}$ Treg cells and Foxp3 mRNA expression in an asthmatic animal model (20). *Astragalus* was further found to prevent the recurrence of asthma by modulating Th1/Th2 cytokines in asthmatic children (21). *Astragalus* oral solution (AOS) is made by the Affiliated Nanjing Hospital of Nanjing Medical University, and one of active ingredients is Astragaloside A, which regulates immune responses. Despite the high efficacy of AOS, little is known about the changes of IL-10, TGF-β, Th1, and Th2 cytokines, and $CD4^{+}CD25^{high}CD127^{low}$ Treg cells in the children with allergic asthma. Children with allergic asthma were recruited at our hospital from 2016 to 2017, and treated by using AOS. Related indicators and immunological changes were examined to evaluate the value of AOS treatment for the children with allergic asthma.

MATERIALS AND METHODS

Materials

Astragaloside A was purchased from China Pharmaceutical and Biological Laboratory (lot number 11078-200703, Beijing, China). AOS was purchased from Nanjing Hospital of Traditional Chinese Medicine (patches numbers: 100234,100406, 100609, 100815, 100987, and 101009; Nanjing, China). AOS was prepared as follows: AM slices were dried to a constant weight, 450 g. After soaking in 5 liters of distilled water overnight, the main ingredients of AM were extracted by using the ultrasonic constant temperature ultrasonic extractor (Cat. No., Scientz-5TQL4, Ningbo Scientz Biotech., Ningbo, China) twice. The first extract was obtained at 30 min (1000 W), and the second tract at 45 min and 50°C, and the extracts were concentrated to 450 mL. The extracts were further centrifuged at $12,000 \times g$ for 30 min, and supernatants were filtered through a 10 kDa membrane (Millipore, Bedford, MA, USA).

Chromatographic Conditions

The HPLC system consisted of a Kromasil C18 column (4.6×200 mm, id 5 μm) with a guard column (10×4.6 mm, id 5 μm) (Waters Chromatography Division of Millipore Corp., Milford, MA, USA), a Waters 515 HPLC Pump, a full-wavelength UV detector, a Waters 717 plus autosampler injector and an Empower workstation. The mobile phase was composed of acetonitrile-water (35:65, v/v), the determination wavelength was 203 nm, and the column temperature was 30°C. All reagents were of chromatographic grade. To achieve the baseline separation and accurate quantitative analysis, the theoretical plate number of Astragaloside A was not less than 3,000.

Measurement of Astragaloside A in AOS

One-milliliter of AOS was added to a 10 mL volumetric flask and extracted twice with petroleum. The petroleum ether extract was discarded, and the lower solution was extracted four times with saturated n-butanol (20, 15, 15, and 10 mL). The combined n-butanol solution was washed with 5% sodium bicarbonate solution twice, each for 30 mL. The washings were discarded and n-butanol solution was collected, and evaporated to dry. The residue was dissolved in 10-mL ethanol. Approximately 0.05 g Astragaloside A standard was added to a 25 mL volumetric flask, and ethanol was added to achieve 1.967 mg/mL Astragaloside A as a reference. A series of the stock solution (0.2, 0.4, 0.6, 0.8, and 1.0 mL) was added to 10 mL volumetric flask, and ethanol was added to achieve a series of Astragaloside A standards with different concentrations (0.0393, 0.0786, 0.118, 0.157, 0.196 mg/mL). Ten microliter of solution was injected into HPLC and the peak area of Astragaloside A was determined. The measurements were repeated twice. The peak area was used as the ordinate, Astragaloside A concentration was used as abscissa, and the standard curve was plotted. The regression equation was $y = 1.245x + 7.526C$, $r = 0.9996$. The standard was repeated for five times with RSD 0.7% to ensure the method was accurate. AOS was measured by using the same situation and the results showed perfect repeatability. The average content of Astragaloside A was 0.216% with RSD 1.5%. The tests were stable at 0, 2, 4, 6, and 8 h.

Patients

Before the experiment, all procedures were approved by the human research ethical committee of the Affiliated Hospital of Changchun University of Traditional Chinese Medicine (Changchun, China, approval no. 20170128x). A written consent form approved by our committee and signed by all subjects. Eighty children with allergic asthma, were recruited at the Department of Pediatrics, Affiliated Hospital of Changchun University of Traditional Chinese Medicine. The clinical diagnostic criteria of the "Children's Asthma Diagnosis and Prevention Guide" was used to examine allergic asthma in children (22), and the children had the following symptoms: wheezing, shortness of breath, chest pain or cough, and allergic asthma caused by cold air, physical and chemical stimulation, viral upper respiratory tract infection and exercise. Wheezing episodes in the lungs could be heard and the expiratory phase was prolonged. The typical clinical manifestations, such as no clear wheezing or signs should have at least the following positive test: bronchial provocation test or motor positive test, and or bronchial diastolic positive test (forced expiratory volume in 1 s FEV1 increased).

Allergy Skin Test

The hypersensitivity response of each patient was assessed by using conventional skin prick tests against 16 common aeroallergens according to an earlier report (23). Skin prick tests were performed according to the methods introduced by Gislason (24). The test would be regarded as clinically significant if the allergen reactions were more than 10.

Measurement of Total IgE

Serum IgE levels were measured by using the Human IgE ELISA Kit from Abcam (Shanghai, China). Serum IgE levels were positively associated with the color intensity of the test and calibrated against the WHO standard for IgE (25).

The Test for Allergen-Specific IgE

Allergen-specific IgE was detected in the patients' serum against HD, *D. pteronyssinus* (DP), *D. farinae* (DF), and *B. tropicalis* (BT) by using the AllergyScreen system and ImmunoCAP 100 system (Amersham Pharmacia Biotech, Uppsala, Sweden). The test was calibrated against the WHO Standard for IgE ranging from 0.35 to 100 KU/L for specific IgE.

Inclusion Criteria

The following inclusion criteria were used:

(1) Male or female patients between the ages of 3–12 years; (2) Allergens reactions more than 10. (3)Total serum IgE levels more than 350 IU/mL; (4) competency to perform pulmonary function tests and pulmonary function FEV1 <80% predictive value; (5) children not taking the medicine such as aspirin and other drugs that may trigger asthma symptoms within 4 weeks before enrollment; (6) children able to receive treatment under the guardianship of a parent who signed an informed consent form.

Exclusion Criteria

Children who had the following conditions were excluded: (1) various psychiatric disorders; (2) severe congenital heart disease; (3) pneumothorax, pleural effusion, active pulmonary tuberculosis, acute exacerbation within the past month and received emergency treatment; (5) infectious rhinitis and sinusitis; (6) anaphylactic shock or eczema of unknown etiology; (7) received immunotherapy and (8) adverse reactions after enrollment.

Patients Grouping

The extracts of AM were evaporated to dry, and the residue was dissolved in 10 mL ethanol. AOS was prepared by the 10-fold dilution of AM ethanol solution. Residual petroleum and n-butanol compounds were measured by gas chromatography (Agilent 6890, Agilent Tech., USA) with a flame ionization detecting system. None of the residual compounds were found in the AOS solution.

Based on inclusion and exclusion criteria, 80 children with allergic asthma caused by dust mites were recruited at our hospital from February 2016 to June 2017. The sample size was analyzed by using PASS version 13 (NCSS Statistical Software, Kaysville, UT, USA), and the power of sample size was 85%. The children were evenly and randomly assigned into two groups: the AOS group, where the patients received 10 mL AOS daily and the control group, where the patients received placebo (0.1% quinine chloride in deionized water) daily. The duration of the experiment was 6 months.

Evaluation of Allergic Asthma Symptoms

Lung function was measured by using FEV1, which was compared with predicted values. Most symptoms of allergic asthma were investigated by using Pediatric Asthma Quality of Life Questionnaire (PAQLQ) scores as shown in **Table 1** (26).

The severity of asthma was classified into four levels according to previous report (27): mild intermittent, mild persistent, moderate persistent, and severe persistent based on symptom frequency and either spirometric (FEV_1) or peak expiratory flow (PEF). The primary outcome was also measured according to asthma-related clinical events, including cough, wheeze, and need of intervention. Allergic sensitization to common dietary and respiratory allergens were measured according to an earlier report (28). Serum IgE of 0.2 or 0.35 IU/mL were regarded as positive and predictive for allergic asthma. Eosinophils (29) and serum levels of ECP (30) are increased in allergic asthma.

Measurement of Serum Levels of IL-10 and TGF-β

Five millimeters of venous blood was obtained from each patient. Two millimeters of blood was placed at room temperature for 1 h. The serum was isolated via centrifugation at 5000 × *g* for 10 min. The serum levels of IL-10 and TGF-β were measured by using the

TABLE 1 | The Pediatric Asthma Quality of life questionnaire (PAQLQ score).

Scores	Aspects
LIMITED ACTIVITY	
1	Strong physical activity
2	Medium physical activity
3	Social activity
4	Work-related activities
5	Sleepiness
SYMPTOMS	
8	Shortness of breath
14	Dull aching chest
18	Expiratory or inspiratory difficulties, early morning symptoms of asthma
24	Night arousal
ENVIRONMENT	
9	Smoke,
17	Dust
23	Air pollution environment
26	Strong smell symptoms,
25	Air pollution of the environment
28	Strong smell had to be avoided
EMOTION	
6	Chest tightness caused by the degree of discomfort
7	Worried about suffering from asthma
12	Cough caused by discomfort
13	Asthma and worry
15	Medication
16	Clear throat
21	Worry about no asthma medication
22	Heavy breathing
27	Fear of breathlessness
29	Remuneration,
30	Desperately breathing,
10	Limitation of conscious activities

ELISA kits from R & D Systems, Inc. (Minneapolis, MN, USA). The serum Th1 cytokines (IL-2 and IFN-γ), and Th2 cytokines (IL-4 and IL-6) (31) were measured by using the kits from Abcam (Shanghai office, China).

Measurement of the Percentage of Gated $CD4^+$ T Cells, $CD4^+CD25^+$ T Cells, $CD4^+CD25^{high}$ Treg Cells, $CD4^+CD25^+$ $FoxP3^+$ Treg Cells and $CD4^+CD25^{high}$ $CD127^{low}$ Treg Cells

Three millimeters of blood was added to an anticoagulant-containing (EDTA-K2) tube. Peripheral blood mononuclear cells (PBMCs) were isolated from human peripheral blood via Ficoll-Hypaque (Sigma, St. Louis, MO, USA) density gradient centrifugation. Mouse anti-human CD4 monoclonal antibody was purchased from Zhongshan Golden Bridge Biotechnology (Beijing, China) CD127 (BD Pharmingen #558598, San Jose, CA) was conjugated to ALEXA FLUOR 488. Goat-anti-mouse FITC IgG was purchased from Kangwei (Beijing, China). CD25 PE-Cy7 (BD, clone M-A251), CD25 APC (clone 2A3), and FoxP3 PE (clone PCH101) were purchased from BD Biosciences (Franklin, NJ, USA). CD4+ T cells were gated on side scatter height vs. CD4. The percentage of $CD4^+CD25^+$ T cells, $CD4^+CD25^{high}$ Treg cells, $CD4^+CD25^+$ $FoxP3^+$ Treg cells and $CD4^+CD25^{high}CD127^{low}$ Treg cells in PBMCs was measured by using FACSCalibur flow cytometer (Becton Dickinson, Mountain View, CA, USA).

Statistical Analysis

SPSS20.0 statistical software was used to perform statistical analyses. All data were expressed as mean values ± standard deviation (S.D.). Normal distribution and variance homogeneity were analyzed by a paired *t*-test. Normal distribution was analyzed by ANOVA between groups. Non-normal distribution was analyzed by Wilcoxon rank test. Count data were compared by using contingency χ^2 test. The statistical differences were significant if $P < 0.05$.

RESULTS

Recovery Rate of Astragaloside A

AOS was taken from six different batches. With two copies per group, each group was added to a concentration of 0.197 mg/mL Astragaloside A control solution 0.8, 1.0, and 1.2 mL. The average recovery rate of Astragaloside A was 96.2% with RSD 2.65% (**Table 2**).

Average Contents of Astragaloside A in AOS

Table 3 showed that the contents of Astragaloside A were 0.216 ± 0.027 mg/mL from six batches of AOS.

Clinical Demographic Characteristics

The AOS and control groups were composed of 80 cases with 43 males and 37 females, and aged 3–12 years. Age is associated with the risk of allergic asthma (32, 33). In our study, age distribution (5-7, 8-10, and 11-12) was similar between the two groups ($P > 0.05$). The experimental group comprised 23 males and 17 females, with an average age of 8.7 ± 3.3 years. The control group comprised 22 males and 18 females, with an average age of 8.9 ± 2.7 years. The statistical difference was not statistically significant in all parameters (**Table 4**, $P > 0.05$). The most allergic responses to common inhalants included *Cocos nucifera, Brassica nigra*, cat dander, HD, DP, DF, and BT. The statistical difference for these inhalants was insignificant between two groups (**Table 5**, $P > 0.05$). The total serum IgE levels were 428.49 ± 58.61 and 431.27± 60.45 IU/mL between two groups. The statistical difference for allergen-specific IgE reactivity against HD, DP, DF, and BT was insignificant between the two groups (**Table 6**, $P > 0.05$).

No significant differences were found for symptoms of allergic asthma and biochemical characterization of allergic asthma between the two groups (**Tables 7**, **8**). Significant differences of asthma-related events were found after 6-month follow-up (**Table 7**). The severity of allergic asthma was significantly

TABLE 2 | Recovery rate of Astragaloside A.

Times	Sampling volume/ml	Sample content/mg	Addition/mg	Measured values/mg	Recovery rate	Average value	RSD/%
1	10	0.215	0.1574	0.35420	0.9511	0.962	2.65
2	10	0.215	0.1574	0.36540	0.9812		
3	10	0.215	0.1967	0.39870	0.9684		
4	10	0.215	0.1967	0.37540	0.9118		
5	10	0.215	0.2360	0.44670	0.9905		
6	10	0.215	0.2360	0.43650	0.9678		

TABLE 3 | The average contents of Astragaloside A from 6 batches of AOS.

Batches	1	2	3	4	5	6
Contents of Astragaloside A, mg/ml	0.203	0.242	0.213	0.189	0.243	0.204

AOS, astragalus oral solution.

TABLE 4 | Clinical demographic characteristics.

	AOS group	Control group	χ^2 values or *t* values	*P*-values
Age, years	8.7 ± 3.3	8.9 ± 2.7	0.124	0.658
5-7 year, *n* (%)	6	4	0.630	0.730
8-10 year, *n* (%)	26	29		
11-12 year, *n* (%)	8	7		
Male/Female	23/17	22/18	0.051	0.822
BMI	22.67 ± 3.18	23.98 ± 2.75	0.578	0.209
Disease duration, months	36.90 ± 4.28	38.91 ± 5.27	2.397	0.009
Respiratory rate, times/min	19.74 ± 1.54	20.33 ± 1.49	−1.908	0.153
Heart rate, time/min	76.82 ± 3.77	77.02 ± 3.03	−0.292	0.768
Systolic pressure, mmHg	121.68 ± 9.35	123.83 ± 11.55	−1.039	0.326
Diastolic pressure, mmHg	77.04 ± 7.11	75.46 ± 6.51	1.127	0.235

BMI, body mass index = weight (kg)/height (m^2).

lower in the experimental group than in the control group ($P < 0.05$).Similarly, biochemical indices of allergic asthma were significantly lower in the experimental group than in the control group (**Table 8**, $P < 0.05$).

AOS Treatment Improved the Allergic Asthma Symptoms in Children

Before treatment, the FEV1% in the AOS group was comparable with that in the control group ($P > 0.05$, **Figure 1A**). After treatment, the FEV1% were significantly increased in the AOS group than in the control group ($P < 0.05$, **Figure 1A**). Similarly, PAQLQ scores were comparable between two groups before treatment ($P > 0.05$, **Figure 1B**). After treatment, PAQLQ scores were increased significantly in the AOS group when compared with those in the control group ($P < 0.05$, **Figure 1B**). The results suggest that AOS reduces the symptoms of allergic asthma by improving FEV1% and PAQLQ.

TABLE 5 | Allergic response to common inhalants.

	AOS group	Control group	*P*-values
Pollens			0.936
Cocos nucifera	31 (77.5)	33 (82.5)	
Brassica nigra	20 (50)	24 (60)	
Delonix sp.	19 (47.5)	17 (42.5)	
Azadirachta indica	17 (42.5)	15 (37.5)	
Caesalpinia sp	15 (37.5)	18 (45)	
Molds			0.915
Aspergillus fumigatus	11 (27.5)	12 (30)	
Aspergillus niger	8 (20)	9 (22.5)	
Candida albicans	5 (12.5)	4 (10)	
Cladosporium sp.	6 (15)	7 (17.5)	
Alternaria lternate	4 (10)	2 (5)	
Others			0.623
Dog dander	6 (15)	9 (22.5)	
Cat dander	20 (50)	21 (52.5)	
House dust	40 (100)	32 (80)	
Dermatophagoides pteronyssinus	32 (80)	39 (97.5)	
Dermatophagoides farinae	21 (52.5)	19 (47.5)	
Blomia tropicalis	24 (60)	22 (55)	

Chi-square test was performed and there will be significant difference if P < 0.05 between two groups.

TABLE 6 | Allergen-specific IgE reactivity against HD, DP, DF, and BT Allergens.

	AOS group	Control group	*P*-values
HD	28 (70)	25 (62.5)	0.478
DP	24 (60)	20 (50)	0.369
DF	30 (75)	33 (82.5)	0.412
BT	35 (87.5)	28 (70)	0.056

HD, House dust; DP, D. pteronyssinus; DF, D. farinae; BT, B. tropicalis. Chi-square test was performed and there will be significant difference if P < 0.05 between two groups.

AOS Increased the Serum Level of IL-10 and Reduced the Level of TGF-β

The serum levels of IL-10 were comparable between the AOS (24.12 ± 3.68 pg/mL) and control groups (26.25 ± 3.79 pg/mL) (**Figure 2A**, $P > 0.05$). Comparatively, the serum levels of TGF-β were same between the AOS (932.67 ± 148.43 pg/mL) and

TABLE 7 | Comparison of symptoms of allergic asthma between two groups.

	AOS group, $n = 40$	Control group, $n = 40$	*P*-values
BEFORE THERAPY			
No. of wheezing episodes	1.10 (0.7–1.6)	1.08 (0.6–1.5)	0.85
Days with wheeze	7.58 (1.36–13.9)	6.95 (0.90–12.3)	0.25
Days on inhalative betamimetics	13.8 (3.37–24.6)	13.2 (8.18–17.2)	0.78
Days on inhalative steroids	10.0 (7.23–24.9)	9.80 (6.99–17.5)	0.89
No. of rescue-free days	128.7 (108.4–158.6)	121.5 (112.0–163.0)	0.93
No. of symptom-free days	123.0 (126.4–162.6)	128.5 (115.7–160.3)	0.71
Allergic Asthma Classification, Cases (%)			
Mild intermittent	13 (32.5)	15 (37.5)	0.968
Mild persistent	12 (30)	11 (27.5)	
Moderate persistent	8 (20)	7 (17.5)	
Severe persistent	7 (17.5)	7 (17.5)	
AFTER THERAPY			
No. of wheezing episodes	0.51 (0.3–1.9)	1.10 (0.6–1.9)	0.03
Days with wheeze	5.26 (3.03–13.7)	11.3 (7.15–14.8)	0.01
Days on inhalative betamimetics	10.7 (6.3–30.2)	13.9 (2.68–18.9)	0.02
Days on inhalative steroids	10.5 (6.3–22.7)	14.8 (4.6–25.6)	0.01
No. of rescue-free days	148.5 (108.9–168.1)	126.0 (99.6–172.4)	0.02
No. of symptom-free days	142.5 (102.6–152.5)	104.0 (86.2–141.8)	
Allergic Asthma Classification, Cases (%)			
Mild intermittent	21 (52.5)	12 (30)	0.02
Mild persistent	10 (2.5)	6 (1.5)	
Moderate persistent	4 (10)	14 (3.5)	
Severe persistent	5 (12.5)	8 (20)	

The statistical difference was significant if $P < 0.05$.

TABLE 8 | Comparison of biochemical characterization of allergic asthma between two groups.

	AOS group, $n = 40$	Control group, $n = 40$	*P*-values
BEFORE THERAPY			
Total IgE (IU/mL)	416.7 (312.8–556.4)	412.2 (310.0–560.6)	0.86
Eosinophils (%)	2.6 (2.3–3.9)	2.8 (2.3–3.5)	0.32
ECP (μg/mL)	22.3 (14.9–29.9)	21.9 (12.6–28.2)	0.69
AFTER THERAPY			
Total IgE (IU/mL)	214.7 (162.3–290.5)	420.2 (316.2–481.3)	0.01
Eosinophils (%)	2.2 (1.5–4.0)	3.0 (2.5–3.6)	0.01
ECP (μg/mL)	16.7 (9.89–23.8)	24.8 (16.6–32.4)	0.01

The statistical difference was significant if $P < 0.05$.

control groups (968.27 ± 150.64 pg/mL) (**Figure 2B**, $P > 0.05$). After treatment, the serum level of IL-10 in the experimental group was significantly increased and the level of TGF-β was significantly decreased compared with those in the control group (**Figure 2**, $P < 0.05$). The results suggest that AOS treatment increases the serum levels of IL-10 and reduces the levels of TGF-β.

AOS Treatment Reduced Serum Level of Th1 (IL-2 and IFN-γ) and Th2 Cytokines (IL-4 and IL-6)

Before the treatment, the statistical difference for the serum level of Th1 (IL-2, **Figure 3A**, and IFN-γ, **Figure 3D**) and Th2 cytokines (IL-4, **Figure 3B** and IL-6, **Figure 3C**) was insignificant between AOS and control groups ($P > 0.05$). After the treatment, the serum levels of Th1 (IL-2, **Figure 3A**, and IFN-γ, **Figure 3D**) and Th2 cytokines (IL-4, **Figure 3B** and IL-6, **Figure 3C**) were lower in the AOS group than the control group ($P < 0.05$).

Percentage of Gated $CD4^+$ T Cells, $CD4^+CD25^+$ T cells, $CD4^+CD25^{high}$, $CD4^+CD25^+FoxP3^+$ Treg Cells and $CD4^+CD25^{high}CD127^{low}$ Treg Cells

Before treatment, the percentage of gated $CD4^+$ T cells (14.26 ± 3.51%, **Figure 4A**), $CD4^+CD25^+$ T cells (9.15 ± 2.28%, **Figure 4B**), $CD4^+CD25^{high}$ (5.67 ± 0.75%, **Figure 4C**), $CD4^+CD25^+FoxP3^+$ Treg cells (1.53 ± 0.21%, **Figure 4D**), and $CD4^+CD25^{high}CD127^{low}$ (0.72 ± 0.28%, **Figure 4E**) Treg cells in the AOS group were comparable with those in the control group, gated $CD4^+$ T cells (13.89 ± 4.01%, **Figure 4A**), $CD4^+CD25^+$ T cells (9.29 ± 2.37%, **Figure 4B**), $CD4^+CD25^{high}$ (5.38 ± 0.64%, **Figure 4C**), $CD4^+CD25^+FoxP3^+$ Treg cells (1.62 ± 0.30%, **Figure 4D**), and $CD4^+CD25^{high}CD127^{low}$ (0.79 ± 0.25%, **Figure 4E**) ($P > 0.05$). After treatment, the percentage of gated $CD4^+$ T cells (18.63 ± 6.27%, **Figure 4A**), $CD4^+CD25^+$ T cells (12.34 ± 4.61%, **Figure 4B**), $CD4^+CD25^{high}$ (9.65 ± 0.83%, **Figure 4C**), $CD4^+CD25^+FoxP3^+$ Treg cells (2.46 ± 0.37%, **Figure 4D**) and $CD4^+CD25^{high}CD127^{low}$ (1.34 ± 0.31%, **Figure 4E**) Treg cells in the AOS group were significantly higher than those in the control group, gated $CD4^+$ T cells (13.99 ± 4.22%, **Figure 4A**), $CD4^+CD25^+$ T cells (9.12 ± 2.05%, **Figure 4B**), $CD4^+CD25^{high}$ (5.63 ± 0.47%, **Figure 4C**), $CD4^+CD25^+FoxP3^+$ Treg cells (1.58 ± 0.24%, **Figure 4D**), and $CD4^+CD25^{high}CD127^{low}$ (0.81 ± 0.28%, **Figure 4E**) ($P < 0.05$) ($P < 0.05$). The results suggest that AOS consumption increases the percentage of gated $CD4^+$ T cells, $CD4^+CD25^+$ T cells, $CD4^+CD25^{high}$, $CD4^+CD25^+FoxP3^+$ Treg cells, and $CD4^+CD25^{high}CD127^{low}$ Treg cells in children with allergic asthma.

DISCUSSION

The results showed that the content of Astragaloside A in AOS varied from 0.19 to 0.24 mg/mL. The quality of the different batches of the mixture was influenced by the quality of the decoction pieces, processing and other factors. HPLC was an effective method to detect the quality of AOS and provided a basis for high-quality standards.

Allergic asthma is caused by a variety of cells, including inflammatory cells (neutrophils, T lymphocytes, eosinophils, and mast cells) (34), airway structural cells (airway smooth muscle cells and epithelial cells) (35), and cell components. AR is the most common symptoms of allergic asthma after individuals come in contact with allergens. Many inflammatory cells and

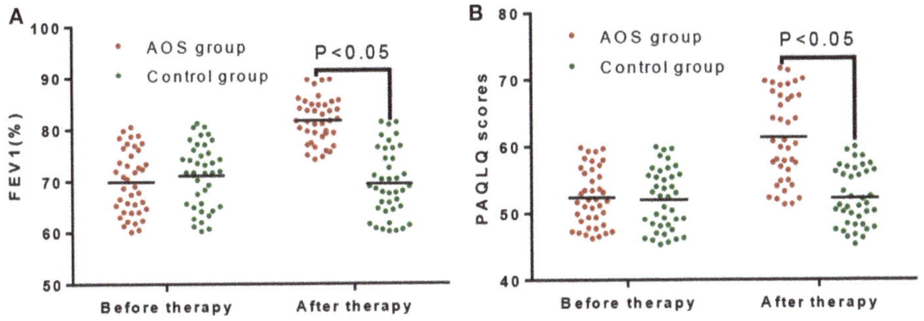

FIGURE 1 | The effects of AOS on FEV1% and PAQLQ scores in the children with allergy asthma. **(A)** The effects of AOS on FEV1% in the children with allergy asthma. **(B)** The effects of AOS on PAQLQ scores in the children with allergy asthma. FEV1, forced expiratory volume in 1 s; PAQLQ, Pediatric Asthma Quality of Life Questionnaire. $n = 40$ for each group. The statistical difference was significant for $P < 0.05$.

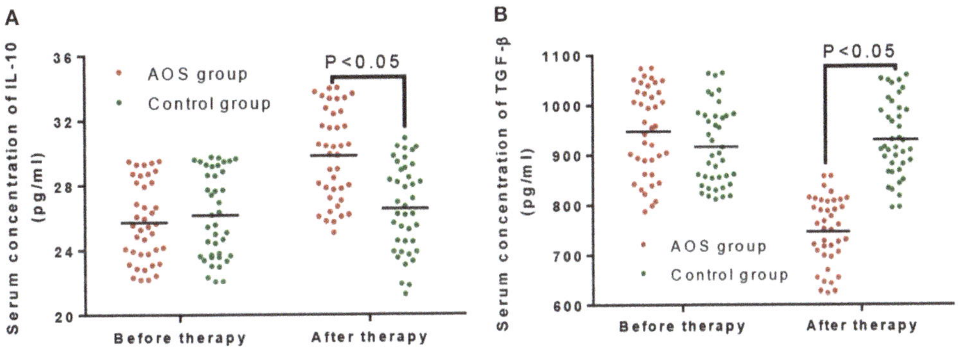

FIGURE 2 | The effects of AOS on the serum levels of IL-10 and TGF-β in the children with allergy asthma. **(A)** The effects of AOS on serum level of IL-10 in the children with allergy asthma. **(B)** The effects of AOS on TGF-β in the children with allergy asthma. $n = 40$ for each group. The statistical difference was significant for $P < 0.05$.

cytokinesare involved in the inflammatory responses, including nasal itching, sneezing, running nose, and stuffy nose. The incidence of childhood allergic asthma has been increasing, but its pathogenesis is not yet clear. The traditional Thl/Th2 imbalance theory cannot explain all the pathogenesis. Presently, a number of studies have focused on Treg cells to investigate the pathognesis (36, 37). Our findings demonstrated that AOS treatment reduced the serum levels of Thl and Th2 cytokines (**Figure 3**). Analyses of childhood allergic asthma by using $CD4^{+}CD25^{high}CD127^{low}$ Treg cells will have important clinical values.

IL-10 regulates allergic asthma and is directly involved in the regulation of inflammatory cells. IL-10 factor can inhibit the proliferation, secretion of Th cells, and the proliferation and differentiation of antigen-presenting cells (38). IL-10 cells inhibit T cells, antigen presentation (39), and the expression of IL-8 (40). IL-10 was reported to inhibit eosinophil-induced inflammatory effects of asthma, suggesting that IL-10 plays a key negative regulatory role in the development of allergic asthma (41). The level of IL-10 was found to be reduced significantly in T cells of peripheral blood during the onset of allergic asthma (42). In our study, the IL-10 level in the AOS group was comparable with that in control group before treatment ($P > 0.05$, **Figure 2**). After treatment, the level of IL-10 in the AOS group was significantly increased ($P < 0.05$). After AOS treatment, IL-10 may inhibit the antigen-presenting process and T cells response and play a critical role in the prevention of asthma.

TGF-β is a kind of stimulating factor with many biological effects, and it plays a critical role in regulating inflammation in various organs and tissues. Thus, TGF-β is widely studied in the transforming growth factor family and involved in the fibrosis formation of tissues and organs. Its overexpression in cardiac tissue can cause cardiac hypertrophy or myocardial fibrosis, which is involved in the process of ventricular remodeling (43, 44).TGF-β is a multifunctional cytokine that can participate in the process of cell proliferation, apoptosis and differentiation (45). In the immune system, TGF-β is a regulator of immunity with both pro- and anti-inflammatory effects and is involved in a variety of airway inflammation and immune responses. Many studies on TGF-β in the pathogenesis of asthma have been performed. However, t many controversies at different stages of development are still present. Most of researchers think that TGF-β can inhibit or promote inflammation (46, 47).

Elevated levels of TGF-β were reported in patients with atopic asthma (48, 49), which may be caused by the continued stimulation of allergens and airway remodeling. TGF-β also has a chemotactic function and can promote the proliferation

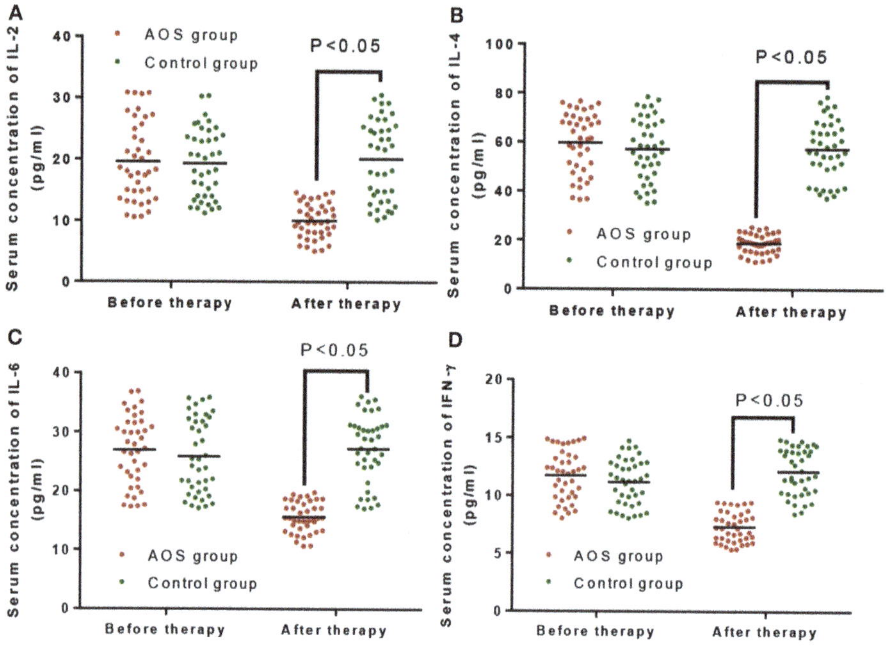

FIGURE 3 | The effects of AOS on the serum levels of Serum Th1 cytokines (IL-2 and IFN-γ), and Th2 cytokines (IL-4 and IL-6). **(A)** The effects of AOS on serum level of IL-2. **(B)** The effects of AOS on serum level of IL-4. **(C)** The effects of AOS on serum level of IL-2. **(B)** The effects of AOS on serum level of IL-6. **(D)** The effects of AOS on serum level of IFN-γ. $n = 40$ for each group. The statistical difference was significant for $P < 0.05$.

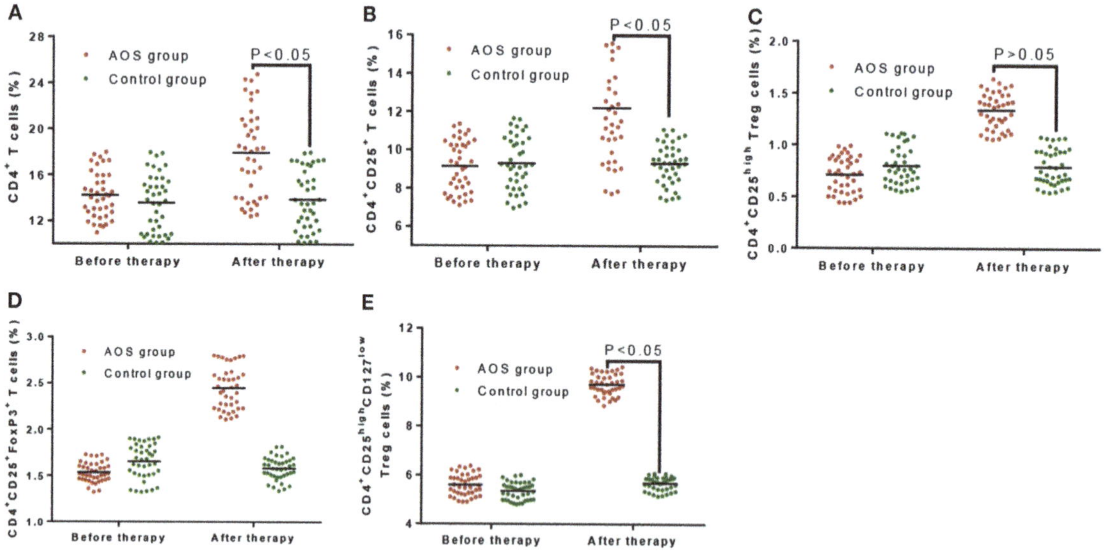

FIGURE 4 | The effects of AOS on the contents of T cells in the children with allergy asthma. **(A)** The effects of AOS on the contents of gated $CD4^+$ T cells in the children with allergy asthma. **(B)** The effects of AOS on the contents of $CD4^+CD25^+$ T cells in the children with allergy asthma. **(C)** The effects of AOS on the contents of $CD4^+CD25^{high}$ Treg cells in the children with allergy asthma. **(D)** The effects of AOS on the contents of $CD4^+CD25^+$FoxP3 Treg cells in the children with allergy asthma. **(E)** The effects of AOS on the contents of $CD4^+CD25^{high}CD127^{low}$ Treg cells in the children with allergy asthma. $n = 40$ for each group. The statistical difference was significant for $P < 0.05$.

and differentiation of inflammatory cytokines (50). In previous studies, the severity of asthma was found to be related to the concentration of TGF-β in the peripheral blood (51). In the present study, the serum level of TGF-β in the experimental group was comparable with that in the control group ($P > 0.05$). After AOS consumption, the level of TGF-β was significantly decreased ($P < 0.05$), suggesting that AOS ameliorates allergic asthma by reducing the serum level of TGF-β.

Treg cells are a subset of T-cells that control the autoimmune reactivity *in vivo* and play a key role in the inhibition of autoimmunity (52, 53). They exert immunosuppressive effects through the specific binding of their surface molecules (CTLA-4, CD25) to the corresponding ligands on the cells (54). IL-10 can inhibit the proliferation of T cells, the synthesis of cytokines such as IL-2 by Th1 and Th2 cells, and the expression of MHCII in macrophages (55). Immune regulatory T cells may maintain the immune tolerance via several mechanisms. $CD4^{+}CD25^{+}$ Treg cells are able to bind to target cells and participate in immune regulation. In previous studies, $CD4^{+}CD25^{+}$ Treg cells and $CD4^{+}CD25^{+}$ T cells were increased simultaneously with $CD4^{+}CD25^{+}$ Treg proliferation (56). The percentage of $CD4^{+}CD25^{+}$ T cells and $CD4^{+}CD25^{high}CD127^{low}$ was decreased during acute episode of childhood allergic asthma (57). In the present study, the percentage was comparable for $CD4^{+}CD25^{+}$ T cells, $CD4^{+}CD25^{high}$, $CD4^{+}CD25^{+}FoxP3^{+}$ Treg cells and $CD4^{+}CD25^{high}CD127^{low}$ Treg cells between two groups before the treatment (**Figure 4**, $P > 0.05$). After the treatment, AOS consumption increased the percentage of $CD4^{+}CD25^{+}$ T cells, $CD4^{+}CD25^{high}$, $CD4^{+}CD25^{+}FoxP3^{+}$ Treg cells and $CD4^{+}CD25^{high}CD127^{low}$ Treg cells (**Figure 4**, $P < 0.05$). The results suggest AOS consumption reduces the risk of allergic asthma by increasing the percentage of $CD4^{+}CD25^{+}$ T cells, $CD4^{+}CD25^{high}$, $CD4^{+}CD25^{+}FoxP3^{+}$ Treg cells and $CD4^{+}CD25^{high}CD127^{low}$ Treg cells in PBMCs.

Th2 cytokines are associated with allergic airway inflammation (2) while Th1 cells inhibit Th2 immune activities (3). The imbalance of Th1/Th2 cytokines indicates the risk of asthma (58). Peripheral blood eosinophils increase the levels of Th1 and Th2 cytokines (4). By contrast, AOS therapy will reduce the levels of peripheral blood eosinophils and may result in the down-regulation of Th1 and Th2 cytokines. AOS may also increase the level of Treg cells, which will suppress the level of blood eosinophils (5).

The present study has some limitations to. For the side effects of AOS were still unclear. According to previous reports, *Astragalus* induces some side effects, including anemia, neutropenia, thrombocytopenia, fatigue, poor appetite, nausea, and vomiting (1). However, these side effects were not found in the present study. Although Astragaloside A is the main bioactive component in AOS, other components were not analyzed in AOS. The functions of certain components should be confirmed in the future work. In this experiment, we only explored the effects of AOS on the serum levels of IL-10, TGF-β and the percentage of $CD4^{+}CD25^{+}$ T cells, $CD4^{+}CD25^{high}$, $CD4^{+}CD25^{+}FoxP3^{+}$ Treg cells and $CD4^{+}CD25^{high}CD127^{low}$ Treg cells in PBMCs. However, modern studies show that the expression level of Treg cells is associated with a variety of autoimmune diseases. The study of Treg alone cannot fully explain the exact mechanism for its action. In recent years, the research on the immune balance between Treg/Th17 has been increased. In the future, further work is highly demanded to reveal the relationship between the impact of the balance and allergic asthma in children.

CONCLUSIONS

The average contents of Astragaloside A were 0.216 ± 0.027 mg/mL from six batches of AOS. After 6-month therapy, AOS treatment was more effective in the experimental group than in the control group ($P < 0.05$). AOS reduced the symptoms of allergy asthma in children group by improving FEV1% and PAQLQ scores. The children with allergic asthma have a lower level of serum IL-10 and higher level of TGF-β. AOS consumption increased the level of serum IL-10 and reduced the level of TGF-β. AOS can be effective in the treatment of allergic asthma in children by increasing the percentage of $CD4^{+}CD25^{+}$ T cells, $CD4^{+}CD25^{high}$, $CD4^{+}CD25^{+}FoxP3^{+}$ Treg cells, and $CD4^{+}CD25^{high}CD127^{low}$ Treg cells.

AUTHOR CONTRIBUTIONS

WW conceived, designed the study, and wrote the manuscript. QL and WJ performed the experiments, analyzed the data, and contributed reagents, materials, analysis tools.

ACKNOWLEDGMENTS

We are very grateful to two reviewers for their critical and strategic comments, which have significantly improved the quality of our paper.

REFERENCES

1. Lin YD, Fan XL, Zhang H, Fang SB, Li CL, Deng MX, et al. The genes involved in asthma with the treatment of human embryonic stem cell-derived mesenchymal stem cells. *Mol Immunol.* (2018) 95:47–55. doi: 10.1016/j.molimm.2018.01.013
2. Normansell R, Kew KM, Bridgman AL. Sublingual immunotherapy for asthma. *Cochrane Database Syst Rev.* (2015) 8:CD011293. doi: 10.1002/14651858.CD011293.pub2
3. Powell C, Milan SJ, Dwan K, Bax L, Walters N. Mepolizumab versus placebo for asthma. *Cochrane Database Syst Rev.* (2015) 7:CD010834. doi: 10.1002/14651858.CD010834.pub2
4. Marple BF. Allergic rhinitis and inflammatory airway disease: interactions within the unified airspace. *Am J Rhinol Allergy* (2010) 24:249–54. doi: 10.2500/ajra.2010.24.3499
5. Bousquet J, Van Cauwenberge P, Khaltaev N, World Heath Organization. Allergic rhinitis and its impact on asthma. *J Allergy Clin Immunol.* (2001) 108:S147–334. doi: 10.1067/mai.2001.118891
6. Rahman MA, Chakraborty R, Ferdousi KR, Alam A, Chowdhury MK, Paul BK. New therapeutic approach to treat allergic rhinitis & bronchial asthma, considering these two as one united airway disease. *Mymensingh Med J.* (2017) 26:216–21.
7. Calus L, Devuyst L, Van Zele T, De Ruyck N, Derycke L, Bachert C, et al. The response to nasal allergen provocation with grass pollen is reduced in patients with chronic rhinosinusitis with nasal polyposis and grass sensitization. *Clin Exp Allergy* (2016) 46:555–63. doi: 10.1111/cea.12687
8. Svendsen ER, Gonzales M, Commodore A. The role of the indoor environment: residential determinants of allergy, asthma and pulmonary

function in children from a US-Mexico border community. *Sci Total Environ.* (2018) 616:1513–23. doi: 10.1016/j.scitotenv.2017.10.162
9. Scanlon ST, McKenzie AN. Type 2 innate lymphoid cells: new players in asthma and allergy. *Curr Opin Immunol.* (2012) 24:707–12. doi: 10.1016/j.coi.2012.08.009
10. Amin K. Allergic respiratory inflammation and remodeling. *Turkish Thor J.* (2015) 16:133–40. doi: 10.5152/ttd.2015.4942
11. Hui C, McNagny K, Denburg J, and Siracusa M. *In situ* hematopoiesis: a regulator of T H 2 cytokine-mediated immunity and inflammation at mucosal surfaces. *Mucosal Immunol.* (2015) 8:701. doi: 10.1038/mi.2015.17
12. MacDonald SM. History of histamine-releasing factor (HRF)/translationally controlled tumor protein (TCTP) including a potential therapeutic target in asthma and allergy. *Results Probl Cell Differ.* (2017) 64:291–308. doi: 10.1007/978-3-319-67591-6_16
13. Coquet JM, Schuijs MJ, Smyth MJ, Deswarte K, Beyaert R, Braun H, et al. Interleukin-21-producing CD4+ T cells promote type 2 immunity to house dust mites. *Immunity* (2015) 43:318–30. doi: 10.1016/j.immuni.2015.07.015
14. Kawayama T, Kinoshita T, Matsunaga K, Naito Y, Sasaki J, Tominaga Y, et al. Role of regulatory T cells in airway inflammation in asthma. *Kurume Med J.* (2018) 64:45–55. doi: 10.2739/kurumemedj.MS6430001
15. Shu Y, Hu Q, Long H, Chang C, Lu Q, Xiao R. Epigenetic variability of CD4+CD25+ tregs contributes to the pathogenesis of autoimmune diseases. *Clin Rev Allergy Immunol.* (2017) 52:260–72. doi: 10.1007/s12016-016-8590-3
16. Tian Y, Liang X, Wu Y. The alternation of autophagy/apoptosis in CD4+CD25+Foxp3+ Tregs on the developmental stages of atherosclerosis. *Biomed Pharmacother.* (2018) 97:1053–60. doi: 10.1016/j.biopha.2017.11.013
17. Agarwal A, Singh M, Chatterjee BP, Chauhan A, Chakraborti A. Interplay of T helper 17 cells with CD4(+)CD25(high) FOXP3(+) Tregs in regulation of allergic asthma in pediatric patients. *Int J Pediatr.* (2014) 2014:636238. doi: 10.1155/2014/636238
18. Zhuge Z, Dong Y, Li L, Jin T. Effects of astragalus polysaccharide on the adhesion-related immune response of endothelial cells stimulated with CSFV *in vitro*. *Peer J.* (2017) 5:e3862. doi: 10.7717/peerj.3862
19. Lin SM, Jiang Y, Chen YJ, Luo L, Doolgindachbaporn S, Yuangsoi B. Effects of Astragalus polysaccharides (APS) and chitooligosaccharides (COS) on growth, immune response and disease resistance of juvenile largemouth bass, Micropterus salmoides. *Fish Shellfish Immunol.* (2017) 70:40–47. doi: 10.1016/j.fsi.2017.08.035
20. Jin H, Luo Q, Zheng Y, Nurahmat M, Wu J, Li B, et al. CD4+ CD25+ Foxp3+ T cells contribute to the antiasthmatic effects of Astragalus membranaceus extract in a rat model of asthma. *Int Immunopharmacol.* (2013) 15:42–49. doi: 10.1016/j.intimp.2012.11.009
21. Lin Y, Wang B, Luo X. Clinical study of astragalus's preventing the recurrence of asthma in children. *Zhongguo Zhong xi yi jie he za zhi Zhongguo Zhongxiyi jiehe zazhi* (2011) 31:1090–92.
22. Larenas Linnemann DES, Del Rio Navarro BE, Luna Pech JA, Romero Lombard J, Villaverde Rosas J, Cano Salas MC, et al. Recommendations for the prevention and diagnosis of asthma in children: evidence from international guidelines adapted for Mexico. *Allergol Immunopathol.* (2017) 46:291–303. doi: 10.1016/j.aller.2017.05.011
23. Podder S, Gupta SK, Saha GK. Incrimination of *Blomia tropicalis* as a potent allergen in house dust and its role in allergic asthma in Kolkata Metropolis, India. *World Allergy Organization J.* (2010) 3:182. doi: 10.1097/WOX.0b013e3181df4d4f
24. Gislason D, Gislason T. IgE-mediated allergy to Lepidoglyphus destructor in an urban population–an epidemiologic study. *Allergy* (1999) 54:878–83. doi: 10.1034/j.1398-9995.1999.00996.x
25. Platts-Mills TA, de Weck AL, Aalberse R, Bessot J, Bjorksten B, Bischoff E, et al. Dust mite allergens and asthma—a worldwide problem. *J Allergy Clin Immunol.* (1989) 83:416–27. doi: 10.1016/0091-6749(89)90128-0
26. Sousa KH, West SG, Moser SE, Harris JA, Cook SW. Establishing measurement invariance: english and spanish paediatric asthma quality of life questionnaire. *Nurs Res.* (2012) 61:171–80. doi: 10.1097/NNR.0b013e3182544750
27. Stout JW, Visness CM, Enright P, Lamm C, Shapiro G, Gan VN, et al. Classification of asthma severity in children: the contribution of pulmonary function testing. *Arch Pediatr Adolesc Med.* (2006) 160:844–50. doi: 10.1001/archpedi.160.8.844
28. Rose MA, Stieglitz F, Koksal A, Schubert R, Schulze J, Zielen S. Efficacy of probiotic Lactobacillus GG on allergic sensitization and asthma in infants at risk. *Clin Exp Allergy* (2010) 40:1398–405. doi: 10.1111/j.1365-2222.2010.03560.x
29. Tang W, Smith SG, Du W, Gugilla A, Du J, Oliveria JP, et al. Interleukin-25 and eosinophils progenitor cell mobilization in allergic asthma. *Clin Transl Allergy* (2018) 8:5. doi: 10.1186/s13601-018-0190-2
30. Sin A, Terzioglu E, Kokuludag A, Sebik F, Kabakci T. Serum eosinophil cationic protein (ECP) levels in patients with seasonal allergic rhinitis and allergic asthma. *Allergy Asthma Proc.* (1998) 19:69–73. doi: 10.2500/108854188778607228
31. Yan Y, Wang J, Qu B, Zhang Y, Wei Y, Liu H, et al. CXCL13 and TH1/Th2 cytokines in the serum and cerebrospinal fluid of neurosyphilis patients. *Medicine* (2017) 96:e8850. doi: 10.1097/MD.0000000000008850
32. Henckel E, Svenson U, Nordlund B, Berggren Brostrom E, Hedlin G, Degerman S, et al. Telomere length was similar in school-age children with bronchopulmonary dysplasia and allergic asthma. *Acta Paediatr.* (2018) 107:1395–401. doi: 10.1111/apa.14294
33. Wang P, Wu L, Ju Y, Fu M, Shuang T, Qian Z, et al. Age-Dependent allergic asthma development and cystathionine gamma-lyase deficiency. *Antioxid Redox Signal* (2017) 27:931–44. doi: 10.1089/ars.2016.6875
34. Tschopp CM, Spiegl N, Didichenko S, Lutmann W, Julius P, Virchow JC, et al. Granzyme B, a novel mediator of allergic inflammation: its induction and release in blood basophils and human asthma. *Blood* (2006) 108:2290–9. doi: 10.1182/blood-2006-03-010348
35. Lv J, Xiong Y, Li W, Cui X, Cheng X, Leng Q, et al. IL-37 inhibits IL-4/IL-13-induced CCL11 production and lung eosinophilia in murine allergic asthma. *Allergy* (2018) 73:1642–52. doi: 10.1111/all.13395
36. Dugger KJ, Chrisman T, Sayner SL, Chastain P, Watson K, Estes R. Beta-2 adrenergic receptors increase TREG cell suppression in an OVA-induced allergic asthma mouse model when mice are moderate aerobically exercised. *BMC Immunol.* (2018) 19:9. doi: 10.1186/s12865-018-0244-1
37. Datta A, Moitra S, Das PK, Mondal S, Omar Faruk SM, Hazra I, et al. Allergen immunotherapy modulates sensitivity of Treg cells to apoptosis in a rat model of allergic asthma. *Immunotherapy* (2017) 9:1239–51. doi: 10.2217/imt-2017-0038
38. Wu HY, Maron R, Tukpah A-M, Weiner HL. Mucosal anti-CD3 monoclonal antibody attenuates collagen-induced arthritis that is associated with induction of LAP+ regulatory T cells and is enhanced by administration of an emulsome-based Th2-skewing adjuvant. *J Immunol.* (2010) 185:3401–07. doi: 10.4049/jimmunol.1000836
39. Fiorentino DF, Zlotnik A, Vieira P, Mosmann TR, Howard M, Moore KW, O'Garra A. IL-10 acts on the antigen-presenting cell to inhibit cytokine production by Th1 cells. *J Immunol.* (1991) 146:3444–51.
40. Wang P, Wu P, Anthes JC, Siegel MI, Egan RW, Billah MM. Interleukin-10 inhibits interleukin-8 production in human neutrophils. *Blood* (1994) 83:2678–83.
41. Ogawa Y, Duru EA, Ameredes BT. Role of IL-10 in the resolution of airway inflammation. *Curr Mol Med.* (2008) 8:437–45. doi: 10.2174/156652408785160907
42. Wang Y-H, Voo KS, Liu B, Chen C-Y, Uygungil B, Spoede W, et al. A novel subset of CD4+ TH2 memory/effector cells that produce inflammatory IL-17 cytokine and promote the exacerbation of chronic allergic asthma. *J Exp Med.* (2010) 207:2479–91. doi: 10.1084/jem.20101376
43. Rathinavel A, Sankar J, Mohammed Sadullah SS, Niranjali Devaraj S. Oligomeric proanthocyanidins protect myocardium by mitigating left ventricular remodeling in isoproterenol-induced postmyocardial infarction. *Fundam Clin Pharmacol.* (2018) 32:51–59. doi: 10.1111/fcp.12325
44. Sheu JJ, Ali HEE, Cheng BC, Chiang HJ, Sung PH, Chen KH, et al. Extracorporeal shock wave treatment attenuated left ventricular dysfunction and remodeling in mini-pig with cardiorenal syndrome. *Oncotarget* (2017) 8:54747–63. doi: 10.18632/oncotarget.18287
45. Blomhoff R. Retinoids may increase fibrotic potential of TGF-beta: crosstalk between two multi-functional effectors. *Hepatology* (1997) 26:1067–8. doi: 10.1053/jhep.1997.v26.ajhep0261067

46. Wang W, Koka V, Lan HY. Transforming growth factor-β and Smad signalling in kidney diseases. *Nephrology* (2005) 10:48–56. doi: 10.1111/j.1440-1797.2005.00334.x
47. Bira Y, Tani K, Nishioka Y, Miyata J, Sato K, Hayashi A, Nakaya Y, Sone S. Transforming growth factor β stimulates rheumatoid synovial fibroblasts via the type II receptor. *Modern Rheumatol.* (2005) 15:108–13. doi: 10.3109/s10165-004-0378-2
48. Manuyakorn W, Kamchaisatian W, Atamasirikul K, Sasisakulporn C, Direkwattanachai C, Benjaponpitak S. Serum TGF-beta1 in atopic asthma. *Asian Pac J Allergy Immunol.* (2008) 26:185–9.
49. Datau EA, Mewengkang H, Matheos JC, Purnawan I, Wibisono M, Wongdjaja K, et al. Clinical efficacy and laboratory improvement of bacillus calmette-guerin vaccination on adult atopic asthma: a cohort study. *World Allergy Organ J.* (2008) 1:63–9. doi: 10.1097/WOX.0b013e31816c8b85
50. Li Y, Liu Y, Fu Y, Wei T, Le Guyader L, et al. The triggering of apoptosis in macrophages by pristine graphene through the MAPK and TGF-beta signaling pathways. *Biomaterials* (2012) 33:402–11. doi: 10.1016/j.biomaterials.2011.09.091
51. Hong JG, Dong WF, Zhou XJ. Effect of montelukast sodium on TGF-beta(1) of peripheral blood mononuclear cells from children with mild persistent asthma. *Zhonghua Er Ke Za Zhi* (2011) 49:679–84.
52. Sprouse ML, Scavuzzo MA, Blum S, Shevchenko I, Lee T, Makedonas G, et al. High self-reactivity drives T-bet and potentiates Treg function in tissue-specific autoimmunity. *JCI Insight* (2018) 3:97322. doi: 10.1172/jci.insight.97322.
53. Dash B, Shapiro MJ, Chung JY, Romero Arocha S, Shapiro VS. Treg-specific deletion of NKAP results in severe, systemic autoimmunity due to peripheral loss of Tregs. *J Autoimmun.* (2018) 89:139–48. doi: 10.1016/j.jaut.2017.12.013
54. von Boehmer H. Mechanisms of suppression by suppressor T cells. *Nat Immunol.* (2005) 6:338–44. doi: 10.1038/ni1180
55. Taylor A, Verhagen J, Blaser K, Akdis M, Akdis CA. Mechanisms of immune suppression by interleukin-10 and transforming growth factor-beta: the role of T regulatory cells. *Immunology* (2006) 117:433–42. doi: 10.1111/j.1365-2567.2006.02321.x
56. Sasaki Y, Sakai M, Miyazaki S, Higuma S, Shiozaki A, Saito S. Decidual and peripheral blood CD4+ CD25+ regulatory T cells in early pregnancy subjects and spontaneous abortion cases. *MHR* (2004) 10:347–53. doi: 10.1093/molehr/gah044
57. Huarong H, Tiantian L, Xiandi M. The changes of CD4~+ CD25~+ regulatory T cells in peripheral blood and their significance in the disease severity of asthmatic children. *New Med.* (2009) 4:005. doi: 10.1111/j.1365-2249.2007.03329.x
58. Ramirez-Velazquez C, Castillo EC, Guido-Bayardo L, Ortiz-Navarrete V. IL-17-producing peripheral blood CD177+ neutrophils increase in allergic asthmatic subjects. *Allergy Asthma Clin Immunol.* (2013) 9:23. doi: 10.1186/1710-1492-9-23

21

The Differences in Acute Management of Asthma in Adults and Children

Richard Chavasse [1†] *and Stephen Scott* [2,3*†]

[1] *Consultant Respiratory Paediatrician, St George's University Hospitals NHS Foundation Trust, St George's University of London, London, United Kingdom,* [2] *Consultant in Respiratory Medicine, The Countess of Chester Hospital NHS Foundation Trust, Cheshire, United Kingdom,* [3] *Chester Medical School, The University of Chester, Chester, United Kingdom*

Correspondence:
Stephen Scott
stephenscott2@nhs.net

[†] *These authors have contributed equally to this work*

Acute asthma or wheeze is a common presentation to emergency services for both adults and children. Although there are phenotypic differences between asthma syndromes, the management of acute symptoms follow similar lines. This article looks at the similarities and differences in approaches for children and adults. Some of these may be age dependent, such as the physiological parameters used to define the severity of the attack or the use of age appropriate inhaler devices. Other differences may reflect the availability of evidence. In other areas there is conflicting evidence between adult and pediatric studies such as a temporary increase in dose of inhaled corticosteroids during an acute attack. Overall there are more similarities than differences.

Keywords: asthma, attack, adults, children, treatment

INTRODUCTION

Asthma is the commonest chronic condition in the UK with a UK lifetime prevalence of patient-reported clinician-diagnosed asthma of 15.6%. In 1 year asthma results in 6.3 million primary care consultations and 93,000 hospital in-patient episodes. The costs of asthma are estimated at £1.1 billion 12% of which is accounted for by hospital care and 14% for primary care consultations (1). Many physicians in both adult and pediatric medicine across the whole healthcare economy will therefore be expected to manage patients who may present with an acute attack of their disease so knowledge of this area is very important for good patient care. Guidelines for the management of an acute asthma attacks are documented in a number of national and international publications (2–4). Management of an acute attack may start with treatment at home and may progress to treatment in primary care, the emergency department and on the hospital wards including intensive care. This article looks at similarities and differences in the management of acute management between adults and children of varying ages.

The definition of asthma is difficult and there is no gold standard, and it is increasingly recognized that asthma as a condition is made up of a number of phenotypes (5, 6). The use of phenotypic variations is more likely to inform and modify chronic management, rather than the acute management of a crisis at the present time. The first recognized presentation of asthma is not uncommonly an acute attack, particularly in children, and therefore may present a diagnostic challenge.

The British Thoracic Society and Scottish Intercollegiate Guidelines Network (BTS/SIGN) asthma guideline precis the definitions of asthma as the presence of more than one symptom of wheeze, breathlessness, chest tightness and cough associated with variable airflow obstruction. Other definitions of asthma, in both children and adults, include airway hyper-responsiveness and airway inflammation as components of the disease (BTS/SIGN) (2). The National Institute of Clinical Effectiveness (NICE) have suggested a diagnosis should not be made without objective evidence of airway obstruction or inflammation (3).

In younger children, particularly those <5 years of age, the diagnosis of asthma (or phenotypes of wheeze) is difficult and often controversial (7). Acute wheeze is however a very common presenting complaint to both primary and secondary care and may frequently be recurrent and troublesome. Whilst the intricacies of diagnosis is beyond the context of this piece, recognition of this difficulty is important. Asthma diagnosis and phenotypes are subjects covered elsewhere in this series of articles. As is not uncommon, the evidence for different treatments are less well studied in the younger age groups. For the purpose of this review it will be assumed that the diagnosis of asthma is secure and we will be comparing / contrasting the differences in children and adult asthma.

DEFINITION OF ADULTS AND CHILDREN

The definition of an adult will be taken as a person over 18 years, accepting there is a considerable cross over in the adolescent age group. In most hospital emergency departments, adolescents under 18 are usually managed in the pediatric area, and if necessary by pediatricians, although it is recognized that different healthcare systems may have different policies. Guidelines and clinical trials vary in their cut off ages with many studies including adolescents over 12 in "adult" studies. Age cut offs are clearly not as relevant to provision of care in primary care and the home environment, however the age and maturity of the individual patient should be considered when agreeing a management plan. For children there are differences in the approach to the young, preschool child (<5 years) and there is very little evidence for the management of asthma symptoms in children under 1 year of age.

DEFINITIONS & ASSESSMENT OF ACUTE ASTHMA

An acute asthma attack represents a deterioration in symptoms and lung function from the patient's normal status. Distinguishing between a lower respiratory tract infection and an asthma attack can be challenging, particularly in young children. This can include shortness of breath, wheezing, cough, and chest tightness (4). Attacks are marked by a decrease from baseline in objective measures of pulmonary function, such as peak expiratory flow rate and FEV1. Objective measures, such as FEV1 are less easy to perform in children and young persons, and PEFR can be unreliable in children and young persons if they have not used the technique before and are highly unlikely to be achieved in children <5 years of age (8). In some individuals, in particular those with poor adherence and/or more severe asthma, there can be a challenge in distinguishing between a mild asthma attack and long-standing poorly controlled asthma; the challenge in in part due to symptoms being common to both a mild asthma attack and poorly controlled asthma and in part due to guidelines not defining criteria for a mild asthma attack.

Pharmacological management is entirely dependent upon the severity of the attack which in turn is defined by a number of objective and subjective findings. These differ between adults and children, reflecting the age-related physiologic differences and the reliability of pulmonary function testing in children. Definitions from the BTS/SIGN and Global Initiative for Asthma (GINA) guidelines are outlined in **Table 1**.

PRE-HOSPITAL MANAGEMENT OF ACUTE ASTHMA

Adults are encouraged to have a personalized asthma action plan (PAAP) in place which empowers them to increase treatments in response to increasing symptoms or decreasing PEFR (9). The PAAP should advise them when to seek medical assistance. In children PAAPs advice only recommends increasing short acting beta agonist. A Cochrane database systematic review of 4 clinical trials in children concluded that symptom-based PAAPs are superior to peak flow PAAPs for preventing acute care visits (10). There was insufficient data to firmly conclude how symptom-based PAAPs were superior of the two. For example the observed superiority of symptom-based PAAPs may have been due to greater adherence to the monitoring strategy, earlier identification of onset of deteriorations, higher threshold for presentation to acute care settings, or the specific treatment recommendations (10).

Most adult PAAPs recommend the increased use short acting beta agonists at the onset of acute symptoms (11). Most pediatric management plans suggest a titrated increased dose of beta-2 agonist using doses between 2 and 10 puffs of a salbutamol (pressure dose metered dose inhaler and spacer device) up to every 4 h (12). Safety net advice to seek medical advice and call an ambulance if not responding to treatment should be included. Judicial use of rescue oral steroids at home is sometimes included, although there is no consistent evidence of benefit for this practice (13).

A second approach in adults may be the use of a single combination inhaler for both preventer and relief [Maintenance and Reliever Therapy: (MART)] which patients may titrate in accordance to their symptoms (14). Preparations are not currently licensed or in formulations for younger adolescents or children in the UK.

A recent study in adults suggested a 4-fold increase in inhaled steroid dose used early during an attack resulted in fewer severe asthma exacerbations than a plan in which the dose was not increased and this would be a reasonable self-management strategy in this situation (15). A similar pediatric paper suggesting a quintupled dose of ICS in children however showed no benefit (16). This may reflect a difference in causation of an attack, different responses by age or methodological differences between the studies.

Any patients with features of acute severe or life-threatening asthma should be referred to hospital immediately.

TABLE 1 | Comparison of symptoms and signs associated with levels of acute asthma severity in adults and children the BTS/SIGN (1) and GINA (4) asthma guidelines.

	BTS/SIGN		GINA	
	Adult	**Children**	**Adult & Children >5years**	**Children (0-5)**
Moderate	Increasing symptoms PEFR >50–75% best or predicted No "severe" symptoms	Able to talk in sentences $SpO_2 \geq 92\%$ HR-≤140/min* or 125/min** RR-≤40/min* or 30/min** PEFR ≥50%** best or predicted No "severe" symptoms	Talks in phrases Prefers sitting to lying Not agitated Respiratory rate increased Accessory muscles not used Pulse rate 100-120 bpm SaO_2 in air 90-95% PEF >50% predicted or best	Breathless Agitated Pulse rate ≤200 bpm (0–3), ≤180 (4–5 years) $SaO_2 \geq 92\%$
Severe	Any one of: Inability to complete sentences in one breath PEFR: 33–50% best or predicted HR ≥ 110/min RR ≥ 25/min	Can't complete sentences in one breath or too breathless to talk or feed $SpO_2 < 92\%$ HR ≥ 140/min* or 125/min** RR ≥ 40/min* or 30/min** PEFR 33–50%** best or predicted	Talks in words Sits hunched forwards Agitated Respiratory rate >30 bpm Accessory muscles in use Pulse rate >120 bpm SaO_2 <90% in air PEFR ≤50% predicted or best	Unable to speak or drink Central cyanosis Confusion or drowsiness Marked subcostal and/or sub-glottic retractions SaO_2 <92% Silent chest on auscultation Pulse rate >200 (0–3 years) or >180 bpm (4–5 years)
Life threatening	Severe attack with any of: Altered conscious level Exhaustion Arrhythmia Hypotension Cyanosis Silent Chest Poor respiratory effort PEFR <33% best or predicted SpO_2 <92% PaO_2 <8 kPa Normal $PaCO_2$ 4.6–6 kPa	Severe attack with any of:Silent Chest Cyanosis Poor respiratory effort Hypotension Confusion Exhaustion SpO_2 <92% PEFR <33%** best or predicted	Drowsy Confused Silent chest	
Near fatal	Raised $PaCO_2$ and/or requiring mechanical ventilation			

*children 1–5 years; **children over 5 years.*

MEDICAL MANAGEMENT OF ACUTE ASTHMA IN HEALTHCARE FACILITIES

Oxygen

It is essential to monitor oxygen saturations when assessing an asthma attack. In adults there is evidence that hyperoxia may be detrimental plus there is also a possibility that the patient may have chronic obstruction so that the delivery of oxygen should be controlled to maintain an SpO2 level of 94–98% (17).

In children with saturations <92% in air after initial bronchodilator treatment it is advised that inpatient hospital treatment will be required as this reflects more severe asthma (18, 19). Oxygen should be administered to any child with acute asthma with SpO2 <94% via a tight fitting face mask or nasal cannula at sufficient flow rates to achieve normal saturations of 94–98%.

Short Acting Bronchodilators

The initial management of an acute asthma attack is usually given by the inhaled route. In adults it is recommended that in non-life threatening acute asthma, beta agonists can be given through repeated actuations of a pMDI via an appropriate large volume spacer. The recommendation is to give 4 puffs (400 mcg) as the initial dose and increase by 2 puffs every 2 min up to 10 puffs if needed. In life threatening asthma however wet nebulization of beta agonists with oxygen is preferable. Adult patients who do not respond to initial nebulization of beta agonist may be considered for repeated doses at 15–30 min intervals or continuous nebulization at 5–10 mg/h (2).

In Children, a pMDI and age-appropriate spacer device is the preferred option for delivering inhaled beta agonists with mild to moderate asthma as this is less likely to produce a tachycardia and hypoxia than using a nebulizer (20, 21). A facemask connected to the mouthpiece of a spacer is recommended in children <3 years old. In children drug dosing should be escalated as required from two puffs of salbutamol suitable for mild attacks up to 10 puffs for more severe attacks with 30–60 s between puffs. The inhalers should be activated into the spacer in in individual puffs and inhaled immediately by tidal breathing (for five breaths). In the hospital setting, with appropriate monitoring, doses can be repeated every 20 min over an hour if necessary. In children with severe or life-threatening asthma should receive nebulized bronchodilators driven by oxygen. These can be given in combination with ipratropium bromide which is recommended if there is a poor response to salbutamol alone (22). Repeated doses can be given every 20 min over a 1–2 h period. In contrast to adult recommendations continuous nebulized beta agonists are of no greater benefit than the use of frequent intermittent doses in the same hourly dosage (2, 23, 24).

After the first few hours salbutamol can be tapered down to one to two hourly and ipratropium tapered to four to six hourly or discontinued. In adults ipratropium bromide is recommended in acute severe or life-threatening asthma but is not necessary in milder asthma attacks or after stabilization.

Steroids

For adults and children it is important to give steroids early during an acute attack. Steroid tablets are as effective as injected steroids and should be given for at least 5 days in adults or until recovery. Evidence for the ideal duration of oral steroid treatment is still required (25). Once recovery is achieved, steroids can be stopped abruptly and do not need to be tapered unless the patient is on maintenance steroids or if they have received a prolonged course of three or more weeks (26). Inhaled steroid treatment should continue during prescription of oral steroids (2).

In children, oral prednisolone is the steroid of choice for asthma attacks and intravenous corticosteroids are only indicated for children who are vomiting or who have very severe symptoms which prevent swallowing (27). Some studies using dexamethasone have shown potential equivalence to prednisolone with the potential to reduce the number of doses and therefore potentially improving treatment adherence (28). The use of oral steroids is more controversial in preschool children (age 1–5). This may reflect the presence of common symptoms in asthma and lower respiratory tract infection in this age group. Additionally there may be more than one acute asthma phenotype, but one study considered this and found no difference in outcome between children with "viral induced wheeze" with and without atopy (29). Different prednisolone dose schedules have been recommended from 0.5–2 mg /kg (30) and others recommend an age related dose schedule (2). In children recommendations are usually for 3 days of treatment but may need to be extended from 5 to 10 days to bring about recovery. Tapering is not necessary unless the course exceeds 14 days.

There is no evidence to support the use of Inhaled steroids as an alternative to oral steroids during an asthma attack of this severity but it is good practice to continue the usual maintenance inhaled steroids during an attack (2).

Second Line Treatments

Magnesium

There is some evidence that intravenous magnesium sulfate has bronchodilator effect during an acute asthma attack (31). In adults there is limited evidence that a single dose of iv magnesium may be some benefit in adults with a PEF <50%. This is felt to be safe and may improve lung function and reduce intubation rates in those with acute severe asthma. It may also reduce admission to hospital with asthma from ED in adults who have had little or no response to standard treatment. It should only be used following consultation with senior medical staff (2).

The use of IV magnesium has become more frequent in children with acute asthma. There is relatively little evidence compared to other intravenous therapies although there is one comparative study showing a more rapid improvement compared to IV salbutamol or aminophylline (32). It is generally safe with few side effects. It should be used if there is a poor response to first line therapies and is not recommended in mild to moderate asthma attacks.

The use of nebulized magnesium has been studied in one large UK based trial (33). Overall the benefits were small although did seem to offer some benefit when added to nebulized salbutamol and ipratropium in the first hour of hospital treatment in children presenting with a short duration of acute severe asthma symptoms presenting with an $SpO2 <92\%$ (34). At the time of writing, the role of nebulized magnesium in both adults and children is uncertain.

Aminophylline

In adults evidence suggests that the addition of intravenous aminophylline is unlikely to add any additional bronchodilation compared to standard care and side effects such as arrhythmias and vomiting are increased (35). However, patients with near fatal asthma with a poor response to initial therapy may gain additional benefit from IV aminophylline. It is advised that before its use consultation should take place with a senior member of medical staff as these patients are likely to be rare (2).

In children, aminophylline was previously considered the first line IV treatment following a poor response to initial management (bronchodilators and steroids) but now intravenous magnesium is recommended as first line due to reduced side effects and equal efficacy (2). There is some evidence of benefit in severe or life threatening asthma (36). The risk of side effects is high and ECG monitoring is recommended with the patient monitored in an HDU/PICU environment.

IV Salbutamol

There may be some benefit for the use of IV salbutamol in both adults and children who have not responded to first line treatments and IV magnesium (37).

In children an initial bolus dose (15 mcg/kg) may be given. In comparison with IV aminophylline (bolus and infusion) this has been shown to give equivalent results. Initially it was thought to cause fewer side effects compared to aminophylline but more recently nausea, tachycardia and lactic acidosis have been frequently recognized. There is very limited evidence for the use of a salbutamol infusion in children but is sometimes utilized in the PICU environment.

Antibiotics

In adults an infection precipitating an attack is most likely to be viral and therefore routine prescription of antibiotics is not indicated. Objective measures such as serum procalcitonin where available should be used to guide decisions on using antibiotics (2).

TABLE 2 | Summary of similarities and differences in the diagnoses, assessment and treatment of acute asthma in adults and children.

	Similarities	Differences
Diagnosis	Same symptoms	Challenge in distinguishing from lower respiratory tract infection may be greater in children
Assessment	The same physiological parameters are used in assessment (i.e., Respiratory rate, Heart rate, Oxygen saturations)	Physiological parameters differ numerically between adults and children. Achievability and reliability of PEFR and FEV_1 in children is lower than in adults
Stepping up treatment	Actions plans recommend using short acting beta agonists when symptoms occur	Only adult personal action plans (based on good evidence) recommend MART of quadroupling ICS dose for worsening control/minor asthma attacks
Supplemental oxygen treatment	Required when oxygen saturation are below 92% in all age groups	Aim for ceiling 98% in adults due to potential overlap with COPD
First line treatment	Same medications used	Doses differ in children and adults, e.g., initial short acting beta agonist 400 microg in adults but in children is 200 microg increasing to 1,000 microg
Second line treatment	Same medications used (i.e., intravenous magnesium, salbutamol and aminophylline)	No major differences at this level

In children the role of bacterial infection is also less common than a viral trigger. Antibiotics are not recommended. Procalcitonin is not routinely used at present in children. CRP is more frequently used but less specific.

Critical Care

In both adults and children with acute asthma and a poor response to standard therapy it is important to involve clinicians with the appropriate skills in airway management and critical care support early. There is little good quality evidence to guide treatment at this stage and a national audit of treatment for acute asthma in adults in the UK found a wide variation in clinical practice (38).

In adults admission to critical care is recommended in those requiring ventilator support and acute severe life-threatening asthma indicated by: deteriorating PEF, persisting or worsening hypoxia, hypercapnia, arterial blood gas analysis showing fall in pH or rising hydrogen concentration, exhaustion, feeble respiration, drowsiness, confusion, altered conscious state or respiratory arrest (2).

In children admitted to hospital with status asthmaticus two small studies have reported the use of non-invasive ventilation suggesting that it is safe and feasible but there was insufficient evidence of its effectiveness. In adults there has also been suggestions that the use of NIV can be safe and effective however the evidence is limited and inconclusive. One trial of NIV in a small number of patients showed improvement in hospitalization rates, discharge from emergency departments and lung function. Other trials have shown safety and feasibility of using NIV in treating acute exacerbations of asthma but little evidence of benefit in comparison with standard care. It is recommended that NIV should only be considered in adults in a critical care or equivalent setting (2).

Invasive ventilation strategies are beyond the scope of this article.

The BTS asthma guidelines are able to recommend the following advice for therapies at this stage. In both adults and children Ketamine may be considered as a potential bronchodilator although further prospective trials are required before conclusions about effectiveness can be drawn (39, 40).

In children the anesthetic gas Sevoflurane is potentially an option for correcting high levels of $PaCO_2$ in mechanically ventilated children however its use would be limited to areas where appropriate scavenging facilities to extract gas are available (41).

There is an increasing trend in the use of Recombinant DNase in pediatric intensive care in children with acute asthma due to airway plugging. There is little or no published evidence to support this practice. A study in non-intubated adults with severe asthma showed no improvement in FEV_1 (42).

Extracorporeal Membrane Oxygenation (ECMO)

ECMO is a form of cardiopulmonary life-support, where blood is drained from the vascular system, circulated outside the body by a mechanical pump, and then reinfused into the circulation. While outside the body, hemoglobin becomes fully saturated with oxygen and CO_2 is removed. Oxygenation is determined by flow rate, and CO_2 elimination can be controlled by adjusting the rate of countercurrent gas flow through the oxygenator. It is a highly specialized form of treatment and available in only a few centers in the UK. It has been shown to be useful and an option in severe asthma refractory to mechanical ventilation in both children and adults by providing adequate gas exchange and preventing lung injury. However, careful management is required to avoid complications (43).

Discharge and Follow Up

In adults it is recommended discharge can be considered when clinical signs are compatible with home management i.e., medical therapy can continue safely at home. Patients with PEF <75% best or predicted and diurnal variability of PEF >25% are at greater risk of early relapse and readmission therefore this should be borne in mind when deciding on timing of discharge. This is also true in children (2).

In both adults and children it is important to assess and attend to correct risk factors that may have lead to a loss of control of asthma leading to admission e.g., smoking or exposure to smoke in the household in children. Education prior to discharge is important including advice on inhaler technique, a review of the personal asthma plan and, if used, PEF record keeping. Tools such as the BTS asthma discharge bundle are available to provide help with this process (44).

All patients both adult and children should have an appointment arranged with their primary care team within 48 h of hospital discharge. Secondary care review should be arranged within a few weeks.

CONCLUSION/SUMMARY

There are similarities and differences in the diagnoses, assessment and treatment of acute asthma in adults and children, and these are summarized in **Table 2**. The mainstay of management is to ensure early assessment of severity with appropriate use of bronchodilators with corticosteroids. There are some differences in the recommendations of how these medications are given and their associated doses but because the pathological processes are essentially the same the general principles of treatment are also the same. The more cautious use of oral corticosteroids in children may reflect concern over longer term side effects as well as questionable response in preschool children. The use of variable dose regimes of inhaled steroids may reflect the availability of suitable drug preparations and the difference between an individual feeling their own innate symptoms and a parent recognizing their child's symptoms.

AUTHOR CONTRIBUTIONS

All authors listed have made a substantial, direct and intellectual contribution to the work, and approved it for publication.

REFERENCES

1. Mukherjee M, Stoddart A, Gupta RP, Nwaru BI, Farr A, Heaven M, et al. The epidemiology, healthcare and societal burden and costs of asthma in the UK and its member nations: analysis of standalone and linked national databases. *BMC Med.* (2016) 14:113.doi: 10.1186/s12916-016-0657-8
2. Health improvement Scotland. *BTS/SIGN British Guideline for the Management of Asthma.* SIGN 153 (2016).
3. NICE NG80. *Asthma: Diagnosis, Monitoring and Chronic Asthma Management, NICE NG80* (2017). Available online at: https://www.nice.org.uk/guidance/ng80 (Accessed October 25, 2018).
4. Global Initiative for Asthma. *Global Strategy for Asthma Management and Prevention.* Available online at: http://ginasthma.org/ginareports/ (Accessed October 25, 2018).
5. Haldar P, Pavord ID, Shaw DE, Berry MA, Thomas M, Brightling CE., et al. Cluster analysis and clinical asthma phenotypes. *Am J Respir Crit Care Med.* (2008) 178:218–24. doi: 10.1164/rccm.200711-1754OC
6. Moore WC, Meyers DA, Wenzel SE, Teague WG, Li H, Li X., et al. Identification of asthma phenotypes using cluster analysis in the Severe Asthma Research Program. *Am J Respir Crit Care Med.* (2010) 181:315–23. doi: 10.1164/rccm.200906-0896OC
7. Lenney W, Bush A, Fitzgerald DA, Fletcher M, Ostrem A, Pedersen S, et al. Improving the global diagnosis and management of asthma in children. *Thorax.* (2018) 73:662–9. doi: 10.1136/thoraxjnl-2018-211626
8. Beydon N, Davis SD, Lombardi E, Allen JL, Arets HG, Aurora P, et al. An official American Thoracic Society/European Respiratory Society Statement: pulmonary function testing in preschool children. *Am J Respir Crit Care Med.* (2007) 175:1304–45. doi: 10.1164/rccm.200605-642ST
9. Gibson PG, Powell H. Written action plans for asthma: an evidence-based review of the key components. *Thorax.* (2004) 59:94–9. doi: 10.1136/thorax.2003.011858
10. Bhogal SK, Zemek RL, Ducharme F. Written action plans for asthma in children. *Cochrane Database Syst Rev.* (2006) 3:CD005306. doi: 10.1002/14651858.CD005306.pub2
11. Available online at: https://www.asthma.org.uk/globalassets/health-advice/resources/adults/adult-asthma-action-plan.pdf (Accessed October 25, 2018).
12. Available online at: https://www.asthma.org.uk/globalassets/health-advice/resources/children/child-asthma-action-plan.pdf (Accessed October 25, 2018).
13. Ganaie MB, Munavvar M, Gordon M, Lim HF, Evans DJ. Patient- and parent-initiated oral steroids for asthma exacerbations (Review). *Cochrane Database Syst Rev.* (2016) 12:CD012195. doi: 10.1002/14651858.CD012195.pub2
14. Kew KM, Karner C, Mindus SM, Ferrara G. Combination formoterol and budesonide as maintenance and reliever therapy versus combination inhaler maintenance for chronic asthma in adults and children. *Cochrane Database Syst Rev.* (2013) 12:CD009019. doi: 10.1002/14651858.CD009019.pub2
15. McKeever T, Mortimer K, Wilson A, Walker S, Brightling C, Skeggs A., et al. Quadrupling inhaled glucocorticoid dose to abort asthma exacerbations. *N Engl J Med.* (2018) 378:902–10. doi: 10.1056/NEJMoa1714257
16. Jackson DJ, Bacharier LB, Mauger DT, Boehmer S, Beigelman A, Chmiel JF., et al. Quintupling inhaled glucocorticoids to prevent childhood asthma exacerbations. *N Engl J Med.* (2018) 378:891–901. doi: 10.1056/NEJMoa1710988
17. Perrin K, Wijesinghe M, Healy B, Wadsworth K, Bowditch R, Bibby S., et al. Randomised controlled trial of high concentration versus titrated oxygen therapy in severe exacerbations of asthma. *Thorax.* (2011) 66:937–41. doi: 10.1136/thx.2010.155259
18. Connett GJ, Lenney W. Use of pulse oximetry in the hospital management of acute asthma in childhood. *Paediatr Pulmonol.* (1993) 15:345–9. doi: 10.1002/ppul.1950150606
19. Wright R, Santucchi K, Jay G, Steele D. Evaluation of pre- and post-treatment pulse oximetry in acute childhood asthma. *Acad Emerg Med.* (1997) 4:114–7. doi: 10.1111/j.1553-2712.1997.tb03716.x
20. Leversha AM, Campanella SG, Aickin RP, Asher MI. Costs and effectiveness of spacer versus nebulizer in young children with moderate and severe acute asthma. *J Pediatr.* (2000) 136:497–502. doi: 10.1016/S0022-3476(00)90013-1
21. Cates C, Rowe B. Holding chambers versus nebulisers for beta-agonist treatment of acute asthma. *Cochrane Database Syst Rev.* (2000) 9:CD000052. doi: 10.1002/14651858.CD000052.pub3
22. Plotnick LH, Ducharme FM. Combined inhaled anticholinergic agents and beta-2-agonists for initial treatment of acute asthma in children. *Cochrane Database Syst Rev.* (2000) 8:CD000060. doi: 10.1002/14651858.CD000060
23. Khine H, Fuchs SM, Saville AL. Continuous vs intermittent nebulized albuterol for emergency management of asthma. *Acad Emerg Med.* (1996) 3:1019–24. doi: 10.1111/j.1553-2712.1996.tb03346.x
24. Papo M, Frank J, Thompson A. A rospective randomised study of continuous versus intermittent nebulized albutarol for severe status asthmaticus in children. *Crit Care Med.* (1993) 21:1479–86. doi: 10.1097/00003246-199310000-00015
25. Normansell R, Kew KM, Mansour G. Different oral corticosteroid regimens for acute asthma. *Cochrane Database Syst Rev.* (2016) 5:CD011801. doi: 10.1002/14651858.CD011801.pub2
26. Hatton MQ, Vathenen AS, Allen MJ, Davies S, Cooke NJ. A comparison of 'abruptly stopping' with 'tailing off' oral corticosteroids in acute asthma. *Respir Med.* (1995) 89:101–4. doi: 10.1016/0954-6111(95)90191-4
27. Rowe B, Spooner C, Ducharme F, Bretzlaff JA, Bota GW. Early emergency department treatment of acute asthma with systemic corticosteroids. *Cochrane Database Syst Rev.* (2001) CD002178. doi: 10.1002/14651858.CD002178
28. Greenberg R, Kerby G, RooseveltG. A comparison of oral dexamethasone with oral prednisolone in paediatric asthma exacerbations treated in the emergency department. *Clin Pediatr.* (2008) 47:817–23. doi: 10.1177/0009922808316988

29. Panickar J, Lakhanpaul M, Lambert PC, Kenia P, Stephenson T, Smyth A., et al. Oral prednisolone for preschool children with acute virus-induced wheezing. *NEJM.* (2009) 360:329–38. doi: 10.1056/NEJMoa0804897
30. Langton Hewer S, Hobbs J, Reid F, Lenney W. Prednisolone in acute asthma: clinical response to three dosages. *Respir Med.* (1998) 92:541–6. doi: 10.1016/S0954-6111(98)90305-5
31. Mohammed S, Goodacre S. Intravenous and nebulised magnesium sulphate for acute asthma: systematic review and meta-analysis. *Emerg Med J.* (2007) 24:823–30. doi: 10.1136/emj.2007.052050
32. Singhi S, Grover S, Bansal A, Chopra K. Randomised comparison of intravenous magnesium sulphate, terbutaline and aminophylline for children with acute severe asthma. *Acta Paediatr.* (2014) 103:1301–6. doi: 10.1111/apa.12780
33. Powell C, Dwan K, Milan SJ, Beasley R, Hughes R, Knopp-Sihota JA, et al. Inhaled magnesium sulfate in the treatment of acute asthma. *Cochrane Database Syst Rev.* (2012) 11:CD003898. doi: 10.1002/14651858.CD003898.pub6
34. Powell C, Kolamunnage-Dona R, Lowe J, Boland A, Petrou S, Doull I., et al. Magnesium sulphate in acute severe asthma in children (MAGNETIC): a randomised placebo-controlled trial. *Lancet.* (2013) 1:301–8. doi: 10.1016/S2213-2600(13)70037-7
35. Parameswaran K, Belda J, Rowe BH. Addition of intravenous aminophylline to beta2-agonists in adults with acute asthma. *Cochrane Database Syst Rev.* (2000) CD002742. doi: 10.1002/14651858.CD002742
36. Yung M, South M. Randomised controlled trial of aminophylline for severe acute asthma. *Arch Dis Child.* (1998) 79:405–10. doi: 10.1136/adc.79.5.405
37. Travers A, Jones AP, Kelly K, Barker SJ, Camargo CA, Rowe BH. Intravenous beta2-agonists for acute asthma in the emergency department. *Cochrane Database Syst Rev.* (2001) 1:CD002988. doi: 10.1002/14651858.CD002988
38. *BTS 2016 UK Asthma Audit Report.* Available online at: https://www.brit-thoracic.org.uk/document-library/audit-and-quality-improvement/audit-reports/bts-adult-asthma-report-2016/ (Accessed October 25, 2018).
39. Goyal S, Agrawal A. Ketamine in status asthmaticus: a review. *Indian J Crit Care Med.* (2013) 17:154–61. doi: 10.4103/0972-5229.117048
40. Jat KR, Chawla D. Ketamine for management of acute exacerbations of asthma in children. *Cochrane Database Syst Rev.* (2012) 11:CD009293. doi: 10.1002/14651858.CD009293.pub2
41. Schutte D, Zwitserloot AM, Houmes R, de Hoog M, Draaisma JM, Lemson J. Sevoflurane therapy for life-threatening asthma in children. *Br J Anaesth.* (2013) 111:967–70. doi: 10.1093/bja/aet257
42. Silverman RA, Foley F, Dalipi R, Kline M, Lesser M. The use of rhDNAse in severely ill, non-intubated adult asthmatics refractory to bronchodilators: a pilot study. *Respir Med.* (2012) 106:1096–102. doi: 10.1016/j.rmed.2012.04.002
43. Yeo HJ, Kim D, Jeon D, Kim YS, Rycus P, Cho WH. Extracorporeal membrane oxygenation for life-threatening asthma refractory to mechanical ventilation: analysis of the Extracorporeal Life Support Organization registry. *Crit Care.* (2017) 21:297. doi: 10.1186/s13054-017-1886-8
44. Available online at: https://www.brit-thoracic.org.uk/document-library/audit-and-quality-improvement/asthma-care-bundle/care-bundle-statement/ (Accessed October 25, 2018).

22

Measuring Airway Obstruction in Severe Asthma in Children

*Claudia Calogero, Grazia Fenu and Enrico Lombardi**

Pediatric Pulmonary Unit, "Anna Meyer" Pediatric University Hospital, Florence, Italy

***Correspondence:**
Enrico Lombardi
enrico.lombardi@meyer.it

Lung function is an important tool in the diagnosis and monitoring of patients with asthma at all ages. Airway obstruction is a typical feature of asthma and it can be assessed with several lung function techniques. Spirometry, respiratory resistance and reactance, and lung volumes are available to measure it at different ages and in children. The assessment of a bronchodilator response is always recommended to show the reversibility of the obstruction. Poor lung function is a predictor of poor asthma outcome and a low Forced Expiratory Volume in the first second of expiration percent predicted measured with spirometry, has been shown to be associated with a higher risk of having an exacerbation during the following year independently of the presence of asthma symptoms. In severe asthma lung function assessment is used to distinguish different phenotypes, children with severe asthma have worse airflow limitation prior to administration of a bronchodilator than children with non severe asthma. Airway resistance and reactance are indirect measurements of airway obstruction and they can be measured with the forced oscillation technique, which is feasible also in non-collaborative children. This technique can be more informative in discriminating patients with asthma from healthy controls and is able to indicate a more peripheral involvement of the airways. The role of this technique in severe asthma is still debated. In conclusion lung function is useful in the clinical management of children with severe asthma.

Keywords: severe asthma, lung function, children, respiratory resistance, reactance

INTRODUCTION

Lung function measurements are very important in the diagnosis and monitoring of patients with asthma, especially those with severe asthma. Several techniques are available for children and adults to measure airway obstruction, which is a typical feature of asthma. Furthermore, tracking of lung function, from childhood to adulthood, has been shown in several studies, highlighting that reduced lung function at young age is associated with the development of chronic obstructive pulmonary disease (COPD) in adulthood (1–3). This article will cover the main pulmonary function techniques used in children to detect airway obstruction and their clinical utility in the diagnosis and management of severe asthma in children.

SPIROMETRY

Spirometry indices are obtained with a forced expiratory maneuver according to the technical European Respiratory Society (ERS)/American Respiratory Society (ATS) recommendations (4). Modified acceptability criteria for spirometry in preschool children (2–5 years) have also been published (5). The Forced Expiratory Volume in the first second of expiration (FEV_1) and its ratio to Forced Vital Capacity (FEV_1/FVC) are considered the gold standard to assess airway obstruction in adults and children (6). These indices are sufficient to grade the severity of obstruction, which is very important in the evaluation of subjects with severe asthma. Obstruction is shown by an abnormal FEV_1/FVC (<80%) and is defined as mild when FEV_1 is >70% predicted, moderate 60–69%, moderately severe 50–59%, severe 35–49%, very severe <35% (7).

Once a baseline measure is obtained, the evaluation of the reversibility of the obstruction with the assessment of the bronchodilator response (BDR) is recommended, as this is a typical feature of asthma. A positive BDR is defined by the ERS/ATS recommendations as an increase in $FEV_1 \geq 12\%$ and ≥ 200 mL with respect to baseline after administration of 400 mcg of salbutamol given by metered dose inhaler via a spacer (7). However, it has been described by Tse et al. that in children this cut-off can be not enough sensitive to detect airway obstruction and can lead to a misdiagnosis of asthma (8), suggesting that a lower cut-off (8%) should be used in children.

Regarding the clinical utility of spirometry, the American Academy of Asthma, Allergy and Immunology states in the list of the Choosing Wisely Initiative "do not diagnose or manage asthma without spirometry"[1]. Also, according the most recent update of the GINA Guidelines (9) the diagnosis of asthma should be made not only based on the clinical features of the patient, such as clinical history and symptoms, but also using pulmonary function testing to detect the presence of airflow limitation. Furthermore, the NICE guidelines (10) recommend to perform spirometry in children and adults with a diagnosis of asthma to show an obstructive pattern on the test. The assessment of a bronchodilator response is also recommended to show the reversibility of the obstruction. Several guidelines on asthma also recommend to perform spirometry for monitoring asthma at each visit (10) or at least after 3 or 6 months from the beginning of treatment and on a regular basis afterwards (1–2 years) (9).

Measuring lung function is also useful as a predictor of asthma exacerbations. In the GINA guidelines (9) a low value of FEV_1 is mentioned as a predictor of poor asthma outcome. In a retrospective study in children with asthma, a low FEV_1 percent predicted (particularly when <60%) has been shown to be associated with a higher risk of having an exacerbation during the following year independently of the presence of symptoms (11). Also, Schifano et al. have described in a population of 894 asthmatic children a low concordance between symptoms and lung function results and a higher grade of asthma severity was given when spirometry was taken into account (12). This is very important in children especially when a poor awareness of symptoms is detected.

Spirometry is able to measure flows at low lung volumes that are considered to be more representative of the small airways such as the forced expiratory flow between 25 and 75% of FVC (FEF_{25-75}), at 50% of FVC ($FEF_{50,}$), and at 75% of FVC (FEF_{75}). The role of these indices in detecting airway obstruction in clinical practice is however controversial. Some authors have shown that these indices are more sensitive than FEV_1 in detecting peripheral obstruction [(13)], while others have shown that they do not affect the clinical decision more than FEV_1/FVC (14). For this reason, a recent ATS Technical Statement recommends that FEF_{25-75} should not be shown in the pulmonary function report (15).

The definition of severe asthma, according to an ERS/ATS Task Force (16), is the presence of uncontrolled symptoms despite high dose of corticosteroids and includes difficult to treat asthma and asthma resistant to therapy. Lung function assessment is necessary for confirming the diagnosis of severe asthma and to establish the phenotype. From a practical point of view, spirometry is useful in confirming the diagnosis of severe asthma in children and it should be always performed with the administration of a bronchodilator to detect airway obstruction and its reversibility. The aspect of the Flow-Volume inspiratory and expiratory loops can be also useful in the differential diagnosis of other causes of obstruction, intrathoracic or extrathoracic airway obstruction (17).

Different phenotypes of severe asthma have been described (18, 19). These phenotypes change according to age and are different in children and adults (20). Assessing airway obstruction is useful to identify the phenotypes at all age (21). Airway obstruction however, can be not present or only mild in children with severe asthma especially in between exacerbations (22–24). In respect to adults with severe asthma, children tend to have better lung function, but a greater decline overtime (25). It has been recently reported that children with severe asthma have worse airflow limitation prior to administration of a bronchodilator than children with non-severe asthma, but have similar values after BD showing an increased BDR (20).

In the TENOR Study, that included also children and adolescents, the authors have shown that acute asthmatic exacerbations can have a role in the decline of lung function, as the inflammation cascade can lead to airway remodeling and a fixed non reversible bronchoconstriction (26). In children this mechanism can be different and especially when there is eosinophilic inflammation remodeling of airways is not always present (27). Contrarily, a recent study published by Ortega et al. on lung function data retrospectively collected from the DREAM and MENSA studies on mepolizumab in severe asthmatics with eosinophilic inflammation (mainly adults with a very small proportion of adolescents), shows that a higher number of exacerbations is associated with a worsening of lung function measurements over time (28). These features can identify a more severe phenotype of asthma and each exacerbation can contribute with a loss in FEV_1 of about 50 mL/year (28). The mechanism involved is hypothesized to be a reduced elasticity of the lung as a result of airway narrowing and remodeling associated to deposition of collagen.

Lung function measurements can be used to monitor response to therapy but few data are available on severe asthma in children. Deschildre et al. published data on 1 year of real life experience on 104 children with severe asthma treated with omalizumab showing an increase of 4.9% predicted of FEV_1 at the end of the 12 months (29). A recent longitudinal study on lung function in severe asthma conducted in Brazil on 65 severe asthmatic

[1]http://choosingwisely.org/wp-content/uploads/2015/02/AAAAI-Choosing-Wisely-List.pdf

patients (between 6 and 18 years of age) receiving high dose of corticosteroids showed only a small improvement of airway reversibility (FEV_1 after bronchodilator) (30).

BODY PLETHYSMOGRAPHY

Lung function obtained with the body plethysmography allows to measure airway resistance and lung volumes, with particular interest to Total Lung Capacity (TLC) and Residual Volume (RV). RV is a good index of air trapping and is a marker of hyperinflation when the value is greater than 120% predicted. This measure can add information to the conventional spirometry especially in severe asthmatic patients. It has been shown that 49% of children having airflow obstruction with an FEV_1/FVC <80% have a significant hyperinflation (31). Sorkeness et al. in the SARP cohort, showed that children with severe asthma were more hyperinflated and air-trapped in respect to children with non severe asthma that had normal RV and TLC (32).

RESPIRATORY RESISTANCE AND REACTANCE

Airway resistance, which is an indirect measurement of airway obstruction, can be evaluated with the body plethysmograph, but its measurement requires the panting maneuver which is substantially infeasible in preschool children. Several techniques have been developed, such as the interrupter technique (Rint), the forced oscillation technique (FOT), and the measurement of specific airway resistance (sRaw) using the body plethysmograph, which are performed during tidal breathing. These techniques require only minimal collaboration and are feasible also in preschool children when spirometry cannot be performed or other techniques cannot be used. In addition to respiratory resistance, FOT offers the advantage of also measuring respiratory reactance, which can be thought of as the distensibility of the respiratory system. Technical recommendations for each technique are available (5, 33) and several reference equations have been published (34–36).

The evaluation of the bronchodilator response is also possible and different cut-off values have been reported in the literature (35, 37, 38). Those techniques, with particular regard to FOT has been suggested to be more sensitive in detecting airway obstruction because of no "deep inspiration" effect on bronchial tone that is required with a forced maneuver (39, 40).

In a study conducted from Heijkenskjold Rentzhog et al. (41), the authors showed that FOT measurements were more informative in discriminating patients with asthma from healthy controls. FOT measurements were able to indicate a more peripheral involvement of the airways. Similar results are also available form previous studies on BDR in FOT resistance measurements and spirometry in children (39, 42) and adults (43). IOS results compared to spirometry have been shown to be able to predict loss of control in a group of 54 children with asthma (44). Data from 252 children with mild to moderate persistent asthma, demonstrated that the area under the reactance curve measured with IOS, was able to detect changes in airway mechanics after weeks of treatment in respect to other oscillations indices or spirometry results (45). There are some data that show that sRaw measured at preschool age correlates with mild obstruction measured with low volumes (6), also in a recent study, although on a small number of asthmatic children, sRaw is a better indices of bronchoconstriction in respect to FEV1 after a challenge test (46).

The role of these techniques in severe asthma in children remains to be assessed and further studies are needed.

MULTIPLE BREATH WASHOUT (MBW)

The Multiple Breath Washout technique measures the Lung Clearance Index (LCI), which is the cumulative expired volume required to clear an inert gas from the lungs, divided by FRC or the number of times the lung volume has to be "turned over" to wash out an inert gas such as nitrogen (N_2) or sulfur hexafluoride (SF_6). LCI is an index of inhomogeneity of ventilation and it has been demonstrated to be able to detect early lung damage in particular in children chronic lung disease such as Cystic Fibrosis (47), however it has some limits in measuring airway obstruction. In severe asthma with severe obstruction some areas of the lung can be excluded from ventilation giving a false value of LCI that can even appear within the normal range. S_{cond} is another index measured with MBW that refers to the inhomogeneity of the conducting airways and this might be more useful in asthmatic patients. The limits of this technique are also related to the lack of extended reference equations with particular respect to the pediatric population.

BRONCHIAL HYPERRESPONSIVENESS

Bronchial hyperresponsiveness (BHR) can be considered as the variation of the bronchial tone that can vary after exposition to different stimuli. The stimuli that can be used as provocation test can be direct (chemicals such as histamine or methacholine, or inhaled allergens) or indirect (physical exercise, mannitol, inhaled cold air or hyperventilation with dry cold air). After a brochoprovocation test a fall in FEV_1 of 20 or 15%, depending on the test used, is considered as a cut off value. A maximal fall of FEV_1 between 10 or more in respect to the baseline value on two consecutive measurements after a maximal effort is considered diagnostic for exercised induced bronchoconstriction (48). In children exercise testing can be very important for the assessment of asthma in the diagnostic process but also in monitoring the response to therapy, especially when exercise symptoms are reported or there is a poor perception of symptoms (9). Methacholine bronchoprovocation test is more sensitive but less specific than exercise testing in asthmatics (49).

In a prospective study Part et al, showed in 1,041 children, the CAMP Cohort, that the percent recovery index (the percent increase in FEV_1 after bronchodilator) in response to a bronchial challenge with methacholine was able to predict an asthmatic exacerbation in the following year (50). In severe asthma, both methacholine and exercise tests can be used to asses BHR when the diagnosis is not clear in difficult cases (16). The role of BHR in the clinical evaluation of the child with severe asthma is debatable and it is not safe to evaluate when baseline FEV_1 is low (51).

CONCLUSION

In conclusion, pulmonary function testing assessing airway obstruction is important in the clinical management of children with asthma and severe asthma during diagnosis, monitoring and evaluating response to treatment.

AUTHOR CONTRIBUTIONS

All authors listed have made a substantial, direct and intellectual contribution to the work, and approved it for publication.

REFERENCES

1. Krishnan JK, Martinez FJ. Lung function trajectories and chronic obstructive pulmonary disease: current understanding and knowledge gaps. *Curr Opin Pulm Med.* (2018) 24:124–9. doi: 10.1097/MCP.0000000000000456
2. Bui DS, Lodge CJ, Burgess JA, Lowe AJ, Perret J, Bui MQ et al. Childhood predictors of lung function trajectories and future COPD risk: a prospective cohort study from the first to the sixth decade of life. *Lancet Respir Med.* (2018). doi: 10.1016/S2213-2600(18)30100-0. [Epub ahead of print].
3. Belgrave DCM, Granell R, Turner SW, Curtin JA, Buchan IE, Le Souëf PN et al. Lung function trajectories from pre-school age to adulthood and their associations with early life factors: a retrospective analysis of three population-based birth cohort studies. *Lancet Respir Med.* (2018). doi: 10.1016/S2213-2600(18)30099-7. [Epub ahead of print].
4. Miller MR, Hankinson J, Brusasco V, Burgos F, Casaburi R, Coates A, et al. Standardisation of spirometry. *Eur Respir J.* (2005) 26:319–38. doi: 10.1183/09031936.05.00034805
5. Beydon N, Davis SD, Lombardi E, Allen JL, Arets HGM, Aurora P et al. An official american thoracic society/European respiratory society statement: pulmonary function testing in preschool children. *Am J Respir Crit Care Med.* (2007) 175:1304–45. doi: 10.1164/rccm.200605-642ST
6. Moeller A, Carlsen KH, Sly PD, Baraldi E, Piacentin G, Pavord I et al. Monitoring asthma in childhood: lung function, bronchial responsiveness and inflammation. *Eur Respir Rev.* (2015) 24:204–15. doi: 10.1183/16000617.00003914
7. Pellegrino R, Viegi G, Brusasco V, Crapo F, Burgos F, Casaburi R et al. Interpretative strategies for lung function tests. *Eur Respir J.* (2005) 26:948–68. doi: 10.1183/09031936.05.00035205
8. Tse SM, Gold DR, Sordillo JE, Hoffman EB, Gillman MW, Rifas-Shiman SL et al. Diagnostic accuracy of the bronchodilator response in children. *J Allergy Clin Immunol.* (2013) 132:554–9.e5. doi: 10.1016/j.jaci.2013.03.031
9. Global Initiative for Asthma. *Global Strategy for Asthma Management and Prevention.* (2017). Available online at: www.ginasthma.org
10. *NICE Guideline.* (2017). Available online at: www.nice.org.uk/guidance/ng80
11. Fuhlbrigge AL, Kitch BT, Paltiel AD, Kuntz KM, Neumann PJ, Dockery DW et al. FEV1 is associated with risk of asthma attacks in a pediatric population. *J Allergy Clin Immunol.* (2001) 107:61–7. doi: 10.1067/mai.2001.111590
12. Schifano ED, Hollenbach JP, Cloutier MM. Mismatch between asthma symptoms and spirometry: implications for managing asthma in children. *J Pediatr* (2014) 165:997–1002. doi: 10.1016/j.jpeds.2014.07.026
13. Francisco B, Ner Z, Ge B, Hewett J, König P. Sensitivity of different spirometric tests for detecting airway obstruction in childhood asthma. *J Asthma* (2015) 52:505–11. doi: 10.3109/02770903.2014.984842
14. Quanjer PH, Weiner DJ, Pretto JJ, Brazzale DJ, Boros PW. Measurement of FEF25-75% and FEF75% does not contribute to clinical decision making. *Eur Respir J.* (2014) 43:1051–8. doi: 10.1183/09031936.00128113
15. Culver BH, Graham BL, Coates AL, Wanger J, Berry CE, Clarke PK et al. Recommendations for a standardized pulmonary function report. an official American thoracic society technical statement. *Am J Respir Crit Care Med.* (2017) 196:1463–72. doi: 10.1164/rccm.201710-1981ST
16. Chung KF, Wenzel SE, Brozek JL, Bush A, Castro M, Sterk PJ et al. International ERS/ATS guidelines on definition, evaluation and treatment of severe asthma. *Eur Respir J.* (2014) 43:343–73. doi: 10.1183/09031936.00202013
17. Barsky EE, Giancola LM, Baxi SN, Gaffin JM. A Parctical Approach to Severe Asthma in Children. *Ann Am Thorac Soc.* (2017) 15:399–408. doi: 10.1513/AnnalsATS.201708-637FR
18. Guilbert TW, Bacharier LB, Fitzpatrick AM. Severe asthma in children. *J Allergy Clin Immunol Pract.* (2014) 2:489–500. doi: 10.1016/j.jaip.2014.06.022
19. Fitzpatrick AM. Severe asthma in children: lessons learned and future di- rections. *J Allergy Clin Immunol Pract.* (2016) 4:11–9; quiz 20–1. doi: 10.1016/j.jaip.2015.10.008
20. Teague WG, Phillips BR, Fahy JV, Wenzel SE, Fitzpatrick AM, Moore WC, et al. Baseline features of the Severe Asthma Research Program (SARP III) cohort: differences with age. *J Allergy Clin Immunol Pract.* (2018) 6:545–54.e4. doi: 10.1016/j.jaip.2017.05.032
21. Fitzpatric AM, Moore CW. Severe asthma phenotypes – How should they guide evaluation and treatment? *J Allergy Clin Immunol Pract.* (2017) 5:901–8. doi: 10.1016/j.jaip.2017.05.015
22. Fitzpatrick AM, Teague WG, Meyers DA, Peters SP, Li X, Li H, et al. Heterogeneity of severe asthma in childhood: confirmation by cluster analysis of children in the National Institutes of Health/National Heart, Lung, and Blood Institute Severe Asthma Research Program. *J Allergy Clin Immunol.* (2011) 127:382–89.e1–13. doi: 10.1016/j.jaci.2010.11.015
23. Coverstone A, Bacharier LB, Fitzpatrick AM. Severe asthma in school-age children: evaluation and phenotypic advances. *Curr Allergy Asthma Rep.* (2015) 15:20. doi: 10.1007/s11882-015-0521-5
24. Fitzpatrick AM, Gaston BM, Erzurum SC, Teague WG, National Institutes of Health/National Heart, Lung, and Blood Institute Severe Asthma Research Program. Features of severe asthma in school-age children: atopy and increased exhaled nitric oxide. *J Allergy Clin Immunol.* (2006) 118:1218–25. doi: 10.1016/j.jaci.2006.08.019
25. Jenkins HA, Cherniack R, Szefler SJ, Covar R, Gelfand EW, Spahn JD. A comparison of the clinical characteristics of children and adults with severe asthma. *Chest* (2003) 124:1318–24. doi: 10.1378/chest.124.4.1318
26. Calhoun WJ, Haselkorn T, Miller DP, Omachi TA. Asthma exacerbations and lung function in patients with severe or difficult-to-treat asthma. *J Allergy Clin Immunol.* (2015) 136:1125–7.e4. doi: 10.1016/j.jaci.2015.05.014
27. Castro-Rodriguez JA, Saglani S, Rodriguez-Martinez CE, Oyarzun MA, Fleming L, Bush A. The relationship between inflammation and remodeling in childhood asthma: a systematic review. *Pediatr Pulmonol.* (2018) 53:824–35. doi: 10.1002/ppul.23968
28. Ortega H, Yancey SW, Keene ON, Gunsoy NB, Albers FC, Howarth PH. Asthma exacerbations associated with lung function decline in patients with severe eosinophilic asthma. *J Allergy Clin Immunol Pract.* (2018) 6:980–6.e1. doi: 10.1016/j.jaip.2017.12.019
29. Deschildre A, Marguet C, Salleron J, Pin I, Rittié JL, Dorelle J et al. Add-on omalizumab in children with severe allergic asthma: a 1-year real life survey. *Eur Respir J.* (2013) 42:1224–33. doi: 10.1183/09031936.00149812
30. Versiani Nunes Pinheiro de Queiroz M, Gonçalves AC, Cruz AA, de Lima Belizario Facury Lasmar LM. Lung function in severe pediatric asthma: a longitudinal study in children and adolescents in Brazil. *Clin Transl Allergy* (2017) 7:48. doi: 10.1186/s13601-017-0183-6

31. Labbe G, Merlin E, Kauffman C, Fauquert JL, Héraud MC, Labbé A. The role of lung volume measurements by plethysmography in the follow-up of asthma in children. *Rev Mal Respir* (2010) 27:42–8. doi: 10.1016/j.rmr.2009.11.002
32. Sorkness RL, Teague WG, Penugonda M, Fitzpatrick AM, National Institutes of Health/National Heart, Lung, and Blood Institute Severe Asthma Research Program. Sex dependence of airflow limitation and air trapping in children with severe asthma. *J Allergy Clin Immunol.* (2011) 127:1073–4. doi: 10.1016/j.jaci.2010.12.1079
33. Bisgaard H, Nielsen KG. Plethysmographic measurements of specific airway resistance in young children. *Chest* (2005) 128:355–62. doi: 10.1378/chest.128.1.355
34. Merkus PJFM, Stocks J, Beydon N, Lombardi E, Jones M, McKenzie SA et al. Reference ranges for interrupter resistance technique: the Asthma UK Initiative. *Eur Respir J* (2010) 36:157–63. doi: 10.1183/09031936.00125009
35. Calogero C, Simpson SJ, Lombardi E, Parri N, Cuomo B, Palumbo M et al. Respiratory impedance and bronchodilator responsiveness in healthy children aged 2–13 years. *Pediatr Pulmonol.* (2013) 48:707–15. doi: 10.1002/ppul.22699
36. Kirkby J, Stanojevic S, Welsh L, Lum S, Badier M, Beardsmore C et al. Reference equations for specific airway resistance in children: the Asthma UK initiative. *Eur Respir J.* (2010) 36:622–9. doi: 10.1183/09031936.00135909
37. Nielsen KG, Bisgaard H. Discriminative capacity of bronchodilator response measured with three different lung function techniques in asthmatic and healthy children aged 2 to 5 years. *Am J Respir Crit Care Med.* (2001) 164:554–9. doi: 10.1164/ajrccm.164.4.2006119
38. Thamrin C, Gangell CL, Udomittipong K, Kusel MM, Patterson H, Fukushima T et al. Assessment of bronchodilator responsiveness in preschool children using forced oscillations. *Thorax* (2007) 62:814–9. doi: 10.1136/thx.2006.071290
39. Marotta A, Klinnert MD, Price MR, Larsen GL, Liu AH. Impulse oscillometry provides an effective measure of lung dysfunction in 4-year- old children at risk for persistent asthma. *J Allergy Clin Immunol.* (2003) 112:317–22. doi: 10.1067/mai.2003.1627
40. Song TW, Kim KW, Kim ES, Park JW, Sohn MH, Kim KE. Utility of impulse oscillometry in young children with asthma. *Pediatr Allergy Immunol.* (2008) 19:763–768. doi: 10.1111/j.1399-3038.2008.00734.x
41. Heijkenskjöld Rentzhog C, Janson C, Berglund L, Borres MP, Nordvall L, Alving K et al. Overall and peripheral lung function assessment by spirometry and forced oscillation technique in relation to asthma diagnosis and control. *Clin Exp Allergy* (2017) 47:1546–54. doi: 10.1111/cea.13035
42. Komarow HD, Skinner J, Young M, Gaskins D, Nelson C, Gergen PJ et al. A study of the use of impulse oscillometry in the evaluation of children with asthma: analysis of lung parameters, order effect, and utility compared with spirometry. *Pediatr Pulmonol.* (2012) 47:18–26. doi: 10.1002/ppul.21507
43. Saadeh C, Cross B, Gaylor M, Griffith M. Advantage of impulse oscillometry over spirometry to diagnose chronic obstructive pulmonary disease and monitor pulmonary responses to bronchodilators: an observational study. *SAGE Open Med.* (2015) 3:2050312115578957. doi: 10.1177/2050312115578957
44. Shi Y, Aledia AS, Galant SP, George SC. Peripheral airway impairment measured by oscillometry predicts loss of asthma control in children. *J Allergy Clin Immunol.* (2013) 131:718–23. doi: 10.1016/j.jaci.2012.09.022
45. Larsen GL, Morgan W, Heldt GP, Mauger DT, Boehmer SJ Chinchilli VM. Impulse oscillometry versus spirometry in a long-term study of controller therapy for pediatric asthma. *J Allergy Clin Immunol.* (2009) 123:861–7.e1. doi: 10.1016/j.jaci.2008.10.036
46. Van Nederveen-Bendien SA, Vahl J, Heijerman HGM. Specific airway resistance is a better outcome parameter in bronchial provocation testing compared to FEV1 in patients with bronchial asthma. *J Asthma* (2018) 17:1–5. doi: 10.1080/02770903.2017.1414238
47. Ramsey KA, Rosenow T, Turkovic L, Skoric B, Banton G, Adams AM et al. Lung clearance index and structural lung disease on computed tomography in early cystic fibrosis. *Am J Respir Crit Care Med.* (2016) 193:60–7. doi: 10.1164/rccm.201507-1409OC
48. Weiler JM, Brannan JD, Randolph CC, Hallstrand TS, Parsons J, Silvers W et al. Exercise-induced bronchoconstriction update-2016. *J Allergy Clin Immunol.* (2016) 138:1292–95.e36. doi: 10.1016/j.jaci.2016.05.029
49. Coates AL, Wanger J, Cockcroft DW, Culver BH, Carlsen K-H, Diamant Z et al. ERS technical standard on bronchial challenge testing: general considerations and performance of methacholine challenge tests. *Eur Respir J.* (2017) 49:1601526. doi: 10.1183/13993003.01526-2016
50. Park HW, Song WJ, Chang YS, Cho SH, Datta S, Weiss ST et al. Bronchodilator response following methacholine-induced bronchoconstriction predicts acute asthma exacerbations. *Eur Respir J.* (2016) 48:104–14. doi: 10.1183/13993003.00182-2016
51. Hedlin G. Management of severe asthma in childhood-state of the art and novel perspectives. *Pediatr Allergy Immunol.* (2014) 25:111–21. doi: 10.1111/pai.12112

23

Genetics and Gene-Environment Interactions in Childhood and Adult Onset Asthma

Eva Morales [1,2*†] *and David Duffy* [3†]

[1] Biomedical Research Institute of Murcia (IMIB-Arrixaca), University of Murcia, Murcia, Spain, [2] CIBER Epidemiología y Salud Pública (CIBERESP), Madrid, Spain, [3] QIMR Berghofer Medical Research Institute, Brisbane, QLD, Australia

***Correspondence:**
Eva Morales
embarto@hotmail.com;
evamorales@um.es

† These authors have contributed equally to this work

Asthma is a heterogeneous disease that results from the complex interaction between genetic factors and environmental exposures that occur at critical periods throughout life. It seems plausible to regard childhood-onset and adult-onset asthma as different entities, each with a different pathophysiology, trajectory, and outcome. This review provides an overview about the role of genetics and gene-environment interactions in these two conditions. Looking at the genetic overlap between childhood and adult onset disease gives one window into whether there is a correlation, as well as to mechanism. A second window is offered by the genetics of the relationship between each type of asthma and other phenotypes e.g., obesity, chronic obstructive pulmonary disease (COPD), atopy, vitamin D levels, and inflammatory and immune status; and third, the genetic-specific responses to the many environmental exposures that influence risk throughout life, and particularly those that occur during early-life development. These represent a large number of possible combinations of genetic and environmental factors, at least 150 known genetic loci *vs.* tobacco smoke, outdoor air pollutants, indoor exposures, farming environment, and microbial exposures. Considering time of asthma onset extends the two-dimensional problem of gene-environment interactions to a three-dimensional problem, since identified gene-environment interactions seldom replicate for childhood and adult asthma, which suggests that asthma susceptibility to environmental exposures may biologically differ from early life to adulthood as a result of different pathways and mechanisms of the disease.

Keywords: asthma, genetics, environmental exposures, gene environment interactions, childhood, adulthood

INTRODUCTION

Asthma is characterized by a significant heterogeneity in relation to age of onset, clinical manifestations, genetics, environmental risk factors, response to treatments, and prognosis. Asthma affects as many as 339 million people worldwide (1), of whom 33% are under the age of 14, 27% are adults who first experienced symptoms in childhood (2), and 40% adult-onset cases. What proportion of this last group has the same underlying disease processes acting as in the first two groups? Is the "Dutch" hypothesis of a continuum from asthma to chronic obstructive pulmonary disease (COPD) a better description? (3). Similarly, there is much current interest in the relationship between childhood asthma and obesity. It has been suggested that obesity might affect childhood and adult-onset asthma by separate pathways (4), but evidence for this is still patchy. Allergy plays a key role in childhood-onset asthma, and these subjects more frequently have atopic dermatitis, hay fever and a family history of atopy in comparison to those who develop asthma in adulthood (5). Adult-onset asthma is characterized by reduced lung function and poor prognosis (6). So what proportion of adult-onset asthma has an atopic contribution? Our current understanding is that we need to comprehend both genetic factors, environmental exposures and their interactions.

Asthma runs strongly in families and estimates of its heritability range from 35 to 70%, showing higher estimates among boys and early-onset cases (7, 8). The study of asthma genetics has offered the possibility of understanding the causes and biological mechanisms of the disease as well as the identification of potential targets for treatment, although identified multiple loci only explain a limited proportion of asthma heritability (9).

Differences in rates of asthma between countries and its increasing prevalence in the past few decades clearly suggest that environmental exposures have an important role on asthma occurrence. Environmental risk factors of asthma include exposure to tobacco smoke, farm animals and related products, domestics cats, respiratory viral infections, microbial exposures, dietary factors, breastfeeding, medication, occupational exposures, indoor and outdoor air pollution, and diverse allergens (10). Environmental exposures, including those beginning in early life, play a pivotal role and the exact timing of exposure at critical windows of development influences genetic specific responses and individual risk trajectories that ultimately lead to the development of asthma (11, 12). Gene-environment interaction studies aim to explain how the strength and direction of associations between certain genetic variants and asthma may depend on given environmental exposures, and *vice versa*, and might explain in part the hidden heritability of asthma.

In the light of clinical and epidemiological importance of asthma and the potential benefits of further research into its etiology, this review will provide an overview on current understanding of genetics and gene-environment interactions in childhood and adult onset of the disease.

GENETICS OF CHILDHOOD AND ADULT ONSET ASTHMA

We first examine evidence from: (a) multivariate family based studies, where two traits e.g., childhood-onset asthma and adult-onset asthma are measured in the same family and the correlations between family members (who might be twins) across traits are interpreted; (b) the counting of overlapping genome-wide significant simple nucleotide polymorphism (SNPs) regression results from genome-wide association studies (GWAS) of each trait; (c) the accuracy of a genetic risk score generated from a GWAS of one trait in predicting the second trait in a second GWAS; (d) methods combining all SNPs from two GWAS to estimate the genetic correlation between traits; and (e) Mendelian Randomization (MR) studies of asthma risk factors, where genetic variants affecting the risk factor are tested for an association for asthma, thus increasing evidence of causation between the risk factor and asthma.

Childhood-onset asthma is most commonly accompanied by atopy. We know from a myriad of family-based studies, and now from large genotyping studies of unrelated individuals, that the diseases of the atopic triad are strongly heritable, and genetically correlated. Heritability is a measure of what proportion of trait differences between individuals in a given population are due to causative genetic differences between those individuals (13). Being a proportion, interpretation must be fastidious. For example, in developed countries asthma incidence has increased several-fold over the last 100 years, which must be due to changing environmental exposures. However, heritability estimates have remained roughly constant (14), which implies that average difference between individuals in environmental exposures has not greatly changed (else the genetic proportion of difference would be diluted), and that these exposures affect all genotypes equally at the first approximation. This puts an upper limit on the importance of gene-environment interactions at the population level, but the niceties would take too long to explain. A genetic correlation is also a proportion, comparing the genetic contribution (in the sense above) shared by two traits to those that are unshared. The correlation may well be via a mechanistically uninteresting causative chain e.g., the genetic correlation ($r_g = +0.21$, SE = 0.03) (15) between asthma and depression in the UK Biobank population might be mediated by atopy genes predisposing to chronic asthma, which is depressing for some individuals due to limiting effects on lifestyle. The latter might be suggested by the fact that the genetic correlations for Type 2 diabetes and depression, BMI and depression, myocardial infarction and depression, and schizophrenia and depression are all of a similar magnitude.

The concepts of heritability and genetic correlation come from the theory of inheritance for quantitative traits which are assumed to be (roughly) normally distributed. The extension to binary traits such as asthma requires modification of this model for use in a logistic or probit regression framework.

These methods deal easily with the usual case for complex diseases of very many contributing genes and can be calculated via trait correlations in pedigrees (including monozygotic—MZ, and dizygotic—DZ twins), as well as by measuring genotype-trait association directly (i.e., genome-wide association studies). They have a straightforward mathematical relationship to other measures such as the MZ twin recurrence risk ratio—the expected risk of disease of individuals genetically the same as asthma cases vs. whole population baseline risk (**Figure 1**).

Recently, we have seen the development of statistical methods to estimate heritability and genetic correlations in genome-wide association studies (GWAS) of multiple traits within the same study population, and even by combining separate univariate analyses of different populations using just summary data. These include the GCTA-COJO (16), LDAK Sumher (17), HESS (18) and LD score regression approaches (19). These approaches model contributions of loci of small effect that will not reach genome-wide statistical significance ($P < 5 \times 10^{-8}$) when tested one SNP at a time. Family-based methods will better estimate contributions of rare alleles, or alleles that are not well-measured

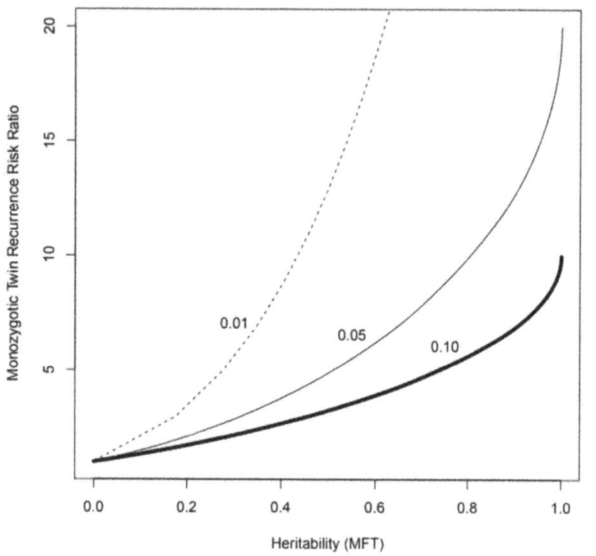

FIGURE 1 | MZ twin recurrence risk ratio vs. heritability under the multifactorial threshold model (probit-normal mixed model, MFT) for three levels of population prevalence (1 to 10%), which might represent asthma of different levels of severity. Note that the recurrence risk ratio is bounded by the trait prevalence (e.g., cannot exceed 10 if the prevalence is 10%). The recurrence risk to an ordinary sibling will correspond to the value for half the heritability (the kinship coefficient for sibs is 0.5).

by a particular set of genetic markers e.g., on a given SNP array, but sample sizes will usually be smaller when compared to genotyping studies of unrelated individuals.

In the case of Mendelian Randomization (MR) and related methods, the pattern of correlations between two traits and a measured SNP is interpreted knowing that genotype is both fixed at birth and largely unaffected by external confounders (ethnic confounding can be controlled for). MR analyses can involve one SNP at a time, a set of known associated SNPs from other studies, or whole genome; they can be bidirectional; and one of the traits can be gene transcript or expressed protein levels, simultaneously confirming the SNP to have biological effects on an intermediate trait and pointing to biological mechanisms for the trait-SNP correlation.

Family Based Studies

A variety of recent studies generally confirm that the heritability of childhood-onset asthma is high, and that this tends to be higher than that of later-onset asthma (**Table 1**). The classical twin studies of children, where the family members being utilized are exactly the same age and birth cohort, tend to give the highest estimates. It should be noted that studies do not find an increased prevalence of asthma in twins, particularly MZ twins, especially after adjusting for covariates such as birth weight (20). Thomsen et al. (21) were able to break down that twin sample by age at onset of asthma, and found the heritability for onset after age 20 to be 60%, compared to 80% in younger twins. And data reported by Paaso et al. (5) can be reanalyzed to estimate the genetic correlations between parental allergy and adult-onset and childhood-onset offspring asthma (first two entries of

TABLE 1 | Heritabilities of asthma from different studies using different designs and statistical methods.

Trait	Heritability	References	Study type
Asthma (<12 y.o.)	0.82 (0.79–0.85)	(20)	Twin study (12635 pairs)
Asthma (<20 y.o.)	0.78 (0.72–0.84)	(21)	Twin study (9051 pairs)
Asthma (>20 y.o.)	0.58 (0.58–0.82)	(8)	Twin study (11147 pairs)
Asthma (<13 y.o.)	0.46 (0.4–0.5)	(5)	Family study (1623 families?)
Asthma	0.42 (0.41–0.43)	(22)	Family study (128989 families, 481657 individuals).
Asthma	0.47 (0.23–0.72)	(23)	GWAS Bayesian mixture linear mixed model
Asthma (UKBB)	0.38 (0.35–0.41)	(24)	GWAS linear mixed model (GCTA)
Asthma (UKBB)	0.34 (0.32–0.36)	(25)	GWAS moment-matching LMM
Asthma (UKBB)	0.07 (0.05–0.08)	(26)	GWAS LD regression
Childhood-onset Asthma (UKBB)	0.004 (0.001–0.007)	Neale, 2018[a]	GWAS LD regression
Asthma onset (UKBB)	0.0 (−0.009 – 0)	Neale, 2018[a]	GWAS LD regression

[a] *http://www.nealelab.is/uk-biobank/.*

Table 2). These give a consistent pattern, where the allergy early-asthma correlation is higher, but there is still a significant genetic correlation between atopy and later-onset asthma.

The heritability estimates based on GWAS (**Table 1**) tend to be lower, given they only represent the contributions of common measured SNPs ("array," "chip," or "SNP" heritability). Even so, the estimates from LD regression seem to be lower again.

Overlap of Identified Causative Loci

The Trans-national Asthma Genetic Consortium (30) compared SNP allele frequencies in 24,000 asthma cases and 119,000 controls to detect 22 asthma associated loci. The locus of greatest effect was that on chromosome 17q21 in the region of *GSDMB* and *ORMDL3* genes. It has been known since 2008 (31) that this locus is associated with childhood onset asthma. Despite the association with early onset disease, these SNPs are not associated with atopy, and the asthma-increasing alleles probably reduce risk of other immunological conditions such as inflammatory bowel disease and Type 1 diabetes. If we take one of the functional 17q21 SNPs rs12936231 (actually within ZPBP2), in the UK BioBank the C allele increases "all" asthma OR = 1.1 ($P = 1 \times 10^{-59}$) and self-reported "emphysema/chronic bronchitis" OR = 1.07 ($P = 1 \times 10^{-8}$, but not doctor-diagnosed emphysema, $P = 0.5$), as well as neutrophil count ($P = 7 \times 10^{-142}$), but less strongly with eosinophil count ($P = 3 \times 10^{-5}$) (32). The effect sizes of these alleles are not large,

TABLE 2 | Genetic correlations between asthma and related traits.

Trait 1	Trait 2	Genetic correlation	References	
Allergy (Espoo)	Childhood Asthma (Espoo)	~0.75	(5)	Family study
Allergy (Espoo)	Later Asthma (Espoo) >13 y.o.	~0.5	(5)	Family study
All Adult Asthma (UKBB)	Asthma (GABRIEL)	0.66	(26)	GWAS based LD regression
All Adult Asthma (UKBB)	Allergic Diseases (UKBB)	0.75	(26)	GWAS based LD regression
Asthma (GABRIEL)	Allergic Rhinitis	0.60	(27)	GWAS based LD regression
All Adult Asthma (UKBB)	Eosinophil count (UKBB)	0.45	(15)	GWAS based LD regression
All Adult Asthma (UKBB)	BMI (UKBB)	0.21	(15)	GWAS based LD regression
Childhood Asthma (GABRIEL)	BMI (GIANT Consortium)	0.19	(28)	GWAS based MoM method
All Adult Asthma (UKBB)	FEV_1/FVC (UKBB)	−0.30	(15)	GWAS based LD regression
Adult Asthma	COPD	0.38	(29)	GWAS based LD regression

so general inferences about childhood vs. adult asthma must be based on aggregated effects of multiple loci.

Demenais et al. (30) also confirmed the association of rs9272346 and rs9273349 in the region of HLA-DQ with asthma. These SNPs were reported more strongly correlated with adult-onset than childhood-onset disease (9, 33), but still exhibiting detectable association in early-onset cases. Like the 17q21 locus, are unrelated (or only weakly associated) to atopy. In the UKBB (32), the rs9272346*A allele increases incidence of asthma, coeliac disease, Type 1 diabetes, hypothyroidism, rheumatoid arthritis, and diminishes risk of multiple sclerosis and ulcerative colitis. It has no association with self-reported COPD. Pividori et al. (34), see below, classify it as shared by childhood and adult onset asthma in UKBB.

Ferreira et al. (35) carried out a GWAS meta-analysis (13 studies, total $N = 360838$) to detect 99 loci (136 peak SNPs) for atopic disease, defined as any of asthma, hayfever or atopic dermatitis. Of these, 49 were novel. Several loci were disease-specific, such as Filaggrin (FLG) for atopic dermatitis, or a SNP near IL18R1, where the effect allele was increased in asthma and hayfever, but not atopic dermatitis. Several variants were associated earlier onset of asthma (7445 asthma-only cases)—the strongest being rs921650 in GSDMB (17q21 region).

Pividori et al. (34) and Ferreira et al. (36) have recently reported on childhood and adult onset asthma within the UK Biobank (UKBB) sample. Pividori et al. were able to detect 61 independent asthma loci comparing 9433 childhood-onset cases, 21564 adult-onset cases, and 318237 controls. Of these, "23 were childhood onset specific, one was adult onset specific, and 37 were shared." Ferreira and coworkers supplemented the UKBB data with data from 23andMe (further 32,000 childhood-onset cases and 215,000 controls) and reported 123 childhood-onset (age <20 years) asthma loci, of which 98 were reproducible in the second dataset. Five of these loci did not affect risk of adult-onset asthma. For adult-onset asthma, they found 34 replicable loci, of which 3 were significantly weaker as predictors of childhood disease. They estimated the genetic correlation between adult and childhood-onset asthma as 0.67. They further tested for loci specifically for age at diagnosis within their childhood-onset sample (defined as < 20 years old) and concluded that such effects were relatively small (5% of variance, $P = 0.02$; but N was only 14,000, so power was low). There were 25 novel childhood-onset asthma loci detected, in or near biologically important genes such as *NOD2*, *IL4R*, *IL2RA*, and *IRF4*. Because the UKBB dataset is generally available, we can contrast these findings to those published by Zhu et al. (26) who reported a total of 38 loci for "doctor diagnosed" asthma detectable using an earlier available version of the dataset containing 7908 cases and 76768 controls, and Johansson et al. (24) who reported 52 loci defined via 41934 cases and 239773 controls (**Figure 2**). The "pure" adult-onset SNP reported by Pividori et al. was rs12617922 on chromosome 2 near *TEX41*, which decreased risk of tobacco smoking ($P = 5 \times 10^{-24}$), as commented on by Ferreira et al. (36). **Figure 3** shows that such a strong negative association is not seen for any of the other asthma loci from Zhu et al. (26). A SNP in the same region near *TEX41*, rs10193706, was previously highlighted as associated with tobacco use in the subset of UKBB used for the BiLEVE study of COPD (37). In European populations, it is in moderate linkage disequilibrium with rs12617922 ($r^2 = 0.37$), but not associated with self-reported asthma in the full UKBB sample.

An even more intriguing observation is that the peak SNP for this region in terms of "any" asthma and smoking (and suggestively with caffeine intake as well) is rs10427255, previously flagged as a locus for the photic sneeze reflex ($P = 1 \times 10^{-11}$) by Eriksson et al. (38) in the 23andMe dataset (see **Table 3**). These SNPs (rs12617922, rs10427255) are not associated with serum eosinophil level or atopy. Of the 32 SNPs known to be associated with photic sneeze reflex, only these near *TEX41* predict asthma, so there is no general relationship between these two phenotypes.

Hobbs et al. (29) examined COPD in 25000 cases and 58000 controls. There were 22 associated loci (13 novel), none overlapping with asthma loci from the GABRIEL study or the NCBI GWAS catalog. Examining the UK BioBank via the GeneAtlas web site (32), one does find that five of their top COPD SNPs are associated with self-reported asthma at $P < 1 \times 10^{-5}$. The strongest association of these five is for rs2070600 (a protein coding change Gly82Ser in AGER on chromosome 6, $P = 4 \times 10^{-29}$), where the T (Serine) allele (European frequency 5–10%) increases asthma (OR = 1.15). The Hobbs et al. (29) result for COPD is OR = 1.21 ($P = 6 \times 10^{-10}$) for the C (Glycine) allele, so (if replicable) this would lead to a negative genetic correlation between asthma and COPD due to this locus. The Ser82 allele reduces sRAGE levels and increases FEV1 (39).

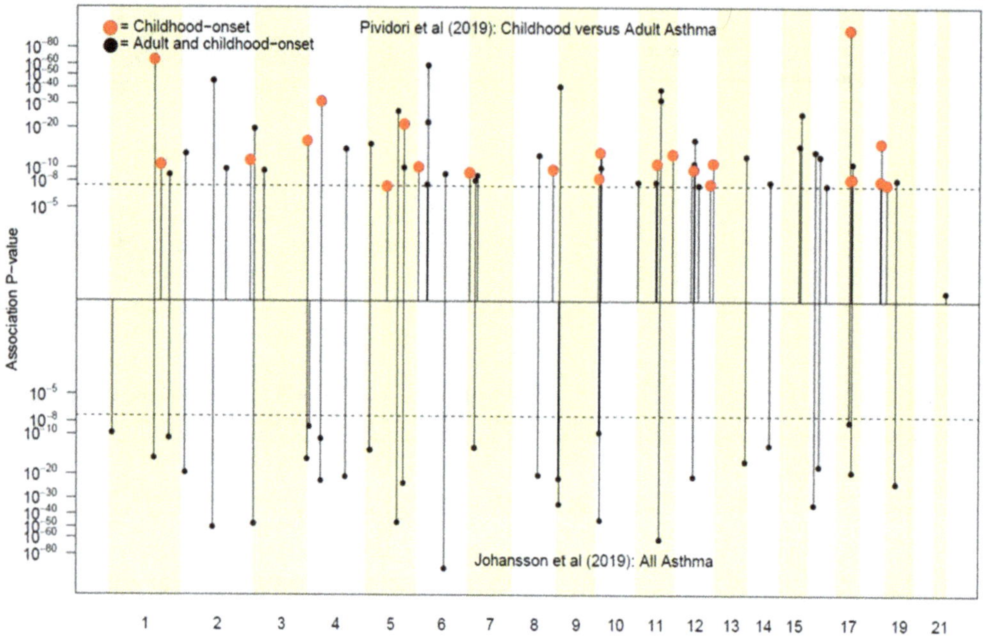

FIGURE 2 | Top association peaks from Pividori et al. (34) and Johansson et al. (24).

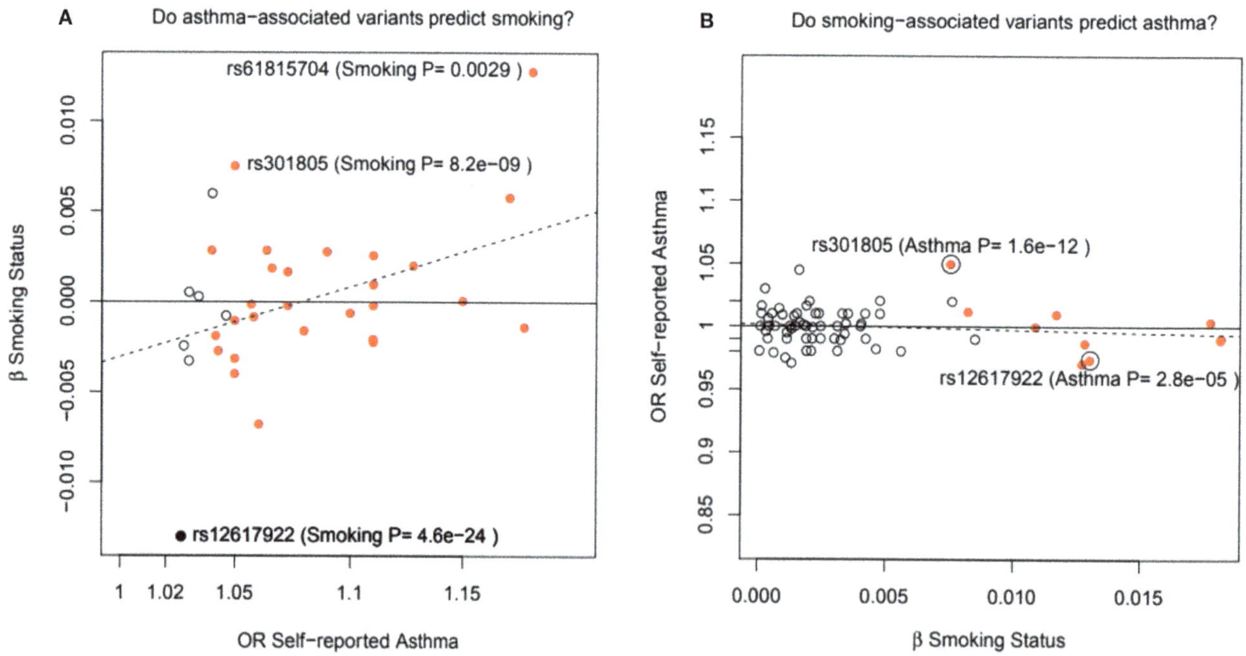

FIGURE 3 | In **(A)**, the adult asthma SNP, rs12617922, from Pividori et al. (34), and all top asthma SNPs from Zhu et al. (26) vs. their relationship to smoking status in the UK Bio Bank analysis of Canela-Xandri et al. (32). Red color denotes an asthma association *P*-value in Canela-Xandri et al. (32) $<5 \times 10^{-8}$. For smoking status, only the *P*-values for rs12617922 and rs301805 are $<5 \times 10^{-8}$. The rs301805 SNP also shows a strong association with eosinophil count, and was flagged by Ferreira et al. (35) as an allergy locus. In **(B)**, smoking-associated SNPs [GWAS Catalog 2018] are tested—red color now denotes a smoking association *P*-value in Canela-Xandri et al. (32) $< 5 \times 10^{-8}$.

Hayden et al. (40) describe the COPDGene study of 10200 current and former adult smokers. The GWAS analysis found known childhood asthma risk SNPs were associated with asthma, and childhood asthma (7% of the sample) increased the risk of later COPD 3.4-fold, and also reduced lung function.

TABLE 3 | Association between SNPs on chromosome 2q22.3 with self-reported asthma, tobacco use and coffee intake in the UK Biobank (32).

SNP	Build 37 position	Allele	LD in Europeans (r^2)				Smoking status		Current smoking		Coffee drinking		Self-reported asthma	
							Beta	*P*-value	Beta	*P*	Beta	*P*	OR	*P*
rs1533426	146119018	G	1				−0.013	1.0e-22	−0.0050	4.9e-06	−0.015	3.9e-05	1.03	8.4e-06
rs10427255	146125523	T	0.74	1			−0.013	9.5e-23	−0.0051	4.0e-06	−0.018	4.0e-05	1.03	6.9e-06
rs12617922	146156679	A	0.55	0.48	1		−0.013	4.6e-24	−0.0053	1.5e-06	−0.019	3.2e-06	1.03	2.8e-05
rs10193706	146316319	C	0.32	0.18	0.37	1	−0.013	8.9e-24	−0.0056	3.6e-07	−0.025	1.6e-09	1.02	0.01

Both rs1533426 and rs10427255 (38) are associated with the photic sneeze reflex and rs10193706 was previously associated to heavy cigarette smoking (37).

TABLE 4 | Application of SNP-based Risk Scores derived for one trait to predict a second trait from http://mrcieu.mrsoftware.org/PRS_atlas/ (41).

PRS trait	Second trait	N SNPs	Beta	*P*-value
Cigarettes/d	Asthma	44	0.004	0.43
Asthma	Cigarettes/d	42	−0.001	0.82
BMI	Asthma	251	0.025	4.1×10^{-6}
Asthma	BMI	42	0.002	0.23
Asthma	"Chronic bronchitis/ emphysema"	42	0.050	2.6×10^{-4}
Major depression	Asthma	37	−0.005	0.37
Asthma	Depression	42	0.004	0.62

The P-values test significance of the regression of the PRS on the second trait.

Genetic Risk Scores

The components of the polygenic risk score (PRS) approach have already been presented (e.g., **Figure 3**), in that the PRS for a trait is merely the weighted sum of the regression coefficients for a number of significantly associated SNPs. Richardson et al. (41) have made available a web site presenting results of such cross-trait analyses (162 PRS, 551 outcomes) using the UK Biobank dataset (see **Table 4**). For example, while the BMI PRS predicts asthma, the asthma PRS does not predict BMI, a finding we can interpret as implying BMI is causative of asthma risk.

A table of results for COPD PRS (spirometric phenotypes including FEV1/FVC were used to define COPD) has been presented by Shrine et al. (42) in yet another preprint. This score (294 SNPs) is a significantly predictor of self-reported asthma ($P = 10^{-41}$). Examining the individual SNPs, we can see that 20 are significant ($P < 1 \times 10^{-5}$) independent predictors of UKBB self-reported asthma, and three are associated with hayfever/rhinitis (in *IL1RL1, SUOX* and *LRP1*).

GWAS Genome-Wide Estimates of Genetic Correlations

The most widely used approach for this is the LD score regression method, and results from this are listed in **Table 2**. Speed and Balding (17) suggest that magnitude of estimates of genetic correlations tend to relatively similar across different methods, which is less true of heritability estimates, as seen above. We see that "any" asthma is more strongly correlated with atopic diseases such as allergic rhinitis (r_g 0.6–0.7) than it is with COPD (r_g 0.4).

Mendelian Randomization Studies

Chen et al. (43) carried out a bidirectional MR analysis of the direction of causation between obesity and childhood asthma in Taiwan. While the obesity genetic risk score was a significant predictor of asthma, the asthma genetic risk score did not predict obesity. Granell et al. (44) similarly estimated the causal relative risk for the effect of BMI on asthma at 1.55 per kg/m^2, slightly more strongly for non-atopic childhood asthma. In 162124 adults from European studies (45), the causal OR for BMI on asthma was 1.07 (−9 ml FEV1, 16 ml FVC). There was no causal effect on allergic sensitization or serum IgE level—despite a positive phenotypic correlation between IgE and overweight in their study population. After all the above, however, Contreras et al. (46) found in a traditional longitudinal study that asthma diagnosis by age 4 was associated with obesity at age 8, which would seem consistent with the idea that asthma causes obesity, or at the very least that genes causative of asthma also cause obesity via a different pathway (acting at a different age) than that by which they cause asthma. Does this give an insight into adult-onset asthma? Multiple longitudinal studies in adults have found that overweight precedes and predisposes to asthma. Burgess et al. (47) showed BMI at age 7 years predicted development of asthma with an onset after age 21 years. So, in this case a causal pathway from overweight to asthma would be supported by both genetic and non-genetic studies.

Finally, the relationship between vitamin D deficiency and childhood and adult asthma is still unclear, with both cross-sectional epidemiological and animal model evidence making this plausible but results from supplementation studies unsupportive (48). MR studies (49, 50) have showed no relationship between vitamin D level SNPs and asthma or atopy.

GENE-ENVIRONMENT INTERACTIONS IN CHILDHOOD AND ADULT ONSET ASTHMA

The most frequently evaluated genetic-environment interactions on asthma include early-life and lifelong exposure to tobacco smoking, outdoor air pollutants, indoor exposures, a farming environment, and microbial exposures. The vast majority of the studies have applied a candidate gene approach and generally examined genes involved in antioxidant defenses, detoxification, inflammation, innate immunity, lung development, and epithelial function. Some investigations are based on family studies and few hypothesis-free studies, also called genome-wide interaction studies (GWISs), are available yet (**Table 5**).

Tobacco Smoking Exposure

This is the most well-studied environmental exposure with respect to genetic interactions in asthma in humans. Family studies have shown regions of linkage to asthma phenotypes to differ by environmental tobacco smoke (ETS) exposure in childhood (51–54). A study in 144 US families suggested that genes in chromosomal regions 1p, 5q, and 17p might interact with ETS to confer asthma risk in the exposed groups (51). The evidence for linkage for asthma and bronchial hyperresponsiveness (BHR) for chromosome 5q in the passive smoke-exposed groups during childhood was subsequently replicated in 200 Dutch families (52). A French study conducted in 295 families reported four regions, 1q43-q44, 4q34, 5p15, and 17p11, potentially involved in genetic susceptibility to BHR interacting with ETS in early life (53); however, none of these regions had been reported by previous genomes scans on gene-ETS interaction, except for the region in the 1q43-q44. Moreover, an interaction has been described between 17q21 variants and early-life exposure to ETS in early-onset asthma (54). The interaction between *ORMDL3* variants and early-life exposure to ETS in childhood-onset asthma was later replicated (94, 95).

Most candidate gene studies have focused on examining variants in genes coding for antioxidant defenses and xenobiotic-metabolizing enzymes and childhood-onset asthma susceptibility to tobacco smoking, especially the glutathione-S transferase (GST) family of antioxidant enzymes. Childhood-onset asthma risk has been shown to differ by *GSTM1* genotype in relation to both maternal smoking in pregnancy (55, 56) and childhood ETS exposure (57), with effects largely restricted to children with *GSTM1* null genotype. Results from other studies have suggested an interaction between *GSTP1* rs1695 A (Ile105) is a risk allele for childhood wheeze illness in relation to maternal smoking in early life, with an effect most clearly seen in children who are exposed to maternal smoking (59, 60). Most of the studies looking at interactions with *GSTM1* and *GSTP1* genetic variants have shown a positive finding, but not always in the same direction for *GSTP1* (58).

Given the importance of inflammation in asthma, genes related to inflammation responses and innate immunity have also been examined. Genetic variation in tumor necrosis factor (*TNF-α*) may contribute to childhood asthma and that associations may be modified by parental smoking (60, 61). Ramadas et al. (62) showed interaction of the interleukin-1 receptor antagonist (*IL1RN*) gene polymorphism rs2234678 and maternal smoking during pregnancy increased the risk for childhood asthma. Salam et al. (63) found that children with the transforming growth factor beta-1 (*TGFB1*)−509TT genotype are at increased risk of asthma when they are exposed to maternal smoking *in utero*; however, no interaction was found for parental tobacco smoke exposure in childhood (96). Household ETS and interleukin-13 gene (*IL-13*) variants may have interactive effects on childhood asthma phenotypes (64). Interactions between the human intercellular adhesion molecule 1 (*ICAM1*) polymorphisms and ETS have also been associated with risk of childhood-onset asthma (65). In adults, Miyake et al. revealed that the combination of ever smoking with interleukin 3 (*IL-3*) genetic variants was significantly positively associated with adult asthma in Japanese women (66).

Several studies have focused on genes related to epithelial function. Reijmerink et al. (67) first reported gene–environment interaction of *ADAM33* genotypes, the first identified asthma gene by positional cloning, and *in utero* tobacco smoke exposure with respect to childhood-onset asthma risk; however, no interaction was detected with postnatal ETS exposure (97). Moreover, Wang et al. (68) reported joint effects of ETS exposure and E-cadherin *CDH1* genotypes associated with the development of childhood asthma.

To date, two GWIS on tobacco smoke exposure and asthma are available. Scholtens et al. (69) conducted the first GWIS specifically aiming to identify genetic polymorphisms that interact with two well-known environmental risk factors for childhood-onset asthma: *in utero* and childhood tobacco smoke exposure. The authors found that genes reported previously to interact with tobacco smoke exposure with respect to asthma development (i.e., *GSTP1, TNF* and *ADAM33*) were not among the most significant hits and showed suggestive interactions between rs8094633 near erythrocyte membrane protein band 4.1 like 3 (*EPB41L3*) and exposure to *in utero* tobacco smoke,

TABLE 5 | Summary of the most relevant examples of gene-by-environment interaction identified in asthma in epidemiological studies.

Exposure	Study design	Gene/region (variant)	Gene/region functionality	Asthma onset	References
Tobacco smoking					
Childhood ETS	Family study	Chr. 1p, 5q, and 17p	–	Childhood/adult	(51)
Childhood ETS	Family study	Chr. 5q	–	Childhood/adult	(52)
Childhood ETS	Family study	Chr. 1q43-q44, 4q34, 5p15, and 17p11	–	Childhood/adult	(53)
Childhood ETS	Family study	Chr. 17q21	Transcriptional activity of ZPBP2, GSDML and ORMDL3 genes	Childhood	(54)
Maternal smoking *in utero*	Candidate gene	*GSTM1 (deletion)*	Antioxidant defenses/detoxification	Childhood	(55) (56)
Childhood ETS	Candidate gene	*GSTM1 (deletion)*	Antioxidant defenses/detoxification	Childhood	(57)
Household ETS	Candidate gene	*GSTP1(Ile105Val)*	Antioxidant defenses/detoxification	Childhood	(58)
Maternal smoking during childhood	Candidate gene	*GSTP1 (Ile105Val)*	Antioxidant defenses/detoxification	Childhood	(59)
Maternal *in utero* smoking or first 2 months of age	Candidate gene	*GSTP1(Ile105Val)* *TNF-α(−857)*	Antioxidant defenses/detoxification Inflammation	Childhood	(60)
Parental smoking	Candidate gene	*TNF-α (−208, −308)*	Inflammation	Childhood	(61)
Maternal smoking *in utero*	Candidate gene	*IL1RN (rs2234678)*	Inflammation	Childhood	(62)
In utero ETS	Candidate gene	*TGFB1 (−509)*	Airway inflammation and remodeling	Childhood	(63)
Household ETS	Candidate gene	*IL-13*	Inflammation	Childhood	(64)
Childhood ETS	Candidate gene	*ICAM1 (rs5491, rs5498)*	Inflammation	Childhood	(65)
Ever smoking	Candidate gene	*IL-3 (rs40401)*	Leukotrienes, IL-4 and TNF-α release	Adult	(66)
In utero ETS	Candidate gene	*ADAM33*	Lung development Endothelial celldifferentiation	Childhood	(67)
Childhood ETS	Candidate gene	*CDH1 (−160)*	Epithelial function	Childhood	(68)
In utero ETS ChildhoodETS	GWIS	Chr. 18 near *EPB4IL3 (rs8094633)* *PACRG(rs1575472)*	Cell-cell junctions and lung development Motile cilia function andmorphogenesis	Childhood	(69)
Active tobacco smoking	GWIS	Intergenic regions on Chr. 9 and 12	Gene expression regulation in lungs	Adult	(70)
Outdoor air pollutants					
NOx and SO_2	Candidate gene	*GSTP1 (Ile105Val)*	Antioxidant defenses/detoxification	Childhood	(71)
Ozone	Candidate gene	*GSTP1 (Ile105Val)* *GSTM1(deletion)*	Antioxidant defenses/detoxification	Childhood	(72)
Ozone and PM2.5	Candidate gene	*GSTP1 (Ile105Val)*	Antioxidant defenses/detoxification	Childhood	(73)
PM10	Candidate gene	*GSTP1 (Ile105Val)*	Antioxidant defenses/detoxification	Childhood	(74)
NO_2	Candidate gene	*GSTP1 (Ile105Val, rs1138272)*	Antioxidant defenses/detoxification	Childhood	(75)
Major road length in 100-m buffer	Candidate gene	*GSTM1 (deletion)* *GSTT1(deletion)*	Antioxidant defenses/detoxification	Childhood	(76)
Living <200 m from a major road	Candidate gene	*GSTT1 (deletion)*	Antioxidant defenses/detoxification	Adult	(77)
NO2	Candidate gene	*NQO1 (rs2917666)*	Antioxidant defense	Adult	(78)
Ozone	Candidate gene	*TNF-α (−308)*	Inflammation	Childhood	(79)
PM2.5	Candidate gene	*TLR2 (rs4696480)* *TLR4 (rs2770150, rs10759931, rs6478317,rs1927911)*	Innate immunity	Childhood	(80)

(Continued)

TABLE 5 | Continued

Exposure	Study design	Gene/region (variant)	Gene/region functionality	Asthma onset	References
NO_2	GWIS	*BMGALT5* *ADCY2* *DLG2*	Glycosphingolipids synthesis Lung function Epithelialstructure	Childhood	(81)
Indoor exposures					
Mold/dampness	Candidate gene	*IL-4*	Humoral and adaptative immunity	Childhood	(82)
Gas cooking	Candidate gene	*GSTM1 (deletion)*	Antioxidant defenses/detoxification	Adult	(83)
Household carpet use	Candidate gene	*IL-13 (h1011 haplotype)*	Airway inflammation	Childhood	(84)
Farming-related exposures					
Farm milk consumption	Candidate gene	*CD14 (−1721)*	Innate immunity	Childhood	(85)
Living on farm	Candidate gene	*TLR2 (−16934)*	Innate immunity	Childhood	(86)
Farm environment	Candidate gene	*TLR6 (rs1039559, rs5743810)*	Innate immunity	Childhood	(87)
Farming exposures	GWIS	*GRM1*	Immunologic synapsis Th1 cytokineproduction	Childhood	(88)
Microbial exposure					
Early respiratory infections	Candidate gene	Chr. *17q21*	Transcriptional activity of ZPBP2, GSDML and ORMDL3	Childhood	(89)
Endotoxins	Candidate gene	*TLR4 (−299, −399)*	Innate immunity	Adult	(90)
Dust endotoxins	Candidate gene	*CD14 (−260)*	Innate immunity	Childhood/adult	(91)
Endotoxins	Candidate gene	*CD14 (−260)* *MD2(rs10808798)*	Innate immunity	Adult	(92)
Endotoxins	Candidate gene	*CD14 (−260)*	Innate immunity	Childhood	(93)

and between rs1575472 in parkin coregulated gene (*PACRG*) and childhood ETS. Interestingly, these two SNPS had not been identified previously in GWAS on childhood asthma. Subsequently, Vonk et al. conducted the first hypothesis-free genome-wide study to identify SNPs that interact with active tobacco smoking with respect to adult-onset asthma using data of the GABRIEL consortium, showing suggestive evidence for an interaction with two intergenic markers (rs9969775 on chromosome 9 and rs5011804 on chromosome 12) with potential regulatory functions linked to gene expression regulation in lung tissue (70).

Overall, existing literature has shown that prenatal and postnatal exposure to maternal/paternal smoking interacts with genetic variants to increase the risk of childhood-onset asthma; interestingly these genes are related to regions of linkage to asthma phenotypes and coding for antioxidant defenses and xenobiotic-metabolizing enzymes, inflammation responses and innate immunity and epithelial function. However, GWIS approaches have failed to replicate those findings revealing additional loci.

Outdoor Air Pollutants

Interactions between outdoor air pollution and genetic variants have been focused on candidate genes related to antioxidative stress and detoxification systems, inflammation, and innate immunity as pathogenic pathways for asthma. Interactive effects of variants in genes belonging to the GST family (*GSTP1* Ile105Val, *GSTM1* deletion) with levels of different outdoor air pollutants (e.g., NO_2, ozone, and particulate matter PM_{10} and $PM_{2.5}$) have been described for childhood asthma (71–75) and traffic-related air pollution (76). Bowatte et al. (76) first reported significant effect modification of *GSTT1* polymorphisms for the association of traffic-related air pollution exposure and childhood-onset asthma, in contrast to previous studies that found no evidence of interaction (73, 74). In addition, Bowatte et al. also first demonstrated effect modification by *GSTT1* genetic variation, but not by *GSTM1* or *GSTP1* polymorphisms, on the association between traffic-related exposure and asthma in adults (77), in contrast to the study by Castro-Giner et al. that only detected an interaction with common polymorphisms in the *NQO1* gene (78).

Genetic variation in few genes related to inflammation and innate immunity have also been investigated as effect modifiers between outdoor air pollution and asthma. In the study of Li et al., the common TNF-α−308 GG genotype was found to interact with annual average levels of ozone in childhood onset asthma (79); although results were not replicated (75). Polymorphisms in toll-like receptor genes (*TLR2* and *TLR4*) have also been identified as potential effect modifiers of the association between outdoor PM2.5 levels and childhood asthma (80).

Recently, a GWIS of air pollution exposure and childhood asthma showed supportive evidence for interaction with outdoor NO_2 levels for the novel loci *B4GALT5* and the previously lung disease associated loci *ADCY2* and *DLG2* (81).

In summary, results on interactions between exposure to outdoor air pollution and genetic variants on genes related to antioxidative stress, detoxification system, inflammation, and innate immunity on childhood and adult onset asthma are inconsistent across studies.

Indoor Exposures

Several studies have investigated interaction between candidate genes and diverse indoor exposures. Gene-environment interactions between the IL-4 promoter and an indoor mold may play an important role in childhood asthma (82). Increased BHR in adults was associated with gas cooking (a major indoor source of NO2), but only among subjects with the *GSTM1* null genotype (83). IL-13 variants were found to interact with household carpet use on the risk of asthma in Taiwanese children (84).

Farming-Related Exposures

The number of gene interactions with a farming environment remains very limited, focusing primarily genes related to innate immunity. Bieli et al. reported an interaction between early farm milk consumption and a polymorphism in the *CD14* gene (CD14/-1721) on the risk of childhood asthma (85). Effect modification by farm exposure in childhood on the association between polymorphism in *TLR* genes and asthma have been shown. Being exposed to a farm environment in childhood was protective against childhood-onset asthma for those with *TLR2*/-16934 T-allele (86), *TLR6*-rs1039559 T-allele and *TLR6*-rs5743810 C-allele (87). The most comprehensive GWIS in 1708 children from 4 rural regions of Central Europe for childhood asthma in relation to farm-related exposures did not reveal any significant interaction with common SNPs (88); however, strong interactions were found for rarer variants in 15 genes, particularly of the glutamate receptor, metabotropic 1 gene (*GRM1*).

Microbial Exposures

Respiratory viral infections in the first few years of life increase risk of childhood asthma; however, not all children develop the disease, suggesting an interaction with the host genetic factors (98). Smit et al. (89) found that 17q21 genetic variants enhance the association between early respiratory infections and childhood-onset asthma. The presence of two common polymorphisms in the extracellular domain of the *TLR4* has been found to modify the effect of endotoxins on asthma in adults (90). Moreover, multiple studies have characterized a similar interaction between asthma, *CD14* variants and environmental endotoxin exposure, a marker of microbial exposure capable of inducing severe airway inflammation. Zambelli-Weiner et al. found CD14/260 polymorphism to interact with dust endotoxin on the risk of childhood-onset asthma (91). Similarly, in adults, Smit et al. showed occupational endotoxin exposure and wheeze in agricultural workers to be significantly modified by genetic variants in *CD14* and *MD2* (92). A recent systematic-review has highlighted the apparent modification of the effect of early life endotoxin exposure on risk of asthma in childhood, but not in adults, by the CD14/260 polymorphism (93).

Literature on inhaled exposures such as indoor air pollution and farming-related is scarce and mostly focused on genetic interactions with genes related to innate immunity and childhood onset asthma. Host innate immunity genetic variation might play a key role in childhood and adult onset asthma susceptibility in relation to microbial exposures including endotoxins.

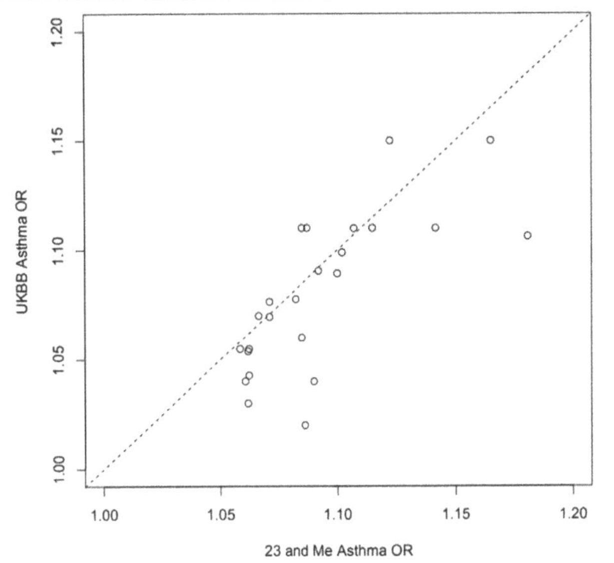

FIGURE 4 | Estimated odds ratios for 24 independent top self-reported "any" asthma associated SNPs from 23 and Me (99) and the UK Biobank (32) samples: exact same SNP in or near *RORA*, *ZBTB10*, *ZPBP2*, *GATA3*, *ID2*, *IL33*, *CD247*, *TSLP*, *RAD50*, *HLAC*, *STAT6*, *D2HGDH*, *RAD51B*, *ADAMTS4*, *SMAD3*, *TLR1*, *BACH2*, *PEX14*, *ADORA1*, *TNFSF4*, *CDHR3*, *CLEC16A*, *LPP*, *LRRC32*.

CONCLUSIONS

There are relatively few large genetic studies examining adult-onset asthma. Studies often rely on relatively simple questionnaire based diagnostic criteria which are validated by the consistency of genetic associations detected (that is, diagnostic looseness is trumped by statistical power, see **Figure 4**), but might be less useful when trying to make fine distinctions about disease onset and persistence. In the present review we have attempted to triangulate via large studies of disorders that will overlap to greater and lesser extents with this condition. Specifically, this has been via the known fact that atopy is more strongly genetically correlated with childhood onset, and the likely fact that COPD overlap will be stronger for adult-onset asthma. In some cases, we can fix pathways of causation by using other types of study, such as traditional longitudinal studies, thus testing and constraining possible interpretations of the genetic evidence. Roughly, it seems that genetic causes of adult-onset asthma tend to affect childhood asthma to the same extent, which in hindsight seems very plausible. Childhood asthma has a larger contribution from atopy loci, while non-atopic immune-related genetic variants seem to be shared by adult-onset and childhood asthma. There are a few loci that might be specific to adult-onset disease, which may overlap with COPD e.g., AGER, but childhood asthma does seem to be a risk factor for adult COPD. Some constitutional risk factors such as increased BMI affect childhood-onset and adult-onset disease equally, and others such as vitamin D level do not show any genetic correlation with asthma.

Most of available studies on gene-environment interaction are focused on childhood-onset asthma, and few studies are based on adult subjects. Gene-environment interactions have revealed novel genes that have previously not been implicated in the pathogenesis of asthma; however, inconsistencies between studies and differences in direction of effects with specific genetic variants have been reported. These issues may likely be due to chance, insufficient power, different populations or ethnic origins, variation in study design and characterization of both exposures and disease phenotypes. Available GWISs have not replicated gene by environment interactions previously reported between common genetic variants and tobacco smoking, outdoor air pollutants, and farming-related exposures. Considering time of asthma onset extends the two-dimensional problem of gene-environment interactions to a three-dimensional problem, since identified gene-environment interactions seldom reproduce for childhood and adult asthma (e.g., endotoxin exposure and CD14/260 genotype). Therefore, evidence suggests that susceptibility of asthma to environmental exposures may biologically differ from early life to adulthood resulting in different pathways and mechanisms of the disease.

FUTURE DIRECTIONS AND RECOMMENDATIONS

- Genetic contributions are higher for childhood-onset asthma.
- The genetic overlap between childhood and adult onset asthma is large.
- The usually small size of the contribution of a single locus to heritability in the population does not preclude a large effect of a drug targeting that pathway. This is the justification given for these larger and larger studies that can detect smaller and smaller effects.
- Mendelian Randomization is a useful tool to investigate pathogenesis—if variation in a gene altering a putative intermediate variable is associated with risk, then environmental exposures affecting that same pathway are supported as truly causative.
- Lacking gene-environmental studies on important risk factors for asthma phenotypes such as diet, medication, microbiota, emerging pollutants, climate change and extreme weather conditions merit consideration.
- Despite methodological challenges, GWIS studies through collaboration hold promise for identifying unexpected gene environment interactions and improving our understanding of asthma phenotypes during a lifetime, beyond candidate studies based on our knowledge of biological processes and/or pathways.

AUTHOR CONTRIBUTIONS

All authors listed have made a substantial, direct and intellectual contribution to the work, and approved it for publication.

REFERENCES

1. The Global Asthma Report 2018. Auckland, New Zealand: Global Asthma Network, 2018.
2. Rhodes L, Moorman JE, Redd SC. Sex differences in asthma prevalence and other disease characteristics in eight states. *J Asthmha.* (2005) 42:777–82. doi: 10.1080/02770900500308387
3. Pavord I, Bush A. Two lovely black eyes; Oh, what a surprise! *Thorax.* (2015)70:609–10. doi: 10.1136/thoraxjnl-2015-207228
4. Bates JHT, Poynter ME, Frodella CM, Peters U, Dixon AE, Suratt BT. Pathophysiology to phenotype in the asthma of obesity. *Ann Am Thorac Soc.* (2017) 14:S395–8. doi: 10.1513/AnnalsATS.201702-122AW
5. Paaso EM, Jaakkola MS, Rantala AK, Hugg TT, Jaakkola JJ. Allergic diseases and asthma in the family predict the persistence and onset-age of asthma: a prospective cohort study. *Respir Res.* (2014) 15:152. doi: 10.1186/s12931-014-0152-8
6. ten Brinke A. Risk factors associated with irreversible airflow limitation in asthma. *Curr Opin Allergy Clin Immunol.* (2008) 8:63–9. doi: 10.1097/ACI.0b013e3282f3b5b5
7. Polderman TJ, Benyamin B, de Leeuw CA, Sullivan PF, van Bochoven A, Visscher PM, et al. Meta-analysis of the heritability of human traits based on fifty years of twin studies. *Nat Genet.* (2015) 47:702–9. doi: 10.1038/ng.3285
8. Thomsen SF, Duffy DL, Kyvik KO, Backer V. Genetic influence on the age at onset of asthma: a twin study. *J Allergy Clin Immunol.* (2010) 126:626–30. doi: 10.1016/j.jaci.2010.06.017
9. Moffatt MF, Gut IG, Demenais F, Strachan DP, Bouzigon E, Heath S, et al. A large-scale, consortium-based genomewide association study of asthma. *N Engl J Med.* (2010) 363:1211–21. doi: 10.1056/NEJMoa0906312
10. Beasley R, Semprini A, Mitchell EA. Risk factors for asthma: is prevention possible? *Lancet.* (2015) 386:1075–85. doi: 10.1016/S0140-6736(15)00156-7
11. Ober C, Vercelli D. Gene-environment interactions in human disease: nuisance or opportunity? *Trends Genet.* (2011) 27:107–15. doi: 10.1016/j.tig.2010.12.004
12. Bønnelykke K, Ober C. Leveraging gene-environment interactions and endotypes for asthma gene discovery. *J Allergy Clin Immunol.* (2016) 137:667–79. doi: 10.1016/j.jaci.2016.01.006
13. Visscher PM, Hill WG, Wray NR. Heritability in the genomics era–concepts and misconceptions. *Nat Rev Genet.* (2008) 9:255–66. doi: 10.1038/nrg2322
14. Thomsen SF. Exploring the origins of asthma: lessons from twin studies. *Eur Clin Respir J.* (2014) 1:25535. doi: 10.3402/ecrj.v1.25535
15. O'Connor LJ, Price AL. Distinguishing genetic correlation from causation across 52 diseases and complex traits. *Nat Genet.* (2018) 50:1728–34. doi: 10.1038/s41588-018-0255-0
16. Yang J, Ferreira T, Morris AP, Medland SE, Genetic Investigation of ANthropometric Traits (GIANT) Consortium, DIAbetes Genetics Replication And Meta-analysis (DIAGRAM) Consortium, et al. Conditional and joint multiple-SNP analysis of GWAS summary statistics identifies additional variants influencing complex traits. *Nat Genet.* (2012) 44:369–75. doi: 10.1038/ng.2213

17. Speed D, Balding DJ. SumHer better estimates the SNP heritability of complex traits from summary statistics. *Nat Genet.* (2019) 51:277–84. doi: 10.1038/s41588-018-0279-5
18. Shi H, Mancuso N, Spendlove S, Pasaniuc B. Local genetic correlation gives insights into the shared genetic achitecture of complex traits. *Am J Hum Genet.* (2017) 101:737–51. doi: 10.1016/j.ajhg.2017.09.022
19. Bulik-Sullivan BK, Loh PR, Finucane HK, Ripke S, Yang J, Schizophrenia Working Group of the Psychiatric Genomics Consortium, et al. LD Score regression distinguishes confounding from polygenicity in genome-wide association studies. *Nat Genet.* (2015) 47:291–5. doi: 10.1038/ng.3211
20. Ullemar V, Lundholm C, Almqvist C. Twins' risk of childhood asthma mediated by gestational age and birthweight. *Clin Exp Allergy.* (2015) 45:1328–36. doi: 10.1111/cea.12547
21. Thomsen SF, van der Sluis S, Kyvik KO, Skytthe A, Backer V. Estimates of asthma heritability in a large twin sample. *Clin Exp Allergy.* (2010) 40:1054–61. doi: 10.1111/j.1365-2222.2010.03525.x
22. Wang K, Gaitsch H, Poon H, Cox NJ, Rzhetsky A. Classification of common human diseases derived from shared genetic and environmental determinants. *Nat Genet.* (2017) 49:1319–25. doi: 10.1038/ng.3931
23. Zhang Y, Qi G, Park JH, Chatterjee N. Estimation of complex effect-size distributions using summary-level statistics from genome-wide association studies across 32 complex traits. *Nat Genet.* (2018) 50:1318–26. doi: 10.1038/s41588-018-0193-x
24. Johansson Å, Rask-Andersen M, Karlsson T, Weronica E Ek. Genome-wide association analysis of 350 000 Caucasians from the UK Biobank identifies novel loci for asthma, hay fever and eczema. *Hum Mol Genet.* (2019) doi: 10.1093/hmg/ddz175. [Epub ahead of print].
25. Ge T, Chen CY, Neale BM, Sabuncu MR, Smoller JW. Phenome-wide heritability analysis of the UK Biobank. *PLoS Genet.* (2017) 13:e1006711. doi: 10.1371/journal.pgen.1006711. Erratum in: *PLoS Genet.* (2018) 14:e1007228.
26. Zhu Z, Lee PH, Chaffin MD, Chung W, Loh PR, Lu Q, et al. A genome-wide cross-trait analysis from UK Biobank highlights the shared genetic architecture of asthma and allergic diseases. *Nat Genet.* (2018) 50:857–64. doi: 10.1038/s41588-018-0121-0
27. Waage J, Standl M, Curtin JA, Jessen LE, Thorsen J, Tian C, et al. Genome-wide association and HLA fine-mapping studies identify risk loci and genetic pathways underlying allergic rhinitis. *Nat Genet.* (2018) 50:1072–80. doi: 10.1038/s41588-018-0157-1. Erratum in: *Nat Genet.* (2018) 50:1343.
28. Lu Q, Li B, Ou D, Erlendsdottir M, Powles RL, Jiang T, et al. A powerful approach to estimating annotation-stratified genetic covariance via GWAS summary statistics. *Am J Hum Genet.* (2017) 101:939–64. doi: 10.1016/j.ajhg.2017.11.001
29. Hobbs BD, de Jong K, Lamontagne M, Bossé Y, Shrine N, Artigas MS, et al. Genetic loci associated with chronic obstructive pulmonary disease overlap with loci for lung function and pulmonary fibrosis. *Nat Genet.* (2017) 49:426–32. doi: 10.1038/ng.3752
30. Demenais F, Margaritte-Jeannin P, Barnes KC, Cookson WOC, Altmüller J, Ang W, et al. Multiancestry association study identifies new asthma risk loci that colocalize with immune-cell enhancer marks. *Nat Genet.* (2018) 50:42–53. doi: 10.1038/s41588-017-0014-7
31. Stein MM, Thompson EE, Schoettler N, Helling BA, Magnaye KM, Stanhope C, et al. A decade of research on the 17q12-21 asthma locus: piecing together the puzzle. *J Allergy Clin Immunol.* (2018) 142:749–64. doi: 10.1016/j.jaci.2017.12.974
32. Canela-Xandri O, Konrad Rawlik K, Tenesa A. An atlas of genetic associations in UK Biobank. *Nat Genet.* (2018) 50:1593–9. doi: 10.1038/s41588-018-0248-z
33. Lasky-Su J1, Himes BE, Raby BA, Klanderman BJ, Sylvia JS, Lange C, et al. HLA-DQ strikes again: genome-wide association study further confirms HLA-DQ in the diagnosis of asthma among adults. *Clin Exp Allergy.* (2012) 42:1724–33. doi: 10.1111/cea.12000
34. Pividori M, Schoettler N, Nicolae DL, Ober C, Hae Kyung IM. Shared and distinct genetic risk factors for childhood onset and adult onset asthma: genome- and transcriptome-wide Studies. *Lancet Resp Med.* (2019) 7:509–22. doi: 10.1016/S2213-2600(19)30055-4
35. Ferreira MA, Vonk JM, Baurecht H, Marenholz I, Tian C, Hoffman JD, et al. Shared genetic origin of asthma, hay fever and eczema elucidates allergic disease biology. *Nat Genet.* (2017) 49:1752–7. doi: 10.1038/ng.3985
36. Ferreira MAR, Mathur R, Vonk JM, Szwajda A, Brumpton B, Granell R, et al. Genetic architectures of childhood- and adult-onset asthma are partlydistinct. *Am J Hum Genet.* (2019) 104:665–84. doi: 10.1016/j.ajhg.2019.02.022
37. Wain LV, Shrine N, Miller S, Jackson VE, Ntalla I, Soler Artigas M, et al. Novel insights into the genetics of smoking behaviour, lung function, and chronic obstructive pulmonary disease (UK BiLEVE): a genetic association study in UK Biobank. *Lancet Respir Med.* (2015) 3:769–81. doi: 10.1016/S2213-2600(15)00283-0
38. Eriksson N, Macpherson JM, Tung JY, Hon LS, Naughton B, Saxonov S, et al. Web-based, participant-driven studies yield novel genetic associations for common traits. *PLoS Genet.* (2010) 6:e1000993. doi: 10.1371/journal.pgen.1000993
39. Miller S, Henry AP, Hodge E, Kheirallah AK, Billington CK, Rimington TL, et al. The Ser82 RAGE variant affects lung Function and serum RAGE in smokers and sRAGE production *in vitro*. *PLoS ONE.* (2016) 11:e0164041. doi: 10.1371/journal.pone.0164041
40. Hayden LP, Cho MH, Raby BA, Beaty TH, Silverman EK, Hersh CP, et al. Childhood asthma is associated with COPD and known asthma variants in COPDGene: a genome-wide association study. *Respir Res.* (2018) 19:209. doi: 10.1186/s12931-018-0890-0
41. Richardson TG, Harrison S, Hemani G, Davey Smith G. An atlas of polygenic risk score associations to highlight putative causal relationships across the human phenome. *Elife.* (2019) 8:e43657. doi: 10.7554/eLife.43657
42. Shrine N, Portelli MA, John C, Soler Artigas M, Bennett N, Hall R, et al. Moderate-to-severe asthma in individuals of European ancestry: a genome-wide association study. *Lancet Respir Med.* (2019) 7:20–34. doi: 10.1016/S2213-2600(18)30389-8
43. Chen YC, Fan HY, Huang YT, Huang SY, Liou TH, Lee YL. Causal relationships between adiposity and childhood asthma: bi-directional mendelian randomization analysis. *Int J Obes.* (2019) 43:73–81. doi: 10.1038/s41366-018-0160-8
44. Granell R, Henderson AJ, Evans DM, Smith GD, Ness AR, Lewis S, et al. Effects of BMI, fat mass, and lean mass on asthma in childhood: a mendelian randomization study. *PLoS Med.* (2014) 11:e1001669. doi: 10.1371/journal.pmed.1001669
45. Skaaby T, Taylor AE, Thuesen BH, Jacobsen RK, Friedrich N, Møllehave LT, et al. Estimating the causal effect of body mass index on hay fever, asthma and lung function using Mendelian randomization. *Allergy.* (2018) 73:153–64. doi: 10.1111/all.13242
46. Contreras ZA, Chen Z, Roumeliotaki T, Annesi-Maesano I, Baïz N, von Berg A, et al. Does early onset asthma increase childhood obesity risk? A pooled analysis of 16 European cohorts. *Eur Respir J.* (2018) 52:1800504. doi: 10.1183/13993003.00504-2018
47. Burgess JA, Walters EH, Byrnes GB, Giles GG, Jenkins MA, Abramson MJ, et al. Childhood adiposity predicts adult-onset current asthma in females: a 25-yr prospective study. *Eur Respir J.* (2007) 29:668–75. doi: 10.1183/09031936.00080906
48. Hall SC, Agrawal DK. Vitamin D and bronchial asthma: an overview of data from the past 5 years. *Clin Ther.* (2017) 39:917–29. doi: 10.1016/j.clinthera.2017.04.002
49. Hysinger EB, Roizen JD, Mentch FD, Vazquez L, Connolly JJ, Bradfield JP, et al. Mendelian randomization analysis demonstrates that low vitamin D is unlikely causative for pediatric asthma. *J Allergy Clin Immunol.* (2016) 138:1747–49.e4. doi: 10.1016/j.jaci.2016.06.056
50. Manousaki D, Paternoster L, Standl M, Moffatt MF, Farrall M, Bouzigon E, et al. Vitamin D levels and susceptibility to asthma, elevated immunoglobulin E levels, and atopic dermatitis: a mendelian randomization study. *PLoS Med.* (2017) 14:e1002294. doi: 10.1371/journal.pmed.1002294
51. Colilla S, Nicolae D, Pluzhnikov A, Blumenthal MN, Beaty TH, Bleecker ER, et al. Evidence for gene-environment interactions in a linkage study of asthma and smoking exposure. *J Allergy Clin Immunol.* (2003) 111:840–6. doi: 10.1067/mai.2003.170
52. Meyers DA, Postma DS, Stine OC, Koppelman GH, Ampleford EJ, Jongepier H, et al. Genome screen for asthma and bronchial hyperresponsiveness: interactions with passive smoke exposure. *J Allergy Clin Immunol.* (2005) 115:1169–75. doi: 10.1016/j.jaci.2005.01.070
53. Dizier MH, Bouzigon E, Guilloud-Bataille M, Siroux V, Lemainque A, Boland A, et al. Evidence for gene x smoking exposure interactions in a genome-wide

linkage screen of asthma and bronchial hyper-responsiveness in EGEA families. *Eur J Hum Genet.* (2007) 15:810–5. doi: 10.1038/sj.ejhg.5201830
54. Bouzigon E, Corda E, Aschard H, Dizier MH, Boland A, Bousquet J, et al. Effect of 17q21 variants and smoking exposure in early-onset asthma. *N Engl J Med.* (2008) 359:1985–94. doi: 10.1056/NEJMoa0806604
55. Gilliland FD, Li YF, Dubeau L, Berhane K, Avol E, McConnell R, et al. Effects of glutathione S-transferase M1, maternal smoking during pregnancy, and environmental tobacco smoke on asthma and wheezing in children. *Am J Respir Crit Care Med.* (2002) 166:457–63. doi: 10.1164/rccm.2112064
56. Rogers AJ, Brasch-Andersen C, Ionita-Laza I, Murphy A, Sharma S, Klanderman BJ, et al. The interaction of glutathione S-transferase M1-null variants with tobacco smoke exposure and the development of childhood asthma. *Clin Exp Allergy.* (2009) 39:1721–9. doi: 10.1111/j.1365-2222.2009.03372.x
57. Kabesch M, Hoefler C, Carr D, Leupold W, Weiland SK, von Mutius E. Glutathione S transferase deficiency and passive smoking increase childhood asthma. *Thorax.* (2004) 59:569–73. doi: 10.1136/thx.2003.016667
58. Lee YL, Lee YC, Guo YL. Associations of glutathione S-transferase P1, M1, and environmental tobacco smoke with wheezing illness in school children. *Allergy.* (2007) 62:641–7. doi: 10.1111/j.1398-9995.2007.01380.x
59. Wu J, Hankinson J, Kopec-Harding K, Custovic A, Simpson A. Interaction between glutathione S-transferase variants, maternal smoking and childhood wheezing changes with age. *Pediatr Allergy Immunol.* (2013) 24:501–8. doi: 10.1111/pai.12086
60. Panasevich S, Lindgren C, Kere J, Wickman M, Pershagen G, Nyberg F, et al. Interaction between early maternal smoking and variants in TNF and GSTP1 in childhood wheezing. *Clin Exp Allergy.* (2010) 40:458–67. doi: 10.1111/j.1365-2222.2010.03452.x
61. Wu H, Romieu I, Sienra-Monge JJ, del Rio-Navarro BE, Anderson DM, Dunn EW, et al. Parental smoking modifies the relation between genetic variation in tumor necrosis factor-alpha (TNF) and childhood asthma. *Environ Health Perspect.* (2007) 115:616–22. doi: 10.1289/ehp.9740
62. Ramadas RA, Sadeghnejad A, Karmaus W, Arshad SH, Matthews S, Huebner M, et al. Interleukin-1R antagonist gene and pre-natal smoke exposure are associated with childhood asthma. *Eur Respir J.* (2007) 29:502–8. doi: 10.1183/09031936.00029506
63. Salam MT, Gauderman WJ, McConnell R, Lin PC, Gilliland FD. Transforming growth factor- 1 C-509T polymorphism, oxidant stress, and early-onset childhood asthma. *Am J Respir Crit Care Med.* (2007) 176:1192–9. doi: 10.1164/rccm.200704-561OC
64. Sadeghnejad A, Karmaus W, Arshad SH, Kurukulaaratchy R, Huebner M, Ewart S. IL13 gene polymorphisms modify the effect of exposure to tobacco smoke on persistent wheeze and asthma in childhood, a longitudinal study. *Respir Res.* (2008) 9:2. doi: 10.1186/1465-9921-9-2
65. Li YF, Lin CC, Tai CK. Interaction of intercellular adhesion molecule 1 (ICAM1) polymorphisms and environmental tobacco smoke on childhood asthma. *Int J Environ Res Public Health.* (2014) 11:6504–16. doi: 10.3390/ijerph110606504
66. Miyake Y, Tanaka K, Arakawa M. IL3 rs40401 polymorphism and interaction with smoking in risk of asthma in Japanese women: the Kyushu Okinawa Maternal and child health study. *Scand J Immunol.* (2014) 79:410–4. doi: 10.1111/sji.12171
67. Reijmerink NE, Kerkhof M, Koppelman GH, Gerritsen J, de Jongste JC, Smit HA, et al. Smoke exposure interacts with ADAM33 polymorphisms in the development of lung function and hyperresponsiveness. *Allergy.* (2009) 64:898–904. doi: 10.1111/j.1398-9995.2009.01939.x
68. Wang MF, Kuo SH, Huang CH, Chen YJ, Lin SH, Lee CJ, et al. Exposure to environmental tobacco smoke, human E-cadherin C-160A polymorphism, and childhood asthma. *Ann Allergy Asthma Immunol.* (2013) 111:262–7. doi: 10.1016/j.anai.2013.07.008
69. Scholtens S, Postma DS, Moffatt MF, Panasevich S, Granell R, Henderson AJ, et al. Novel childhood asthma genes interact with *in utero* and early-life tobacco smoke exposure. *J Allergy Clin Immunol.* (2014) 133:885–8. doi: 10.1016/j.jaci.2013.08.049
70. Vonk JM, Scholtens S, Postma DS, Moffatt MF, Jarvis D, Ramasamy A, et al. Adult onset asthma and interaction between genes and active tobacco smoking: the GABRIEL consortium. *PLoS ONE.* (2017) 12:e0172716. doi: 10.1371/journal.pone.0172716
71. Lee YL, Lin YC, Lee YC, Wang JY, Hsiue TR, Guo YL. Glutathione S-transferase P1 gene polymorphism and air pollution as interactive risk factors for childhood asthma. *Clin Exp Allergy.* (2004) 34:1707–13. doi: 10.1111/j.1365-2222.2004.02099.x
72. Islam T, Berhane K, McConnell R, Gauderman WJ, Avol E, Peters JM, et al. Glutathione-S-transferase (GST) P1, GSTM1, exercise, ozone and asthma incidence in school children. *Thorax.* (2009) 64:197e202. doi: 10.1136/thx.2008.099366
73. Hwang BF, Young LH, Tsai CH, Tung KY, Wang PC, Su MW, et al. Fine particle, ozone exposure, and asthma/wheezing: effect modification by glutathione S-transferase P1 polymorphisms. *PLoS ONE.* (2013) 8:e52715. doi: 10.1371/journal.pone.0052715
74. Su MW, Tsai CH, Tung KY, Hwang BF, Liang PH, Chiang BL, et al. GSTP1 is a hub gene for gene-air pollution interactions on childhood asthma. *Allergy.* (2013) 68:1614–7. doi: 10.1111/all.12298
75. MacIntyre EA, Brauer M, Melén E, Bauer CP, Bauer M, Berdel D, et al. GSTP1 and TNF gene variants and associations between air pollution and incident childhood asthma: the traffic, asthma and genetics (TAG) study. *Environ Health Perspect.* (2014) 122:418–24. doi: 10.1289/ehp.1307459
76. Bowatte G, Lodge CJ, Lowe AJ, Erbas B, Dennekamp M, Marks GB, et al. Do variants in GSTs modify the association between traffic air pollution and asthma in adolescence? *Int J Mol Sci.* (2016) 17:485. doi: 10.3390/ijms17040485
77. Bowatte G, Lodge CJ, Knibbs LD, Lowe AJ, Erbas B, Dennekamp M, et al. Traffic-related air pollution exposure is associated with allergic sensitization, asthma, and poor lung function in middle age. *J Allergy Clin Immunol.* (2017) 139:122–9.e1. doi: 10.1016/j.jaci.2016.05.008
78. Castro-Giner F, Künzli N, Jacquemin B, Forsberg B, de Cid R, Sunyer J, et al. Traffic-related air pollution, oxidative stress genes, and asthma (ECHRS). *Environ Health Perspect.* (2009) 117:1919–24. doi: 10.1289/ehp.0900589
79. Li YF, Gauderman WJ, Avol E, Dubeau L, Gilliland FD. Associations of tumor necrosis factor G-308A with childhood asthma and wheezing. *Am J Respir Crit Care Med.* (2006) 173:970–6. doi: 10.1164/rccm.200508-1256OC
80. Kerkhof M, Postma DS, Brunekreef B, Reijmerink NE, Wijga AH, de Jongste JC, et al. Toll-like receptor 2 and 4 genes influence susceptibility to adverse effects of traffic-related air pollution on childhood asthma. *Thorax.* (2010) 65:690–7. doi: 10.1136/thx.2009.119636
81. Gref A, Merid SK, Gruzieva O, Ballereau S, Becker A, Bellander T, et al. Genome-wide interaction analysis of air pollution exposure and childhood asthma with functional follow-up. *Am J Respir Crit Care Med.* (2017) 195:1373–1383. doi: 10.1164/rccm.201605-1026OC
82. Hwang BF, Liu IP, Huang TP. Gene-environment interaction between interleukin-4 promoter and molds in childhood asthma. *Ann Epidemiol.* (2012) 22:250–6. doi: 10.1016/j.annepidem.2012.01.008
83. Amaral AF, Ramasamy A, Castro-Giner F, Minelli C, Accordini S, Sørheim IC, et al. Interaction between gas cooking and GSTM1 null genotype in bronchial responsiveness: results from the European community respiratory health survey. *Thorax.* (2014) 69:558–64. doi: 10.1136/thoraxjnl-2013-204574
84. Tsai CH, Tung KY, Su MW, Chiang BL, Chew FT, Kuo NW, Lee YL. Interleukin-13 genetic variants, household carpet use and childhood asthma. *PLoS ONE.* (2013) 8:e51970. doi: 10.1371/journal.pone.0051970
85. Bieli C, Eder W, Frei R, Braun-Fahrländer C, Klimecki W, Waser M, et al. A polymorphism in CD14 modifies the effect of farm milk consumption on allergic diseases and CD14 gene expression. *J Allergy Clin Immunol.* (2007) 120:1308–15. doi: 10.1016/j.jaci.2007.07.034
86. Eder W, Klimecki W, Yu L, von Mutius E, Riedler J, Braun-Fahrländer C, et al. Toll-like receptor 2 as a major gene for asthma in children of European farmers. *J Allergy Clin Immunol.* (2004) 113:482–8. doi: 10.1016/j.jaci.2003.12.374
87. Lau MY, Dharmage SC, Burgess JA, Win AK, Lowe AJ, Lodge C, et al. The interaction between farming/rural environment and TLR2, TLR4, TLR6 and CD14 genetic polymorphisms in relation to early- and late-onset asthma. *Sci Rep.* (2017) 7:43681. doi: 10.1038/srep43681
88. Ege MJ, Strachan DP, Cookson WO, Moffatt MF, Gut I, Lathrop M, et al. Gene-environment interaction for childhood asthma and exposure to farming in Central Europe. *J Allergy Clin Immunol.* (2011) 127:138–44. doi: 10.1016/j.jaci.2010.09.041

89. Smit LA, Bouzigon E, Pin I, Siroux V, Monier F, Aschard H, et al. 17q21 Variants modify the association between early respiratory infections and asthma. *Eur Respir J*. (2010) 36:57–64. doi: 10.1183/09031936.00154509
90. Werner M, Topp R, Wimmer K, Richter K, Bischof W, Wjst M, et al. TLR4 gene variants modify endotoxin effects on asthma. *J Allergy Clin Immunol*. (2003) 112:323e30. doi: 10.1067/mai.2003.1648
91. Zambelli-Weiner A, Ehrlich E, Stockton ML, Grant AV, Zhang S, Levett PN, et al. Evaluation of the CD14/-260 polymorphism and house dust endotoxin exposure in the Barbados Asthma genetics study. *J Allergy Clin Immunol*. (2005) 115:1203–9. doi: 10.1016/j.jaci.2005.03.001
92. Smit LA, Heederik D, Doekes G, Koppelman GH, Bottema RW, Postma DS, et al. Endotoxin exposure, CD14 and wheeze among farmers: a gene—environment interaction. *Occup Environ Med*. (2011) 68:826–31. doi: 10.1136/oem.2010.060038
93. Lau MY, Dharmage SC, Burgess JA, Lowe AJ, Lodge CJ, Campbell B, et al. CD14 polymorphisms, microbial exposure and allergic diseases: a systematic review of gene-environment interactions. *Allergy*. (2014) 69:1440–53. doi: 10.1111/all.12454
94. Flory JH, Sleiman PM, Christie JD, Annaiah K, Bradfield J, Kim CE, et al. 17q12-21 variants interact with smoke exposure as a risk factor for pediatric asthma but are equally associated with early-onset versus late-onset asthma in North Americans of European ancestry. *J Allergy Clin Immunol*. (2009) 124:605–7. doi: 10.1016/j.jaci.2009.05.047
95. van der Valk RJ, Duijts L, Kerkhof M, Willemsen SP, Hofman A, Moll HA, et al. Interaction of a 17q12 variant with both fetal and infant smoke exposure in the development of childhood asthma-like symptoms. *Allergy*. (2012) 67:767–74. doi: 10.1111/j.1398-9995.2012.02819.x
96. Li H, Romieu I, Wu H, Sienra-Monge JJ, Ramírez-Aguilar M, del Río-Navarro BE, et al. Genetic polymorphisms in transforming growth factor beta-1 (TGFB1) and childhood asthma and atopy. *Hum Genet*. (2007) 121:529–38. doi: 10.1007/s00439-007-0337-z
97. Schedel M, Depner M, Schoen C, Weiland SK, Vogelberg C, Niggemann B, et al. The role of polymorphisms in ADAM33, a disintegrin and metalloprotease 33, in childhood asthma and lung function in two German populations. *Respir Res*. (2006) 7:91. doi: 10.1186/1465-9921-7-91
98. Calişkan M, Bochkov YA, Kreiner-Møller E, Bønnelykke K, Stein MM, Du G, et al. Rhinovirus wheezing illness and genetic risk of childhood-onset asthma. *N Engl J Med*. (2013) 368:1398–407. doi: 10.1056/NEJMoa1 211592
99. Hinds DA, McMahon G, Kiefer AK, Do CB, Eriksson N, Evans DM, et al. A genome-wide association meta-analysis of self-reported allergy identifies shared and allergy-specific susceptibility loci. *Nat Genet*. (2013) 45:907–11. doi: 10.1038/ng.2686

24

Asthma: Differential Diagnosis and Comorbidities

Nicola Ullmann, Virginia Mirra, Antonio Di Marco, Martino Pavone, Federica Porcaro, Valentina Negro, Alessandro Onofri and Renato Cutrera*

Paediatric Pulmonology & Respiratory Intermediate Care Unit, Sleep and Long Term Ventilation Unit, Department of Paediatrics, Paediatric Hospital "Bambino Gesù" Research Institute, Rome, Italy

***Correspondence:**
Nicola Ullmann
nicola.ullmann@opbg.net

Childhood asthma remains a multifactorial disease with heterogeneous clinical phenotype and complex genetic inheritance. The primary aim of asthma management is to achieve control of symptoms, in order to reduce the risk of future exacerbations and progressive loss of lung function, which results especially challenging in patients with difficult asthma. When asthma does not respond to maintenance treatment, firstly, the correct diagnosis needs to be confirmed and other diagnosis, such as cystic fibrosis, primary ciliary dyskinesia, immunodeficiency conditions or airway and vascular malformations need to be excluded. If control remains poor after diagnostic confirmation, detailed assessments of the reasons for asthma being difficult-to-control are needed. Moreover, all possible risk factors or comorbidities (gastroesophageal reflux, rhinosinusitis, dysfunctional breathing and/or vocal cord dysfunction, obstructive sleep apnea and obesity) should be investigated. At the same time, the possible reasons for poor symptom control need to be find in all modifiable factors which need to be carefully assessed. Non-adherence to medication or inadequate inhalation technique, persistent environmental exposures and psychosocial factors are, currently, recognized as the more common modifiable factors. Based on these premises, investigation and management of asthma require specialist multidisciplinary expertise and a systematic approach to characterizing patients' asthma phenotypes and delivering individualized care. Moreover, since early wheezers are at higher risk of developing asthma, we speculate that precocious interventions aimed at early diagnosis and prevention of modifiable factors might affect the age at onset of wheezing, reduce the prevalence of persistent later asthma and determine long term benefits for lung health.

Keywords: differential diagnosis, asthma, diagnosis, comorbidities, wheeze, asthma mimics

INTRODUCTION

Childhood asthma is a multifactorial disease with heterogeneous clinical phenotype and complex genetic inheritance. The primary aim of asthma management is to make an early diagnosis and to achieve a prompt control of symptoms, in order to reduce the risk of future exacerbations and progressive loss of lung function (1). When asthma is correctly diagnosed, low-dose inhaled corticosteroids can easily control symptoms in most of patients. When asthma does not respond to usual treatment and higher maintenance doses are needed or not sufficient, we enter in the "problematic severe asthma" field (2, 3). However, in some cases, we would probably better define it as "problematic respiratory symptoms unresponsive to prescribed asthma therapy" (4). Nowadays, all pediatricians feel probably confident in clinically diagnose a child with asthma and functional respiratory tests, as a simple spirometry, are often not even performed before starting the basic treatment. Pediatric asthma increased in numbers due to a greater awareness, however, lately we moved from the problem of under diagnosing to a possibly worse condition of over diagnosing asthma (4). The known expression: "Not all that wheezes is asthma" continues to be relevant. In front of a child with ongoing symptoms despite correct treatment, the first consideration is to ensure if the diagnosis of asthma is in fact correct. Depending on the clinical signs and symptoms, alternative diagnosis needs to be taken into consideration, a new correct diagnosis might be made and a different management followed. Differently, when the detailed re-evaluation confirms the diagnosis of asthma, all possible risk factors or comorbidities need to be considered and, sometimes treated, to ensure the maximal effort to obtain symptoms control. At the same time, doctors should verify that basic asthma management strategies are in place. Often the poor symptom control is a consequence of modifiable factors which need to be carefully assessed such as: (1) non-adherence to medication, (2) inadequate inhalation technique, (3) persistent environmental exposures and (4) psychosocial factors. Anytime our asthma management is not satisfying and we categorize our patient as "difficult to treat asthmatic," we need to remember that the first step is always to go right back to square one, instead of keep increasing the corticosteroid treatment: the differential diagnosis, with the most positive attitude of looking for our possible own "mistakes."

The main aim of this paper is to offer a clinical overview of all possible asthma mimickers which need to be taken into consideration and of the comorbidities that might contribute at the poor symptoms control.

PROBLEMATIC SEVERE ASTHMA OR PROBLEMATIC RESPIRATORY SYMPTOMS

As respiratory pediatricians we all experienced that low-dose inhaled corticosteroids can easily control asthma symptoms in most of patients. Moreover, exacerbations in children are often concentrated in some periods of the year due to viral trigger or aeroallergens, and some little patients can even stop their treatment in summer time without clinical deterioration. Nevertheless, children and their parents sometimes keep complaining of recurrent respiratory symptoms despite the correct and continuous treatment, and various courses of antibiotics, beta-2 agonists and oral corticosteroids are frequently prescribed by pediatrician. As a consequence of the poor symptoms control, asthma treatment is often increased and the patient categorized as "problematic severe asthmatic." However, an earlier step could be identified and this condition better defined as "problematic respiratory symptoms unresponsive to prescribed asthma therapy" (4). In fact, the known expression: "Not all that wheezes is asthma" continues to be relevant and the asthma diagnosis should be clinically reconsidered. In the last few decades, we possibly moved from under diagnosing to over diagnosing asthma. Nowadays, a thriving child with history of recurrent cough and a need of frequent beta-2 and inhaled corticosteroid (ICS) treatment is often diagnosed with "probable asthma" and ICS in ever increasing doses immediately prescribed. The initial suspected diagnosis, made with insufficient features and no spirometry testing, gradually, and with no evidence, becomes a definitive diagnosis rarely questioned in the future. Over diagnosis of asthma is a significant problem both in primary and secondary care (5, 6). With this new concept, before an unjustified referral for difficult asthma is made, all the components of the airway disease need to be reconsidered and atypical signs or symptoms which point to an alternate diagnosis recognized. "False asthmas" are often diagnosed years after the onset of clinical symptoms, leading to excessive use of anti-asthmatic medications other than dangerous progression of the misdiagnosed chronic primary disease (7). As often suggested, the first step is to go back to the beginning and take a really detailed history and perform a complete physical examination.

THE HISTORY AND PHYSICAL EXAMINATION

Asthma diagnosis is often suspected when a constellation of typical features is present, however, as most guidelines highlight, diagnosis has to be confirmed either by objective tests or an objective response to treatment. One of the initial major error that occurs is that insufficient features of the asthma pattern are sought before the diagnosis is made. Patient's history should always give enough answers to the following question: "Does the child have any or all of cough, wheeze and breathlessness?." A persistent cough (especially if non-productive) alone in an otherwise well-child is highly unlikely be due to asthma (8). The medical term wheezing is often used by parents to describe different sounds and care should be taken to be sure what they actually mean (9, 10). The habit to ask the family to try to demonstrate the sound of wheezing yourself, could help to avoid misunderstanding. It is also important to understand if the child is noisy and breathless at the same time and to assess the severity of symptoms. After an intense exercise, breathlessness is common but a formal diagnosis of asthma or exercise-induced laryngeal obstruction (EILO) is correct only in about half of those complaining of symptoms. The rest of adolescents are just deconditioned or exaggerating their symptoms (11). The possibility of fabricated and induced illness should be also excluded and possible personal or family psychological factors should be investigated. If symptoms are not clear and an uncontrolled symptomatic asthma need to be ruled out, instead of an extra increase of ICS or of a useless beta-2 prescription, an exercise test may be useful. One of the most "typical" asthma symptoms, such as cough is often present but, at the same time, is definitively a non-specific symptom. In fact, a cough may be the first symptom of many diseases or conditions affecting the respiratory tract. Almost all diseases of the respiratory tract, and in some cases of the extra-respiratory tract, can cause cough (12).

If symptoms are referred just during daytime (no cough or wheezing at night or first hours of morning) and with a sudden onset of symptoms in the absence of obvious triggers, asthma cannot be definitively excluded but other possible diagnosis should be seriously considered. Finally, pattern of symptoms need to be explored with important implications for therapy. For example, of particular importance is distinguishing children only with asthma induced by viral symptoms from those with elapsing symptoms between colds, the latter being more compatible with a chronic disease. At this stage, the atopic status of the family and of the patient should already being stated or it would be necessary to do so, in fact, non-atopic pediatric severe asthma exists but it is rare.

Moreover, history should always include specific questions on parents' smoking habits, pets and home environment. Information on pregnancy, delivery and neonatal period could lead our attention to rule out different diseases: persistent symptoms from birth or first weeks of life are rarely due to an asthmatic condition (13).

A careful physical examination is as important as a careful history. Examination is usually normal, however atypical signs and symptoms need to be identified to think of alternative possible diseases. The diagnosis of asthma should be reconsidered in case of the following: (1) presence of clubbing, cyanosis, significant anemia or nasal polyps; (2) failure to thrive (13).

The presence of symptoms "typical" of asthma plus the finding on physical examination of wheezing strongly point to a diagnosis of asthma. Confirmation of the diagnosis of asthma is based on three key additional elements:

- The demonstration of variable expiratory airflow limitation, preferably by spirometry, when possible.
- Documentation of reversible obstruction.
- Exclusion of alternative diagnoses (see "Alternative Diagnosis" below).

Evidence of airway obstruction on spirometry, especially if reversible with a bronchodilator, can confirm the diagnosis of asthma or assess the severity (14, 15). However, normal spirometry does not exclude the diagnosis. Moreover, young or non-compliant patients are often unable to perform. Improvement on a trial of medications is often used to confirm the diagnosis in these patients (16).

Measurements of peak expiratory flow using a peak flow meter are more variable and effort dependent. Thus, peak flow measurements alone should not be used to diagnose asthma but is more often used in the follow-up of patients to monitor patients' symptoms and response to therapy.

Since, especially in young patients, there is no gold standard test for asthma diagnosis, other possible tests could be performed such as: allergy testing, done either by skin or *in vitro*. Outdoor aeroallergens are unusual triggers in infants and very young children but may be triggers in older children. In addition, when indicated testing reveals the presence of IgE antibody to any allergen, an atopic diathesis is demonstrated, increasing the likelihood that chest symptoms are due to asthma.

In older children bronchoprovocation testing (with methacholine, cold air, or exercise) could be performed when the clinical features are suggestive of asthma but spirometry is normal and there is no response to asthma medications. An exercise challenge of sufficient magnitude may provoke symptoms in children with asthma (17). A negative bronchoprovocation study may also be useful in reducing the likelihood that a child has asthma, although it cannot be used to exclude the diagnosis. Chest radiograph should be performed only in children whit persistent symptoms who do not respond to treatment. In those children, the chest radiograph may display findings suggestive of causes for wheezing other than asthma. Exhaled nitric oxide testing is not recommended as a diagnostic tool but is mostly used in the follow up of asthmatic patients.

TABLE 1 | Clinical clues to alternative diagnosis in children with wheezing.

Clinical clue	Possible diagnosis
PERINATAL AND FAMILY HISTORY	
Symptoms present from birth	Chronic lung disease of prematurity, PCD, CF
Family history of unusual chest disease	CF, Neuromuscular disorders, PCD
Severe upper respiratory tract disease	PCD
SYMPTOMS AND SIGNS	
Persistent moist cough	PBB, Bronchiectasis, Recurrent aspiration, PCD, CF
Excessive vomiting	GERD (w/without aspiration)
Dysphagia	Swallowing problems (w/without aspiration)
Breathlessness with light headedness and peripheral tingling	Dysfunctional breathing, Panic attacks
Inspiratory stridor	Tracheal or laryngeal disorder
Abnormal voice or cry	Laryngeal problems
Focal signs in chest	Developmental anomaly, FB, Post-infective syndrome
Persistent wheeze	Extrinsic intra thoracic airway compression, Airway-malacia, Luminal obstruction, CF, FB
Finger clubbing	CF, Bronchiectasis
Failure to thrive	CF, GERD

CF, cystic fibrosis; FB, foreign body; GERD, gastro-esophageal reflux disease; PBB, protracted bacterial bronchitis; PCD, primary ciliary dyskinesia.

ALTERNATIVE DIAGNOSIS

When to Look for Other Diagnosis

As specified above, the persistent condition of "problematic respiratory symptoms unresponsive to prescribed asthma therapy" need to motivate a clinical full reassessment to exclude that the patient was wrongly labeled with the diagnosis of asthma. To be able to do so, all possible conditions which might mimic asthma need to be considered. Some diseases, better defined as comorbidities, might also coexist with a diagnosis of asthma and will be discussed in a specific section.

Table 1 modified from British Guideline on the Management of Asthma, enlists the clinical clues to alternative diagnosis in asthmatic young children (18). **Table 2** lists alternative diagnosis for "persistent respiratory symptoms not responding to asthma treatment" and the main clinical characteristics for each.

TABLE 2 | When to suspect specific alternative diagnosis and initial useful diagnostic examinations.

Alternative diagnosis	When to suspect	Useful diagnostic examinations
Cystic fibrosis and bronchiectasis	Daily cough productive of sputum, clubbing, malabsorption and failure to thrive, recurrent chest infections, airways bacterial colonization	Sweat chloride test, Genetic tests, Swab culture, Lung Function tests, Chest CT
Immunodeficiency	Recurrent airway infections, Systemic infections (from a few months of age)	Immunoglobulins and specific tests
Primary ciliary dyskinesia	Neonatal upper airway symptoms, Chronic rhinosinusitis, Recurrent otitis media, Daily wet cough, Laterality defects	Nasal NO, HSVM, EM, Genetic tests, Immunofluorescence, Chest CT
Protracted Bacterial Bronchitis	Cronich wet cough, Poor response to Beta-2 agonists, Good response to prolonged course of antibiotics	Often no need of examinations, Swab culture, Bronchoscopy with BAL
Airway malacia	Monophonic wheeze when the child is active, High risk setting (i.e., pt operated for tracheo-esophageal fistula or vascular ring), Presence of associated stridor	Lung function test (truncated expiratory flow in spirometry), Flexible bronchoscopy, Dynamic CT
Airway foreign body	Abrupt onset of symptoms, History of choking, Unilateral monophonic wheeze, Focal hyperinflation of lung	Bronchoscopy, chest x-ray
Habit cough	Prolonged dry, honking cough; Absence of cough during sleep; Absence of any physical findings	Medical investigations should be avoided
Vocal cord dysfunction	Absence of structural abnormalities, Sudden worsening of "asthma" symptoms, No response to asthma medications	Video of an attack, Laryngoscopy during attack
Bronchiolitis obliterans	History of severe viral respiratory infection in the first 3 years of life	CT scan (characteristic mosaic pattern and air trapping)

CT, computed tomography; EM, eletcron microscopy; HSVM, high speed video microscopy; NO, nitric oxide.

Symptoms and clinical signs present from birth, such as: daily productive cough, recurrent upper and lower airway infections could suggest Cystic Fibrosis, Primary Ciliary Dyskinesia or an Immunodeficiency condition. When a chronic wet cough responds to prolonged antibiotic treatment a diagnosis of Protracted Bacterial Bronchitis should be made. Inspiratory sounds or difficult breathing suggest extra-thoracic pathological conditions (tracheal or laryngeal disorders). Respiratory problems combined with significant gastresophageal symptoms should prompt investigations to rule out: GER, recurrent aspiration, swallowing problems. Moreover, the sudden onset of respiratory symptoms with mono lateral thoracic sounds could be indicative for airway foreign body.

Finally, doctors should also remember that a child who presented early on his life one or few episodes of preschool wheeze or dry cough related to colds or upper airway infections should not be labeled with a diagnosis of asthma. Many of these patients in fact are just "healthy" children that will stop experiencing wheezing and respiratory symptoms at school age. This correct medical attitude will possibly avoid overtreatment, medicalization, and anxiety in parents.

Cystic Fibrosis, Non-CF Bronchiectasis and Immunodeficiency

One of the typical symptoms of a patient affected by Cystic Fibrosis (CF) or diffuse non-CF bronchiectasis is chronic cough with the production of abundant sputum which is definitively atypical for a severe asthmatic child. Moreover, CF patients suffer from recurrent chest infections from a very young age and might present episodes of bronchial asthma, which could lead to some diagnostic confusion (19–22).

In non-CF bronchiectasis, the most frequently reported symptoms are productive cough; sputum expectoration; respiratory distress; growth retardation; night sweats (23, 24).

Similarly, respiratory symptoms and complications present a significant cause of morbidity and also mortality among patients suffering from different forms of Primary immunodeficiencies. Frequent and severe infections of either upper (e.g., sinusitis and otitis media) or lower respiratory tract (e.g., pneumonia, bronchitis, bronchiectasis, and interstitial lung diseases) are typical of an immunodeficiency condition. (25–27). Failure to thrive signs and sign of malabsorption could be observed both in CF and immunodeficiency patients.

Primary Ciliary Dyskinesia

Lower airways are commonly involved in Primary Ciliary Dyskinesia (PCD). One of the most common manifestation is chronic asthma, that is generally unresponsive to maintenance treatment, especially at school-age and during adolescence (28). A mild to moderate obstructive pattern is frequently found at spirometry. Possible pathological changes accounting for this include airway smooth muscle hypertrophy and fibrosis, intraluminal secretions and altered lung mechanics secondary to repeated infection (29). Frequently, heterogeneous clinical presentation asthma symptoms let to a challenging diagnosis. More worrying, many patients remain not diagnosed until adulthood when they might already have developed lung bronchiectasis. Lower and upper recurrent respiratory symptoms with no obvious other cause, such as prematurity should suggest to rule out this diagnosis (30). Later in childhood, these children suffer of chronic moist cough often triggered by viral infections, which is one of the reason for years of misdiagnosis with bronchial asthma.

A history of unexplained respiratory distress at birth, recurrent otitis, lower and upper respiratory infections require further examinations. Nasal nitric oxide (nNO) measurement represents a helpful screening tool for PCD diagnosis. nNO levels are extremely low in PCD compared to healthy and disease controls (31). Otherwise, there is no single gold standard diagnostic test for PCD. A complete diagnostic work-up, including high-speed video microscopy analysis, transmission electron microscopy, immunofluorescence, sinus and chest TC is mandatory when PCD is highly suspected (32).

The management of PCD patients involves mainly airway clearance, infection control, and elimination of exposure to inflammatory triggers, also including passive smoke, without which asthma could not improve.

Protracted Bacterial Bronchitis

In children with chronic cough (lasting ≥4 weeks) not responding to asthma treatment, protracted bacterial bronchitis (PBB) should be clinically suspected and a prolonged (minimum of 2 weeks) course of antibiotic should be prescribed. PBB is often misdiagnosed as asthma, resulting in inappropriate and often high doses of inhaled Corticosteroids. Children with PBB were usually young and scarce systemic symptoms, without evidence of sinusitis or ear disease. They typically appeared well, with normal growth and development (33, 34).

Untreated, this condition over time can lead to suppurative lung disease and bronchiectasis. Lung function tests are usually normal (35).

Airway Malacia

Medical awareness for this condition is unfortunately still low and a good number of children are still misdiagnosed as asthmatic after several years of fruitless asthma treatment. (36). Malacic airways (laryngomalacia, tracheomalacia, bronchomalacia) are the most common congenital abnormalities of the pediatric airway and are characterized by excessive softness of tissues leading to increased airway compliance and excessive dynamic collapse during the respiratory cycle (37). Laryngomalacia can be suspected when positional stridor occurs in infants. Even though it is usually a benign condition resolving spontaneously, symptom persistence associated to feeding disturbance, poor weight gain, chest retraction and progressive deformation of rib cage require other investigation to exclude neurologic, genetic and cardiac disorders. When malacia involves intra thoracic airways barking cough, diffuse (tracheomalacia) or unilateral (bronchomalacia) monophonic wheeze, and prolonged expiratory phase expiratory symptoms may occur and must be distinguished from asthma. Sometimes, excessive dynamic collapse can also cause cyanotic spells, apnea and difficulty weaning ventilator support (38).

Congenital tracheomalacia may occur in isolation but has also been associated with other airway abnormalities (tracheoesophageal fistulas, laryngeal clefts, laryngomalacia, and bronchomalacia). Differently, acquired tracheomalacia occurs in the normally developed trachea that undergoes damage from external compression (tumors, cysts, goiter, vascular structures), trauma (tracheostomy), positive pressure ventilation, infection, or inflammation (38). The specific characteristic cough sound often triggered after viral respiratory infection and the flow-volume spirometry pattern (reduction in peak expiratory flow) can help to suspect this condition (39). Other more invasive tests are needed for final diagnosis, such as flexible bronchoscopy and dynamic CT scan with contrast enhancement (40). Observation and conservative management are typically all that are required. However, surgical intervention can be necessary in the most severe cases, and can result in significant improvement in symptoms (37).

Airway Foreign Body

Usually, the sudden onset of respiratory symptoms is more suggestive for a diagnosis of an accidental aspiration of foreign body than of a sudden onset of asthma. Definitively, it is more common in young children (<4 years old). History could be positive for choking and immediate distress but the absence of such history does not certainly rule out the diagnosis. Clinically patient might present persistent cough, unilateral and monophonic wheeze and respiratory distress. However, symptoms depend on the grade of airway obstruction (complete or partial).

Habit Cough

Diagnosis can usually be suspected when the patient coughs repeatedly during the visit, especially when the cough is noising and referred exclusively during daily hours. Usually these children would have received many therapies, including asthma drugs, with no benefit on the honking, brassy cough of many weeks duration, often occurring after a respiratory tract infection. It is more common in children older than 8 years and can cause undue distress to children and both parents. The cough disappears as soon as the child is distracted and always absent during sleep. The origins of the habit cough are often obscure, in some patients can also occur in the background of mild asthma. The diagnosis is made after exclusion of other causes. Some patients might respond to control of breathing exercises from a physiotherapist or speech therapist. Psychological stresses need to be sought in the child's school or home life. The help of a psychologist may be needed to identify and resolve the problem.

Psychological Issues

There is a growing evidence in literature that stress could be a mediator of atopy and that worsens asthma in children. On one hand, asthma control shall be reduced in stressed patients and families due to a poor adherence to treatment; on the other hand, neuroimmunological mechanisms may influence asthma when a psychological distress occurs (41). Lind et al. found that stress, exhaustion, anxiety, depression, were higher than normal in allergic asthma and atopic dermatitis, but not in nonallergic asthma. The vicious circle between psychological issues and symptoms is well-established: inflammatory and non-inflammatory mechanisms contribute to enhance atopy and asthma symptoms (42, 43). Finally, has been demonstrated the strong relationship between panic disorder and asthma. The typical presentation of panic disorder is the hyperventilation:

rapid expiration causes dehydration of the airway contributing to induce asthma by airway narrowing (44).

Vocal Cord Dysfunction

This condition is characterized by inappropriate movement of the vocal cords (adduction during inspiration) induced by: (a) exercise (b) psychological stress (c) local irritation– i.e., reflux. Often vocal cord dysfunction coexists with asthma but it is unresponsive to short-acting beta-2 agonists and it presents with intermittent inspiratory symptoms. The diagnosis of vocal cord dysfunction involves an accurate medical history and specific exams. Patients report air hunger, intermittent aphonia or dysphonia, sensation of choking, chest tightness, chest pain, difficulty swallowing, fatigue and throat clearing. Endoscopic examination with direct visualization of the vocal cords via flexible, transnasal fiber-optic laryngoscopy, possibly after bronchial challenge or during an acute attack, is the gold standard for the diagnosis. Spirometry may show an abnormal shape of inspiratory loop consistent with a variable extrathoracic obstruction (45). Treatment depends on the underlying cause, however, often children are taught breathing control exercises, encouraging nose breathing, and appropriate use of the diaphragm (46). This intervention is often leaded by a respiratory physiotherapist or speech therapist and may help resolving the problem (47–49).

Bronchiolitis Obliterans

Bronchiolitis obliterans (BO) is frequently secondary to influenza, parainfluenza, measles, respiratory syncytial virus, varicella, and Mycoplasma pneumoniae. However, adenovirus is by far the most common agent linked to the development of BO, and can present with persistent wheezing, rather than paroxysmal symptoms. CT scan will show a characteristic mosaic pattern and air trapping (50).

ASTHMA PLUS: CO-MORBIDITIES

In cases where symptoms remain uncontrolled despite maximal guideline-recommended treatment, and all alternate diagnosis have been excluded, possible comorbidities need to be investigated as they may be a coincidental finding or they may contribute directly for the severity of asthma (51).

Establishing the real impact and the causative effect of comorbidities on asthma control it is complicated, and a medical treatment is sometimes necessary to assess their role (52). In most cases, although the ability to improve pediatric severe asthma by treating comorbidities remains unconfirmed, a therapeutic trial should be prescribed.

Obesity

Obesity is a risk factor for poor asthma control, but the relationship between the two conditions is still under debate. It is evident that breathlessness due to simple deconditioning may lead to an erroneous diagnosis of asthma, however, there might be some interesting recent findings. Both, overweight and deconditioning merit treatment in their own right, however weight reduction is known to be very difficult to achieve. Recently, it was found an increased prevalence of asthma in obese children and this group of patients showed more severe exacerbations (greater risk of admission to pediatric intensive care unit) suggesting that asthma in obesity could be a specific disease (53). Moreover, obesity seems to be possible associated with steroid resistance (54). However, we need to be cautious to consider a real association between severe asthma and obesity, as results might be confounded by the known association of obesity with low socio-economic conditions and all what this brings (55). Finally, obesity is known to be associated with variable increased inflammatory phenotypes and airway may be the target of systemic inflammation (56). Obese asthmatic patients probably will also need to be investigated for obstructive sleep apneas and treated appropriately (57). In conclusion, behavioral and weight reduction programs should be offered to asthmatic obese patients to obtain weight reduction. At the same time, it is important to assess airway disease and, before steroid therapy is escalated, look for evidence of uncontrolled airway inflammation (4).

Rhinosinusitis

Pediatric chronic rhinosinusitis (CRS) represent different stages of one chronic inflammatory disease of the mucosa of the nasal cavity and paranasal sinuses, resulting from repeated acute bacterial rhinosinusitis, and leading to a "maladaptive-eosinophilic" stage disease. CRS is a major disease condition with high morbidity and can influence lower airway disease status in adults. In a cross-sectional Korean study, including 17,506 participants, CRS was significantly related to asthma, in particular CRS without nasal polyps was related to childhood-onset asthma (onset before 18 years) or early-onset asthma (onset before 40 years) in adults (58). Given this potential evolution toward more irreversible disease, a more aggressive early intervention it is hoped, to prevent these long-term consequences. Coexistence of chronic rhinosinusitis with nasal polyps and asthma and rather similar characteristics of inflammation support assumption that chronic rhinosinusitis and nasal polyps and asthma may be, at least in part, the same disease process. Chronic rhinosinusitis with nasal polyps is estimated to occur in 7% of all asthmatics, whereas asthma is reported to occur in 26–48% of patients with Chronic rhinosinusitis with nasal polyps (59). Patients with allergic rhinitis and/or chronic rhinosinusitis report poorer asthma control, more exacerbations and emergency visits and have more difficulty achieving symptom control (60), and increased asthma severity has also been shown to be associated with sinonasal inflammation (61). Upper airway symptoms can significantly affect patients' quality of life and should be treated irrespectively of any benefit on asthma control, which could also be obtained (62). A study by Penn et al. examined the efficacy of anti-IgE therapy for the treatment of Chronic rhinosinusitis with nasal polyps. Despite the small number of patients, the nasal polyp scores significantly improved in the anti-IgE group (63, 64). In a recent randomized, double-blind, placebo-controlled trial, Gevaert et al. reported a reduction of nasal polyp size and an improvement of symptoms, compared with placebo in patients with Chronic rhinosinusitis with nasal polyps independent of atopic status (65). Otherwise, despite these promising results, further studies are needed in order to confirm them, as well as of other biologics.

Gastro-Esophageal Reflux

Symptoms of GER often coexist in children with severe asthma. Micro-aspiration, acid stimulation of the esophagus and vagus nerve stimulation are the mechanism proposed to explain how the GER can trigger asthma (66). Furthermore, GER can trigger VCD with consequent laryngeal dysfunction mimicking asthma symptoms. Anyway, it has been proven that GER treatment does not improve asthma control (67). This may suggest that symptoms triggered by GER are mimics of asthma symptoms, rather than exacerbating airway inflammation or airway hyperresponsiveness. Specific examinations assessing for GER, such as impedance-pHmetry and/or gastroesophageal endoscopy must be request in order to exclude this comorbidity (68). A trial of treatment with PPI is recommended as the initial diagnostic step in symptomatic children (69).

Food Allergy

It is still debated whether there is a real relationship between difficult asthma and food allergy, however, there is a higher incidence of food allergy in asthmatic patients admitted to intensive care units and thus it could be considered as a comorbid condition (70). In the literature evidences that support the close relationship between food allergy and asthma as well as the early food sensitization or allergy preceding the development of asthma and other atopic disease can be found (71).

Sometimes patients with food allergy report bronchospasm caused by ingestion or inhalation of the offending food. Even though it is a rare condition (72) linked to an underlying bronchial reactivity, it may develop either in children suffering from asthma or in non-asthmatic patients as part of an allergic reaction to food. When the ingestion of the offending food occurs closely to physical exertion, asthma and anaphylactic symptoms may develop configuring the clinical picture of food-dependent exercise-induced anaphylaxis (73).

It is already showed that symptomatic sensitization to foods is associated with asthma (74) and that the risk of asthma morbidity (daytime symptoms, hospital admissions, lower percent predicted forced expiratory volume in 1-s, asthma persistence, severe asthma exacerbation) is higher in children with food allergy. This risk is especially increased in children with high levels of food specific IgEs and multiple or severe food allergy (75, 76).

When food allergy is diagnosed (suggestive clinical history, positive skin prick tests and specific IgE, positive oral food challenge), the avoidance of the offending food should be suggested, even though specific immunotherapy can be also considered in selected cases to alter the course of atopic march (77).

PROBLEMATIC ASTHMA OR TRUE SEVERE UNCONTROLLED ASTHMA

During the previous process of considering alternative diagnosis and the possible presence of comorbidities that may impact asthma clinical expression and control in childhood, doctors should always verify that basic asthma management strategies are in place (78). Often, the poor symptom control is a consequence of modifiable factors which need to be carefully assessed before proceeding to more invasive investigations. The most frequent conditions that might justify a poor control of symptoms are: non-adherence to medication, inadequate inhalation technique, persistent environmental exposures and psychosocial factors (79). Finally, all patients and carers must be given an individualized written asthma action plan that details current treatment, how to recognize and treat an exacerbation and when to seek appropriate help (47).

SUMMARY AND CONCLUSIONS

In conclusion, since it is known that the majority of asthmatic children can be well-controlled with the basic treatment, if a patient keeps complaining of severe or recurrent respiratory symptoms despite all the basic asthma management strategies are in place, alternative diagnosis need to be considered. Any deviation from common typical patterns should alert one to keep a high index of suspicion for diseases that mimic asthma. Moreover, all possible co-morbidities that might contribute to the uncontrolled clinical condition, need to be excluded and eventually treated. To do so, we need to remember that there is no substitute for a good clinical evaluation that can be performed by all doctors before an unnecessary referral is made.

AUTHOR CONTRIBUTIONS

NU, VM, and FP drafted the initial manuscript, searched for bibliography and revised the final manuscript. VN, AD, and MP were involved in drafting the manuscript, critically revised the manuscript, and approved the final manuscript. RC and NU made substantial contributions to conception and design of the study. RC reviewed and approved the final manuscript. All authors read and approved the final manuscript as submitted.

REFERENCES

1. Global Initiative for Asthma Report. *Global Strategy for Asthma Management and Prevention* (2016). Available online at: www.ginasthma.org (Accessed April 18, 2018).
2. Fitzpatrick AM, Teague WG. Severe asthma in children: insights from the National Heart, Lung, and Blood Institute's Severe Asthma Research Program. *Pediatr Allergy Immunol Pulmonol.* (2010) 23:131–8. doi: 10.1089/ped.2010.0021
3. Chung KF, Wenzel SE, Brozek JL, Bush A, Castro M, Sterk PJ, et al. International ERS/ATS guidelines on definition, evaluation and treatment of severe asthma. *Eur Respir J.* (2014) 43:343–53. doi: 10.1183/09031936.00202013
4. Bush A, Fleming L, Saglani S. Severe asthma in children. *Respirology* (2017) 22:886–97. doi: 10.1111/resp.13085
5. Looijmans-van den Akker I, van Luijn K, Verheij T. Overdiagnosis of asthma in children in primary care: a retrospective analysis. *Br J Gen Pract.* (2016) 66:e152–7. doi: 10.3399/bjgp16X683965

6. Aaron SD, Vandemheen KL, FitzGerald JM, Ainslie M, Gupta S, Lemière C, et al. Canadian Respiratory Research Network. Reevaluation of diagnosis in adults with physician-diagnosed asthma. *JAMA* (2017) 317:269–79. doi: 10.1001/jama.2016.19627
7. Bel EH, Sousa A, Fleming L, Bush A, Chung KF, Versnel J, et al. Unbiased Biomarkers for the Prediction of Respiratory Disease Outcome (U-BIOPRED) Consortium, Consensus Generation. Diagnosis and definition of severe refractory asthma: an international consensus statement from the Innovative Medicine Initiative (IMI). *Thorax* (2011) 66:910–7. doi: 10.1136/thx.2010.153643
8. Kelly YJ, Brabin BJ, Milligan PJ, Reid JA, Heaf D, Pearson MG. Clinical significance of cough and wheeze in the diagnosis of asthma. *Arch Dis Child.* (1996) 75:489–93.
9. Cane RS, Ranganathan SC, McKenzie SA. What do parents of wheezy children understand by "wheeze"? *Arch Dis Child.* (2000) 82:327–32. doi: 10.1136/adc.82.4.327
10. Levy ML, Godfrey S, Irving CS, Sheikh A, Hanekom W, Bush A, et al. Wheeze detection: recordings vs. assessment of physician and parent. *J Asthma* (2004) 41:845–53. doi: 10.1081/JAS-200038451
11. Johansson H, Norlander K, Berglund L, Janson C, Malinovschi A, Nordvall L, et al. Prevalence of exercise-induced bronchoconstriction and exercise-induced laryngeal obstruction in a general adolescent population. *Thorax* (2015) 70:57–63. doi: 10.1136/thoraxjnl-2014-205738
12. Bergamini M, Kantar A, Cutrera R, Interest Group IPC. Analysis of the literature on chronic cough in children. *Open Respir Med J.* (2017) 11:1–9 doi: 10.2174/1874306401711010001
13. Rosenthal M. Differential diagnosis of asthma. *Paediatr Respir Rev.* (2002) 3:148–53. doi: 10.1016/S1526-0550(02)00008-2
14. British Guideline on the Management of Asthma. British Thoracic Society, Scottish Intercollegiate Guidelines Network. *Thorax* (2008) 63(Suppl. 4):iv1–121. doi: 10.1136/thx.2008.097741
15. Papadopoulos NG, Arakawa H, Carlsen KH, Custovic A, Gern J, Lemanske R, et al. International consensus on (ICON) pediatric asthma. *Allergy* (2012) 67:976. doi: 10.1111/j.1398-9995.2012.02865.x
16. National Asthma Education and Prevention Program: Expert panel report 3 (EPR3). *Guidelines for the Diagnosis and Management of Asthma. Bethesda, MD: National Heart, Lung, and Blood Institute* (2007).
17. Jones A, Bowen M. Screening for childhood asthma using an exercise test. *Br J Gen Pract.* (1994) 44:127.
18. SIGN 153 @BULLET *British Guideline on the Management of Asthma* (2016). Available online at: https://www.brit-thoracic.org.uk/document-library/clinical-information/asthma/btssign-asthma-guideline-2016.
19. De Boeck K, Vermeulen F, Dupont L. The diagnosis of cystic fibrosis. *Presse Med.* (2017) 46: e97–108. doi: 10.1016/j.lpm.2017.04.010
20. Paranjape SM, Mogayzel PJ Jr, Cystic fibrosis in the era of precision medicine. *Paediatr Respir Rev.* (2018) 25:64–72. doi: 10.1016/j.prrv.2017.03.001
21. Villanueva G, Marceniuk G, Murphy MS, Walshaw M, Cosulich R, Guideline Committee. Diagnosis and management of cystic fibrosis: summary of NICE guidance. *BMJ* (2017) 359:j4574. doi: 10.1136/bmj.j4574
22. Ren CL, Morgan RL, Oermann C, Resnick HE, Brady C, Campbell A, et al. Cystic fibrosis foundation pulmonary guidelines. Use of cystic fibrosis transmembrane conductance regulator modulator therapy in patients with cystic fibrosis. *Ann Am Thorac Soc.* (2018) 15:271–80. doi: 10.1513/AnnalsATS.201707-539OT
23. Satirer O, Yesil AM, Emiralioglu N, Tugcu GD, Yalcin E, Dogru D, et al. A review of the etiology and clinical presentation of non-cystic fibrosis bronchiectasis: a tertiary care experienceis. *Respir Med.* 137 35–9. doi: 10.1016/j.rmed.2018.02.013
24. Gallucci M, di Palmo E, Bertelli L, Camela F, Ricci G Pession A. A pediatric disease to keep in mind: diagnostic tools and management of bronchiectasis in pediatric age. *Ital J Pediatr.* (2017) 43:117. doi: 10.1186/s13052-017-0434-0
25. JesenakM, Banovcin P, Jesenakova B Babusikova E. Pulmonary manifestations of primary immunodeficiency disorders in children. *Front Pediatr.* (2014) 2:77. doi: 10.3389/fped.2014.00077
26. Owayed A, Al-Herz W. Sinopulmonary complications in subjects with primary immunodeficiency. *Respir Care* (2016) 61:1067–72. doi: 10.4187/respcare.04479
27. Yazdani R, Abolhassani H Asgardoon M, Shaghaghi M, Modaresi M, Azizi G, et al. Infectiousand noninfectious pulmonary complications in patients with primary immunodeficiency disorders. *J Invest Allergol Clin Immunol.* (2017) 27:231–24. doi: 10.18176/jiaci.0166
28. Sagel SD, Davis SD, Campisi P, Dell SD. Update of respiratory tract disease in children with primary ciliary dyskinesia. *Proc Am Thorac Soc.* (2011) 8:438–43. doi: 10.1513/pats.201103-024SD
29. Patella V, Bocchino M, Steinhilber G. Asthma is associated with increased susceptibility to infection. *Miner Med.* (2015) 106(4 Suppl. 3):1–7.
30. Mirra V, Werner C, Santamaria F. Primary ciliary dyskinesia: an update on clinical aspects, genetics, diagnosis, and future treatment strategies. *Front Pediatr.* (2017) 5:135. doi: 10.3389/fped.2017.00135
31. Marthin JK, Nielsen KG. Choice of nasal nitric oxide technique as first-line test for primary ciliary dyskinesia. *Eur Respir J.* (2011) 37:559–65. doi: 10.1183/09031936.00032610
32. Lucas JS, Dimitrov BD, Behan L, Kuehni CE. Diagnostic testing in primary ciliary dyskinesia. *Eur Respir J.* (2016) 48:960–1. doi: 10.1183/13993003.00909-2016
33. Kantar A, Chang AB, Shields MD, Marchant JM, Grimwood K, Grigg J, et al. ERS statement on protracted bacterial bronchitis in children. *Eur Respir J.* (2017) 50:1602139. doi: 10.1183/13993003.02139-2016
34. Di Filippo P, Scaparrotta A, Petrosino MI, Attanasi M, Di Pillo S, Chiarelli F, et al. An underestimated cause of chronic cough: the protracted bacterial bronchitis. *Ann Thorac Med.* (2018) 13:7–13 doi: 10.4103/atm.ATM_12_17
35. Chang AB, Upham JW, Masters IB, Redding GR, Gibson PG, Marchant JM, et al. Protracted bacterial bronchitis: the last decade and the road ahead. *Pediatr Pulmonol.* (2016) 51:225–42. doi: 10.1002/ppul.23351
36. Petreschi F, Ullmann N, Bottero S, Tomà P, Inserra A, Francalanci P, et al. A young girl with apparent treatment-resistant asthma treated at Bambino Gesù children's hospital. *Thorax* (2014) 69:396–8. doi: 10.1136/thoraxjnl-2013-204880
37. Hysinger EB. Laryngomalacia, tracheomalacia and bronchomalacia.*Curr Probl Pediatr Adolesc Health Care* (2018) 48:113–8. doi: 10.1016/j.cppeds.2018.03.002
38. Fraga JC, Jennings RW, Kim PC. Pediatric tracheomalacia. *Semin Pediatr Surg.* (2016) 25:156–64. doi: 10.1053/j.sempedsurg.2016.02.008
39. Boogaard R, Huijsmans SH, Pijnenburg MW, Tiddens HA, de Jongste JC, Merkus PJ. Tracheomalacia and bronchomalacia in children: incidence and patient characteristics. *Chest* (2005) 128:3391–7. doi: 10.1378/chest.128.5.3391
40. Ullmann N, Secinaro A, Menchini L, Caggiano S, Verrillo E, Santangelo TP, et al. Dynamic expiratory CT: an effective non-invasive diagnostic exam for fragile children with suspected tracheo-bronchomalacia. *Pediatr Pulmonol.* (2018) 53:73–80. doi: 10.1002/ppul.23831
41. Hedlin G, Bush A, Lødrup Carlsen K, Wennergren G, De Benedictis FM, Melén E, et al. Problematic severe asthma in children, not one problem but many: a GA2LEN initiative. *Eur Respir J.* (2010) 36:196–201. doi: 10.1183/09031936.00104809
42. Lind N, Nordin M, Palmquist E, Nordin S. Psychological distress in asthma and allergy: the västerbotten environmental health study. *Psychol Health Med.* (2014) 19:316–23. doi: 10.1080/13548506.2013.806814
43. Rand CS, Wright RJ, Cabana MD, Foggs MB, Halterman JS, Olson L, et al. Mediators of asthma outcomes. *J Allergy Clin Immunol.* (2012) 129(3 Suppl.):S136–41. doi: 10.1016/j.jaci.2011.12.987
44. Lee YC, Lee CT, Lai YR, Chen VC, Stewart R. Association of asthma and anxiety: a nationwide population-based study in Taiwan. *J Affect Disord.* (2016) 189:98–105. doi: 10.1016/j.jad.2015.09.040
45. Dunn NM, Katial RK, Hoyte FCL. Vocal cord dysfunction: a review. *Asthma Res Pract.* (2015) 1:9. doi: 10.1186/s40733-015-0009-z
46. Cook J, Beresford F, Fainardi V, Hall P, Housley G, Jamalzadeh A, et al. Managing the pediatric patient with refractory asthma: a multidisciplinary approach. *J Asthma Allergy* (2017) 10:123–30. doi: 10.2147/JAA.S129159
47. Lødrup Carlsen KC, Hedlin G, Bush A, Wennergren G, de Benedictis FM, De Jongste JC, et al. PSACI (Problematic Severe Asthma in Childhood Initiative) group. Assessment of problematic severe asthma in children. *Eur Respir J.* (2011) 37:432–40. doi: 10.1183/09031936.00091410

48. Weinberger M, Abu-Hasan M. Pseudo-asthma: when cough, wheezing, and dyspnea are not asthma. *Pediatrics* (2007) 120:855–64. doi: 10.1542/peds.2007-0078
49. de Groot EP, Duiverman EJ, Brand PL. Dysfunctional breathing in children with asthma: a rare but relevant comorbidity. *Eur Respir J.* (2013) 41:1068–73. doi: 10.1183/09031936.00130212
50. Fischer GB, Sarria EE, Mattiello R, Mocelin HT, Castro-Rodriguez JA. Post infectious bronchiolitis obliterans in children. *Paediatr Respir Rev.* (2010) 11:233–9. doi: 10.1016/j.prrv.2010.07.005
51. Bush A, Saglani S. Management of severe asthma in children. *Lancet* (2010) 376:814–5. doi: 10.1016/S0140-6736(10)61054-9
52. Mirra V, Montella S, Santamaria F. Pediatric severe asthma: a case series report and perspectives on anti-IgE treatment. *BMC Pediatr.* (2018) 18:73. doi: 10.1186/s12887-018-1019-9
53. Weinmayr G, Forastiere F, Büchele G, Jaensch A, Strachan DP, Nagel G, ISAAC Phase Two Study Group. Overweight/obesity and respiratory and allergic disease in children: international study of asthma and allergies in childhood (ISAAC) phase two. *PLoS ONE* (2014) 9:e113996. doi: 10.1371/journal.pone.0113996
54. Forno E, Lescher R, Strunk R, Weiss S, Fuhlbrigge A, Celedón JC, Childhood Asthma Management Program Research Group. Decreased response to inhaled steroids in overweight and obese asthmatic children. *J Allergy Clin Immunol.* (2011)127:741–9. doi: 10.1016/j.jaci.2010.12.010
55. Carroll CL, Stoltz P, Raykov N, Smith SR, Zucker AR. Childhood overweight increases hospital admission rates for asthma. *Pediatrics* (2007) 120:734–40. doi: 10.1542/peds.2007-0409
56. Peters MC, McGrath KW, Hawkins GA, Hastie AT, Levy BD, Israel E, et al. Plasma interleukin-6 concentrations, metabolic dysfunction, and asthma severity: a cross-sectional analysis of two cohorts. *Lancet Respir Med.* (2016) 4:574–84. doi: 10.1016/S2213-2600(16)30048-0
57. Kumar S, Kelly AS. Review of childhood obesity: from epidemiology, etiology, and comorbidities to clinical assessment and treatment. *Mayo Clin Proc.* (2017) 92:251–65. doi: 10.1016/j.mayocp.2016.09.017
58. Won HK, Kim YC, Kang MG, Park HK, Lee SE, Kim MH, et al. Age-related prevalence of chronic rhinosinusitis and nasal polyps and their relationships with asthma onset. *Ann Allergy Asthma Immunol.* (2018) 120:389–94. doi: 10.1016/j.anai.2018.02.005
59. Promsopa C, Kansara S, Citardi MJ, Fakhri S, Porter P, Luong A. Prevalence of confirmed asthma varies in chronic rhinosinusitis subtypes. *Int Forum Allergy Rhinol.* (2016) 6:373–7. doi: 10.1002/alr.21674
60. Valovirta E, Pawankar R. Survey on the impact of comorbid allergic rhinitis in patients with asthma. *BMC Pulm Med.* (2006) 6:S3. doi: 10.1186/1471-2466-6-S1-S3
61. Lin DC, Chandra RK, Tan BK, Zirkle W, Conley DB, Grammer LC, et al. Association between severity of asthma and degree of chronic rhinosinusitis. *Am J Rhinol Allergy* (2011) 25:205–8. doi: 10.2500/ajra.2011.25.3613
62. de Groot EP, Nijkamp A, Duiverman EJ, Brand PL. Allergic rhinitis is associated with poor asthma control in children with asthma. *Thorax* (2012) 67:582–7. doi: 10.1136/thoraxjnl-2011-201168
63. Penn R, Mikula S. The role of anti-IgE immunoglobulin therapy in nasal polyposis: a pilot study. *Am J Rhinol.* (2007) 21:428–32. doi: 10.2500/ajr.2007.21.3060
64. Gevaert P, Calus L, Van Zele T, Blomme K, De Ruyck N, Bauters W, et al. Omalizumab is effective in allergic and nonallergic patients with nasal polyps and asthma. *J Allergy Clin Immunol.* (2013) 131:110-6.e1. doi: 10.1016/j.jaci.2012.07.047
65. Denlinger LC, Phillips BR, Ramratnam S, Ross K, Bhakta NR, Cardet JC, et al. Inflammatory and co-morbid features of patients with severe asthma and frequent exacerbations. *Am J Respir Crit Care Med.* (2017) 195:302–13. doi: 10.1164/rccm.201602-0419OC
66. Gibson PG, Henry R, Coughlan JJ. Gastro-oesophageal reflux treatment for asthma in adults and children. In: Gibson PG, editor. *Cochrane Database of Systematic Reviews.* Chichester: John Wiley & Sons, Ltd (2003).
67. Writing Committee for the American Lung Association Asthma Clinical Research Centers, Holbrook JT, Wise RA, Gold BD, Blake K, Brown ED, et al. Lansoprazole for children with poorly controlled asthma: a randomized controlled trial. *JAMA* (2012) 307:373–81. doi: 10.1001/jama.2011.2035
68. Naik RD, Vaezi MF. Extra-esophageal gastroesophageal reflux disease and asthma: understanding this interplay. *Expert Rev Gastroenterol Hepatol.* (2015) 9:969–82. doi: 10.1586/17474124.2015.1042861
69. Roberts G, Patel N, Levi-Schaffer F, Habibi P, Lack G. Food allergy as a risk factor for life-threatening asthma in childhood: a case-controlled study. *J Allergy Clin Immunol.* (2003) 112:168–74. doi: 10.1067/mai.2003.1569
70. de Groot EP, Kreggemeijer WJ, Brand PL. Getting the basics right resolves most cases of uncontrolled and problematic asthma. *Acta Paediatr.* (2015) 104:916–21. doi: 10.1111/apa.13059
71. Illi S, von Mutius E, Lau S, Nickel R, Grüber C, Niggemann B, et al. The nat-ural course of atopic dermatitis from birth to age 7 years and the association with asthma. *J Allergy Clin Immunol.* (2004) 113:925–31. doi: 10.1016/j.jaci.2004.01.778
72. James JM. Respiratory manifestations of food allergy. *Pediatrics* (2003) 111:1625–30.
73. Bock SA, Atkins FM. The natural history of peanut allergy. *J Allergy Clin Immunol.* (1989) 83:900–4.
74. Brown SJ, Asai Y, Cordell HJ, Campbell LE, Zhao Y, Liao H, et al. Loss-of-function variants in the filaggrin gene are a significant risk factor for peanut allergy. *J Allergy Clin Immunol.* (2011) 127:661–7. doi: 10.1016/j.jaci.2011.01.031
75. Chan SM, Turcanu V, Stephens AC, Fox AT, Grieve AP, Lack G. Cutaneous lymphocyte antigen and alpha4-beta7 T-lymphocyte responses are associated with peanut allergy and tolerance in children. *Allergy* (2012) 67:336–42. doi: 10.1111/j.1398-9995.2011.02765.x
76. Caffarelli C, Garrubba M, Greco C, Mastrorilli C, Dascola CP. Asthma and food allergy in children: is there a connection or interaction? *Front Pediatr.* (2016) 4:34. doi: 10.3389/fped.2016.00034
77. Porcaro F, Corsello G, Pajno GB. SLIT's prevention of the allergic march. *Curr Allergy Asthma Rep.* (2018) 18:31. doi: 10.1007/s11882-018-0785-7
78. Saglani S, Fleming L. How to manage a child with difficult asthma? *Expert Rev Respir Med.* (2016) 10:873–9. doi: 10.1080/17476348.2016.1191355
79. Levy ML. The national review of asthma deaths: what did we learn and what needs to change? *Breathe (Sheff).* (2015) 11:14–24. doi: 10.1183/20734735.008914

Permissions

All chapters in this book were first published by Frontiers; hereby published with permission under the Creative Commons Attribution License or equivalent. Every chapter published in this book has been scrutinized by our experts. Their significance has been extensively debated. The topics covered herein carry significant findings which will fuel the growth of the discipline. They may even be implemented as practical applications or may be referred to as a beginning point for another development.

The contributors of this book come from diverse backgrounds, making this book a truly international effort. This book will bring forth new frontiers with its revolutionizing research information and detailed analysis of the nascent developments around the world.

We would like to thank all the contributing authors for lending their expertise to make the book truly unique. They have played a crucial role in the development of this book. Without their invaluable contributions this book wouldn't have been possible. They have made vital efforts to compile up to date information on the varied aspects of this subject to make this book a valuable addition to the collection of many professionals and students.

This book was conceptualized with the vision of imparting up-to-date information and advanced data in this field. To ensure the same, a matchless editorial board was set up. Every individual on the board went through rigorous rounds of assessment to prove their worth. After which they invested a large part of their time researching and compiling the most relevant data for our readers.

The editorial board has been involved in producing this book since its inception. They have spent rigorous hours researching and exploring the diverse topics which have resulted in the successful publishing of this book. They have passed on their knowledge of decades through this book. To expedite this challenging task, the publisher supported the team at every step. A small team of assistant editors was also appointed to further simplify the editing procedure and attain best results for the readers.

Apart from the editorial board, the designing team has also invested a significant amount of their time in understanding the subject and creating the most relevant covers. They scrutinized every image to scout for the most suitable representation of the subject and create an appropriate cover for the book.

The publishing team has been an ardent support to the editorial, designing and production team. Their endless efforts to recruit the best for this project, has resulted in the accomplishment of this book. They are a veteran in the field of academics and their pool of knowledge is as vast as their experience in printing. Their expertise and guidance has proved useful at every step. Their uncompromising quality standards have made this book an exceptional effort. Their encouragement from time to time has been an inspiration for everyone.

The publisher and the editorial board hope that this book will prove to be a valuable piece of knowledge for researchers, students, practitioners and scholars across the globe.

List of Contributors

Amelia Licari, Ilaria Brambilla, Alessia Marseglia, Maria De Filippo, Valeria Paganelli and Gian L. Marseglia
Department of Pediatric, Fondazione IRCCS Policlinico San Matteo, University of Pavia, Pavia, Italy

Louise Fleming
National Heart and Lung Institute, Imperial College, London and Royal Brompton Hospital, London, United Kingdom

Liam Heaney
Centre for Experimental Medicine, School of Medicine, Dentistry and Biomedical Sciences, Institute for Health Sciences, Queens University Belfast, Belfast, United Kingdom

Stefania Arasi and Alessandro G. Fiocchi
Pediatric Allergology Unit, Bambino Gesù Hospital (IRCCS), Rome, Italy

Federica Porcaro
Pediatric Pulmonology & Respiratory Intermediate Care Unit, Sleep and Long-Term Ventilation Unit, Department of Pediatrics, Bambino Gesù Children's Hospital, Rome, Italy

Adelaide LIndsay Withers
Department of Respiratory Medicine, Perth Children's Hospital, Perth, WA, Australia

Ruth Green
Glenfield Hospital, Leicester, United Kingdom

Giuliana Ferrante
Department of Science for Health Promotion and Mother and Child Care, University of Palermo, Palermo, Italy

Stefania La Grutta
Department of Science for Health Promotion and Mother and Child Care, University of Palermo, Palermo, Italy
National Research Council of Italy, Institute of Biomedicine and Molecular Immunology, Palermo, Italy

Shyamali C. Dharmage
Allergy and Lung Health Unit, School of Population and Global Health, University of Melbourne, Melbourne, VIC, Australia

Jennifer L. Perret
Allergy and Lung Health Unit, School of Population and Global Health, University of Melbourne, Melbourne, VIC, Australia
Institute for Breathing and Sleep, Melbourne, VIC, Australia

Adnan Custovic
Department of Paediatrics, Imperial College London, London, United Kingdom

Maria A. Tosca and Roberta Olcese
Department of Pediatrics, Allergy Center, Istituto Giannina Gaslini (IRCCS), Genoa, Italy

Gianluigi Marseglia
Department of Pediatrics, Ospedale San Matteo (IRCCS), Pediatrics Clinic, University of Pavia, Pavia, Italy

Oliviero Sacco
Pediatric Pulmonology and Endoscopy, Istituto Giannina Gaslini (IRCCS), Genoa, Italy

Giorgio Ciprandi
Allergy Clinic, Ospedale San Martino (IRCCS), Genoa, Italy

Marcella Gallucci, Emanuela di Palmo and Giampaolo Ricci
Department of Pediatrics, S. Orsola-Malpighi Hospital, University of Bologna, Bologna, Italy

Paolo Carbonara, Angela Maria Grazia Pacilli and Stefano Nava
Department of Specialistic, Diagnostic and Experimental Medicine (DIMES), University of Bologna, Alma Mater Studiorum, Bologna, Italy

Ceyda Oksel, Sadia Haider, Sara Fontanella and Adnan Custovic
Section of Paediatrics, Department of Medicine, Imperial College London, London, United Kingdom

Clement Frainay
Department of Epidemiology and Biostatistics, Faculty of Medicine, School of Public Health, Imperial College London, London, United Kingdom
INRA, UMR1331, Toxalim, Research Centre in Food Toxicology, Toulouse, France

Alan Kaplan
Department of Family and Community Medicine, University of Toronto, Toronto, ON, Canada

Antony Hardjojo and Shaylynn Yu
Observational and Pragmatic Research Institute, Singapore, Singapore

David Price
Observational and Pragmatic Research Institute, Singapore, Singapore
Division of Applied Health Sciences, Centre of Academic Primary Care, University of Aberdeen, Aberdeen, United Kingdom
Optimum Patient Care, Cambridge, United Kingdom

Laura Tenero, Marco Zaffanello, Michele Piazza and Giorgio Piacentini
Department of Surgical Sciences, Dentistry, Gynecology and Pediatrics, University of Verona, Verona, Italy

Gary J. Connett and Mike Thomas
University Hospital Southampton NHS Foundation Trust, Southampton, United Kingdom

Riccardina Tesse, Giorgia Borrelli, Giuseppina Mongelli, Violetta Mastrorilli and Fabio Cardinale
Allergy, Immunology and Pediatric Pulmonology Unit, Ospedale Pediatrico Papa Giovanni XXIII, Bari, Italy

Sejal Saglani
National Heart & Lung Institute, Imperial College London, London, United Kingdom
Department of Respiratory Paediatrics, Royal Brompton Hospital, London, United Kingdom

Andrew N. Menzie-Gow
National Heart & Lung Institute, Imperial College London, London, United Kingdom
Department of Respiratory Medicine, Royal Brompton Hospital, London, United Kingdom

Barbara Boutopoulou, Kostas N. Priftis and Konstantinos Douros
Respiratory and Allergy Unit, 3rd Pediatric Department of National and Kapodistrian University of Athens, University General Hospital "Attikon," Athens, Greece

Despoina Koumpagioti
2nd Pediatric Department of National and Kapodistrian University of Athens, "P & A Kiriakou" Children Hospital, Athens, Greece

Vasiliki Matziou
Faculty of Nursing, National and Kapodistrian University of Athens, Athens, Greece

Li Ping Chung
Department of Respiratory Medicine, Fiona Stanley Hospital, Perth, WA, Australia

James Y. Paton
School of Medicine, College of Medical, Veterinary, and Life Sciences, University of Glasgow, Glasgow, United Kingdom

Neeta Kulkarni
Department of Infection, Immunity and Inflammation, Institute for Lung Health, University of Leicester, Leicester, United Kingdom

Ahmad Kantar
Pediatric Cough and Asthma Center, Istituti Ospedalieri Bergamaschi, University and Research Hospitals, Bergamo, Italy

Silvia Costella
High Altitude Paediatric Asthma Centre in Misurina, Pio XII Institute, Belluno, Italy

Vincenzo Ragazzo
Department of Pediatrics, Versilia Hospital, Lido di Camaiore, Italy

Giorgio Piacentini and Attilio Boner
Pediatrics Section, Department of Surgery, Dentistry, Paediatrics, and Gynaecology, University of Verona, Verona, Italy

Christopher O'Callaghan
Respiratory, Critical Care and Anaesthesia, UCL Great Ormond Street Institute of Child Health, NIHR Great Ormond Street Hospital Biomedical Research Centre, Great Ormond Street Children's Hospital, London, United Kingdom

Marco Maglione, Marco Poeta and Francesca Santamaria
Department of Translational Medical Sciences, Federico II University, Naples, Italy
Department of Pediatrics, Federico II University, Naples, Italy

Andrew Bush
Departments of Paediatrics and Paediatric Respiratory Medicine, Royal Brompton Harefield NHS Foundation Trust and Imperial College, London, United Kingdom

Wei Wang, Wei Jing and Qingbin Liu
Department of Pediatric, Affiliated Hospital of Changchun University of Chinese Medicine, Changchun, China

Richard Chavasse
Consultant Respiratory Paediatrician, St George's University Hospitals NHS Foundation Trust, St George's University of London, London, United Kingdom

Stephen Scott
Consultant in Respiratory Medicine, The Countess of Chester Hospital NHS Foundation Trust, Cheshire, United Kingdom
Chester Medical School, The University of Chester, Chester, United Kingdom

Claudia Calogero, Grazia Fenu and Enrico Lombardi
Pediatric Pulmonary Unit, "Anna Meyer" Pediatric University Hospital, Florence, Italy

Eva Morales
Biomedical Research Institute of Murcia (IMIB-Arrixaca), University of Murcia, Murcia, Spain
CIBER Epidemiología y Salud Pública (CIBERESP), Madrid, Spain

David Duffy
QIMR Berghofer Medical Research Institute, Brisbane, QLD, Australia

Nicola Ullmann, Virginia Mirra, Antonio Di Marco, Martino Pavone, Federica Porcaro, Valentina Negro, Alessandro Onofri and Renato Cutrera
Paediatric Pulmonology & Respiratory Intermediate Care Unit, Sleep and Long Term Ventilation Unit, Department of Paediatrics, Paediatric Hospital "Bambino Gesù" Research Institute, Rome, Italy

Index

www.ingramcontent.com/pod-product-compliance
Lightning Source LLC
LaVergne TN
LVHW082127200926
848484LV00008B/2015